THIRD EDITION

Medical Terminology
Language for Health Care

Nina Thierer, CMA, BS, CPC, CCAT
Ivy Tech Community College of Indiana, Fort Wayne, IN

Deborah Nelson, MS, CMA (AAMA), RMA (AMT)
Baker College of Flint and Cass City, Flint, MI

Judy K. Ward, CMA (AAMA), PBT (ASCP), NREMT-P
Ivy Tech Community College of Indiana, Indianapolis, IN

LaTanya Young, RMA (AMT), MMSc, MPH, PA-C
Clayton State University, Morrow, GA

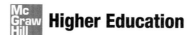

Higher Education

Boston   Burr Ridge, IL   Dubuque, IA   New York   San Francisco   St. Louis
Bangkok   Bogotá   Caracas   Kuala Lumpur   Lisbon   London   Madrid   Mexico City
Milan   Montreal   New Delhi   Santiago   Seoul   Singapore   Sydney   Taipei   Toronto

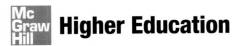

MEDICAL TERMINOLOGY: LANGUAGE FOR HEALTH CARE

Published by McGraw-Hill, a business unit of The McGraw-Hill Companies, Inc., 1221 Avenue of the Americas, New York, NY, 10020. Copyright © 2010 by The McGraw-Hill Companies, Inc. All rights reserved. Previous editions © 2006 and 2002. No part of this publication may be reproduced or distributed in any form or by any means, or stored in a database or retrieval system, without the prior written consent of The McGraw-Hill Companies, Inc., including, but not limited to, in any network or other electronic storage or transmission, or broadcast for distance learning.

Some ancillaries, including electronic and print components, may not be available to customers outside the United States.

This book is printed on acid-free paper.

1 2 3 4 5 6 7 8 9 0 WCK/WCK 0 9 8

ISBN 978-0-07-337472-7
MHID 0-07-337472-5

Vice president/Editor in chief: *Elizabeth Haefele*
Vice president/Director of marketing: *John E. Biernat*
Senior sponsoring editor: *Debbie Fitzgerald*
Director of development, Allied Health: *Patricia Hesse*
Developmental editor: *Bonnie Hemrick*
Executive marketing manager: *Roxan Kinsey*
Lead media producer: *Damian Moshak*
Media developmental editor: *Marc Mattson*
Director, Editing/Design/Production: *Jess Ann Kosic*
Lead project manager: *Rick Hecker*
Senior production supervisor: *Janean A. Utley*
Senior designer: *Srdjan Savanovic*
Senior photo research coordinator: *Lori Hancock*
Media project manager: *Mark A. S. Dierker*
Outside development house: *Myrna Breskin, Chestnut Hill Enterprises, Inc.*
Cover design: *Jessica M. Lazar*
Interior design: *Jenny EI-Shamy*
Typeface: *10/13 Goudy*
Compositor: *Laserwords Private Limited*
Printer: *Quebecor World Dubuque Inc.*
Cover credit: © *3D4Medical.com/Gettyimages*
Credits: *The credits section for this book begins on page 729 and is considered an extension of the copyright page.*

Library of Congress Cataloging-in-Publication Data

Medical terminology: language for healthcare/Nina Thierer . . . [et al.]. —3rd ed.
p.; cm.
Includes index.
ISBN-13: 978-0-07-337472-7 (alk. paper)
ISBN-10: 0-07-337472-5 (alk. paper)
1. Medicine—Terminology—Handbooks, manuals, etc. I. Thierer, Nina.
[DNLM: 1. Medicine—Terminology—English. W 15 M4885 2010]
R123.T45 2010
610.1'4—dc22   2008047096

www.mhhe.com

Brief Contents

Contents

CHAPTER 1

Learning Terminology   1

CHAPTER 2

Prefixes and Suffixes in Medical Terms   23

CHAPTER 7 The Respiratory System   209

CHAPTER 8 The Nervous System   249

CHAPTER 9 — The Urinary System   290

CHAPTER 10 — The Female Reproductive System   324

CHAPTER
11

The Male Reproductive System   358

UROLOGY

CHAPTER
12

The Blood System   378

HEMATOLOGY

CHAPTER
13

The Lymphatic and Immune Systems   413

CHAPTER
14

The Digestive System   439

CHAPTER
15

The Endocrine System   482

ENDOCRINOLOGY

CHAPTER
16

The Sensory System   523

OPHTHALMOLOGY, OTOLOGY

CHAPTER
17

Human Development   556

PEDIATRICS, GERONTOLOGY

CHAPTER 18

Terms in Oncology—Cancer and Its Causes   569

CHAPTER 19

Diagnostic Imaging, Radiation Oncology, and Surgery   593

CHAPTER 20

Terms in Psychiatry   615

CHAPTER 21

Terms in Dental Practice   631

CHAPTER 22

Terms in Pharmacology   646

CHAPTER
23

Terms in Complementary and Alternative Medicine   665

Acknowledgments

Reviewers

Reviewers for Third Edition

Yvonne Beth Alles, MBA, RMT
Davenport University

Dominica Austin, BSN
Lincoln College of Technology

Diana Alagna, RN, RMA
Branford Hall Career Institute

Alecia C. Blake, MD
Medical Careers Institute at ECPI College of Technology

Cynthia Boles, BS, MBA
Bradford School

Deborah Briones, MS
Medical Careers Academy, Taller San Jose
Argosy University Orange County

Tamra Brown, MEPD, RHIA
Western Technical College

Jean M. Chenu, MS, BS
Genesee Community College

Stephen M. Coleman, NCMA
Central Florida Institute

Tiffany Cooper, AAS, BS
Isothermal Community College

Sheronda Cooper, BSD, BSN, MSFN, RMA (AMT), NRCPT(NAHP)
Director of Medical Assisting
Bradford School of Business

Linda Demain LPN, BS, MS
Wichita Technical Institute

Patricia Dudek, RN
McCann School of Business and Technology

Jane W. Dumas, MSN
Remington College-Cleveland West Campus

Cynthia A. Ebert, LPN
Brown Mackie Merrillville

Rhonda K. Epps, AS
National College of Business and Technology

Thomas F. Finnegan IV, DC, FABDA
Minnesota School of Business, Globe University

Terri Fleming, BSN, MS
Ivy Tech Community College

Walter E. Flowers, MA & LAB
Lamson Institute

Ron Gaines, BS, MS
Cameron University

Janette Gallegos, RMA
ECPI College of Technology

Darlene S. Grayson Harmon, BS
Remington College

Elizabeth A. Hoffman, MA Ed., CMA, (AANMA), CPT, (ASPT)
Baker College of Clinton Township

Susan Horn, AAS, CMA (AAMA)
Indiana Business College

Jacqueline M. Johnson, BA
Brown Mackie College

Pam Kowalski, MA
Ross Medical Education Center

Naomi Kupfer, CMA
Heritage College

Kathy Locke, BA, CMA, RMA
Northwestern Business College

Leigh Ann Long, RN
Brookstone College of Business

Roger K. Oatman, DC
Pinnacle Career Institute

Darlene Owen
SE School for Career Development

Rosemarie Scaringella, BA
Hunter Business School

Lynn G. Slack, BS CMA
Kaplan Career Institute-ICM Campus

Donna J. Slovensky, PhD, RHIA
School of Health Professions, University of Alabama at Birmingham

Catherine A. Teel, AST, RMA, CMA
Allied Health Programs Director, McCann School of Business and Technology

Lynn Ward, BS
MSU-GF College of Technology

Mindy Wray, BS, CMA, RMA
ECPI College of Technology

Reviewers for Second Edition

Dr. Judy Adams
Department of Public and Allied Health; Bowling Green State University

Barbara G. Brice, Ph.D., RHIA
Associate Professor, Clark Atlanta University

Mona M. Burke, RHIA
Bowling Green State University—Firelands College

Barbara Desch, LVN, AHI
San Jeaquin Valley College

Jennifer M. Evans
South Seattle Community College

Shawnie Haas, RN, CCRN, MBA
Yakima Valley Community College

JoAnne E. Habenicht, MPA, RT (RTM)
Manhattan College

Georgia D. Hammill
Vatterott College

Judy Johnson, RN
Nashville State Community College

Patricia Kalvelage, MS
Governors State University

Judith Karls
Madison Area Technical College

Paula LaGrass, J.D.
Ohio Business College, Sandusky Campus

Vicki Legg, MS, ATC
Marietta College

Anne M. Loochtan
Columbus State Community College

Nelly Mangarova
Heald College

Evelyn Kay Mayer
Tri-State Business Institute

Ann Minks
Medical Terminology & Transcription
Instructor
Lake Washington Technical College

Neil H. Penny, MS, OTR/L
Alvernia College

Ellen J. Rarick
EduTek College

Donna J. Slovensky, PhD, RHIA,
FAHIMA
University of Alabama at Birmingham

Deborah M. Sulkowski, CMA
Pittsburgh Technical Institute

Marilu Vazquez, M.D., M.S.
University of Texas Health Sciences Center

Lela Weaver, Health Educator
Northwestern College

Kathryn L. Whitley, MSN, FNP
Associate Professor
Patrick Henry Community College

CD-ROM Reviewers

Shawnie Haas, RN, CCRN, MBA
Yakima Valley Community College

Judy Johnson, RN
Nashville State Community College

Judith Karls
Madison Area Technical College

Anne Loochtan
Columbus State Community College

Nelly Mangarova
Heald College

Ann Minks
Lake Washington Technical College

David Lee Sessoms, Jr., M.Ed.,
CMA
Miller-Motte Technical College

Deborah M. Sulkowski, CMA
Pittsburgh Technical Institute

Sharion Thompson
Sanford Brown Institute

Dyan Whitlow Underhill,
MHA, BS
Miller-Motte Technical College

Lela Weaver, Health Educator
Northwestern College

Spanish Language Audio CD Reviewer

Lilia Torres, CMA
Florida Career College

Medical Terminology Symposium Participants

Betty Chong-Menard
UT-Brownsville/Texas Southmost
College

Shawnie Haas, RN, CCRN, MBA
Yakima Valley Community College

Judy Johnson, RN
Nashville State Community College

Judith Karls
Madison Area Technical College

Anne Loochtan
Columbus State Community College

Nelly Mangarova
Heald College

Ann Minks
Lake Washington Technical College

Irma Rodriguez
South Texas Community College

Sue Shellman
Gaston College

Nina Thierer
Ivy Tech State College

Sharion Thompson
Sanford Brown Institute

Lilia Torres, CMA
Florida Career College

Mary Worsley
Miami-Dade College, Medical Center
Campus

To the Student

Medical Terminology: Language for Health Care, Third Edition, is designed for you, the students in the allied health curriculum, who need to know the language of health care. Its purpose is to help you succeed in your chosen health care careers by familiarizing you with how medical words are formed and by providing a systematic learning structure.

Before this section takes you through a short, instructive journey on how the book is set up and how it will work best for you, take the time to go through some general tips for success in school.

How Can I Succeed in This Class?

If you're reading this, you're on the right track.

> *"You are the same today that you are going to be five years from now except for two things: the people with whom you associate and the books you read."*
>
> Charles Jones

Right now, you're probably leafing through this book feeling just a little overwhelmed. You're trying to juggle several other classes (which probably are equally daunting), possibly a job, and on top of it all, a life.

This special section —To the Student—has been designed specifically to help you focus. It's here to help you learn how to manage your time and your studies to succeed.

Start Here

It's true—you are what you put into your studies. You have a lot of time and money invested in your education; you've been planning since high school, working an extra job or through summer vacations to save your money. Don't blow it now by only putting in half of the effort this class requires. Succeeding in this class (and life) requires:

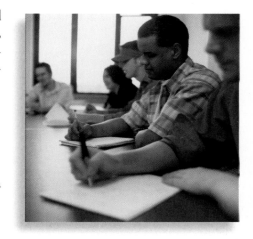

- a commitment—of time and perseverance
- knowing and motivating yourself
- getting organized
- managing your time

This specially designed section will help you learn how to be effective in these areas, as well as offer guidance in:

- getting the most out of your class
- thinking through—and applying—the material
- getting the most out of your textbook
- finding extra help when you need it

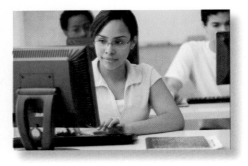

A Commitment—of Time and Perseverance

Learning—and mastering—takes time and patience. Nothing worthwhile comes easily. Be committed to your studies and you will reap the benefits in the long run.

Consider this: your education is building the foundation for your future—a future in your chosen profession. Sloppy and hurried work now will only lead to lack of success later. Two or four years of committed education time now is nothing compared to the lifetime that awaits you.

Note: A good rule of thumb is to allow a minimum of 2 hours of study time each week for every hour you spend in class.

For instance, 3 hours of class deserve 6 hours of weekly study time. If you set aside time each day to study, you will be investing a little time every day, including the weekend. Study time includes completing exercises, reading the text, practicing words, listening to recordings, and reviewing notes.

Why Study Medical Terminology?

If you were moving to a foreign country where very few people spoke English, you would make every effort to learn the language of that country. You have chosen a course of study in allied health or health care and you will need to know the language that is used in that discipline. Medical terminology covers the specifics words and phrases you will need to learn to function effectively and understand the "language" of health care.

Whether you deal with the clinical side or the administrative side, everyone involved in health care uses various terms to describe certain diseases, procedures, and office practices. Many of the terms used in health care are "built up," which means they are formed from word parts. In this text, you will learn how to understand words by breaking them down into parts. Although learning a new "language" basically involves memorization, this text gives you tools to help you learn large numbers of terms without memorizing each one. Take advantage of all the study elements within the text, on the student CD-ROM, and on the Web site to help you become a proficient participant in allied health.

Knowing and Motivating Yourself

What type of a learner are you? When are you most productive? Know yourself and your limits and work within them. Know how to motivate yourself to give your all to your studies and achieve your goals. Quite bluntly, you are the one who will benefit most from your success. If you lack self-motivation and drive, you will be the first person to suffer.

Know yourself: There are many types of learners, and no right or wrong way of learning. Which category do you fall into?

Visual Learner—You respond best to "seeing" processes and information. Particularly focus on text illustrations and charts, course handouts. Check to see if there are animations on the course or text Web site to help you. Also, consider drawing diagrams in your notes to illustrate concepts.

Auditory Learner—You work best by listening to—and possibly tape recording—the class lecture and by talking information through with a study partner. Your study sessions should include a flash card drill with a study partner or family member.

Tactile/Kinesthetic Learner—You learn best by being "hands on." You'll benefit by applying what you've learned during class time. Think of ways to apply your critical thinking skills in a variety of situations. Perhaps a text Web site or interactive CD-ROM will also help you.

Identify your own personal preferences for learning and seek out the resources that will best help you with your studies. Also, learn by recognizing your weaknesses and try to compensate for them while you work to improve them.

Getting Organized

It's simple, yet it's fundamental. It seems the more organized you are, the easier things come. Take the time before your course begins to look around and analyze your life and your study habits. Get organized now and you'll find you have a little more time—and a lot less stress.

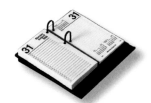

- Find a calendar system that works for you. The best kind is one that you can take with you everywhere. To be truly organized, you should integrate all aspects of your life into this one calendar—school, work, leisure. Some people also find it helpful to have an additional monthly calendar posted by their desk for "at a glance" dates and to have a picture of what's to come. If you do this, be sure you are consistently synchronizing both calendars so you don't miss anything. More tips for organizing your calendar can be found in the time management discussion on the next page.
- By the same token, keep everything for your course or courses in one place—and at your fingertips. A three-ring binder works well because it allows you to add or organize handouts and notes from class in any order you prefer. Incorporating your own custom tabs helps you flip to exactly what you need at a moment's notice.
- Find your space. Find a place that helps you be organized and focused. If it's your desk in your room or elsewhere in your home, keep it clean. Clutter adds confusion, stress, and wastes time. Or perhaps your "space" is at the library. If that's the case, keep a backpack or bag that's fully stocked with what you might need—your text, binder or notes, pens, highlighters, Post-its, phone numbers of study partners (hint: a good place to keep phone numbers is in your "one place for everything calendar").

A Helpful Hint—add extra "padding" into your deadlines to yourself. If you have a test on Friday, set a goal for yourself to have most of the studying done by Wednesday. Then, take time on Thursday to look over the work again, with a fresh eye. Review anything you had trouble remembering and be ready for the test on Friday.

Managing Your Time

Managing your time is the single most important thing you can do to help yourself. And, it's probably one of the most difficult tasks to successfully master.

You are taking this course because you want to succeed in life. You are preparing for a career. In school, you are expected to work much harder and to learn much more than you ever have before. To be successful you need to invest in your education with a commitment of time.

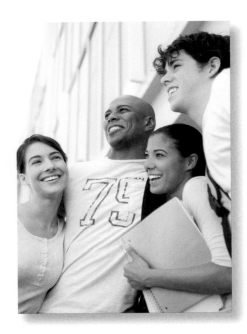

How Time Slips Away

People tend to let an enormous amount of time slip away from them, mainly in three ways:

1. **Procrastination,** putting off chores simply because you don't feel in the mood to do them right away
2. **Distraction,** getting sidetracked by the endless variety of other things that seem easier or more fun to do, often not realizing how much time they eat up
3. **Underestimating the value of small bits of time,** thinking it's not worth doing any work because you have something else to do or somewhere else to be in 20 minutes or so.

We all lead busy lives. But we all make choices as to how we spend our time. Choose wisely and make the most of every minute you have by implementing these tips.

- **Know yourself and when you'll be able to study most efficiently.** When are you most productive? Are you a late nighter? Or an early bird? Plan to study when you are most alert and can have some uninterrupted time. This could include a quick 5-minute review before class or a one-hour problem solving study session with a friend.
- **Create a set study time for yourself daily.** Having a set schedule for yourself helps you commit to studying, and helps you plan instead of cram.
- **Organize *all* of your activities in one place.** Find—and use—a planner that is small enough to carry with you everywhere. This can be a $2.50 paper calendar or a more expensive electronic version. They all work on the same premise.
- **Less is more. Schedule study time using shorter, focused blocks with small breaks.** Doing this offers two benefits:
  1. You will be less fatigued and gain more from your effort, and
  2. Studying will seem less overwhelming and you will be less likely to procrastinate.
- **Do plan time for leisure, friends, exercise, and sleep.** Studying should be your main focus, but you need to balance your time—and your life.
- Make sure you log your projects and homework deadlines in your personal calendar.
- "Plot" your assignments on your calendar or task list. If you have a report, for instance, break the assignment down into smaller targets. For example, set a goal for a first draft, second draft, and final copy.
- Try to complete tasks ahead of schedule. This will give you a chance to carefully review your work before you hand it in (instead of at 1 a.m. when you are half awake). You'll feel less stressed in the long run.
- Prioritize! In your calendar or planner, highlight or number key projects; do them first, and then cross them off when you've completed them. Give yourself a pat on the back for getting them done!
- Review your calendar and reprioritize daily.
- Try to resist distractions by setting and sticking to a designated study time (remember your commitment!). Distractions may include friends, surfing the Internet, or even a pet lizard.
- Multitask when possible—You may find a lot of extra time you didn't think you had. Review material in your head while walking to class, doing laundry, or during "mental down time." (Note—mental down time does NOT mean in the middle of lecture.)

Note: Plan to study and plan for leisure. Being well balanced will help you focus when it is time to study.

Tip: Try combining social time with studying (a study partner) or social time with mealtime or exercise (dine or work out with a friend). Being a good student doesn't mean you have to be a hermit. It does mean you need to know how to smartly budget your time.

Learn to Manage or Avoid Time Wasters

DON'T
- Don't let friends manage your time

Tip: Kindly ask, "Can we talk later?" when you are trying to study; this will keep you in control of your time without alienating your friends.

- Don't get sucked into the Internet

It's easy to lose hours in front of the computer surfing the web. Set a time limit for you self and stick to it.

DO
- Do use small bits of time to your advantage

Example: Arrive to class five minutes early and review notes. Review your personal calendar for upcoming due dates and events while eating meals or waiting for appointments.

- Do balance your life—sleep, study, and leisure are all important. Keep each in balance.

Getting the Most out of Classes

Believe it or not, instructors want you to succeed. They put a lot of effort into helping you learn and preparing their classes. Attending class is one of the simplest, most valuable things you can do to help yourself. But it doesn't end there; getting the most out of your classes means being organized. Here's how:

Prepare Before You Go to Class

Really! You'll be amazed at how much better you understand the material when you preview the chapter before you go to class. Don't feel overwhelmed by this suggestion. One tip that may help you—plan to arrive to class 5-15 minutes before lecture. Bring your text with you and skim the chapter before class begins. This will at the very least give you an overview of what may be discussed.

Be a Good Listener

Most people think they are good listeners, but few really are. Are you?

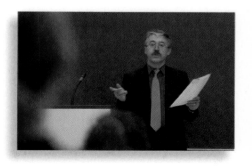

Obvious, but important points to remember:

- You can't listen if you are talking.
- You aren't listening if you are daydreaming.
- Listening and comprehending are two different things. If you don't understand something your instructor is saying, ask a question or jot a note

and visit the instructor after hours. Don't feel dumb or intimidated; you probably aren't the only person who "doesn't get it."

Take Good Notes

- Use a standard size notebook, or better yet, a three-ring binder with loose leaf notepaper. The binder will allow you to organize and integrate your notes and handouts, make use of easy-to-reference tabs, etc.
- Use a standard black or blue ink pen to take your initial notes. You can annotate later using a pencil, which can be erased if need be.
- Start a new page for each class or note-taking session (yes—you can and should also take notes from your textbook).
- Label each page with the date and a heading for each day.
- Focus on main points and try to use an outline format to take notes to capture key ideas and organize sub-points.
- Leave lots of white space in your note-taking. A solid page of notes is difficult to study.
- Review and edit your notes shortly after class—at least within 24 hours to make sure they make sense and that you've recorded core thoughts. You may also want to compare your notes with a study partner later to make sure neither of you have missed anything.

Get a Study Partner

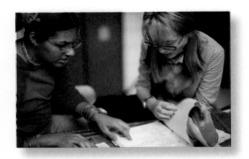

Having a study partner has so many benefits. First, he/she can help you keep your commitment to this class. By having set study dates, you can combine study and social time, and maybe even make it fun! In addition, you now have two sets of eyes and ears and two minds to help digest the information from class and from the text. Talk through concepts, compare notes, and quiz each other.

An Obvious Note: Don't take advantage of your study partner by skipping class or skipping study dates. You soon won't have a study partner—or a friend!

Helpful Hint: Take your text to class, and keep it open to the topics being discussed. You can take brief notes in your textbook margin or reference textbook pages in your notebook to help you study later.

How to Study for an Exam

- rereading is not studying
- be an active learner—
  - Read.
  - Be an active participant in class; ask questions.
  - Finish reading all material—text, notes, handouts—at least three days prior to the exam.
  - Three days prior to the exam, set aside time each day to do self-testing, practice problems, review notes, and use critical thinking skills to understand the material.
  - Analyze your weaknesses, and create an "I don't know this yet" list. Focus on strengthening these areas and narrow your list as you study.
  - Create your own study tools such as flash cards and checklists and practice defining key terms.

- Make up a mock test. If you were the instructor, what questions would you put on the test? You will be surprised at how accurate you will be.

Useful tools to help: the end-of-chapter reviews, questions and practice problems; text Web site; student CD-ROM; and your study partner.

Very Important

Be sure to sleep and eat well before the exam.
If you are determined to fail, just follow these few simple instructions:

1. Skip class, or if you do attend, arrive fashionably late.
2. Don't buy the book, or if you buy it, don't read it.
3. Don't bother studying if you have to be somewhere else in 20 minutes; that's not enough time to get anything done.
4. Big test coming up? Beat the stress by relaxing with friends, going out for a few beers, or hanging out in an Internet chat room. Be sure to complain to your chat room friends about how there's not way you can pass the test tomorrow.
5. Don't ask questions in class; you're probably the only one who doesn't know the answer, and everyone else will think you're stupid.
6. Don't visit the instructor in his or her office; instructors don't want to be bothered.
7. If you miss a class, trust your friends' notes to be complete and accurate.
8. Be sure to pull an all-nighter before the exam; you don't have time to sleep.
9. Don't strain your brain trying to do the chapter review. Look up the answers and fill them in. You can fool your friends into thinking you're really smart (as long as they don't see your test grade).
10. When you study with friends, have a good time—chat about things unrelated to your study topic.
11. The time to begin studying for an exam is the day before the test. Four hours ought to be plenty.

Getting the Most Out of Your Textbook

McGraw-Hill and the authors of this book have invested their time, research, and talents to help you succeed as well. The goal is to make learning easier for you.

What's New This Edition

- The material in various chapters has been expanded to include new procedures, more on electronic health records, and more on use of the Internet.
- This edition of the textbook features more than DOUBLE the number of practice exercises with heavy emphasis on the building up and deconstructing of word parts.
- By the end of studying this text, students will be able to understand a wide range of medical vocabulary.

McGraw-Hill LearnSmart: Medical Terminology

McGraw-Hill LearnSmart is a diagnostic learning system that determines the level of student knowledge, then feeds the student appropriate content. Students learn faster and study more efficiently.

As a student works within the system, LearnSmart develops a personal learning path adapted to what the student has learned and retained. Learn-Smart is also able to recommend additional study resources to help the student master topics.

In addition to being an innovative, outstanding study tool, LearnSmart has features for instructors. There is a Course Gauge where the instructor can see exactly what students have accomplished as well as a built-in assessment tool for graded assignments.

Students and instructors will be able to access LearnSmart anywhere via a web browser. And for students on the go, it will also be available through any iPhone or iPod Touch.

McGraw-Hill Connect Allied Health

McGraw-Hill *Connect Allied Health* is a web-based assignment and assessment platform that gives students the means to better connect with their coursework, with their instructors, and with the important concepts that they will need to know for success now and in the future. With *Connect Allied Health*, instructors can deliver assignments, quizzes and tests easily online. Students can practice important skills at their own pace and on their own schedule. With *Connect Allied Health Plus*, students also get 24/7 online access to an eBook–an online edition of the text–to aid them in successfully completing their work, wherever and whenever they choose.

Here's How

Throughout the pages of *Medical Terminology: Language for Health Care*, you'll find an organized learning system. Follow it throughout your course and you will become a proficient "speaker" of the language of health care.

A Journey Through *Medical Terminology: Language for Health Care*

Forming Medical Terms

The first three chapters of the book introduce the way that most medical terms are formed. Most medical terms are built from word parts, often derived from Latin and Greek terms. These three chapters introduce many of the major word parts used in the formation of medical terms.

Chapter 1 gives the major combining forms used in medical terminology except for the combining forms that are more specific to each body part. Those combining forms are learned in each chapter that covers a different body system.

Chapter 2 provides the majority of general prefixes and suffixes that are used to form medical terms. Learning these prefixes and suffixes will enable you to break apart built-up terms that you are not familiar with and understand their meanings by knowing the meaning of the parts.

Chapter 3 introduces you to the body systems you will be studying throughout this book. It also covers the most commonly used body system word parts, which are then repeated in the individual body system chapters. This concentrated repetition is designed to reinforce the body system approach to medical word building.

Using the Systematic Learning Approach

Chapters 4 through 16 are the body system chapters. The format of these chapters is designed to acquaint you with an overview of each body system, including coverage of its basic anatomy and physiology. At the same time, each chapter teaches the specific terms and word parts used in the medical terminology. Each body system chapter is presented in the following format:

A. Objectives
B. Structure and Function
C. Combining Forms and Abbreviations
D. Diagnostic, Procedural, and Laboratory Terms
E. Pathological Terms
F. Surgical Terms
G. Pharmacological Terms
H. Terminology in Action and Challenge Section
I. Using the Internet
J. Section Exercises
K. Chapter Review
L. Answers to Chapter Exercises

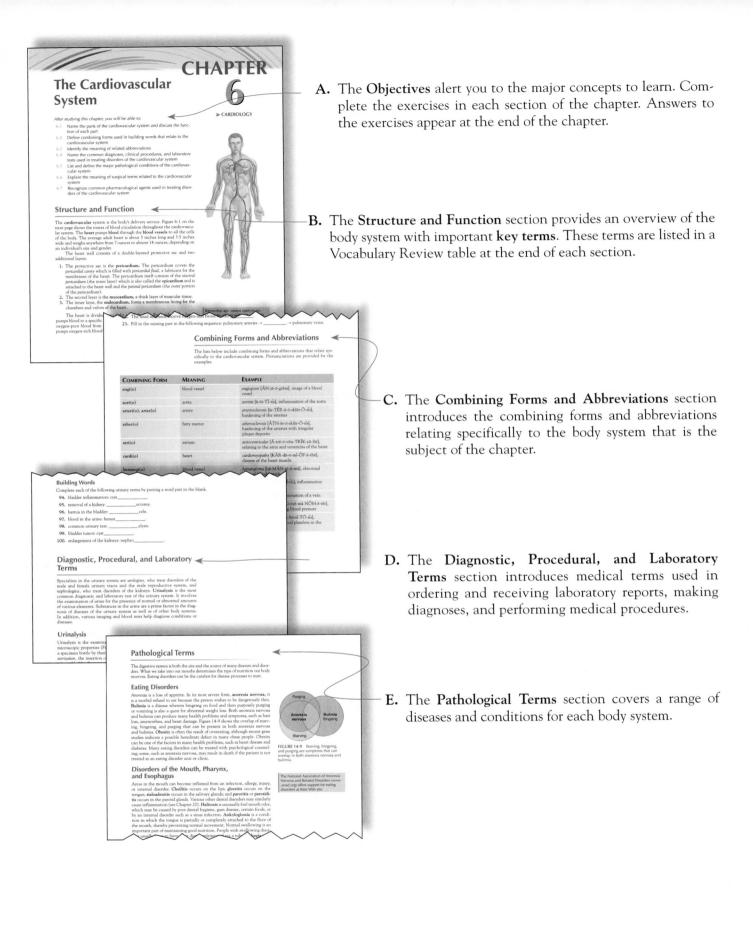

A. The **Objectives** alert you to the major concepts to learn. Complete the exercises in each section of the chapter. Answers to the exercises appear at the end of the chapter.

B. The **Structure and Function** section provides an overview of the body system with important **key terms**. These terms are listed in a Vocabulary Review table at the end of each section.

C. The **Combining Forms and Abbreviations** section introduces the combining forms and abbreviations relating specifically to the body system that is the subject of the chapter.

D. The **Diagnostic, Procedural, and Laboratory Terms** section introduces medical terms used in ordering and receiving laboratory reports, making diagnoses, and performing medical procedures.

E. The **Pathological Terms** section covers a range of diseases and conditions for each body system.

F. The **Surgical Terms** section provides an overview of common surgical procedures performed for each body system.

G. The **Pharmacological Terms** section covers the classes of drugs used to treat illnesses of the system being discussed and provides examples of both generic and trade name medications.

H. The **Terminology in Action** and **Challenge Sections** are an additional opportunity for critical thinking.

I. Using the Internet offers you an opportunity to gather information from a medical Web site and familiarize yourself with medical offerings on the Internet.

J. Section Exercises provide review of each section.

K. The **Chapter Review** gives a complete listing of key terms, combining forms, and abbreviations learned in the chapter.

L. Answers to Chapter Exercises allow self-study and instant feedback so you can determine how well you learned the material.

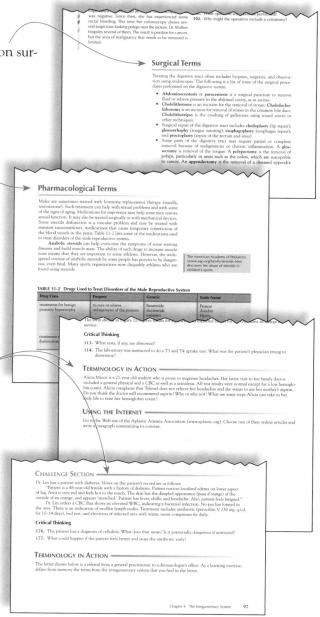

Special Features

Each chapter contains some special features that reinforce learning, provide additional information, or expose you to realistic situations that you may encounter in your chosen allied health profession.

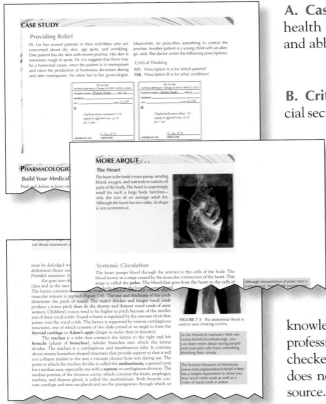

A. Case Studies throughout the text provide you with realistic health care situations. The case studies shows you how terminology and abbreviations are used in a realistic context.

B. Critical Thinking following the case studies and in some other special sections, you are asked critical thinking questions. Critical thinking skills are essential to the development of your decision-making skills as a future allied health care professional.

C. More About boxes throughout the book provide some medical information that would not normally appear within a medical terminology text.

D. Internet References appear in many places in the margin of the text. These references direct you to the Internet to learn more about the material being studied and to familiarize yourself with using the Internet to enhance your knowledge—something that will be helpful to you both personally and professionally throughout your life. Although all Web sites have been checked, some Web sites become inactive. In such cases, if the Web site does not work, use a search engine on your computer to find another source. Simply insert a related word and go to some suggested sites to find more information.

Warning: Using the Internet can be helpful but it may also be harmful. Some people are posting false and even damaging or misleading medical information on the Internet. Check the source of the site to make sure it is a trustworthy medical resource. Avoid advertisements, clubs, and articles written by anyone asking for a donation. Use common sense—if it sounds too good to be true, it usually is false. Also, if someone is trying to sell you something, beware of buying medical items on the Internet without sound medical advice. Never substitute the advice of someone you don't know on the Internet for the advice you can get from a medical professional.

Specialized Chapters

Chapters 17 through 23 cover general and special areas of health care.

Additional Study Resources

In addition to the textbook, McGraw-Hill offers the following study resources to enhance your learning of medical terminology:

- An interactive student CD-ROM. The next section gives instructions for using the CD-ROM.
- A set of English audio CDs. The two English audio CDs are organized by chapter sections. You can use these to test your ability to spell and pronounce all key terms in the book.
- An Online Learning Center (OLC) Web site. The Web site (www.mhhe.com/medterm3e) includes an Information Center with general information about the medical terminology program. It includes an instructor's side with resources for classroom testing and management. For you, the student, it includes major checkpoints from the text along with additional learning activities. These additional activities will reinforce what you learned in the text and what you practiced on the student CD-ROM.
- A Spanish-English audio CD (available for purchase). To use this audio CD effectively, listen to the Spanish words while you look at the selected Spanish terms in the appropriate body system chapter. If you want to read the definition in Spanish, refer to the Spanish Glossary on the Online Learning Center (www.mhhe.com/medterm3e).

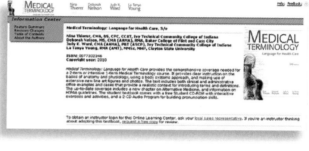

Using the CD-ROM

The Medical Terminology: Language for Health Care, Third Edition Student CD-ROM is an interactive tutorial designed to complement the student textbook. In it you will find key terms, flashcards, drag and drop word building and labeling exercises, and games (such as Hangman and That's Epidemic!) that are designed to challenge you.

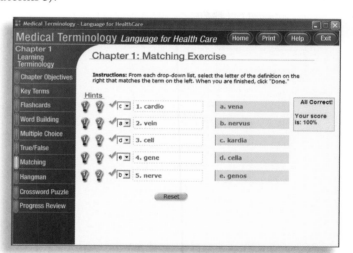

System Requirements

To run this product, your computer must meet the following minimum specifications:
- Pentium II or higher processor
- Microsoft Vista 2000, or XP (Windows XP recommended)
- 64 MB of RAM or higher (128 required for Windows XP)
- 800x600 or higher desktop display
- 16-bit or higher desktop color (24-bit or 32-bit highly recommended)
- Internet Explorer 5.5 or higher required (6.0 or higher recommended)
- Windows Media Player 7.1 or higher required (9.0 or higher recommended)

Installation

The installation and setup program checks your computer to make sure it meets the minimum specifications to run the Medical Terminology: Language for Health Care, Second Edition Student CD-ROM.

To run the installation program:
1. Insert the CD-ROM into your CD-ROM drive.
2. In the Run: box, type D:/Start_Here.exe (where D is the letter of your CD-ROM drive).

- If you have already installed the program, AutoRun will ask if you want to run the program instead.
- If AutoRun does not start automatically, you will need to follow these steps:
1. Click the Windows Start menu and go to Run.
2. In the Run: box, type D:\autorun.exe (where D is the letter of your CD-ROM drive).
3. Click OK.
4. To run the program after it is installed, go to the Windows Start menu, point your mouse to Programs (or All Programs), point your mouse to Medical Terminology, and click the icon for Medical Terminology.

The Help Section

Once you have installed the software, you are strongly encouraged to read and review the Help section of this software. The Help section will explain in detail all of the features and activities. It will also discuss frequently asked questions and offer troubleshooting tips. To access help, click on the Help button found on the top right of your computer screen.

Software Support

If you are experiencing difficulties with this product, please contact our Digital CARE team at http://www.mhhe.com/support.

Learning Terminology

After studying this chapter, you will be able to:

1.1 Explain how medical terms are developed
1.2 Describe the process of pluralizing terms
1.3 Describe how to interpret pronunciation marks
1.4 Define the four word parts used to build medical terms
1.5 Define common medical combining forms
1.6 List basic legal and ethical issues for health-related professionals
1.7 Describe how medical documentation is compiled
1.8 Describe HIPAA in relation to allied health

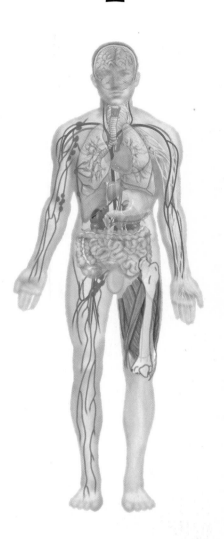

The Language of Medicine

Many everyday terms that we use to describe our health and our medical care go back to the early history of civilization. The language of medicine dates to the time when people had only spoken language, not written. Like all people who followed after them, they gave names to parts of their bodies, to illnesses, and to the cures they used. Some of these names survive in the roots and words still used today in medical terminology. For example, the ancient Greeks thought of the disease we call "cancer" as something eating at a person on the inside, and so named the condition *karkinos*, meaning both crab and cancer.

Medical terminology began to become standardized when Hippocrates (460–377 B.C.), a Greek physician, set about to organize an approach to medicine. The Hippocratic oath that is generally attributed to him has been in use for over 2,000 years. The actual Hippocratic oath along with other information about the oath appears in the student online learning center at www.mhhe.com/medterm3e.

Derivation of Medical Terminology

Many medical terms originate directly from ancient Greek or Latin terms. Table 1-1 shows a sampling of words taken directly from those languages. Notice how the terms have retained their meaning over the centuries. Other languages form words in the same way. For example, the word nerve is derived from the Latin *nervus*. In Spanish, the word *nervio* is also derived

TABLE 1–1 Derivations of Terms

Modern Term	Historical Derivation
artery	Latin *arteria;* Greek *arteria*
cardi(o), the heart	Greek *kardia*
cell	Latin *cella,* chamber
gene	Greek *genos,* birth
hernia	Latin *hernia,* rupture
ligament	Latin *ligamentum*
nerve	Latin *nervus*
sinus	Latin *sinus,* cavity
tendon	Latin *tendo*
vein	Latin *vena*

from the same Latin word. (In the student online learning center (www .mhhe.com/medterm3e), you will find a Spanish-English glossary of some of the key terms used in this book. In many cases, you will find the words very similar to their English counterparts.)

Later, people of many cultures used these ancient terms in their languages. Even though the appearance of the words changed, the roots from which the words developed remained the original Greek or Latin terms. Over the ensuing centuries, people involved in medicine and the development of treatments tended to look for Greek or Latin words or roots to describe their newest discoveries. Hence, many medical terms used today are based on ancient Greek and Latin. Word building became and remains the primary way to describe new medical discoveries.

The study of the origin of words is called *etymology.* General language terms tend to change dramatically. It takes a talented word detective to find the actual root of a word that has undergone centuries of change. Remember that most languages, up until the last 500 years, were spoken by most of the population, but were available in written form to only a few. Although books had been around for many centuries, printed material was not available to the general population until the advent of the printing press in the sixteenth century. Even then, it took some time for large numbers of people to become readers of newspapers, journals, and books. As spoken words are passed down through generations, pronunciations (and even meanings) often change. An example is the word *heart.* It is derived from Old English *heorte,* which ultimately comes from an early Germanic word, related to Greek *kardia,* meaning heart, and found in words like *cardiac, cardiology,* and *cardiogram.*

The change in medical terms has generally been less drastic. Most people who have studied medicine since Greek and Roman times have also studied the Latin and Greek languages as part of learning medical terminology. So, a suffix, *-tomy,* which means "cutting," may be used in modern types of surgery (*phlebotomy,* incision into a vein), but the basic meaning is still the original one, "cutting." Throughout this text, you will learn the parts of words that enable you to understand many medical terms.

HISTORY OF MEDICAL TERMS EXERCISES

Fill in the Blanks

1. If a word is derived from an Old English word, it might also be related to a _____ or _____ word that means the same thing.
2. The first organized approach to medicine was formalized by _____.
3. The word cardiology is derived from a _____ root.
4. Two languages studied throughout the history of medicine are _____ and _____.
5. When a word is passed through spoken language only, it is more likely to be altered than if it is passed through _____ language.

Pluralizing Terms

Most English plurals are formed by adding -s or -es to a word. This is also true of many medical terms (cancer, cancers; abscess, abscesses). However, medical terms derived from ancient Greek and Latin often use the regular plural forms from those languages (bursa, bursae; embolus, emboli). Throughout time, some of these ancient plural forms have been replaced by adding -s or -es. As you study the text, you will learn which plurals are commonly used as well as irregular plurals (foot, feet; tooth, teeth). Table 1-2 shows the formation of plurals.

TABLE 1–2 Formation of Plurals

Singular Words	Plural Words	Pluralizing Rules
joint, face, angioma, cancer, muscle, paraplegic	joints, faces, angiomas, cancers, muscles, paraplegics	Add -s to words ending in any vowel or consonant except s, x, z, or y.
abscess, reflex	abscesses, reflexes	Add -es to words ending in s, x, or z.
vasectomy	vasectomies	Remove the y and add -ies to words ending in -y preceded by a consonant. When an ending -y is preceded by a vowel, the usual plural suffix is -s.
appendix, radix	appendices, radices	Remove the x and add -ces to Latin words ending in x.
fossa	fossae	Add -e to Latin terms ending in -a.
staphylococcus	staphylococci	Remove -us and add -i to Latin words ending in -us.
ganglion, datum	ganglia, data	Remove -on and add -a to Greek words ending in -on; remove -um from and add -a to Latin words ending in -um.
neurosis	neuroses	Change -sis to -ses in Greek words ending in -sis.

Spelling and Pronunciation of Medical Terms

Misspellings and mispronunciations in a medical setting can result in life-threatening situations. A misspelled or a misunderstood abbreviation for a medicine dosage was responsible for the death of several children in a cancer ward. Recently, a famous actor's infant twins were given a potentially fatal dose of a blood thinner because of a misspelled abbreviation. Several new AIDS medications are close enough in sound to other drugs as to make prescribing, particularly by telephone, difficult. A physician ordered a prescription for an AIDS drug, saquinavir, for an AIDS patient. The pharmacy filled a prescription for a sedative, Sinequan, and the patient became critically ill.

Aside from the possibility of written mistakes, people in health care must remain vigilant in checking and rechecking verbal instructions. Misspellings that result in harm to a patient may become legal issues. Patients have the right to expect a certain standard of care. Misunderstandings caused by incorrect or misspelled words may be disastrous in certain circumstances. For example, some hospitals and doctors' offices require that written forms requesting an electrocardiogram include the abbreviation EKG instead of ECG because of the possible confusion of a written "C" with an "E" as in EEG (electroencephalogram).

Learning how to spell and pronounce medical terms is a matter of practice. In this text, spellings and pronunciations are given in both the vocabulary review sections of each chapter and in the end-of-chapter review sections. Familiarizing yourself with correct spellings of terms is a matter of practice and of seeing the terms over and over again. Pronouncing a word out loud each time you see the pronunciation will help familiarize you with the sound of the word. You may also want to write and pronounce terms several terms or work with a partner writing and pronouncing terms to each other. (Note: Not everyone agrees on every pronunciation, and there may be regional variations. If your instructor has a particular preference, follow that preference.) Also, use your own medical dictionary as a reference when you have a question. It is a good idea to know some basic terms in other languages such as Spanish when you work in an area where many people mainly speak that language. Since Spanish is the second most common language spoken in the United States today, this textbook has a Spanish-English glossary for your reference.

For quick checking of terms, you can use www.medical-spell-checker.com, which is not an official Web site but is provided free for Internet users. It is important to note that such sites are supported by advertising, so use them carefully.

For more information on medical errors, go to www.ahrq.gov and search for medical errors.

MORE ABOUT . . .

Medical Errors

Both government and the health care industry are investigating ways to avoid the increasing number of medical errors (mistakes). Several companies have now devised an electronic method for entering prescriptions (known as CPOE, computerized physician order entry) with only doctors having passwords; the amounts and drug names are double-checked by the program. Some health care services centers now require every direction or order given by phone to be read back at least once for confirmation. Some surgeons insist that a patient actually write "yes" on the correct limb to be operated on before they will proceed.

TABLE 1–3 Pronunciation Guide

Vowel	Long (−) or Short (˘)	Examples of Pronunciation
a	long ā	pace, plate, atrium
e	long ē	feline, easy, beat
i	long ī	dine, line, I, bite
o	long ō	boat, wrote, rose
u	long ū	cute, cube
a	short ă	rap, cat, mar
e	short ě	ever, pet
i	short ĭ	pit, kitten
o	short ŏ	pot, hot
u	short ŭ	put, cut

In this text, there are two ways we help you learn to pronounce words. First, we capitalize one syllable of all words with two or more syllables so you can tell where the heaviest accent falls. For example, the word *femoral* is pronounced FEM-or-al, with the accent on the first syllable. Next, we add marks, called *diacritical marks*, to the vowels to guide you in pronouncing them. Vowels are either long or short, as shown in Table 1-3.

Long and short vowels are just a guide to help you pronounce the words correctly. English dictionaries have much more extensive pronunciation systems, with many degrees of vowel sounds. For the purposes of learning medical terminology, long and short marks provide enough guidance.

Some spelling differences occur in different fields of allied health. For example, medical transcriptionists follow AAMT (The American Association for Medical Transcription) style. In this style, diseases, procedures, and conditions that are named after people are spelled without the possessive form. For example, *Alzheimer's disease* is spelled *Alzheimer disease* and *Fontan's operation* is spelled *Fontan operation*. The AMA (American Medical Association) has also adopted this practice. However, U.S. government Websites still use the possessive form, as do most organizations (for example, Alzheimer's Foundation of America). Appendix F gives some examples of these style differences.

Pronunciation Exercises

Saying What You Mean

In the following list of words, the accented syllable is shown in capital letters. The vowels need a long or short mark added. As an exercise in how familiar you already are with medical words, add the diacritical marks to the vowels. Check the answers at the end of the chapter.

6. anemia [a-NE-me-a]
7. angioplasty [AN-je-o-plas-te]
8. bursitis [ber-SI-tis]
9. disease [di-ZEZ]

10. hemoglobin [HE-mo-GLO-bin]
11. lymphoma [lim-FO-ma]
12. neuritis [nu-RI-tis]
13. osteoporosis [OS-te-o-po-RO-sis]

14. paraplegia [par-a-PLE-je-a]
15. pulse [puls]
16. radiation [ra-de-A-shun]
17. reflex [RE-fleks]
18. retina [RET-i-na]
19. rheumatism [RU-ma-tizm]
20. sciatica [si-AT-i-ka]
21. septum [SEP-tum]
22. sinus [SI-nus]
23. therapy [THAR-a-pe]
24. typhoid [TI-foyd]
25. vaccine [VAK-sen]

Forming Medical Terms

Many medical terms are formed from two or more word parts. There are four word parts to learn about in the study of medical terminology.

- A **word root** is the fundamental portion of a word that contains the basic meaning. For example, the word root *cardi* means "heart."
- **Combining forms** are the word root and a combining vowel that enable two parts to be connected. For example, the word root *cardi* + the combining vowel -o- can form words relating to the basic meaning "heart," such as *cardiology*, the practice that studies, diagnoses, and treats disorders of the heart. It is often easier to understand medical terms by looking at the suffix first. Thus, *-logy*, the study of, plus the prefix *cardio-* gives you a quick understanding of the definition.
- **Prefixes** are word parts attached to the beginning of a word or word root that modify the meaning of that word root. For example, the prefix *peri-*, meaning "around, near, surrounding," helps to form the word *pericardium*, meaning "around or surrounding the heart." Common prefixes used in medical terminology are discussed in Chapter 2 as well as in the body systems chapters.
- **Suffixes** are word parts attached to the end of a word or word root that modify the meaning of that word root. For example, the suffix *-oid*, meaning "like or resembling," helps to form the word *fibroid*, meaning "made of fibrous tissue." Common suffixes used in medical terminology are discussed in Chapter 2 as well as in the body systems chapters.

By familiarizing yourself with the word parts in this chapter and in Chapters 2 and 3, you will find the separate chapters about body systems easier to understand. Once you have learned the basic words, combining forms, and word parts in the systems chapters, you will be able to define many of the medical terms you will encounter as a health care professional.

Word Roots and Combining Forms

Most medical word roots come directly from Greek and Latin terms. The history of a word is called its *etymology*. The list that follows includes common medical combining forms with meanings that are not specifically part of a body system or may apply both to general terms and to specific body systems. (Body systems combining forms are discussed in later chapters.) Many of the combining forms in this chapter form medical terms when used with word parts or other terms. In Chapter 2, you will study prefixes and suffixes. Once you master all three basic word parts, along with roots, you will have the basic tools necessary for understanding medical terms.

Combining Form	Meaning	Example
acanth(o)	spiny; thorny	*acanthoid* [ă-KĂN-thŏyd], spine-shaped
actin(o)	light	*actinotherapy* [ĂK-tĭn-ō-THĀR-ă-pē], ultraviolet light therapy used in dermatology
aer(o)	air; gas	*aerogen* [ĀR-ō-jĕn], gas-producing microorganism
alge, algesi, algio, algo	pain	*algospasm* [ĂL-gō-spăzm], pain caused by a spasm
amyl(o)	starch	*amylophagia* [ĂM-ĭ-lō-FĀ-jē-ă], abnormal craving for starch
andro	masculine	*androblastoma* [ĂN-drō-blăs-TŌ-mă], testicular tumor
athero	plaque; fatty substance	*atheroma* [ăth-ĕr-Ō-mă], swelling on the surface of an artery from a fatty deposit
bacill(i)	bacilli; bacteria	*bacilliform* [bă-SĬL-ĭ-fŏrm], rod-shaped like a bacterium
bacteri(o)	bacteria	*bacteriogenic* [băk-TĒR-ē-ō-JĔN-ĭk], caused by bacteria
bar(o)	weight; pressure	*barostat* [BĂR-ō-stăt], pressure-regulating device
bas(o), basi(o)	base	*basophilic* [BĀ-sō-FĬL-ĭk], having an affinity for basic dyes (said of tissue)
bio-	life	*biopsy* [BĪ-ŏp-sē], sampling of tissue from living patients
blasto	immature cells	*glioblastoma* [GLĪ-ō-blăs-TŌ-mă], growth consisting of immature neural cells
cac(o)	bad; ill	*cacomelia* [kăk-ō-MĒ-lē-ă], congenital limb deformity
calc(o), calci(o)	calcium	*calcipenia* [kăl-sĭ-PĒ-nē-ă], calcium deficiency
carcin(o)	cancer	*carcinogen* [kăr-SĬN-ō-jĕn], cancer-producing substance
chem(o)	chemical	*chemolysis* [kĕm-ŎL-ĭ-sĭs], chemical decomposition
chlor(o)	chlorine, green	*chloruresis* [klō-yū-RĒ-sĭs], excretion of chloride in urine
chondrio, chondro	cartilage, grainy, gritty	*chondrocyte* [KŎN-drō-sīt], cartilage cell
chore(o)	dance	*choreoathetosis* [KŌR-ē-ō-ăth-ĕ-TŌ-sĭs], abnormal body movements
chrom, chromat, chromo	color	*chromatogenous* [krō-mă-TŎJ-ĕ-nŭs], producing color
chrono	time	*chronometry* [krō-NŎM-ĕ-trē], measurement of time intervals

COMBINING FORM	MEANING	EXAMPLE
chyl(o)	chyle, a digestive juice	*chylopoiesis* [KĪ-lō-pŏy-Ē-sĭs], production of chyle in the intestine
chym(o)	chyme, semifluid production of chyme in the stomach	*chymopoiesis* [KĪ-mō-pŏy-Ē-sĭs], present during digestion
cine(o)	movement	*cineradiography* [SĬN-ĕ-rā-dē-ŎG-ră-fē], imaging of an organ in motion
coni(o)	dust	*coniometer* [kō-nē-ŎM-ĕ-tĕr], device for measuring dust
crin(o)	secrete	*crinogenic* [krĭn-ō-JĔN-ĭk], causing secretion; *endocrine* [EN-do-krin], a gland that secretes internally into systemic circulation
cry(o)	cold	*cryocautery* [KRĪ-ō-KĂW-tĕr-ē], destruction of tissue by freezing
crypt(o)	hidden; obscure	*cryptogenic* [krĭp-tō-JĔN-ĭk], of obscure origin
cyan(o)	blue	*cyanopsia* [sī-ă-NŎP-sē-ă], condition following a cataract operation in which all objects appear blue
cycl(o)	circle; cycle; ciliary body	*cyclectomy* [sī-KLĔK-tō-mē], removal of a part of a ciliary body
cyst(o), cysti	bladder, cyst, cystic duct	*cystoid* [SĬS-tŏyd], bladder-shaped
cyt(o)	cell	*cytoarchitecture* [SĪ-tō-ĂR-kĭ-tĕk-chūr], arrangement of cells in tissue
dextr(o)	right, toward the right	*dextrocardia* [DĔKS-trō-KĂR-dē-ă], displacement of the heart to the right
dips(o)	thirst	*dipsomania* [dĭp-sō-MĀ-nē-ă], alcoholism
dors(o), dorsi	back	*dorsalgia* [dōr-SĂL-jē-ă], upper back pain
dynamo	force; energy	*dynamometer* [dī-nă-MŎM-ĕ-tĕr], instrument for measuring muscular power
echo	reflected sound	*echocardiogram* [ĕk-ō-KĂR-dē-ō-grăm], ultrasound recording of the heart
electr(o)	electricity; electric	*electrocardiogram* [ē-lĕk-trō-KĂR-dē-ō-grăm], graphic record of heart's electrical currents
eosin(o)	red; rosy	*eosinophilic* [ē-ō-sĭn-ō-FĬL-ĭk], staining readily with certain dyes
ergo	work	*ergograph* [ĔR-gō-grăf], instrument for measuring work of muscular contractions
erythr(o)	red, redness	*erythroclasis* [ĕr-ĭ-THRŎK-lă-sĭs], fragmentation of red blood cells

COMBINING FORM	MEANING	EXAMPLE
esthesio	sensation, perception	*esthesiometry* [ĕs-thē-zē-ŎM-ĕ-trē], measurement of tactile sensibility
ethmo	ethmoid bone	*ethmonasal* [ĕth-mō-NĀ-săl], relating to the ethmoid and nasal bones
etio	cause	*etiopathology* [Ē-tē-ō-pă-THŎL-ō-jē], study of the cause of an abnormality or disease
fibr(o)	fiber	*fibroplastic* [fī-brō-PLĂS-tĭk], producing fibrous tissue
fluor(o)	light; luminous; fluorine	*fluorochrome* [FLŪR-ō-krōm], fluorescent contrast medium
fungi	fungus	*fungicide* [FŬN-jĭ-sīd], substance that destroys fungi
galact(o)	milk	*galactophoritis* [gă-LĂK-tō-fō-RĪ-tĭs], inflammation of the milk ducts
gen(o)	producing; being born	*genoblast* [JĔN-ō-blăst], nucleus of a fertilized ovum
gero, geront(o)	old age	*gerontology* [jār-ŏn-TŎL-ō-jē], study of the problems of aging
gluco	glucose	*glucogenic* [glū-kō-JĔN-ĭk], producing glucose
glyco	sugars	*glycopenia* [glī-kō-PĒ-nē-ă], sugar deficiency
gonio	angle	*goniometer* [gō-nē-ŎM-ĕ-tĕr], instrument for measuring angles
granulo	granular	*granuloma* [grăn-yū-LŌ-mă], small, granular lesion
gyn(o), gyne, gyneco	women	*gynopathy* [gī-NŎP-ă-thē], disease peculiar to women
home(o), homo	same; constant	*homeoplasia* [HŌ-mē-ō-PLĀ-zhē-ă], formation of new, similar tissue
hydr(o)	hydrogen, water	*hydrocephaly* [hī-drō-SĔF-ă-lē], condition characterized by excessive fluid accumulation in the head
hypn(o)	sleep	*hypnogenesis* [hĭp-nō-JĔN-ĕ-sĭs], induction of sleep
iatr(o)	physician; treatment	*iatrogenic* [ī-ăt-rō-JĔN-ĭk], produced or caused by treatment or diagnostic procedure
ichthy(o)	dry; scaly; fish	*ichthyotoxism* [ĬK-thē-ō-TŎK-sĭzm], poisoning by fish
idio	distinct; unknown	*idiopathic* [ĬD-ē-ō-PĂTH-ĭk], of unknown origin (said of a disease)

Combining Form	Meaning	Example
immun(o)	safe; immune	*immunodeficient* [ĬM-yū-nō-dē-FĬSH-ĕnt], lacking in some essential immune function
kal(i)	potassium	*kalemia* [kă-LĒ-mē-ă], presence of potassium in the blood
karyo	nucleus	*karyolysis* [kăr-ē-ŎL-ĭ-sĭs], destruction of a cell nucleus
ket(o), keton(o)	ketone; acetone	*ketogenesis* [kē-tō-JĔN-ĕ-sĭs], metabolic production of ketones
kin(o), kine	movement	*kinesthesia* [KĬN-ĕs-THĒ-zhē-ă], perception of movement
kinesi(o), kineso	motion	*kinesiology* [kĭ-nē-sē-ŎL-ō-jē], study of movement
kyph(o)	humpback	*kyphoscoliosis* [KĬ-fō-skō-lē-Ō-sĭs], kyphosis combined with scoliosis
lact(o), lacti	milk	*lactogen* [LĂK-tō-jĕn], agent that stimulates milk production
latero	lateral, to one side	*lateroduction* [LĂT-ĕr-ō-DŬK-shŭn], movement to one side
lepto	light, frail, thin	*leptomeninges* [lĕp-tō-mĕ-NĬN-jēz], two delicate layers of meninges
leuk(o)	white	*leukoblast* [LŪ-kō-blăst], immature white blood cell
lip(o)	fat	*lipoblast* [LĬ-pō-blăst], embryonic fat cell
lith(o)	stone	*lithotomy* [lĭ-THŎT-ō-mē], operation for removal of stones
log(o)	speech, words, thought	*logopathy* [lŏg-ŎP-ă-thē], speech disorder
lys(o)	dissolution	*lysemia* [lī-SĒ-mē-ă], dissolution of red blood cells
macr(o)	large; long	*macromelia* [măk-rō-MĒ-lē-ă], abnormally sized limb
medi(o)	middle; medial plane	*mediolateral* [MĒ-dē-ō-LĂT-ĕr-ăl], relating to the medial plane and one side of the body
meg(a), megal(o)	large; million	*megaloencephaly* [MĔG-ă-lyō-ĕn-SĔF-ă-lē], abnormally large brain
melan(o)	black; dark	*melanoderma* [MĔL-ă-nō-DĔR-mă], abnormal skin darkening
mes(o)	middle; median	*mesocephalic* [MĔZ-ō-sĕ-FĂL-ĭk], having a medium-sized head
micr(o)	small; one-millionth; tiny	*microorganism* [MĪ-krō-ŌR-găn-ĭzm], tiny organism

Combining Form	Meaning	Example
mio	smaller; less	*miopragia* [mī-ō-PRĀ-jē-ă], lessened functional activity
morph(o)	structure; shape	*morphology* [mōr-FŎL-ō-jē], study of the structure of animals and plants
narco	sleep; numbness	*narcolepsy* [NĂR-kō-lĕp-sē], sleep disorder
necr(o)	death; dying	*necrology* [nĕ-KRŎL-ō-jē], study of the cause of death
noct(i)	night	*nocturia* [nŏk-TŪ-rē-ă], urination at night
normo	normal	*normocyte* [NŌR-mō-sīt], normal red blood cell
nucle(o)	nucleus	*nucleotoxin* [NŪ-klē-ō-TŎK-sĭn], poison that acts upon a cell nucleus
nyct(o)	night	*nyctalopia* [nĭk-tă-LŌ-pē-ă], reduced ability to see at night
oncho, onco	tumor	*oncolysis* [ŏng-KŎL-ĭ-sĭs], destruction of a tumor
orth(o)	straight; normal	*orthodontics* [ōr-thō-DŎN-tĭks], dental specialty concerned with correction of tooth placement
oxy	sharp; acute; oxygen	*oxyphonia* [ŏk-sē-FŌN-nē-ă], shrillness of voice
pachy	thick	*pachyonychia* [PĂK-ē-ō-NĬK-ē-ă], abnormal thickening of the nails
path(o)	disease	*pathogen* [PĂTH-ō-jĕn], disease-causing substance
phago	eating; devouring; swallowing	*phagocyte* [FĂG-ō-sīt], cell that ingests bacteria and other particles
pharmaco	drugs; medicine	*pharmacology* [FĂR-mă-KŎL-ō-jē], the science of drugs, including their sources, uses, and interactions
phon(o)	sound; voice; speech	*phonometer* [fō-NŎM-ĕ-tĕr], instrument for measuring sound
phot(o)	light	*photometer* [fō-TŎM-ĕ-tĕr], instrument for measuring light
physi, physio	physical; natural	*physiotherapy* [FĬZ-ē-ō-THĀR-ă-pē], physical therapy
physo	air; gas; growing	*physocele* [FĬ-sō-sēl], swelling due to gas
phyt(o)	plant	*phytoxin* [fī-tō-TŎK-sĭn], substance from plants that is similar to a bacterial toxin
plasma, plasmo	formative; plasma	*plasmapheresis* [PLĂZ-mă-fĕ-RĒ-sĭs], separation of blood into parts

Combining Form	Meaning	Example
poikilo	varied; irregular	*poikilocyte* [PŎY-kĭ-lō-sīt], irregularly shaped red blood cell
pseud(o)	false	*pseudodiabetes* [SŪ-dō-dī-ă-BĒ-tēz], false positive test for sugar in the urine
pyo	pus	*pyocyst* [PĪ-ō-sĭst], cyst filled with pus
pyreto	fever	*pyretogenous* [pī-rĕ-TŎJ-ĕ-nŭs], causing fever
pyro	fever; fire; heat	*pyrogenic* [pī-rō-JĔN-ĭk], causing fever
radio	radiation; x-ray; radius	*radiography* [RĀ-dē-ŎG-ră-fē], x-ray examination
salping(o)	tube	*salpingectomy* [săl-pĭn-JĔK-tō-mē], removal of the fallopian tube
schisto	split	*schistocytosis* [SKĬS-tō-sī-TŌ-sĭs], bladder fissure
schiz(o)	split; division	*schizophrenia* [skĭz-ō-FRĔ-nē-ă, skĭts-ō-FRĔ-nē-ă], a spectrum of mental disorders often with a disorder in perception
scler(o)	hardness; hardening	*scleroderma* [sklēr-ō-DĔR-mă], thickening and hardness of the skin
scolio	crooked; bent	*scoliometer* [skō-lē-ŎM-ĕ-tĕr], instrument for measuring curves
scoto	darkness	*scotograph* [SKŌ-tō-grăf], appliance for helping the blind to write
sidero	iron	*sideropenia* [SĬD-ĕr-ō-PĒ-nē-ă] abnormally low level of iron in the blood
sito	food; grain	*sitotoxin* [sī-tō-TŎK-sĭn], any food poison
somat(o)	body	*somatogenic* [SŌ-mă-tō-JĔN-ĭk], originating in the body
somn(o), somni	sleep	*somnambulism* [sŏm-NĂM-byū-lĭzm], sleepwalking
sono	sound	*sonomotor* [sŏn-ō-MŌ-tĕr], relating to movements caused by sound
spasmo	spasm	*spasmolytic* [SPĂZ-mō-LĬT-ĭk], agent that relieves spasms
spher(o)	round; spherical	*spherocyte* [SFĒR-ō-sīt], spherical red blood cell
spir(o)	breath; breathe	*spiroscope* [SPĪ-rō-skōp], device for measuring lung capacity
squamo	scale; squamous	*squamofrontal* [SKWĀ-mō-FRŎN-tăl], relating to the squamous part of the frontal bone

Combining Form	Meaning	Example
staphyl(o)	grapelike clusters	*staphylococcus* [STĂF-ĭ-lō-KŎK-ŭs], a common species that is the cause of a variety of infections
steno	narrowness	*stenocephaly* [stĕn-ō-SĔF-ă-lē], narrowness of the head
stere(o)	three-dimensional	*stereology* [STĔR-ē-ŎL-ō-jē], study of three-dimensional aspects of a cell
strepto	twisted chains; streptococci	*streptococcus* [strĕp-tō-KŎK-ŭs], a common organism that can cause various infections
styl(o)	peg-shaped	*styloid* [STĪ-lŏyd], peg-shaped; said of a bony growth
syring(o)	tube	*syringitis* [sĭ-rĭn-JĪ-tĭs], inflammation of the eustachian tube
tel(o), tele(o)	distant; end; complete	*telophase* [TĔL-ō-fāz], final stages of mitosis or meiosis
terato	monster (as a malformed fetus)	*teratogen* [TĔR-ă-tō-jĕn], agent that causes a malformed fetus
therm(o)	heat	*thermometer* [thĕr-MŎM-ĕ-tĕr], an instrument for measuring temperature
tono	tension; pressure	*tonometer* [tō-NŎM-ĕ-tĕr], instrument for measuring pressure
top(o)	place; topical	*topography* [tō-PŎG-ră-fĕ], description of a body part in terms of a specific surface area
tox(i), toxico, toxo	poison; toxin	*toxipathy* [tŏk-SĬP-ă-thē], disease due to poisoning
tropho	food; nutrition	*trophocyte* [TRŎF-ō-sīt], cell that provides nutrition
vivi	life	*viviparous* [vī-VĬP-ă-rŭs], giving birth to living young
xanth(o)	yellow	*xanthoderma* [zăn-thō-DĔR-mă], yellowish skin
xeno	stranger	*xenophobia* [zĕn-ō-FŌ-bē-ă], extreme fear of strangers or foreigners
xer(o)	dry	*xerasia* [zĕ-RĀ-zhē-ă], dry and brittle hair condition
xiph(o)	sword; xiphoid	*xiphocostal* [ZĬF-ō-KŎS-tăl], relating to the xiphoid process and the ribs
zo(o)	life	*zooblast* [ZŌ-ō-blăst], animal cell
zym(o)	fermentation; enzyme	*zymogram* [ZĪ-mō-grăm], strips of paper for testing for location of enzymes

Forming Medical Terms Exercises

Building Medical Words

Using the following word parts, build medical terms for the definitions given in the following questions. Use two word parts for each answer.

cephalic	cyesis	dys	macro
micro	necro	normo	nycto
osis	otic	phobia	phonia
pseudo	scolio	scope	

26. instrument to view small items _____
27. false pregnancy _____
28. fear of night _____
29. condition of difficult speech _____
30. pertaining to a normal size head _____
31. abnormal curvature of the spine _____

Understanding Word Parts

Define each of the following medical terms. Then break each term into word parts and give the definition for each part. If you need help with any suffixes, refer to Chapter 2.

32. cyanosis _____

_____

33. leukocyte _____

_____

34. cytometer _____

_____

35. chrondroma _____

_____

36. adipocele _____

_____

37. fungicide _____

_____

38. glucogenesis _____

_____

39. karyocyte _____

_____

40. hydrotherapy _____

_____

41. homeostasis _____

_____

42. radiology _____

_____

43. necrosis _____

_____

44. dysphagia _____

_____

Completing the Terms

Using one or more of the following combining forms, complete the word that best fits the definition given below. If you have difficulty understanding some of the word parts, refer to Chapter 2.

angi(o)	burs(o)	carcin(o)	cry(o)
cyst(o)	cyt(o)	erythr(o)	fibr(o)
glyc(o)	gynec(o)	hypn(o)	immun(o)
later(o)	lip(o)	lith(o)	lymph(o)
macr(o)	medi(o)	neur(o)	oste(o)

45. condition of red blood cells: _____ osis

46. cancerous tumor: _____ oma

47. ultrasound examination of the bladder: _____ graphy

48. examination of a cell: _____ scopy

49. cold therapy: _____ therapy

50. pertaining to one side: _____ al

51. deficiency of sugar: _____ penia

52. large enough to be examined with the naked eye: _____ scopic

53. breakdown of fats: _____ lysis

54. altered state of consciousness resembling sleep: _____ osis

55. toward the middle: _____ ad

56. impairment or insufficient development of immune response: _____ compromised

57. branch of medicine dealing with the diagnosis of disorders affecting women: _____ ology

58. resembling or made of fibers or fibrous tissue: _____ oid

59. surgical crushing of a stone: _____ tripsy

60. abnormal thinning and degeneration of the bone: _____ porosis

61. inflammation of the bursa: _____ itis

62. nerve inflammation: _____ itis

63. surgical repair of a vessel: _____ plasty

64. mass or tumor made of lymph tissue: _____ oma

Legal and Ethical Issues

Health care workers share some special obligations, both legally and ethically. Many legal decisions have upheld the right of patients to privacy in the health care setting. Patients also have the right to sue over maltreatment. Ethical standards require that patients and their families are treated fairly. "Fair" may include giving the best care, keeping clear records, or respecting patients' rights. The American Hospital Association's Patient's Bill of Rights gives twelve guidelines for medical staff, administrative personnel, and patients. Although these are specifically meant for hospitals, most of the following guidelines provide a clear, ethical standard for patients' rights in all health care settings.

- The right to considerate and respectful care.
- The right to relevant, current, and understandable information about their diagnosis, treatment, and prognosis.
- The right to make decisions about the planned care and the right to refuse care.
- The right to have an advance directive (such as a living will) concerning treatment if they become incapacitated.
- The right to privacy in all procedures, examinations, and discussions of treatment.
- The right to confidential handling of all information and records about their care.
- The right to look over and have all records about their care explained.
- The right to suggest changes in the planned care or to transfer to another facility.
- The right to be informed about the business relationships among the hospital and other facilities that are part of the treatment and care.
- The right to decide whether to take part in experimental treatments.
- The right to understand their care options after a hospital stay.
- The right to know about the hospital's policies for settling disputes and to examine and receive an explanation of all charges.

For more information about the Patient's Bill of Rights, go to the American Hospital Association's Web site (www.aha.org).

As a worker in health care, you may be a clinical worker who provides direct care, or you may be an administrative worker who usually has access to, or responsibility for, patient records. In either case, the adherence to all legal and ethical standards is a fundamental requirement of your job. Many issues are legislated differently around the country. You must follow the rules of the state and institution for which you work. Never take it upon yourself to make medical decisions for which you have not been trained and are not qualified.

HIPAA and Allied Health Professions

In 1996, Congress passed the Health Insurance Portability and Accountability Act of 1996 (HIPAA). This law protects health insurance coverage for workers and their families when they change or lose their jobs. The act also requires the Department of Health and Human Services to

MORE ABOUT . . .

HIPAA and Privacy

The following are examples of possible violations of patient privacy under HIPAA regulations and some suggestions about how to avoid them.

- Telephone conversations with (or regarding) patients should not be held within earshot of the reception room or other patients. This is why phone triage is set apart from patient areas.

- A conversation with the patient being escorted down the hall to the exam or treatment room should not include the reason the patient is being seen, how treatment is progressing, or whether they followed the prep instructions for this visit. Limit the conversation until there is a private environment.

- Patient records, documents, telephone messages, lab reports, etc. should be sorted, processed, and/or filed promptly. If there is a need to retain the documents for processing or reference, the documents should be stored in an area apart from patient flow.

- When scheduling a procedure by phone, it should be done away from areas of high traffic, preferably in a private office.

establish national standards for electronic health care transactions and national identifiers such as personal identification numbers (or PINS) for providers, health plans, and employers. It also addresses the security and privacy of health data. The goal of the law is to improve the efficiency and effectiveness of the nation's health care system by encouraging the widespread use of electronic data interchange in health care.

> There are a number of Web sites where you can learn about HIPAA (www.cms.gov; www.hhs.gov). You can also do a search for the keyword HIPAA and you will come up with many more sites.

CASE STUDY

Working in Health Care

The Crestview Walk-In Medical Center is a nonemergency clinic. It employs three doctors, four nurses, three medical assistants, and two receptionists. All twelve employees have access to the many patient records kept in the files and in the computers at Crestview. The small conference room at the back of the facility doubles as a lunchroom. Most of the staff bring their snacks and lunches to work because Crestview is in a suburban neighborhood that does not have many stores or restaurants nearby.

All the employees have one thing in common—the patients. When they gather in the conference room for meetings, the teams discuss how to handle their cases. However, when the room becomes a lunchroom, all patient discussion stops. The facility has a strict policy that allows discussion of cases only in a professional setting. Everyone observes the ethical and legal codes that forbid staff from discussing cases outside the facility and outside the domain of a work situation.

Critical Thinking

65. Why should the facility have a policy about discussing specific cases among the staff? What should it be?

66. Based on what you understand about the roles of the physicians, nurses, medical assistants, and receptionists, who do you think should have access to patient files?

Using Medical Terminology

Many careers depend on a sound knowledge of medical terminology. Written or electronic records are developed and used by many people involved in health care services. Spoken directions are used to communicate orders for health care and administrative procedures in the health care setting. The role of each health care professional (worker) is usually limited to the skills, procedures, and knowledge outlined by state or federal law for each profession. Usually includes the duties that each person is or is not allowed to do. For example, physicians, nurse practioners, and physician assistants diagnose, treat, and prescribe medications for the treatment of diseases. Nurses and medical assistants administer medications, track vital signs, and give care, but are not allowed to prescribe medication. Other health care employees (such as patient care technicians) may combine administrative and clinical duties in various health care settings. People in health information management perform many of the administrative tasks that allow facilities to get paid or reimbursed in the complicated world of health care. The systems chapters, case studies, and career pages in this text will introduce you to people working in the health care environment.

From the time someone calls or visits a physician's office, that patient's medical record is involved. The medical assistant or receptionist first gathers or updates personal information about the patient, such as name, address, and insurance information, as well as learns the patient's chief complaint, or reason for the visit. The medical documentation continues to grow as the provider (the physician, nurse, nurse-practitioner, and so on) sees the patient, gathers the pertinent medical history and performs a physical examination, reaches a diagnosis, and provides procedures appropriate for the condition or illness. If a patient is hospitalized, or additional laboratory or x-ray services are needed, hospital workers, laboratory technicians, and radiologists may perform procedures, which must be documented. The patient's medical record then provides the basis for payment for these services. Coders and billing clerks then fill out the paperwork necessary to enable the provider to get paid.

Documentation of health care services must be complete for both ethical and legal reasons. Many health care careers require an understanding of documentation. Documentation in the form of medical records typically uses many terms learned in medical terminology courses.

Formats for records depend on state law, the institution's responsibilities, the configuration of its computer systems, and its coding and billing practices. One plan of organization is the SOAP approach. SOAP stands for *subjective, objective, assessment,* and *plan*. When first dealing with a patient, the health care practitioner receives the subjective information from the patient (how the patient feels, what the symptoms are). Next, the health care practitioner performs an examination (takes temperature, blood pressure, pulse) and orders tests (blood and urine tests, allergy tests), thereby getting the objective facts needed for a diagnosis. The assessment stage is the examination of all data and the reaching of a conclusion (the diagnosis). Finally, a plan—treatments, medications, tests, and patient education—is determined and put into action for ongoing evaluation. Figure 1-1 is an

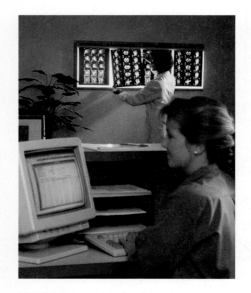

FIGURE 1-1 Medical procedures are documented electronically as in this hospital or on paper as in many medical offices. Sometimes, both types of documentation are used.

example of a SOAP medical record. Another method of documentation is chronological, in which patient interactions are listed in chronological order with the earliest date at the top (Figure 1-2). Figure 1-3 shows documentation for a specific procedure—with the procedure, the person performing it, and what took place. Appendix E gives patient records in several formats.

Do you know the difference between subjective and objective? Subjective information is something that is thought or felt in the mind but may not be observable by others. Objective information is something that can be measured or observed by others.

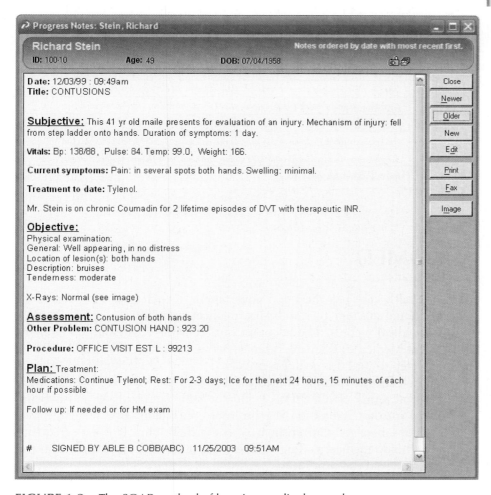

FIGURE 1-2   The SOAP method of keeping medical records.

Patient name _Angela O'Toole_	Age _57_	Current Diagnosis _angina_

DATE/TIME	
10/10/XX	Patient presents with increased chest pain, particularly after meals. Sent to lab for echocardiogram; BP 143/84. Leonard Glasser, M.D.
10/14/XX	Phone consultation with patient—echocardiogram shows status quo. Suspect acid reflux, tell patient to add Tagamet to medications. Leonard Glasser, M.D.
10/21/XX	Patient call—experiencing relief. Continue present medication and Tagamet. Leonard Glasser, M.D.

FIGURE 1-3   A chronological medical record.

FIGURE 1-4 A medical record of a
gastroscopy, a surgical procedure.

PROCEDURE: *Gastroscopy*		PATIENT: *Holly Berger*
STAFF: *Dr. Walker*		ID no.: *888–22–8888*
DATE 9/28/XX	*Instrument—GIF100 video gastroscope*	
	Premedication: 2% Cetacaine spray locally; Demerol 50 mg; Valium 20 mg IV;	
	Atropine 0.4 mg IM.	
	History: 51 year-old white female with longstanding Crohn's disease, status post	
	resection of the terminal ileum and proximal colon in 1971. The patient has been	
	complaining of epigastric and right-sided abdominal pain with occasional	
	nausea, vomiting over the last 3 weeks. Upper GI *series and small bowel follow*	
	through showed narrowing of the duodenal bulb and post-bulbar segment and	
	then approximately 8 cm. irregular stenotic area in the right side of the abdomen,	
	probably at the area of the previous anastomosis and the right proximal	
	jejunal stricture.	
	Procedure: The patient was brought to the endoscopy suite on a gurney. Her	
	oropharynx was sprayed with 2% Cetacaine and then she was placed in the left	
	lateral decubitus position.	

SNOMED

For more information, visit SNOMED's
Web site (www.snomed.org).

Many health care providers and government agencies are involved in an international attempt to standardize medical terminology for use in electronic medical records. The adoption of SNOMED (Systematized Nomenclature of Medicine) Clinical Terms®, better known as SNOMED CT®, is a major step toward this goal. Eventually, it is expected that all medical coding and electronic transfer of medical data will use SNOMED as the basis for medical terms. SNOMED is gradually being standardized and is being uploaded into a database on the Internet continually. It is available in a number of languages. Currently, it is in use in Britain. It is expected that people who do medical coding will be using it for electronic records in the United States in the near future.

ICD-9 and ICD-10

The set of diagnosis codes in the coding reference called *The International Classification of Diseases, 9th Revision, Clinical Modification* is the current standard for coding patient records and death certificates. Eventually, it is thought that ICD will be combined with SNOMED once all healthcare records are electronic.

The World Health Organization (WHO) developed the ICD CM system. The numeric reference indicates what edition is being used within the system. *ICD-10CM* and *ICD-10PCS* (Professional Coding System prepared by the Centers for Medicare and Medicaid) are currently available; however, the United States is not currently using the new updated classifications. More information on ICD-10 can be found at: www.ahima.org.

Abbreviations

Throughout this text, you will learn common medical abbreviations. In recent years, several organizations have come out with recommendations regarding the use of certain abbreviations that have caused confusion. See Appendix for more details on the use of abbreviations in the medical setting.

USING MEDICAL TERMINOLOGY EXERCISES

Analyzing the Record

Write S for subjective, O for objective, A for assessment, and P for plan after each of the following phrases.

67. I feel nauseous _____

68. Allergy medicine prescribed _____

69. Has dermatitis (rash) _____

70. My arm aches _____

71. Has hypertension _____

Check Your Knowledge

Circle T for true of F for false.

72. Nurses never add to a patient's record. T F

73. A medical assistant should be able to decipher the doctor's notes. T F

74. Rules of confidentiality apply to patient records. T F

75. Objective information is always given by the patient. T F

76. A plan for treatment must never be changed. T F

77. HIPAA governs the Patient's Bill of Rights. T F

78. SNOMED is used widely in the United States. T F

79. Privacy in the medical office is the responsibility of everyone who works there. T F

80. Combining forms are the same as prefixes. T F

81. A word's history is called its etymology. T F

USING THE INTERNET

82. At the Electronic Privacy Information Center site (http://epic.org/privacy/medical/), you will find discussions of current cases, articles, and advice on safeguarding medical records. Click one of the site's topics. Write a paragraph explaining the issue being discussed.

83. Using a search engine, find a site that discusses medical errors and gives details of one type of medical error that you find.

Answers to Chapter Exercises

1. Greek, Latin
2. Hippocrates
3. Greek
4. Greek, Latin
5. written
6. ă-NĒ-mē-ă
7. ĂN-jē-ō-plăs-tē
8. bĕr-SĪ-tĭs
9. dĭ-ZĒZ
10. hē-mō-GLŌ-bĭn
11. lĭm-FŌ-mă
12. nū-RĪ-tĭs
13. ŎS-tē-ō-pō-RŌ-sĭs
14. păr-ă-PLĒ-jē-ă
15. pŭls
16. rā-dē-Ā-shŭn
17. RĒ-flĕks
18. RĔT-ĭ-nă
19. RŪ-mă-tĭzm
20. sī-ĂT-ĭ-kă
21. SĔP-tŭm
22. SĪ-nŭs
23. THĀR-ă-pē
24. TĪ-fŏyd
25. VĂK-sēn
26. microscope
27. pseudocyesis
28. nyctophobia
29. dysphonia
30. normocephalic
31. scoliosis
32. abnormal condition of blue (skin): cyan(o), blue + -osis, condition, state, process
33. white blood cell: leuk(o), white + -cyte, cell
34. instrument for counting and measuring cells: cyt(o), cell + -meter, instrument for measuring

35. tumor (or tumor-like growth) of cartilage: chondro, cartilage + -oma, tumor
36. hernia containing fat or fatty tissue: adip(o), fat + -cele, hernia
37. agent that destroys fungi: fungi-, fungus + -cide, destroying or killing
38. the formation/production of glucose: gluco-, glucose + -genesis, production of
39. any cell containing a nucleus: karyo-, nucleus + -cyte, cell
40. therapy using water: hydro-, water + therapy, treatment
41. the ability of the body to remain in a constant state of equilibrium: homeo-, same + -stasis, stopping
42. study of radiation (x-ray) radio-, radiation + -logy, study of
43. abnormal death of tissue: necro-, death + -osis, condition of
44. difficulty swallowing: dys-, difficult + -phagia, swallowing
45. erythrocytosis
46. carcinoma
47. cystography
48. cytoscopy
49. cryotherapy
50. lateral
51. glycopenia
52. macroscopic
53. lipolysis
54. hypnosis
55. mediad
56. immunocompromised

57. gynecology
58. fibroid
59. lithotripsy
60. osteoporosis
61. bursitis
62. neuritis
63. angioplasty
64. lymphoma
65. There needs to be a policy because unsupervised discussion of cases in an informal setting can lead to breaches of confidentiality. The policy should limit discussion to case review (often supervised) and answering of specific questions.
66. Specific members of the staff need access to patient files. Facility policy should make the rules of access clear enough that the staff understands the legal and ethical implications of confidentiality.
67. S
68. P
69. O
70. S
71. A
72. F
73. T
74. T
75. F
76. F
77. F
78. F
79. T
80. F
81. T

Prefixes and Suffixes in Medical Terms

CHAPTER 2

After studying this chapter, you will be able to:

2.1   Define common medical prefixes
2.2   Define common medical suffixes
2.3   Describe how word parts are put together to form words

Medical Prefixes and Suffixes

In Chapter 1, you learned about the four basic word parts—word roots, combining forms, prefixes, and suffixes, and you learned the important medical roots and combining forms. In this chapter, you learn the important medical prefixes and suffixes and how word parts are put together to form medical terms.

Prefixes

Prefixes are word parts that modify the meaning of the word or word root. They attach to the beginning of words. Prefixes tend to indicate size, quantity, position, presence of, and location. When trying to understand a word with a prefix, you can take apart the word, find the meaning of each part, and then determine the meaning of the entire word. For example, terms for paralysis include *paraplegia, hemiplegia,* and *quadriplegia.* By taking apart the three terms, you can deduce the meaning of each of these three medical terms.

para- = abnormal; involving two parts + -plegia = paralysis
hemi- = half
quadri- = four

Sometimes you need to reason out a meaning that is not quite the prefix plus the root but is a meaning that makes sense. *Paraplegia* is paralysis of the two lower limbs; *hemiplegia* is paralysis of one side; and *quadriplegia* is paralysis of all four limbs. The meaning "limbs" is not contained specifically in the prefix but it is understood from the combination of the numbers in the prefix's meaning and the root meaning paralysis—so "two paralysis" is paralysis of the two lower limbs (since you cannot have paralysis of just the upper limbs).

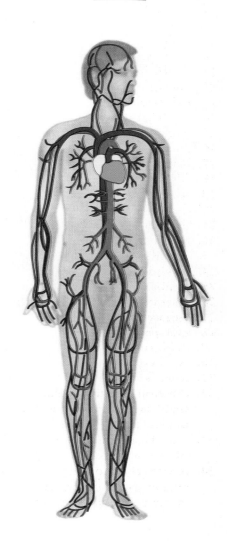

To learn more about paralysis and what is being done to cure it, go to the National Spinal Cord Injury Association's Web site (www.spinalcord.org).

PREFIXES	MEANING	EXAMPLE
a-	without	*asepsis* [ā-SĔP-sĭs], without living organisms
ab-, abs-	away from	*abduct* [ăb-DŬKT], to draw away from a position
ad-	toward, to	*adduct* [ă-DŬKT], to draw toward the body, as a limb
ambi-	both, around	*ambidextrous* [ăm-bē-DĔKS-trŭs], having ability on both the right and left sides (said of the hands)
an-	without	*anencephalic* [ăn-ĕn-sĕ-FĂL-ĭk], without a brain
ana-	up, toward	*anaphylactic* [ĂN-ă-fĭ-LĂK-tĭk], exaggerated reaction to an antigen or toxin
ante-	before	*antemortem* [ĂN-tē-mŏr-tĕm], before death
anti-	against	*antibacterial* [ĂN-tē-băk-TĒR-ē-ăl], preventing the growth of bacteria
apo-	derived, separate	*apobiosis* [ăp-ō-bī-Ō-sĭs], death of a part of a living organism
aut(o)-	self	*autoimmune* [ăw-tō-ĭ-MYŪN], against an individual's own tissue
bi-	twice, double	*biparous* [BĬP-ă-rŭs], bearing two young
brachy-	short	*brachyesophagus* [BRĂK-ē-ĕ-sŏf-ă-gŭs], abnormally short esophagus
brady-	slow	*bradycardia* [brăd-ē-KĂR-dē-ă], abnormally slow heartbeat
cata-	down	*cataplexy* [KĂT-ă-plĕk-sē], sudden extreme muscle weakness
circum-	around	*circumoral* [sĕr-kŭm-ŌR-ăl], around the mouth
co-, col-, com-, con-, cor-	together	*codominant* [kō-DŎM-ĭ-nănt], having an equal degree of dominance (said of two genes)
contra-	against	*contraindicated* [kŏn-tră-ĭn-dĭ-KĀ-tĕd], not recommended
de-	away from	*demyelination* [dē-MĬ-ĕ-lĭ-NĀ-shŭn], loss of myelin
di-, dif-, dir-, dis-,	not, separated	*disarticulation* [dĭs-ăr-tĭk-yū-LĀ-shŭn], amputation of a joint
dia-	through	*diaplacental* [dī-ă-plă-SĔN-tăl], passing through the placenta

PREFIXES	MEANING	EXAMPLE
dys-	abnormal; difficult	*dysfunctional* [dĭs-FŬNK-shŭn-ăl], functioning abnormally
ect(o)-	outside	*ectopic* [ĕk-TŎP-ĭk], occurring outside the normal place, as a pregnancy occurring outside of the uterus
end(o)-	within	*endoabdominal* [ĔN-dō-ăb-DŎM-ĭ-năl], within the abdomen
epi-	over	*epicondyle* [ĕp-ĭ-KŎN-dīl], projection over or near the condyle
eu-	well, good, normal	*eupepsia* [yū-PĔP-sē-ă], normal digestion
ex-	out of, away from	*exhale* [ĔKS-hāl], breathe out
exo-	external, on the outside	*exogenous* [ĕks-ŎJ-ĕ-nŭs], produced outside of the organism
extra-	without, outside of	*extracorporeal* [ĕks-tră-kōr-PŎ-rē-ăl], outside of the body
hemi-	half	*hemiplegia* [hĕm-ĭ-PLĒ-jē-ă], paralysis on one side of the body
hyper-	above normal; overly	*hyperactive* [hī-pĕr-ĂK-tĭv], abnormally restless and inattentive
hypo-	below normal	*hypoglycemia* [hī-pō-glī-SĒ-mē-ă], low blood sugar
infra-	positioned beneath	*infrasternal* [ĭn-fră-STĔR-năl], below the sternum
inter-	between	*interdental* [ĭn-tĕr-DĔN-tăl], between the teeth
intra-	within	*intramuscular* [ĬN-tră-MŬS-kyū-lăr], within the substance of the muscles
iso-	equal, same	*isometric* [ī-sō-MĔT-rĭk], of the same dimensions
mal-	bad; inadequate	*malabsorption* [măl-ăb-SŎRP-shŭn], inadequate absorption
meg(a)-, megal(o)-	large	*megacephaly* [mĕg-ă-SĔF-ă-lē], abnormal enlargement of the head
mes(o)-	middle, median	*mesoderm* [MĔZ-ō-dĕrm], the middle layer of skin
meta-	after	*metacarpus* [MĔT-ă-KĂR-pŭs], bones attached to the carpus

Prefixes	Meaning	Example
micr(o)-	small, microscopic	*microplasia* [mī-krō-PLĀ-zhē-ă], stunted growth, as in dwarfism
mon(o)-	single	*monomania* [mŏn-ō-MĀ-nē-ă], obsession with a single thought or idea
multi-	many	*multiarticular* [MŬL-tē-ăr-TĬK-yū-lăr], involving many joints
olig(o)-	few; little; scanty	*oligospermia* [ŏl-ĭ-gō-SPĔR-mē-ă], low sperm count
pan-, pant(o)-	all, entire	*panarthritis* [păn-ăr-THRĪ-tĭs], arthritis involving all joints
par(a)-	beside; abnormal; involving two parts	*parakinesia* [păr-ă-kĭ-NĒ-zhē-ă], motor abnormality
per-	through, intensely	*peraxillary* [pĕr-ĂK-sĭ-lār-ē], through the axilla
peri-	around, about, near	*periappendicitis* [PĔR-ē-ă-pĕn-dĭ-SĪ-tĭs], inflammation of the tissue surrounding the appendix
pluri-	several, more	*pluriglandular* [plū-rĭ-GLĂN-dū-lăr], of several glands
poly-	many	*polyarteritis* [pŏl-ē-ăr-tĕr-Ī-tĭs], inflammation of a number of arteries
post-	after, following	*postmortem* [pōst-MŌR-tĕm], after death
pre-	before	*prenatal* [prē-NĀ-tăl], before birth
pro-	before, forward	*prodrome* [PRŌ-drōm], a symptom or group of symptoms that occurs before a disease shows up
quadra-, quadri-	four	*quadriplegia* [kwăh-drĭ-PLĒ-jē-ă], paralysis of all four limbs
re-	again, backward	*reflux* [RĒ-flŭks], backward flow
retro-	behind, backward	*retroversion* [rĕ-trō-VĔR-shŭn], a turning backward, as of the uterus
semi-	half	*semicomatose* [sĕm-ē-KŌ-mă-tōs], drowsy and inactive, but not in a full coma
sub-	less than, under, inferior	*subcutaneous* [sŭb-kyū-TĀ-nē-ŭs], beneath the skin
super-	more than, above, superior	*superacute* [sū-pĕr-ă-KYŪT], more acute
supra-	above, over	*supramaxillary* [sū-pră-MĂK-sĭ-lār-ē], above the maxilla

PREFIXES	MEANING	EXAMPLE
syl-, sym-, syn-, sys-	together	*symbiosis* [sĭm-bē-Ō-sĭs], mutual interdependence
tachy-	fast	*tachycardia* [TĂK-i-KAR-de-a], rapid heartbeat
trans-	across, through	*transocular* [trăns-ŎK-yū-lăr], across the eye
ultra-	beyond, excessive	*ultrasonic* [ŭl-tră-SŎN-ĭk], relating to energy waves of higher frequency than sound waves
un-	not	*unconscious* [ŭn-KŎN-shŭs], not conscious
uni-	one	*uniglandular* [yū-nĭ-GLĂN-dū-lăr], involving only one gland

Suffixes

Suffixes can also be combining forms at then end of terms. In the section "Prefixes," the example meaning paralysis, *-plegia*, is both a suffix and a combining form. It both attaches to the end of the word and carries the underlying meaning of the word such as *cardioplegia*, paralysis of the heart.

Many suffixes have several variations that can make the compound word a noun, verb, adjective, or adverb. For example:

an intense fear of closed spaces is *claustrophobia* (noun)

relating to or having such a condition is *claustrophic* (adjective)

Some suffixes form both verbs and nouns so it may be important to look at the sentence in which it appears to determine the exact meaning. For example, *hemorrhage* can mean both "to bleed profusely" (verb) or "profuse bleeding" (noun). In the sentence, "It is possible to hemorrhage profusely from certain injuries," *hemorrhage* is a verb. In the sentence, "The hemorrhage was caused by an injury to his leg," *hemorrhage* is a noun.

SUFFIXES	MEANING	EXAMPLE
-ad	toward	*cephalad* [SĔF-ă-lăd], toward the head
-algia	pain	*neuralgia* [nū-RĂL-jē-ă], nerve pain
-asthenia	weakness	*neurasthenia* [nūr-ăs-THĒ-nē-ă], condition with vague symptoms, such as weakness
-blast	immature, forming	*astroblast* [ĂS-trō-blăst], immature cell
-cele	hernia	*cystocele* [SĬS-tō-sēl], hernia of the urinary bladder
-cidal	destroying, killing	*suicidal* [sū-ĭ-SĪD-ăl], likely to kill oneself
-cide	destroying, killing	*suicide* [SŪ-ĭ-sīd], killing of oneself; *bacteriocide* [băk-TĒR-ē-ō-sīd], agent that destroys bacteria

SUFFIXES	MEANING	EXAMPLE
-clasis	breaking	*osteoclasis* [ŎS-tē-ŎK-lă-sĭs], intentional breaking of a bone
-clast	breaking instrument	*osteoclast* [ŎS-tē-ō-klăst], instrument used in osteoclasis
-crine	secreting	*endocrine* [ĔN-dō-krĭn], gland that secretes hormones into the bloodstream
-crit	separate	*hematocrit* [HĒ-mă-tō-krĭt, HĔM-ă-to-krĭt], percentage of volume of a blood sample that is composed of cells
-cyte	cell	*thrombocyte* [THRŎM-bō-sīt], blood platelet
-cytosis	condition of cells	*erythrocytosis* [ĕ-RĬTH-rō-sī-tō-sĭs], condition with an abnormal number of red blood cells in the blood
-derma	skin	*scleroderma* [sklēr-ō-DĔR-mă], hardening of the skin
-desis	binding	*arthrodesis* [ăr-THRŎD-ĕ-sĭs, ăr-thrō-DĒ-sĭs], stiffening of a joint
-dynia	pain	*neurodynia* [nūr-ō-DĬN-ē-ă], nerve pain
-ectasia	expansion; dilation	*neurectasia* [nūr-ĕk-TĀ-zhē-ă], operation with dilation of a nerve
-ectasis	expanding; dilating	*bronchiectasis* [brŏng-kē-ĔK-tă-sĭs], condition with chronic dilation of the bronchi
-ectomy	removal of	*appendectomy* [ăp-ĕn-DĔK-tō-mē], removal of the appendix
-edema	swelling	*lymphedema* [lĭmf-ĕ-DĒ-mă], swelling as a result of obstructed lymph nodes
-ema	condition	*empyema* [ĕm-pī-Ē-mă], pus in a body cavity
-emesis	vomiting	*hematemesis* [hē-mă-TĔM-ĕ-sĭs], vomiting of blood
-emia	blood	*anemia* [an-N-mē-ă], deficiency of red blood cells or hemoglobin
-emic	relating to blood	*uremic* [yū-RĒ-mĭk], having excess urea in the blood
-esthesia	sensation	*paresthesia* [păr-ĕs-THĒ-zhē-ă], abnormal sensation, such as tingling
-form	in the shape of	*uniform* [YŪ-nĭ-fŏrm], having the same shape throughout
-gen	producing, coming to be	*carcinogen* [kăr-SĬN-ō-jĕn], cancer-causing agent
-genesis	production of	*pathogenesis* [păth-ō-JĔN-ĕ-sĭs], production of disease
-genic	producing	*iatrogenic* [ī-ăt-rō-JĔN-ĭk], induced by treatment

Suffixes	Meaning	Example
-globin	protein	*hemoglobin* [hē-mō-GLŌ-bĭn], protein of red blood cells
-globulin	protein	*immunoglobulin* [ĭm-yū-nō-GLŎB-yū-lĭn], one of certain structurally related proteins
-gram	a recording	*electrocardigram* [e-LEK-tro-kar-de-grăm], brain scan
-graph	recording instrument	*encephalograph* [ĕn-SĔF-ă-lō-grăf], instrument for measuring brain activity
-graphy	process of recording	*echocardiography* [ĔK-ō-kăr-dē-ŎG-ră-fĕ], graphic record of the electric activity of the heart
-iasis	pathological condition or state	*psoriasis* [sō-RĪ-ă-sĭs], chronic skin disease
-ic	pertaining to	*gastric* [GĂS-trĭk], relating to the stomach
-ics	treatment, practice, body of knowledge	*orthopedics* [ōr-thō-PĒ-dĭks], medical-practice concerned with treatment of skeletal disorders
-ism	condition, disease, doctrine	*dwarfism* [DWŌRF-ĭzm], condition characterized by abnormally small size
-itis (pl., -itides)	inflammation	*nephritis* [nĕ-FRĪ-tĭs], kidney inflammation; *neuritides* [nū-RĬT-ĭ-dēz], inflammations of nerves
-kinesia	movement	*bradykinesia* [brăd-ĭ-kĭn-Ē-zhē-ă], decrease in movement
-kinesis	movement	*hyperkinesis* [hĭ-pĕr-kĭ-NĒ-sĭs], excessive muscular movement
-lepsy	condition of	*catalepsy* [KĂT-ă-lĕp-sē], condition characterized by seizures of extreme rigidity
-leptic	having seizures	*cataleptic* [kăt-ă-LĔP-tĭk], person with catalepsy
-logist	one who practices	*dermatologist* [dĕr-mă-TŎL-ō-jĭst], one who practices dermatology
-logy	study, practice	*dermatology* [dĕr-mă-TŎL-ō-jĕ], study and treatment of skin disorders
-lysis	destruction of	*electrolysis* [ē-lĕk-TRŎL-ĭ-sĭs], permanent removal of unwanted hair
-lytic	destroying	*thrombolytic* [thrŏm-bō-LĬT-ĭk], dissolving a thrombus
-malacia	softening	*osteomalacia* [ŎS-tē-ō-mă-LĀ-shē-ă], gradual softening of bone
-mania	obsession	*monomania* [mŏn-ō-MĀ-nē-ă], obsession with one idea
-megaly	enlargement	*cephalomegaly* [SĔF-ă-lō-MĔG-ă-lē], abnormal enlargement of the head
-meter	measuring device	*ophthalmometer* [ŏf-thăl-MŎM-ĕ-tĕr], device for measuring cornea curvature

SUFFIXES	MEANING	EXAMPLE
-metry	measurement	*optometry* [ŏp-TŎM-ĕ-trē], specialty concerned with measurement of eye function
-oid	like, resembling	*cardioid* [KĂR-dē-ŏyd], resembling a heart
-oma (pl., -omata)	tumor, neoplasm	*myoma (pl., myomata)* [mī-Ō-mă (mī-ō-MĂ-tă)], neoplasm of muscle tissue
-opia	vision	*diplopia* [dĭ-PLŌ-pē-ă], double vision
-opsia	vision	*chloropsia* [klō-RŎP-sē-ă], condition of seeing objects as green
-opsy	view of	*biopsy* [BĪ-ŏp-sē], cutting from living tissue to be viewed
-osis (pl., -oses)	condition, state, process	*halitosis* [hăl-ĭ-TŌ-sĭs], chronic bad breath
-ostomy	opening	*colostomy* [kō-LŎS-tō-mē], surgical opening in the colon
-oxia	oxygen	*anoxia* [ăn-ŎK-sē-ă], lack of oxygen
-para	bearing	*primipara* [prī-MĬP-ăr-ă], woman who has given birth once
-paresis	slight paralysis	*monoparesis* [mŏn-ō-pă-RĒ-sĭs], paralysis of only one extremity
-parous	producing; bearing	*viviparous* [vī-VĬP-ă-rŭs], bearing living young
-pathy	disease	*osteopathy* [ŏs-tē-ŎP-ă-thē], bone disease
-penia	deficiency	*leukopenia* [lū-kō-PĒ-nē-ă], condition with fewer than normal white blood cells
-pepsia	digestion	*dyspepsia* [dĭs-PĔP-sē-ă], impaired digestion
-pexy	fixation, usually done surgically	*nephropexy* [NĔF-rō-pĕk-sē], surgical fixation of a floating kidney
-phage, -phagia, -phagy	eating, devouring	*polyphagia* [pŏl-ē-FĀ-jē-ă], excessive eating
-phasia	speaking	*aphasia* [ă-FĀ-zhē-ă], loss of or reduction in speaking ability
-pheresis	removal	*leukapheresis* [lū-kă-fĕ-RĒ-sĭs], removal of leukocytes from drawn blood
-phil	attraction; affinity for	*cyanophil* [SI-ăn-nō-fĭl], element that turns blue after staining
-philia	attraction; affinity for	*hemophilia* [hē-mō-FĬL-ē-ă], blood disorder with tendency to hemorrhage
-phobia	fear	*acrophobia* [ăk-rō-FŌ-bē-ă], fear of heights
-phonia	sound	*neuraphonia* [nūr-ă-FŌ-nē-ă], loss of sounds
-phoresis	carrying	*electrophoresis* [ē-lĕk-trō-FŌR-ē-sĭs], movement of particles in an electric field

SUFFIXES	MEANING	EXAMPLE
-phoria	feeling; carrying	*euphoria* [yū-FŌR-ē-ă], feeling of well-being
-phrenia	of the mind	*schizophrenia* [skĭz-ō-FRĔ-nē-ă, skĭt-sō-FRĔ-nē-ă], term for a common psychosis
-phthisis	wasting away	*hemophthisis* [hē-MŎF-thĭ-sĭs], anemia
-phylaxis	protection	*prophylaxis* [prō-fĭ-LĂK-sĭs], prevention of disease
-physis	growing	*epiphysis* [ĕ-PĬF-ĭ-sĭs], part of a long bone distinct from and growing out of the shaft
-plakia	plaque	*leukoplakia* [lū-kō-PLĀ-kē-ă], white patch on the mucous membrane
-plasia	formation	*dysplasia* [dĭs-PLĀ-zhē-ă], abnormal tissue formation
-plasm	formation	*protoplasm* [PRŌ-tō-plăzm], living matter
-plastic	forming	*hemoplastic* [hē-mō-PLĂS-tĭk], forming new blood cells
-plasty	surgical repair	*rhinoplasty* [RĪ-nō-plăs-tē], plastic surgery of the nose
-plegia	paralysis	*quadriplegia* [KWĂH-drĭ-PLĒ-jē-ă], paralysis of all four limbs
-plegic	one who is paralyzed	*quadriplegic* [kwăh-drĭ-PLĒ-jĭk], person who has quadriplegia
-pnea	breath	*eupnea* [yūp-NĒ-ă], easy, normal respiration
-poiesis	formation	*erythropoiesis* [ĕ-RĬTH-rō-pŏy-Ē-sĭs], formation of red blood cells
-poietic	forming	*erythropoietic* [ĕ-RĬTH-rō-pŏy-ĕt-ĭk], of the formation of red blood cells
-poietin	one that forms	*erythropoietin* [ĕ-RĬTH-rō-pŏy-ĕ-tĭn], an acid that aids in the formation of red blood cells
-porosis	lessening in density	*osteoporosis* [ŎS-tē-ō-pō-RŌ-sĭs], lessening of bone density
-ptosis	falling down; drooping	*blepharoptosis* [blĕf-ă-RŎP-tō-sĭs], drooping eyelid
-rrhage	discharging heavily	*hemorrhage* [HĔM-ō-răj], to bleed profusely
-rrhagia	heavy discharge	*tracheorrhagia* [trā-kē-ō-RĀ-jē-ă], hemorrhage from the trachea
-rrhaphy	surgical suturing	*herniorrhaphy* [HĔR-nē-ŌR-ă-fē], surgical repair of a hernia
-rrhea	a flowing, a flux	*dysmenorrhea* [dĭs-mĕn-ŌR-ē-ă], difficult menstrual flow

SUFFIXES	MEANING	EXAMPLE
-rrhexis	rupture	*cardiorrhexis* [kăr-dē-ō-RĔK-sĭs], rupture of the heart wall
-schisis	splitting	*spondyloschisis* [spŏn-dĭ-LŎS-kĭ-sĭs], failure of fusion of the vertebral arch in an embryo
-scope	instrument (especially one used for observing or measuring)	*microscope* [MĪ-krō-skōp], instrument for viewing small objects
-scopy	use of an instrument for observing	*microscopy* [mĭ-KRŎS-kō-pē], use of microscopes
-somnia	sleep	*insomnia* [ĭn-SŎM-nē-ă], inability to sleep
-spasm	contraction	*esophagospasm* [ĕ-SŎF-ă-gō-spăzm], spasm of the walls of the esophagus
-stalsis	contraction	*peristalsis* [pĕr-ĭ-STĂL-sĭs], movement of the intestines by contraction and relaxation of its tube
-stasis	stopping; constant	*homeostasis* [HŌ-mē-ō-STĀ-sĭs], state of equilibrium in the body
-stat	agent to maintain a state	*bacteriostat* [băk-TĒR-ē-ō-stăt], agent that inhibits bacterial growth
-static	maintaining a state	*hemostatic* [hē-mō-STĂT-ĭk], stopping blood flow within a vessel
-stenosis	narrowing	*stenostenosis* [STĔN-ō-stĕ-NŌ-sĭs], narrowing of the parotid duct
-stomy	opening	*colostomy* [kō-LŎS-tō-mē], surgical opening in the colon
-tome	cutting instrument, segment	*osteotome* [ŎS-tē-ō-tōm], instrument for cutting bone
-tomy	cutting operation	*laparotomy* [LĂP-ă-RŎT-ō-mē], incision in the abdomen
-trophic	nutritional	*atrophic* [ā-TRŌF-ĭk], of a wasting state, often due to malnutrition
-trophy	nutrition	*dystrophy* [DĬS-trō-fē], changes that result from inadequate nutrition
-tropia	turning	*esotropia* [ĕs-ō-TRŌ-pē-ă], crossed eyes
-tropic	turning toward	*neurotropic* [nūr-ō-TRŎP-ĭk], localizing in nerve tissue
-tropy	condition of turning toward	*neurotropy* [nū-RŎT-rō-pē], affinity of certain contrast mediums for nervous tissue
-uria	urine	*pyuria* [pĭ-YŪ-rē-ă], pus in the urine
-version	turning	*retroversion* [rĕ-trō-VĔR-zhŭn], a turning backward (said of the uterus)

Putting It All Together

All medical terms have a word root, which is the element that gives the essential meaning to the word. For example, *card-* is a word root meaning heart. In the word *pericarditis*, the prefix *peri-* and the suffix *-itis* are added to the word root to form the whole word meaning an inflammation (*-itis*) of the area surrounding (*peri-*) the heart (*card-*). The word root can also appear in a combining form, which is the root plus a combining vowel or vowels. For example, *cardiology* is formed from *cardio-* (the word root *card-* plus the combining vowels -i- and -o-) plus the suffix *-logy* meaning the study of the heart.

MORE ABOUT . . .

Detecting Compound Words

An easy way to define compound words is to start at the end of the word, look at the suffix to determine its meaning, and then look at the word root. The word root will contain a combining vowel if the suffix begins with a consonant. If not, the combining vowel (usually "o") will be removed. An example is *neuritis*. The suffix *-itis* means "inflammation of." The word root *neur-*, nerve, does not need a combining vowel because *-itis* begins with a vowel. Therefore, *neuritis* is inflammation of a nerve. To repeat the basic rules: If a suffix begins with a vowel, do NOT use the "o." If the suffix begins with a consonant, retain the "o." Then figure out the meaning of any prefixes.

WORD PARTS EXERCISES

Build Your Medical Vocabulary

Using the lists in this chapter and in Chapter 1, write the appropriate prefix, suffix, or combining form in the blank for each word part. The definition of each word part needed is given immediately under the blank. Item 1 is completed as an example.

1. ____osteo____ myel ____itis____
   (bone)   (inflammation)

2. _____ cardio _____
   (within)   (visual examining)

3. _____ dactyly
   (together)

4. _____ violet
   (beyond)

5. _____ sensitive
   (overly)

6. entero _____ _____
      (disease)   (causing)

7. _____ dermic
   (beneath)

8. _____ therapy
   (sleep)

9. _____ ost _____
   (together)   (condition)

10. _____ tonsillar
    (above)

11. _____ cranio _____
    (half)   (cutting)

12. _____ _____
    (old people)   (fear)

13. _____ glandular
    (within)

14. _____ blast
    (white)

15. _____ _____
     (structure)   (study of)

16. arterio _____
          (suture)

17. dermato _____
         (hemorrhage)

18. _____ flexion
     (half)

19. _____ algesia
     (heat)

20. fibr _____
     (resembling)

21. _____ organism
     (tiny)

22. _____ plasm
     (new)

23. subcost _____
       (pain)

24. blepharo _____
       (paralysis)

25. _____ myx _____
     (fiber)   (tumor)

26. _____ lingual
     (under)

27. _____ meno _____
   (scanty, little)   (a flowing)

28. _____ dipsia
   (many, excessive)

Find a Match

Each of the words in the left-hand column contains a word part that matches one of the definitions in the right-hand column. Write the letter of the answer that best fits into the left-hand column. Exercise 26 is completed as an example.

29. _o_ antipsychotic   **a.** in the shape of

30. ____ polycystic   **b.** without

31. ____ acephaly   **c.** enlargement

32. ____ tenosynovitis   **d.** abnormally low

33. ____ myotrophy   **e.** nutrition

34. ____ laryngoscope   **f.** self

35. ____ dysgnosia   **g.** outside of

36. ____ decontamination   **h.** inflammation

37. ____ chyliform   **i.** instrument for viewing

38. ____ autoinfection   **j.** abnormal

39. ____ cardiomegaly   **k.** between

40. ____ extrasensory   **l.** away from

41. ____ intercerebral   **m.** condition

42. ____ osteoporosis   **n.** many

43. ____ hyposthenia   **o.** against

Find the Word Part

Complete the word for which the definition is given. Add a word part(s) learned in this chapter.

44. Any disease of the hair: tricho _____

45. Repair of a nose defect: rhino _____

46. Removal of the appendix: append _____

47. Having a jaw that protrudes abnormally forward: _____ gnathic

48. Disease of the heart: cardio _____

49. Inflammation of the bronchi: bronch _____

50. Outer layer of a cell: _____ blast

51. Rib-shaped: costi _____

52. Bone-forming cell: osteo _____

53. Above the nose: _____ nasal

54. Study of the skin: dermato _____

55. Loss of the voice: _____ phonia

56. Study of tissue: hist _____

57. Inflammation of the ovary: ovar _____

58. Inflammation of the ear: ot _____

59. Specialist in the treatment of disorders of the nervous system: neuro _____

60. Incision into a vein: phlebo _____

61. Study of the mind: psycho _____

62. Enlargement of the spleen: spleno _____

63. Difficulty speaking: dys _____

64. Cancer of the blood: leuk _____

65. Total or partial loss of sensation or awareness: an _____

66. A person with epilepsy: epi _____

67. Study and treatment of the heart: cardio _____

68. Producing disease: patho _____

69. Moving a part away from the midline of the body: _____ duction

70. Abnormally slow heartbeat: _____ cardia

71. Not recommended: _____ indicated

72. Low blood sugar: _____ glycemia

73. Between the layers of the skin: _____ dermal

74. Abnormal enlargement of the head: _____ cephaly

75. Paralysis on one side of the body: _____ plegia

76. Below the sternum: _____ sternal

77. Abnormally restless and inattentive: _____ active

78. Against an individual's own tissue: _____ immune

Separate the Word Parts

Break apart the following words and define each part in the space allowed. You will want to study the list in Chapter 1 before you do this exercise.

79. exocrine _____

80. endocranium _____

81. antidepressant _____

82. somatotropic _____

83. pseudesthesia _____

84. dextrotropic _____

85. algesic _____

86. xiphoid _____

87. litholysis _____

88. cryolysis _____

89. pericardiorrhaphy _____

90. multigravida _____

91. pancytopenia _____

92. salpingitis _____

93. megalomania _____

94. lithiasis _____

95. chromatopsia _____

96. hemiparesis _____

Find Where Word Parts Come From

Match the word part on the left with its etymology on the right. Remember, some of these word parts are from Chapter 1.

97. _____ xipho-

98. _____ ambi-

99. _____ -graph

100. _____ -kinesia

101. _____ ichthyo-

102. _____ eosino-

103. _____ bio-

104. _____ xantho-

105. _____ -phylaxis

106. _____ -trophy

107. _____ chrono-

108. _____ melano-

109. _____ -clasis

110. _____ -plasia

111. _____ lacto-

a. Greek *xanthos*, yellow

b. Greek *ichthys*, fish

c. Latin *lac*, milk

d. Greek *melas*, black

e. Greek *grapho*, to write

f. Greek *trophe*, nutrition

g. Greek *klastos*, broken

h. Greek *eos*, dawn

i. Greek *plasso*, to form

j. Greek *chronos*, time

k. Greek *xiphos*, sword

l. Greek *phylaxis*, protection

m. Latin *ambi-*, around; about

n. Greek *kinesis*, movement

o. Greek *bios*, life

USING THE INTERNET

Go to the Centers for Disease Control's site (www.cdc.gov). Click on several of the topics on the site and find at least ten combining forms, suffixes, and prefixes that you learned about in this chapter and in Chapter 1.

Answers to Chapter Exercises

1. osteomyelitis
2. endocardiography
3. syndactyly
4. ultraviolet
5. hypersensitive
6. enteropathogenic
7. hypodermic
8. hypnotherapy
9. synostosis
10. supratonsillar
11. hemicraniotomy
12. gerontophobia
13. intraglandular
14. leukoblast
15. morphology
16. arteriorrhaphy
17. dermatorrhagia
18. semiflexion
19. thermalgesia
20. fibroid
21. microorganism
22. neoplasm
23. subcostalgia
24. blepharoplegia
25. fibromyxoma
26. sublingual
27. oligomenorrhea
28. polydipsia
29. o
30. n
31. b
32. h
33. e
34. i
35. j
36. l
37. a
38. f
39. c
40. g
41. k
42. m
43. d
44. trichopathy
45. rhinoplasty
46. appendectomy
47. prognathic
48. cardiopathy
49. bronchitis
50. ectoblast
51. costiform
52. osteoblast
53. supranasal
54. dermatology
55. aphonia
56. histology
57. ovaritis
58. otitis
59. neurologist
60. phlebotomy
61. psychology
62. splenomegaly
63. dysphasia
64. leukemia
65. anesthesia
66. epileptic
67. cardiology
68. pathogenic
69. abduction
70. bradycardia
71. contraindicated
72. hypoglycemic
73. interdermal
74. megacephaly
75. hemiplegia
76. infrasternal
77. hyperactive
78. autoimmune
79. exo-, outside of; crin-, secreting
80. endo-, within; cranium
81. anti-, against; depressant
82. somato-, body; -tropic, turning toward
83. pseud-, false; -esthesia, sensation
84. dextro-, right; -tropic, turning toward
85. alges-, pain; -ic, pertaining to
86. xiph-, sword; -oid, resembling
87. litho, stone; -lysis, destruction of
88. cryo-, cold; -lysis, destruction of
89. peri-, around, near; cardio-, heart; -rrhaphy, surgical suturing
90. multi-, many; -gravida, pregnancy
91. pan-, all; cyto- cell; -penia, deficiency
92. salping-, fallopian tube; -itis, inflammation
93. megalo-, abnormally large; -mania, obsession
94. lith-, stone(s); -iasis, pathological condition or state
95. chromat-, color; -opsia, vision
96. hemi-, half; -paresis, slight paralysis
97. k
98. m
99. e
100. n
101. b
102. h
103. o
104. a
105. l
106. f
107. j
108. d
109. g
110. i
111. c

CHAPTER
3

Body Structure

After studying this chapter, you will be able to:

3.1   Define the elements of human body structure

3.2   Describe the planes of the body

3.3   Locate the body cavities and list organs that are contained within each cavity

3.4   Recognize combining forms that relate to elements and systems of the body

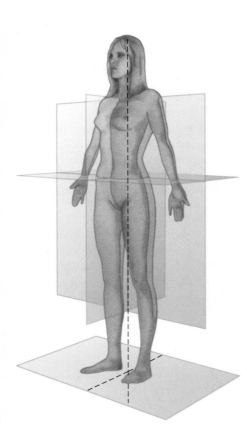

Body Structure and Organization

The body is organized from its smallest element, the **cell,** to the collection of systems, with all its interrelated parts. The entire body is made of cells that vary in size, shape, and function, but all cells have one thing in common: they need food, water, and oxygen to live and function.

Cells

The basic structure of a cell (Figure 3-1) includes three parts:

1. The *cell membrane* is the outer covering of the cell. It holds substances inside the cell while helping the cell maintain its shape. It also regulates substances that are allowed to pass in and out of the cell.

2. The *nucleus* is the central portion of each cell. It directs the cell's activities and contains the *chromosomes*. The chromosomes are the bearers of *genes*—those elements that control inherited traits such as eye color, height, inherited diseases, gender, and so on. The chromosomes are made of deoxyribonucleic acid or DNA, which contains all the genetic information for the cell.

3. Surrounding the nucleus is the *cytoplasm*, a substance that contains the material to instruct cells to perform different essential tasks, such as reproduction and movement. This material, called *organelles*, comes in many different types. Some common examples are *mitochondria* (sing. *mitochondrion*), organelles that provide energy needed for the body's tasks; *ribosomes*, which manufacture proteins; and *lysosomes*, which can break down substances, such as bacteria.

Cell growth can be either normal or abnormal. Later in this book you will learn how normal cell growth takes place so that the body can grow and function. You will also learn about abnormal cell growth, which is a major factor in some diseases.

To see some videos about living cells, go to www.cellsalive.com and click on animal cells.

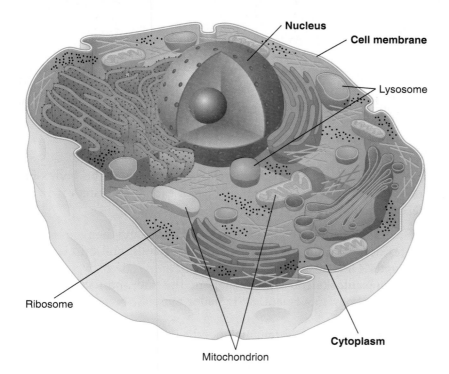

Nucleus

Cell membrane

Lysosome

Ribosome

Mitochondrion

Cytoplasm

FIGURE 3-1 The human body is made up of cells. Cells have three basic parts—a cell membrane, a nucleus, and cytoplasm.

Tissues

Groups of cells that work together to perform the same task are called **tissue.** The body has four types of tissue:

- **Connective tissue** holds and connects body parts together. Examples are bones, ligaments, and tendons.
- **Epithelial tissue** covers the internal and external body surfaces. Skin and linings of internal organs (such as the intestines) are epithelial tissue.
- **Muscle tissue** expands and contracts, allowing the body to move.
- **Nervous tissue** carries messages to and from the brain and spinal cord from all parts of the body.

MORE ABOUT . . .

Cell Types

Cells all have specialized functions. Their shape influences their function. Nerve cells usually have long, thin extensions that can transmit nerve impulses over a distance. Epithelial cells that line the mouth are thin, flat, and tightly packed so that they form a protective layer over underlying cells. Muscle cells are slender rods that attach at the ends of the structures they move. As these types of cells specialize further, their shape and function change to fit a specific need.

Parts of a cell are also important to its function. For example, a cell membrane either allows or prevents passage of nutrients and waste products through it, providing control over what materials move in and out of a cell.

Organs

Groups of tissue that work together to perform a specific function are called **organs.** Examples are the *kidneys,* which maintain water and salt balance in the blood, and the *stomach,* which breaks down food into substances that the circulatory system can transport throughout the body as nourishment for its cells.

Systems

Groups of organs that work together to perform one of the body's major functions form a **system.** The terminology for each body system is provided in a separate chapter.

- The **integumentary system** consists of the skin and the accessory structures derived from it—hair, nails, sweat glands, and oil glands. (See Chapter 4.)
- The **musculoskeletal system** supports the body, protects organs, and provides body movement. It includes muscles, bones, and cartilage. (See Chapter 5.)
- The **cardiovascular system** includes the heart and blood vessels, which pump and transport blood throughout the body. Blood carries nutrients to and removes waste from the tissues. (See Chapter 6.)
- The **respiratory system** includes the lungs and the airways. This system performs respiration. (See Chapter 7.)
- The **nervous system** consists of the brain, spinal cord, and peripheral nerves. The nervous system regulates most body activities and sends and receives messages from the sensory organs. (See Chapter 8.) The two major sensory organs are covered in the sensory system. (See Chapter 16.)
- The **urinary system** includes the kidneys, ureters, bladder, and urethra. It eliminates metabolic waste, helps to maintain acid-base and water-salt balance, and helps regulate blood pressure. (See Chapter 9.)
- The **reproductive system** controls reproduction and heredity. The female reproductive system includes the ovaries, vagina, uterine (fallopian) tubes, uterus, and mammary glands. (See Chapter 10.) The male reproductive system includes the testes, penis, prostate gland, vas deferens, and the seminal vesicles. (See Chapter 11.)
- The **blood system** includes the blood and all its components. (See Chapter 12.)
- The **lymphatic and immune systems** includes the lymph, the glands of the lymphatic system, lymphatic vessels, and the nonspecific and specific defenses of the immune system. (See Chapter 13.)
- The **digestive system** includes all the organs of digestion and excretion of waste. (See Chapter 14.)
- The **endocrine system** includes the glands that secrete hormones for regulation of many of the body's activities. (See Chapter 15.)
- The **sensory system** covers the eyes and ears and those parts of other systems that are involved in the reactions of the five senses. (See Chapter 16.)

Cavities

The body has two main cavities (spaces)—the dorsal and the ventral. The **dorsal cavity,** on the back side of the body, is divided into the **cranial cavity,** which holds the brain, and the **spinal cavity,** which holds the spinal cord. The **ventral cavity,** on the front side of the body, is divided (and separated by a muscle called the **diaphragm**) into the **thoracic cavity,** which holds the heart, lungs, and major blood vessels, and the **abdominal cavity,** which holds the organs of the digestive and urinary systems. The bottom portion of the abdominal cavity is called the **pelvic cavity.** It contains the reproductive system. Figure 3-2 shows the body cavities.

VOCABULARY REVIEW

In the previous section, you learned terms relating to body structure and organization. Before going on to the exercises, review the terms below and refer to the previous section if you have any questions. Pronunciations are provided for certain terms. Sometimes information about where the word came from is included after the term. These etymologies (word histories) are for your information only. You do not need to memorize them.

Term	Definition
abdominal [ăb-DŎM-ĭ-năl] **cavity**	Body space between the abdominal walls, above the pelvis, and below the diaphragm.
blood [blŭd] **system** Old English *blud*.	Body system that includes blood and all its component parts.
cardiovascular [KĂR-dē-ō-VĂS-kyū-lăr] **system**	Body system that includes the heart and blood vessels; circulatory system.
cell [sĕl] Latin *cella*, storeroom	Smallest unit of a living structure.

Term	Definition
connective [kŏn-NĔK-tǐv] **tissue**	Fibrous substance that forms the body's supportive framework.
cranial [KRĀ-nē-ăl] **cavity**	Space in the head that contains the brain.
diaphragm [DĪ-ă-frăm]	Muscle that divides the abdominal and thoracic cavities.
digestive [dī-JĔS-tǐv] **system**	Body system that includes all organs of digestion and waste excretion, from the mouth to the anus.
dorsal [DŌR-săl] **cavity**	Main cavity on the back side of the body containing the cranial and spinal cavities.
endocrine [ĔN-dō-krǐn] **system**	Body system that includes glands which secrete hormones to regulate certain body functions.
epithelial [ĕp-ǐ-THĒ-lē-ăl] **tissue**	Tissue that covers or lines the body or its parts.
integumentary [ǐn-tĕg-yū-MĔN-tă-rē] **system**	Body system that includes skin, hair, and nails.
lymphatic [lǐm-FĂT-ǐk] **and immune** [ǐ-MYŪN] **system**	Body system that includes the lymph, glands of the lymphatic system, lymphatic vessels, and the specific and nonspecific defenses of the immune system.
muscle [MŬS-ĕl] **tissue** Latin *musculus*, muscle, mouse	Tissue that is able to contract and relax.
musculoskeletal [MŬS-kyū-lō-SKĔL-ĕ-tăl] **system**	Body system that includes muscles, bones, and cartilage.
nervous [NĔR-vŭs] **system**	Body system that includes the brain, spinal cord, and nerves and controls most body functions by sending and receiving messages.
nervous tissue	Specialized tissue that forms nerve cells and is capable of transmitting messages.
organ [ŌR-găn]	Group of specialized tissue that performs a specific function.
pelvic [PĔL-vǐk] **cavity**	Body space below the abdominal cavity that includes the reproductive organs.
reproductive [RĒ-prō-DŬK-tǐv] **system**	Either the male or female body system that controls reproduction.
respiratory [RĔS-pǐ-ră-tōr-ē, rĕ-SPĪR-ă-tōr-ē] **system**	Body system that includes the lungs and airways and performs breathing.
sensory [SĔN-sŏ-rē] **system**	Body system that includes the eyes and ears and those parts of other systems involved in the reactions of the five senses.
spinal [SPĪ-năl] **cavity**	Body space that contains the spinal cord.
system [SĬS-tĕm]	Any group of organs and ancillary parts that work together to perform a major body function.
thoracic [thō-RĂS-ǐk] **cavity**	Body space above the abdominal cavity that contains the heart, lungs, and major blood vessels.

Term	Definition
tissue [TĬSH-ū]	Any group of cells that work together to perform a single function.
urinary [YŪR-ĭ-nār-ē] system	Body system that includes the kidneys, ureters, bladder, and urethra and helps maintain homeostasis by removing fluid and dissolved waste.
ventral [VĔN-trăl] cavity	Major cavity in the front of the body containing the thoracic, abdominal, and pelvic cavities.

BODY STRUCTURE AND ORGANIZATION EXERCISES

Find the Match

Match the system to its function.

1. ____ cardiovascular system
2. ____ digestive system
3. ____ endocrine system
4. ____ blood system
5. ____ integumentary system
6. ____ lymphatic and immune system
7. ____ musculoskeletal system
8. ____ nervous system
9. ____ reproductive system
10. ____ respiratory system
11. ____ urinary system

a. performs breathing
b. removes fluid and dissolved waste
c. sends and receives messages
d. pumps and circulates blood to tissues
e. consists of blood and its elements
f. covers the body and its internal structures
g. provides defenses for the body
h. breaks down food
i. regulates through production of hormones
j. controls reproduction
k. supports organs and provides movement

Complete the Sentence

12. The basic element of the human body is a(n) _____.
13. Groups of these basic elements form _____.
14. Tissue that covers the body or its parts is called _____ tissue.
15. The brain is contained within the _____ cavity.
16. The muscle separating the two main parts of the ventral cavity is called the _____.
17. The spinal and cranial cavities make up the _____ cavity.
18. The space below the abdominal cavity is called the _____ cavity.
19. The system that helps eliminate fluids is the _____ system.
20. The system that breaks down food is called the _____ system.

Directional Terms, Planes, and Regions

In making diagnoses or prescribing treatments, health care providers use standard terms to refer to different areas of the body. These terms describe each anatomical position as a point of reference. The anatomical position always means the body is standing erect, facing forward, with upper limbs at the sides and with the palms facing forward. For example, if a pain is described as in the *right lower quadrant* (RLQ), medical personnel immediately understand that to mean the lower right portion of the patient's body. Certain terms refer to a direction going to or from the body or in which the body is placed. Others divide the body into imaginary planes as a way of mapping the body when the person is in the anatomical position. Still others refer to specific regions of the body.

Directional Terms

Directional terms locate a portion of the body or describe a position of the body. The front side (**anterior** or **ventral**) and the back side (**posterior** or **dorsal**) are the largest divisions of the body. Figure 3-3 shows the body regions of the anterior and posterior sections. Each of these regions contain

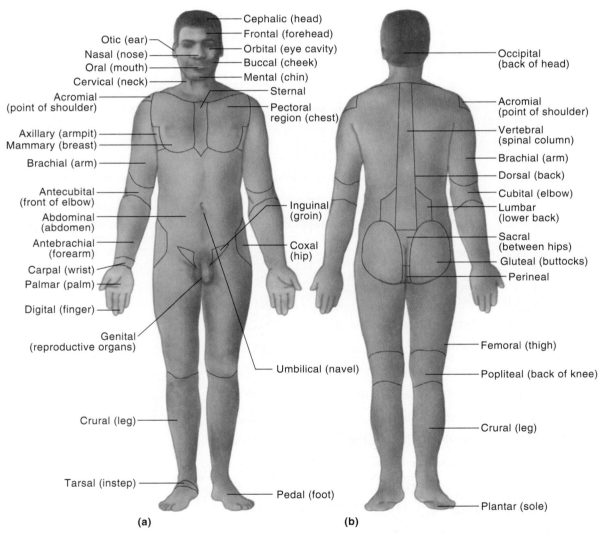

FIGURE 3-3   Anterior (**a**) and Posterior (**b**) regions. The parts shown in each of the regions are discussed in the body systems chapters throughout the book.

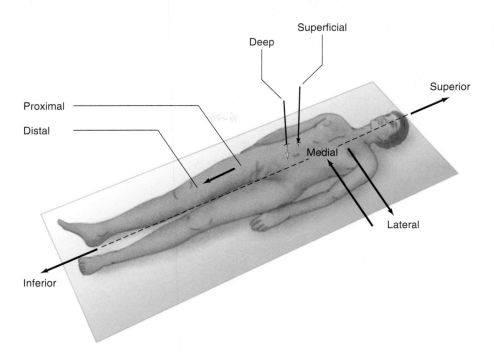

many parts of the body that will be discussed as part of the body systems of which they are a part.

Some terms indicate a position relative to something else. **Inferior** means below another structure; for example, the vagina is inferior to (or below) the uterus. **Superior** means above another structure; for example, the stomach is superior to the large intestine. **Lateral** means to the side; for example, the eyes are lateral to the nose. **Medial** means middle or near the medial plane of the body; for example, the nose is medial to the eyes. **Deep** means through the surface (as in a deep cut), while **superficial** means on or near the surface (as a scratch on the skin). **Proximal** means near the point of attachment to the trunk; for example, the proximal end of the thighbone joins the hip bone. **Distal** means away from the point of attachment to the trunk; for example, the distal end of the thighbone forms the knee. Figure 3-4 shows the directional terms.

For examination purposes, patients are either **supine** (lying on their spine face upward) or **prone** (lying on the abdomen with their face down). Figure 3-5 shows a patient lying in supine position and Figure 3-6 shows one in prone position.

Planes of the Body

For anatomical and diagnostic discussions, some standard terms are used for the planes and positions of the body. The imaginary planes of the body when it is vertical and facing front are: **frontal (coronal) plane,** which divides the body into anterior and posterior positions; **sagittal (lateral) plane,** which is the plane parallel to the medial and divides the body into left and right sections; **medial** or **midsagittal plane,** which divides the body into equal left and right halves; and **transverse (cross-sectional) plane,** which intersects the body horizontally and divides the body into upper and lower sections. Figure 3-7 on page 46 shows the planes of the body.

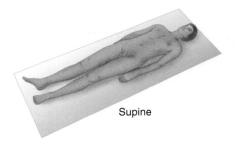

Supine

FIGURE 3-5 A patient lying in a supine position with the spinal cord facing down.

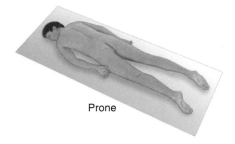

Prone

FIGURE 3-6 A patient lying in a prone position with the spinal cord facing up.

FIGURE 3-7 The planes of and directions from the body.

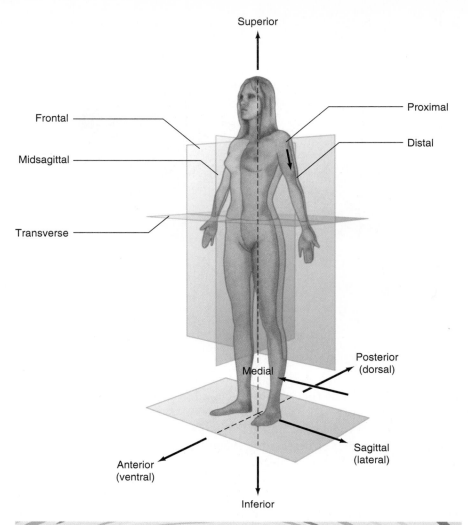

MORE ABOUT . . .

Areas of the Body

Pain is sometimes felt in only one region of the body (as a muscle pull in the RUQ or right upper quadrant). Other times, internal pain is felt in an area that is not the actual source of the pain. This is known as "referred pain" or synalgia. Such pain usually emanates from nerves or other deep structures within the body.

Regions of the Body

Health care practitioners usually refer to a specific organ, area, or bone when speaking of the upper body. In the back, the spinal column is divided into specific regions (cervical, thoracic, lumbar, sacral, and coccygeal). Chapter 5 describes the spinal column in detail. The middle portion of the body (abdominal and pelvic cavities) is often the site of pain. Doctors use two standard sections to describe this area of the body. The larger section is divided into four quarters with the navel being the center point (Figure 3-8).

- **Right upper quadrant** (RUQ): On the right anterior side; contains part of the liver, the gallbladder, and parts of the pancreas and intestinal tract.

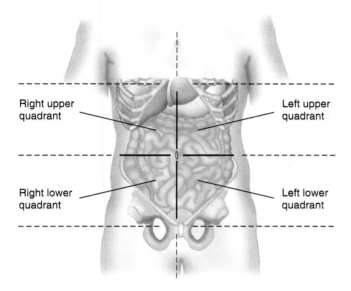

FIGURE 3-8 The four quadrants of the abdominopelvic area.

- **Right lower quadrant** (RLQ): On the right anterior side; contains the appendix, parts of the intestines, and parts of the reproductive organs in the female.
- **Left upper quadrant** (LUQ): On the left anterior side; contains the stomach, spleen, and parts of the liver, pancreas, and intestines.
- **Left lower quadrant** (LLQ): On the left anterior side; contains parts of the intestines and parts of reproductive organs in the female.

The smaller divisions of the abdominal and pelvic areas are the nine regions, each of which correspond to a region near a specific point in the body (Figure 3-9).

FIGURE 3-9 The regions of the abdominopelvic area.

Right hypochondriac region

Left hypochondriac region

Epigastric region

Right lumbar region

Umbilical region

Left lumbar region

Right inguinal (iliac) region

Hypogastric region

Left inguinal (iliac) region

- **Epigastric region:** the area above the stomach.
- **Hypochondriac regions** (left and right): the two regions just below the cartilage of the ribs, immediately over the abdomen.
- **Umbilical region:** the region surrounding the umbilicus (navel).
- **Lumbar regions** (left and right): the two regions near the waist.
- **Hypogastric region:** the area just below the umbilical region.
- **Iliac (inguinal) regions** (left and right): the two regions near the upper portion of the hip bone.

VOCABULARY REVIEW

In the previous section, you learned terms relating to directional terms, planes, and regions of the body. Before going on to the exercises, review the terms below and refer to the previous section if you have any questions. Pronunciations are provided for certain terms. Sometimes information about where the word came from is included after the term.

Term	Definition
anterior [ăn-TĒR-ē-ŏr]	At or toward the front (of the body).
coronal [KŌR-ŏ-năl] **plane**	Imaginary line that divides the body into anterior and posterior positions.
cross-sectional plane	Imaginary line that intersects the body horizontally.
deep	Away from the surface (of the body).
distal [DĬS-tăl]	Away from the point of attachment to the trunk.
dorsal [DŌR-săl]	At or toward the back of the body.
epigastric [ĕp-ĭ-GĂS-trĭk] **region**	Area of the body immediately above the stomach.
frontal [FRŬN-tăl] **plane**	Imaginary line that divides the body into anterior and posterior positions.
hypochondriac [hĭ-pō-KŎN-drē-ăk] **regions**	Left and right regions of the body just below the cartilage of the ribs and immediately above the abdomen.
hypogastric [hĭ-pō-GĂS-trĭk] **region**	Area of the body just below the umbilical region.
iliac [ĬL-ē-ăk] **regions**	Left and right regions of the body near the upper portion of the hip bone.
inferior [ĭn-FĒR-ē-ōr]	Below another body structure.
inguinal [ĬN-gwĭ-năl] **regions**	Left and right regions of the body near the upper portion of the hip bone.
lateral [LĂT-ĕr-ăl]	To the side.
lateral plane	Imaginary line that divides the body perpendicularly to the medial plane.

Term	Definition
left lower quadrant (LLQ)	Quadrant on the lower left anterior side of the patient's body.
left upper quadrant (LUQ)	Quadrant on the upper left anterior side of the patient's body.
lumbar [LŬM-băr] **regions**	Left and right regions of the body near the abdomen.
medial [MĒ-dē-ăl]	At or near the middle (of the body).
medial plane	Imaginary line that divides the body into equal left and right halves.
midsagittal [mĭd-SĂJ-ĭ-tăl] **plane**	See medial plane.
posterior	At or toward the back side (of the body).
prone	Lying on the stomach with the face down.
proximal [PRŎK-sĭ-măl]	At or near the point of attachment to the trunk.
right lower quadrant (RLQ)	Quadrant on the lower right anterior side of the patient's body.
right upper quadrant (RUQ)	Quadrant on the upper right anterior side of the patient's body.
sagittal [SĂJ-ĭ-tăl] **plane**	Imaginary line that divides the body into right and left portions.
superficial [sū-pĕr-FĬSH-ăl]	At or near the surface (of the body).
superior [sū-PĒR-ē-ōr]	Above another body structure.
supine [sū-PĪN]	Lying on the spine facing upward.
transverse plane	Imaginary line that intersects the body horizontally.
umbilical [ŭm-BĬL-ĭ-kăl] **region**	Area of the body surrounding the umbilicus.
ventral [VĔN-trăl]	At or toward the front (of the body).

CASE STUDY

Locating a Problem

Dr. Lena Woodrow checked the chart of the next patient, Darlene Gordon. Darlene had called yesterday with a vague pain in her LUQ. She also experienced some nausea and general discomfort. Dr. Woodrow had suggested she make a morning appointment.

Critical Thinking

21. What organs might be causing pain in the LUQ?
22. Is it possible for the source of the pain to be located elsewhere in the body?

Check Your Knowledge

Circle T for true or F for false.

23. The epigastric region is below the hypogastric region. T F

24. The heart is deeper than the ribs. T F

25. The leg is inferior to the foot. T F

26. The nose is superior to the eyes. T F

27. The right lower quadrant contains the appendix. T F

28. The coronal plane divides the body horizontally. T F

29. The lateral plane is another name for the sagittal plane. T F

30. The wrist is proximal to the shoulder. T F

31. The spleen is in the left upper quadrant. T F

Complete the Diagram

32. Using any of the terms below, fill in the blanks on the following diagram.

    Distal

    Supine

    Inferior

    Deep

    Superficial

    Anterior

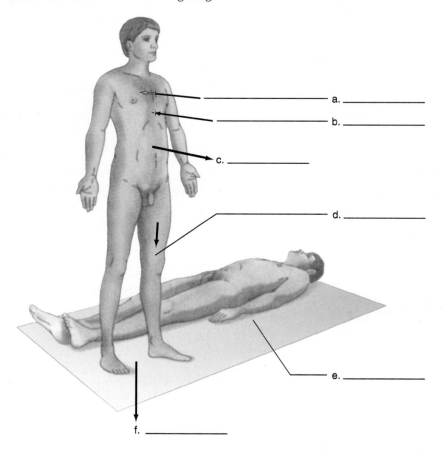

a. _____

b. _____

c. _____

d. _____

e. _____

f. _____

Combining Forms

Chapters 1 and 2 introduced many word roots, combining forms, prefixes, and suffixes used in medical terminology. The combining forms in this chapter relate to elements and systems of the body described here. Once you familiarize yourself with the word parts in Chapters 1, 2, and 3, you will understand many medical terms.

COMBINING FORM	MEANING	EXAMPLE
abdomin(o)	abdomen	*abdominoplasty* [ăb-DŎM-ĭ-nō-plăs-tě], surgical repair of the abdomen
acetabul(o)	cup-shaped hip socket	*acetabulectomy* [ĂS-ě-tăb-yū-LĔK-tō-mē], excision of the acetabulum
aden(o)	gland	*adenitis* [ăd-ě-NĪ-tĭs], inflammation of a gland
adip(o)	fat	*adiposis* [ĂD-ĭ-pōs], condition of excessive accumulation of fat
adren(o)	adrenal glands	*adrenotoxin* [ă-drē-nō-TŎK-sĭn], a substance toxic to the adrenal glands
alveol(o)	air sac, alveolus	*alveolitis* [ĂL-vē-ō-LĪ-tĭs], inflammation of alveoli
angi(o)	vessel	*angiomegaly* [ĂN-jē-ō-MĔG-ă-lē], enlargement of blood vessels
aort(o)	aorta	*aortitis* [ā-ōr-TĪ-tĭs], inflammation of the aorta
appendic(o)	appendix	*appendicitis* [ă-pěn-dĭ-SĪ-tĭs], inflammation of the appendix
arteri(o)	artery	*arteriosclerosis* [ăr-TĒR-ē-ō-sklěr-Ō-sĭs], hardening of the arteries
arteriol(o)	arteriole	*arteriolosclerosis* [ăr-tēr-ē-Ō-lō-sklěr-Ō-sĭs], hardening of the arterioles, often seen in conjunction with chronic high blood pressure
arthr(o)	joint; articulation	*arthralgia* [ăr-THRĂL-jē-ă], severe joint pain
aur(i), auricul(o)	ear	*auriform* [ĂW-rĭ-fǒrm], ear-shaped; *auriculocranial* [ăw-RĬK-yū-lō-KRĀ-nē-ăl], of the ear and cranium
blephar(o)	eyelid	*blepharitis* [BLĔF-ă-RĪ-tĭs], inflammation of the eyelid
brachi(o)	arm	*brachialgia* [brā-kē-ĂL-jē-ă], pain in the arm

COMBINING FORM	MEANING	EXAMPLE
bronch(o), bronchi	bronchus	*bronchomycosis* [BRŎNG-kō-mī-KŌ-sĭs], fungal disease of the bronchi
bucc(o)	cheek	*buccolabial* [bŭk-ō-LĀ-bē-ăl], relating to both the cheeks and lips
burs(o)	bursa	*bursitis* [bĕr-SĪ-tĭs], inflammation of a bursa
calcane(o)	heel bone	*calcaneodynia* [kăl-KĀ-nē-ō-DĬN-ē-ă], heel pain
cardi(o)	heart; esophageal opening of the stomach	*cardiomegaly* [kăr-dē-ō-MĔG-ă-lē], enlargement of the heart; *cardiectomy* [kăr-dē-ĔK-tō-mē], excision of the cardiac portion of the stomach
carp(o)	wrist bones	*carpopedal* [KĂR-pō-PĔD-ăl], relating to the wrist and the foot
celi(o)	abdomen	*celiorrhaphy* [sē-lē-ŌR-ă-fē], suture of an abdominal wound
cephal(o)	head	*cephalomegaly* [SĔF-ă-lō-MĔG-ă-lē], enlargement of the head
cerebell(o)	cerebellum	*cerebellitis* [sĕr-ĕ-bĕl-Ī-tĭs], inflammation of the cerebellum
cerebr(o)	cerebrum	*cerebrotomy* [sĕr-ĕ-BRŎT-ō-mē], incision into the brain
cervic(o)	neck; cervix	*cervicodynia* [SĔR-vĭ-kō-DĬN-ē-ă], neck pain
cheil(o), chil(o)	lip	*cheiloplasty, chiloplasty* [KĪ-lō-plăs-tē], plastic surgery of the lips
chir(o)	hand	*chiropractic* [kī-rō-PRĂK-tĭk], theory that uses manipulation of the spine to restore and maintain health
chol(e), cholo	bile	*cholelith* [KŌ-lē-lĭth], gallstone
chondri(o), chondr(o)	cartilage	*chondromalacia* [KŎN-drō-mă-LĀ-shē-ă], softening of cartilage
col(o), colon(o)	colon	*colonoscopy* [kō-lŏn-ŎS-kō-pē], visual examination of the colon
colp(o)	vagina	*colporrhagia* [kōl-pō-RĀ-jē-ă], vaginal hemorrhage
core(o)	pupil	*coreoplasty* [KŌR-ē-ō-plăs-tē], surgical correction of a pupil
cortic(o)	cortex	*corticectomy* [kōr-tĭ-SĔK-tō-mē], removal of a part of the cortex
costi, costo	rib	*costogenic* [kŏs-tō-JĔN-ĭk], arising from a rib

COMBINING FORM	MEANING	EXAMPLE
crani(o)	cranium	*craniotomy* [krā-nē-ŎT-ō-mē], opening into the skull
cyst(i), cysto	bladder; cyst	*cystoscopy* [sĭs-TŎS-kō-pē], examination of the interior of the bladder
cyt(o)	cell	*cytology* [sī-TŎL-ō-jē], study of cells
dactyl(o)	fingers, toes	*dactylitis* [dăk-tĭ-LĪ-tĭs], finger inflammation
dent(i), dento	tooth	*dentiform* [DĔN-tĭ-fŏrm], tooth-shaped
derm(o), derma, dermat(o)	skin	*dermatitis* [dĕr-mă-TĪ-tĭs], inflammation of the skin
duoden(o)	duodenum	*duodenoscopy* [dū-ō-dĕ-NŎS-kō-pē], examination of the interior of the duodenum
encephal(o)	brain	*encephalomyeloneuropathy* [ĕn-SĔF-ă-lō-MĪ-ĕ-lō-nū-RŎP-ă-thē], disease involving the brain, spinal cord, and nerves
enter(o)	intestines	*enteritis* [ĕn-tĕr-Ī-tĭs], inflammation of the intestine
episi(o)	vulva	*episiotomy* [ĕ-pĭz-ē-ŎT-ō-mē], surgical incision into the vulva at the time of birth to avoid tearing of the perineum
gastr(o)	stomach	*gastritis* [găs-TRĪ-tĭs], inflammation of the stomach
gingiv(o)	gum	*gingivitis* [jĭn-jĭ-VĪ-tĭs], inflammation of the gums
gloss(o)	tongue	*glossodynia* [GLŎS-ō-DĬN-ē-ă], pain in the tongue
gnath(o)	jaw	*gnathoplasty* [NĂTH-ō-plăs-tē], plastic surgery on the jaw
gonad(o)	sex glands	*gonadopathy* [gŏn-ă-DŎP-ă-thē], disease of the gonads
hem(a), hemat(o), hemo	blood	*hematoma* [hē-mă-TŌ-mă], mass of clotted blood
hepat(o), hepatic(o)	liver	*hepatoma* [hĕp-ă-TŌ-mă], malignant cancer of liver cells
hidr(o)	sweat	*hidropoeisis* [HĪ-drō-pŏy-Ē-sĭs], production of sweat
histi(o), histo	tissue	*histolysis* [hĭs-TŎL-ĭ-sĭs], breakdown of tissue
hyster(o)	uterus, hysteria	*hysterectomy* [hĭs-tĕr-ĔK-tō-mē], removal of the uterus

COMBINING FORM	MEANING	EXAMPLE
ile(o)	ileum	*ileocolitis* [ĬL-ē-ō-kō-LĪ-tĭs], inflammation of the colon and the ileum
ili(o)	ilium	*iliospinal* [ĬL-ē-ō-SPĪ-năl], relating to the ilium and the spine
inguin(o)	groin	*inguinoperitoneal* [ĬNG-gwĭ-nō-PĔR-ĭ-tō-NĒ-ăl], relating to the groin and peritoneum
irid(o)	iris	*iridodilator* [ĬR-ĭ-dō-dī-LĀ-tĕr], agent that causes dilation of the pupil
ischi(o)	ischium	*ischialgia* [ĭs-kē-ĂL-jē-ă], hip pain
kary(o)	nucleus	*karyotype* [KĂR-ē-ō-tĭp], chromosomal characteristics of a cell
kerat(o)	cornea	*keratitis* [kĕr-ă-TĪ-tĭs], inflammation of the cornea
labi(o)	lip	*labioplasty* [LĀ-bē-ō-plăs-tē], plastic surgery of a lip
lamin(o)	lamina	*laminectomy* [LĂM-ĭ-NĔK-tō-mē], removal of a bony portion that forms the arch that surrounds the vertebra
lapar(o)	abdominal wall	*laparomyositis* [LĂP-ă-rō-mī-ō-SĪ-tĭs], inflammation of the abdominal muscles
laryng(o)	larynx	*laryngitis* [lăr-ĭn-JĪ-tĭs], inflammation of the larynx
linguo	tongue	*linguocclusion* [lĭng-gwō-KLŪ-zhŭn], displacement of a tooth toward the tongue
lip(o)	fat	*liposuctioning* [LĬP-ō-SŬK-shŭn-ĭng], removal of body fat by vacuum pressure
lymph(o)	lymph	*lymphuria* [lĭm-FŪ-rē-ă], discharge of lymph into the urine
mast(o)	breast	*mastitis* [măs-TĪ-tĭs], inflammation of the breast
maxill(o)	maxilla	*maxillitis* [MĂK-sĭ-LĪ-tĭs], inflammation of the jawbone
medull(o)	medulla	*medulloblastoma* [MĔD-ŭ-lō-blăs-TŌ-mă], tumor having cells similar to those in medullary substances
mening(o)	meninges	*meningitis* [mĕn-ĭn-JĪ-tĭs], inflammation of the membranes of the brain or spinal cord
muco	mucus	*mucolytic* [myū-kō-LĬT-ĭk], agent capable of dissolving mucus

Combining Form	Meaning	Example
my(o)	muscle	*myocarditis* [MĪ-ō-kăr-DĪ-tĭs], inflammation of the muscle tissue of the heart
myel(o)	spinal cord; bone marrow	*myelopathy* [mī-ĕ-LŎP-ă-thē], disease of the spinal cord
nephr(o)	kidney	*nephritis* [nĕ-FRĪ-tĭs], inflammation of the kidneys
neur, neuro	nerve	*neuritis* [nū-RĪ-tĭs], inflammation of a nerve
oculo	eye	*oculodynia* [ŎK-yū-lō-DĬN-ē-ă], eye pain
odont(o)	tooth	*odontalgia* [ō-dŏn-TĂL-jē-ă], toothache
onych(o)	nail	*onychoid* [ŎN-ĭ-kŏyd], resembling a fingernail
oo	egg	*oocyte* [Ō-ō-sīt], immature ovum
oophor(o)	ovary	*oophorectomy* [ō-ŏf-ōr-ĔK-tō-mē], removal of an ovary
ophthalm(o)	eye	*ophthalmoscope* [ŏf-THĂL-mō-skōp], device for examining interior of the eyeball
opto, optico	eye; sight	*optometer* [ŏp-TŎM-ĕ-tĕr], instrument for measuring eye refraction
or(o)	mouth	*orofacial* [ōr-ō-FĀ-shăl], relating to the mouth and face
orchi(o), orchid(o)	testis	*orchialgia* [ōr-kē-ĂL-jē-ă], pain in the testis
osseo, ossi	bone	*ossiferous* [ō-SĬF-ĕr-ŭs], containing or generating bone
ost(e), osteo	bone	*osteochondritis* [ŎS-tē-ō-kŏn-DRĪ-tĭs], inflammation of a bone and its cartilage
ot(o)	ear	*otitis* [ō-TĪ-tĭs], inflammation of the ear
ovari(o)	ovary	*ovariopathy* [ō-văr-ē-ŎP-ă-thē], disease of the ovary
ovi, ovo	egg; ova	*oviduct* [Ō-vĭ-dŭkt], uterine (fallopian) tube through which ova pass
ped(o), pedi	foot; child	*pedicure* [PĔD-ĭ-kyūr], treatment of the feet; *pedophilia* [pĕ-dō-FĬL-ē-ă], abnormal sexual attraction to children
pelvi(o), pelvo	pelvic bone; hip	*pelviscope* [PĔL-vĭ-skōp], instrument for examining the interior of the pelvis
pharyng(o)	pharynx	*pharyngitis* [făr-ĭn-JĪ-tĭs], inflammation of the pharynx

COMBINING FORM	MEANING	EXAMPLE
phleb(o)	vein	*phlebitis* [flĕ-BĪ-tĭs], inflammation of a vein
phren(o), phreni, phrenico	diaphragm; mind	*phrenicocolic* [FRĔN-ĭ-kō-KŎL-ĭk], relating to the diaphragm and colon; *phrenotropic* [FRĔN-ō-TRŎ-pĭk], exerting its principal effect on the mind
pil(o)	hair	*pilonidal* [pī-lō-NĪ-dăl], having hair, as in a cyst
plasma, plasmo, plasmat(o)	plasma	*plasmacyte* [PLĂZ-mă-sīt], plasma cell
pleur(o), pleura	rib; side; pleura	*pleurography* [plūr-ŎG-ră-fē], imaging of the pleural cavity
pneum(a), pneumat(o), pneum(o), pneumon(o)	lungs; air; breathing	*pneumonitis* [nū-mō-NĪ-tĭs], inflammation of the lungs
pod(o)	foot	*podiatrist* [pō-DĪ-ă-trĭst], specialist in diseases of the foot
proct(o)	anus	*proctalgia* [prŏk-TĂL-jē-ă], pain in the anus or rectum
psych(o), psyche	mind	*psychomotor* [sī-kō-MŌ-tĕr], relating to psychological influence on body movement
pulmon(o)	lung	*pulmonitis* [pūl-mō-NĪ-tĭs], inflammation of the lungs
pyel(o)	renal pelvis	*pyelitis* [pī-ĕ-LĪ-tĭs], inflammation of the cavity below the kidneys
rachi(o)	spine	*rachiometer* [rā-kē-ŎM-ĕ-tĕr], instrument for measuring curvature of the spine
rect(o)	rectum	*rectitis* [rĕk-TĪ-tĭs], inflammation of the rectum
reni, reno	kidney	*reniform* [RĔN-ĭ-fŏrm], kidney-shaped
rhin(o)	nose	*rhinitis* [rī-NĪ-tĭs], inflammation of the nasal membranes
sacr(o)	sacrum	*sacralgia* [sā-KRĂL-jē-ă], pain in the sacral area
sarco	fleshy tissue; muscle	*sarcopoietic* [SĂR-kō-pŏy-ĔT-ĭk], forming muscle
scler(o)	sclera	*sclerodermatitis* [SKLĒR-ō-dĕr-mă-TĪ-tĭs], inflammation and thickening of the skin
sial(o)	salivary glands; saliva	*sialism* [SĪ-ă-lĭzm], excessive production of saliva
sigmoid(o)	sigmoid colon	*sigmoidectomy* [sĭg-mŏy-DĔK-tō-mē], excision of the sigmoid colon
somat(o)	body	*somatophrenia* [SŌ-mă-tō-FRĒ-nē-ă], tendency to imagine bodily illnesses

COMBINING FORM	MEANING	EXAMPLE
sperma, spermato, spermo	semen; spermatozoa	*spermatocide* [spĕr-MĂT-ō-sīd, SPĔR-mă-tō-sīd], agent that destroys sperm
splanchn(o), splanchni	viscera	*splanchnolith* [SPLĂNGK-nō-lĭth], stone in the intestinal tract
splen(o)	spleen	*splenectomy* [splē-NĔK-tō-mē], removal of the spleen
spondyl(o)	vertebra	*spondylitis* [spŏn-dĭ-LĪ-tĭs], inflammation of a vertebra
stern(o)	sternum	*sternalgia* [stĕr-NĂL-jē-ă], sternum pain
steth(o)	chest	*stethoscope* [STĔTH-ō-skōp], device for listening to chest sounds
stom(a), stomat(o)	mouth	*stomatopathy* [stō-mă-TŎP-ă-thē], disease of the mouth
ten(o), tendin(o), tendo, tenon(o)	tendon	*tenectomy* [tĕ-NĔK-tō-mē], *tenonectomy* [tĕn-ō-NĔK-tō-mē], removal of part of a tendon
test(o)	testis	*testitis* [tĕs-TĪ-tĭs], inflammation of the testis
thorac(o), thoracico	thorax, chest	*thoracalgia* [thōr-ă-KĂL-jē-ă], chest pain
thym(o)	thymus gland	*thymokinetic* [THĬ-mō-kĭ-NĔT-ĭk], agent that activates the thymus gland
thyr(o)	thyroid gland	*thyrotomy* [thī-RŎT-ō-mē], operation that cuts the thyroid gland
trache(o)	trachea	*tracheotomy* [trā-kē-ŎT-ō-mē], operation to create an opening into the trachea
trachel(o)	neck	*trachelophyma* [TRĂK-ĕ-lō-FĪ-mă], swelling of the neck
trich(o), trichi	hair	*trichoid* [TRĬK-ŏyd], hairlike
varico	varicosity	*varicophlebitis* [VĀR-ĭ-kō-flĕ-BĪ-tĭs], inflammation of varicose veins
vas(o)	blood vessel, duct	*vasoconstrictor* [VĀ-sō-kŏn-STRĬK-tŏr], agent that narrows blood vessels
vasculo	blood vessel	*vasculopathy* [văs-kyū-LŎP-ă-thē], disease of the blood vessels
veni, veno	vein	*venipuncture* [VĔN-ĭ-pŭngk-shūr, VĒ-nĭ-pŭnkg-shūr], puncture of a vein, as with a needle
ventricul(o)	ventricle	*ventriculitis* [vĕn-trĭk-yū-LĪ-tĭs], inflammation of the ventricles in the brain

COMBINING FORM	MEANING	EXAMPLE
vertebro	vertebra	*vertebrosacral* [věr-tě-brō-SĀ-krăl], relating to the vertebra and the sacrum
vesic(o)	bladder	*vesicoprostatic* [VĚS-ĭ-kō-prŏs-TĂT-ĭk], relating to the bladder and the prostate

COMBINING FORMS AND ABBREVIATIONS EXERCISES

Build Your Medical Vocabulary

Match each compound term with its meaning.

33. ____ adrenomegaly   **a.** agent that stops the flow of blood

34. ____ splanchnopathy   **b.** spasm of an artery

35. ____ angiography   **c.** study of the hair and its diseases

36. ____ osteosclerosis   **d.** inflammation of the liver

37. ____ arteriospasm   **e.** destruction of sperm

38. ____ trichology   **f.** relating to the abdomen and thorax

39. ____ hepatitis   **g.** abnormal hardening of bone

40. ____ spermatolysis   **h.** radiography of blood vessels

41. ____ abdominothoracic   **i.** enlargement of the adrenal glands

42. ____ hemostat   **j.** disease of the viscera

Add a Suffix

Add the suffix needed to complete the statement.

43. An inflammation of an artery is called arter _____.

44. Suturing of a tendon is called teno _____.

45. Death of muscle is called myo _____.

46. A name for any disorder of the spinal cord is myelo _____.

47. Cephal _____ means head pain.

48. Angio _____ means repair of a blood vessel.

49. Softening of the walls of the heart is called cardio _____.

50. Incision into the ileum is called an ileo _____.

51. Enlargement of the kidney is called nephro _____.

52. Any disease of the hair is called tricho _____.

USING THE INTERNET

Go to the National Institutes of Health's Web site (http://www.health.nih.gov/) and click on one of the body systems you have learned about in this chapter. Find the name of at least two diseases of that body system.

CHAPTER REVIEW

The material that follows is to help you review all the material in this chapter as well as to challenge you to think critically about the material you have studied. In addition, this would be a good time to review the chapter on the student CD-ROM and to examine any further related material on the book's Web site (www.mhhe.com/medterm3e).

Word Building

Build the Right Term

Using the word lists and vocabulary reviews in Chapters 1, 2, and 3, construct a medical term that fits each of the following definitions. The number following each definition tells you the number of word parts—combining forms, suffixes, or prefixes—you will need to use.

53. Disease of the heart muscle (3) _____

54. Reconstruction of an artery wall (2) _____

55. Muscle pain (2) _____

56. Incision into the intestines (2) _____

57. Study of poisons (2) _____

58. Relating to the bladder, uterus, and vagina (3) _____

59. Inflammation of the tissue surrounding a blood vessel (3) _____

60. Producing saliva (2) _____

61. Morbid fear of blood (2) _____

62. Paralysis of the heart (2) _____

63. Plastic surgery of the skin (2) _____

64. Causing death of an ovum (2) _____

Define the Terms

Using the information you have learned in Chapters 1, 2, and 3, and without consulting a dictionary, give the closest definition you can for each of the following terms.

65. otorhinolaryngology _____

66. tracheomegaly _____

67. cystopyelitis _____

68. onychorrhexis _____

69. fibroma _____

70. oophorrhagia _____

71. antiparasitic _____

72. neopathy _____

73. retropharynx _____

74. lipocardiac _____

Find a Match

Match the combining form with its definition.

75. ____ adip(o)
76. ____ blephar(o)
77. ____ carp(o)
78. ____ celi(o)
79. ____ core(o)
80. ____ costo
81. ____ mening(o)
82. ____ or(o)
83. ____ osseo

a. rib
b. mouth
c. eyelid
d. fat
e. bone
f. wrist
g. abdomen
h. meninges
i. pupil

Find What's Wrong

In each of the following terms, one or more word parts are misspelled.
Replace the misspelled word part(s) and write the correct term in the space provided.

84. meningiitus _____
85. polmonary _____
86. abdomenal _____
87. cardiomagaley _____
88. ensephaloscope _____
89. mielopathy _____
90. larynjectomy _____
91. ooocyte _____
92. optimetrist _____
93. hemoglobine _____
94. athrodesis _____
95. yatrogenic _____
96. carcinsoma _____
97. paraplejic _____
98. mezomorph _____
99. simbiosis _____
100. schizofrenia _____

Find the Specialty

For each of the following diagnoses, name the appropriate specialist who would generally treat the condition. If you do not know the meaning of any of these conditions, look them up in the glossary/index at the back of the book.

101. myocarditis _____
102. dermatitis _____
103. bronchitis _____

104. ovarian cysts _____

105. prostatitis _____

106. cancer _____

107. glaucoma _____

108. colitis _____

109. neuritis _____

110. allergy to bee sting _____

Build Your Medical Vocabulary

Match the directional term with its meaning

111. ____ anterior

112. ____ distal

113. ____ lateral

114. ____ medial

115. ____ posterior

116. ____ superficial

117. ____ proximal

118. ____ prone

119. ____ inferior

120. ____ supine

121. ____ superior

122. ____ deep

a. at or near the surface (of the body)

b. to the side

c. away from the point of attachment to the trunk

d. at or toward the front (of the body)

e. lying on the spine facing upward

f. at or toward the backside (of the body)

g. below another body structure

h. at or near the middle (of the body)

i. away from the surface (of the body)

j. at or near the point of attachment to the trunk

k. lying on the stomach with the face down

l. above another body structure

DEFINITIONS

On a separate sheet of paper, define the following terms and combining forms. Review the chapter before starting. Make sure you know how to pronounce each term as you define it. Check your answers in this chapter or in the glossary/index at the end of the book.

TERM

123. abdominal [ăb-DOM-i-năl] cavity

124. abdomin(o)

125. acetabul(o)

126. aden(o)

127. adip(o)

128. adren(o)

129. alveol(o)

130. angi(o)

131. anterior [ăn-TĒR-ē-ŏr]

132. aort(o)

133. appendic(o)

134. arteri(o)

135. arteriol(o)

136. arthr(o)

137. aur(i), auricul(o)

138. blephar(o)

139. brachi(o)

140. blood [blŭd] system

141. bronch(o), bronchi

142. bucc(o)

143. burs(o)

144. calcane(o)

145. cardi(o)

146. cardiovascular [KĂR-dē-ō-VĂS-kyū-lăr] system

147. carp(o)

148. celi(o)

149. cell [sĕl]

150. cephal(o)

151. cerebell(o)

152. cerebr(o)

153. cervic(o)

154. cheil(o), chil(o)
155. chir(o)
156. chol(e), cholo
157. chondri(o), chondro
158. col(o), colon(o)
159. colp(o)
160. connective [kŏn-NĔK-tĭv] tissue
161. core(o)
162. coronal [KŌR-ō-năl] plane
163. cranial [KRĀ-nē-ăl] cavity
164. cortic(o)
165. costi, costo
166. crani(o)
167. cross-sectional plane
168. cyst(i), cysto
169. cyt(o)
170. dactyl(o)
171. deep
172. dent(i), dento
173. derm(o), derma, dermat(o)
174. diaphragm [DĪ-ă-frăm]
175. digestive [dī-JĔS-tĭv] system
176. distal [DĬS-tăl]
177. dorsal [DŌR-săl]
178. dorsal cavity
179. duoden(o)
180. encephal(o)
181. endocrine [ĔN-dō-krĭn] system
182. enter(o)
183. epigastric [ĕp-ĭ-GĂS-trĭk] region
184. episi(o)
185. epithelial [ĕp-ĭ-THĒ-lē-ăl] tissue

186. frontal plane
187. gastr(o)
188. gingiv(o)
189. gloss(o)
190. gnath(o)
191. gonad(o)
192. hem(a), hemat(o), hemo
193. hepat(o), hepatic(o)
194. hidr(o)
195. histi(o), histo
196. hypochondriac [hī-pō-KŎN-drē-ăk] regions
197. hypogastric [hī-pō-GĂS-trĭk] region
198. hyster(o)
199. ile(o)
200. ili(o)
201. iliac [ĬL-ē-ăk] regions
202. inferior [ĭn-FĒR-ē-ōr]
203. inguin(o)
204. inguinal [ĬN-gwĭ-năl] regions
205. integumentary [ĭn-tĕg-yū-MĔN-tă-rē] system
206. irid(o)
207. ischi(o)
208. kary(o)
209. kerat(o)
210. labi(o)
211. lamin(o)
212. lapar(o)
213. laryng(o)
214. lateral [cf. "inferior" above]
215. lateral plane
216. left lower quadrant
217. left upper quadrant
218. linguo

219. lip(o)
220. lumbar [LŬM-băr] regions
221. lymph(o)
222. lymphatic [lĭm-FĂT-ĭk] and immune [ĭ-MYŪN] system
223. mast(o)
224. maxill(o)
225. medial [MĒ-dē-ăl]
226. medial plane
227. medull(o)
228. mening(o)
229. midsagittal [mĭd-SĂJ-ĭ-tăl] plane
230. muco
231. muscle [MŬS-ĕl] tissue
232. musculoskeletal [mŭs-kyū-lō-SKĔL-ĕ-tăl] system
233. my(o)
234. myel(o)
235. nephr(o)
236. nervous [NĔR-vŭs] system
237. nervous tissue
238. neur, neuro
239. oculo
240. odont(o)
241. onych(o)
242. oo
243. oophor(o)
244. ophthalm(o)
245. opto, optico
246. or(o)
247. orchi(o), orchid(o)
248. organ [ŌR-găn]
249. osseo, ossi
250. ost(e), osteo
251. ot(o)

252. ovari(o)
253. ovi, ovo
254. ped(o), pedi
255. pelvi(o), pelvo
256. pelvic [PĔL-vĭk] cavity
257. pharyng(o)
258. phleb(o)
259. phren(o), phreni, phrenico
260. pil(o)
261. plasma, plasmo, plasmat(o)
262. pleur(o), pleura
263. pneum(a), pneumat(o), pneum(o), pneumon(o)
264. pod(o)
265. posterior
266. proct(o)
267. prone
268. proximal [PRŎK-sĭ-măl]
269. psych(o), psyche
270. pulmon(o)
271. pyel(o)
272. rachi(o)
273. rect(o)
274. reni, reno
275. reproductive [rē-prō-DŬK-tĭv] system

276. respiratory [RĔS-pĭ-ră-tōr-ē, rĕ-SPĪR-ă-tōr-ē] system
277. rhin(o)
278. right lower quadrant
279. right upper quadrant
280. sacr(o)
281. sagittal [SĂJ-ĭ-tăl] plane
282. sarco
283. scler(o)
284. sensory system
285. sial(o)
286. sigmoid(o)
287. somat(o)
288. sperma, spermato, spermo
289. spinal [SPĪ-năl] cavity
290. splanchn(o), splanchni
291. splen(o)
292. spondyl(o)
293. stern(o)
294. steth(o)
295. stom(a), stomat(o)
296. superficial
297. superior
398. supine [sū-PĪN]
399. system [SĬS-tĕm]

300. ten(o), tendin(o), tendo, tenon(o)
301. test(o)
302. thorac(o), thoracico
303. thoracic [thō-RĂS-ĭk] cavity
304. thym(o)
305. thyr(o)
306. tissue [TĬSH-ū]
307. trache(o)
308. trachel(o)
309. transverse plane
310. trich(o), trichi
311. umbilical [ŭm-BĬL-ĭ-kăl] region
312. urinary [YŪR-ĭ-nār-ē] system
313. varico
314. vas(o)
315. vasculo
316. veni, veno
317. ventral [VĔN-trăl]
318. ventral cavity
319. ventricul(o)
320. vertebro
321. vesic(o)

Answers to Chapter Exercises

1. d
2. h
3. i
4. e
5. f
6. g
7. k
8. c
9. j
10. a
11. b
12. cell
13. tissue
14. epithelial
15. cranial
16. diaphragm
17. dorsal
18. pelvic
19. urinary
20. digestive
21. stomach, spleen, intestines, liver, pancreas
22. Yes, pain may be "referred," felt in one part of the body but actually coming from another part.
23. F
24. T
25. F
26. F
27. T
28. F
29. T
30. F
31. T
32.

a. Deep
b. Superficial
c. Anterior
d. Distal
e. Supine
f. Inferior

33. i
34. j
35. h
36. g
37. b
38. c
39. d
40. e
41. f
42. a
43. itis
44. rrhaphy
45. necrosis
46. pathy
47. algia
48. plasty
49. malacia
50. tomy
51. megaly
52. pathy
53. cardiomyopathy
54. arterioplasty
55. myalgia or myodynia
56. enterotomy
57. toxicology
58. vesicouterovaginal
59. periangitis
60. sialogenous
61. hemophobia
62. cardioplegia
63. dermatoplasty
64. ovicidal
65. study of the ear, nose, and throat
66. abnormally enlarged trachea
67. inflammation of the bladder and the renal pelvis
68. abnormal breaking of the nails
69. benign neoplasm in fibrous tissues
70. ovarian hemorrhage
71. destructive to parasites
72. a new disease process
73. back part of the pharynx
74. relating to a fatty heart
75. d
76. c
77. f
78. g
79. i

80. a
81. h
82. b
83. e
84. meningitis
85. pulmonary
86. abdominal
87. cardiomegaly
88. encephaloscope
89. myelopathy
90. laryngectomy
91. oocyte
92. optometrist
93. hemoglobin
94. arthrodesis
95. iatrogenic
96. carcinoma
97. paraplegic
98. mesomorph
99. symbiosis
100. schizophrenia
101. cardiologist
102. dermatologist
103. pulmonologist
104. gynecologist
105. urologist
106. oncologist
107. opthalmologist
108. gastroenterologist
109. neurologist
110. allergist
111. d
112. c
113. b
114. h
115. f
116. a
117. j
118. k
119. g
120. e
121. l
122. i
123–321. Answers are available in the vocabulary reviews in this chapter.

The Integumentary System

▶ DERMATOLOGY

After studying this chapter, you will be able to:

4.1 Name the parts of the integumentary system and discuss the function of each part

4.2 Define the combining forms used in building words that relate to the integumentary system

4.3 Identify the meaning of related abbreviations

4.4 Name the common diagnoses, laboratory tests, and clinical procedures used in testing and treating disorders of the integumentary system

4.5 List and define the major pathological conditions of the integumentary system

4.6 Define surgical terms related to the integumentary system

4.7 List common pharmacological agents used in treating disorders of the integumentary system

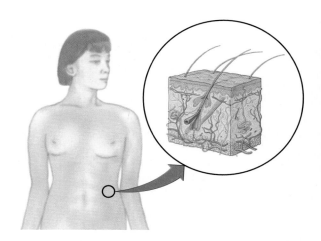

Structure and Function

The integumentary system includes the skin or **integument,** the *hair,* the **nails,** the **sweat glands** (also called the *sudoriferous glands*), and the oil-producing glands (also called the **sebaceous glands**). This system covers and protects the body, helps regulate the body's temperature, excretes some of the body's waste materials, and includes the body's sensors for pain and sensation. Figure 4-1a shows a cross-section of skin with the parts of the integumentary system labeled. Figure 4-1b is a diagram showing the three layers of skin and what they contain.

Skin

The skin is the largest body organ. The average adult has about 21.5 square feet of skin. The four major functions of the skin are:

1. It protects the body from fluid loss and injury and from the intrusion of harmful microorganisms and ultraviolet (UV) rays of the sun.
2. It helps to maintain the proper internal temperature of the body.
3. It serves as a site for excretion of waste materials through perspiration.
4. It is an important sensory organ.

The skin varies in thickness, depending on what part of the body it covers and what its function is in covering that part. For example, the skin on the

FIGURE 4-1a The integumentary system consists of the skin with all its layers, hair, nails, and glands.

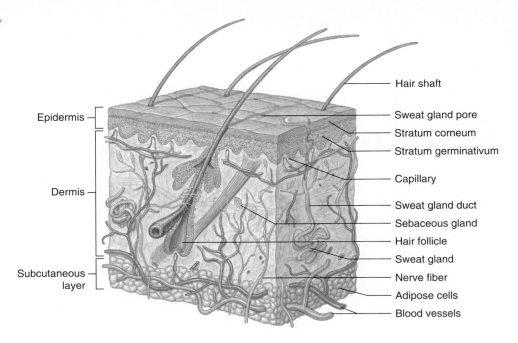

Epidermis

Dermis

Subcutaneous layer

Hair shaft
Sweat gland pore
Stratum corneum
Stratum germinativum
Capillary
Sweat gland duct
Sebaceous gland
Hair follicle
Sweat gland
Nerve fiber
Adipose cells
Blood vessels

FIGURE 4-1b A diagram showing the three layers of skin and what they contain.

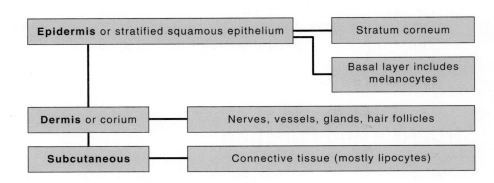

Epidermis or stratified squamous epithelium	Stratum corneum
	Basal layer includes melanocytes
Dermis or corium	Nerves, vessels, glands, hair follicles
Subcutaneous	Connective tissue (mostly lipocytes)

upper back is about ten times thicker than the skin on the eyelid. The eyelid skin must be light, flexible, and movable, so it is thin. The skin on the upper back must cover and move with large muscle groups and bones, so it is thick to provide the necessary strength and protection.

The skin has three main parts or layers—the **epidermis,** the **dermis** or **corium,** and the **subcutaneous layer** or **hypodermis.**

Epidermis

The epidermis, the outer layer of skin, ranges from 1/200 to 1/20 of an inch thick, and consists of several **strata** (sublayers). The epidermis is made up of cells called **squamous epithelium,** a flat, scaly layer of cells. The layers that make up the squamous epithelium are called **stratified squamous epithelium.**

Not all parts of the body's skin contain all the sublayers of epidermis. The top sublayer is called the **stratum corneum.** It consists of a flat layer of dead cells arranged in parallel rows. As new cells are produced, the dead cells are sloughed off. As they die, the cells in the stratum corneum fill with **keratin**—a waterproof barrier to keep microorganisms out and moisture in. The keratin of the epidermis is softer than the hard keratin in nails. Dead skin cells on the suface fall off naturally as replacement cells rise from the base layers. Dead skin can also be removed by *exfoliation* or *desquamation*, the falling off in layers or scales, especially of skin. This is sometimes done for cosmetic reasons as exfoliation of the facial skin using an abrasive cloth or substance.

The bottom sublayer of the epidermis is called the **stratum germinativum.** Here new cells are produced and pushed up to the stratum corneum. The epidermis itself is a nonvascular layer of skin, meaning that it does not contain blood vessels.

Specialized cells called **melanocytes** produce a pigment called **melanin,** which helps to determine skin and hair color. Melanin is essential in screening out ultraviolet rays of the sun that can harm the body's cells.

Dermis

The dermis (also called the corium) contains two sublayers, a thin top one called the **papillary layer,** and a thicker one called the **reticular layer.** The dermis contains connective tissue that holds many capillaries, lymph cells, nerve endings, sebaceous and sweat glands, and hair follicles. These nourish the epidermis and serve as sensitive touch receptors. The connective tissue is composed primarily of **collagen** fibers that form a strong, elastic network. Collagen is a protein substance that is very tough, yet flexible. When the collagen fibers stretch, they form **striae** or stretch marks.

Subcutaneous Layer or Hypodermis

The subcutaneous layer is the layer between the dermis and the body's inner organs. It consists of **adipose** (or fatty) tissue and some layers of fibrous tissue. Within the subcutaneous layers lie blood vessels and nerves. The layer of fatty tissue serves to protect the inner organs and to maintain the body's temperature.

Hair

Hair grows out of the epidermis to cover various parts of the body. Hair serves to cushion and protect the areas it covers. Figure 4-2 shows a detail of hair growing out of the epidermis. Hair has two parts. The **hair shaft** protrudes from the skin, and the **hair root** lies beneath the surface of the skin. The shaft is composed of outer layers of scaly cells filled with inner layers of soft and hard keratin. Hair grows upward from the root through the **hair**

MORE ABOUT . . .

Skin Color

All people have melanin (except those with albinism). The darker the skin, the more melanin is produced. There are many variations in skin color within each racial group, but some overall characteristics are unique to each racial group. For example, African-American people have high melanin levels; Asians have low melanin and high *carotene* (a pigment that is converted to vitamin A in the body) levels; Caucasians have comparatively low melanin levels. The rates of skin cancer go down as the amount of available melanin goes up.

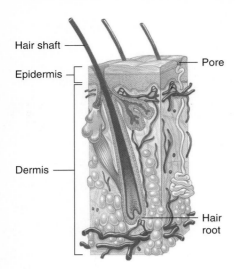

Hair shaft

Epidermis

Dermis

Pore

Hair root

FIGURE 4-2 Detail of hair growing out of the epidermis.

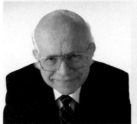
follicles (tubular sacs that hold the hair fibers). The shape of the follicle determines the shape of the hair (straight, curly, or wavy). Hair color is determined by the presence of melanin, which is produced by the melanocytes in the epidermis. Gray hair occurs when melanocytes stop producing melanin. Hair growth, thickness, and curliness are generally determined by heredity. In addition to heredity, baldness or **alopecia** may result from disease, injury, or medical treatment (such as chemotherapy). A general term for removal of hair by the roots is *epilation* or *depilation*. Such removal may be the result of some kind of injury or it may be done voluntarily to remove unwanted hair.

Nails

Nails are plates made of hard keratin that cover the dorsal surface of the distal bone of the fingers and toes. Nails serve as a protective covering, help in the grasping of objects, and allow us to scratch. Healthy nails appear pinkish because the translucent nail covers vascular tissue. At the base of most nails, a **lunula,** or whitish half-moon, is an area where keratin and other cells have mixed with air. Nails are surrounded by a narrow band of epidermis called a **cuticle,** except at the top. The top portion of the nail grows above the level of the finger.

Glands

The integumentary system includes various types of glands. The glands in the skin are:

1. The sweat glands (also called sudoriferous glands) are found almost everywhere on the body surface. Glands that secrete outward toward the surface of the body through ducts are called **exocrine glands.** The excretion of sweat is called **diaphoresis.** Secretions exit the body through **pores** or tiny openings in the skin surface. Sweat (also called *perspiration*) is composed of water and sodium chloride and other compounds

Nail Health

The nails sometimes offer a picture of inner health. In the photo on the left, the normal nails are healthy and pinkish, with no discolorations or white spots. The nail in the photo on the right has been altered by a fungal infection.

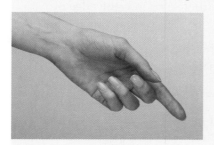
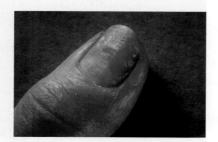

depending on many factors, such as external temperature, fluid intake, level of activity, hormonal levels, and so on.

2. **Eccrine** (or small sweat) **glands** are found on many places of the body. They excrete a colorless fluid that keeps the body at a constant temperature.

3. The **apocrine glands** appear during and after puberty and secrete sweat from the armpits, near the reproductive organs, and around the nipples.

   The female breast, which contains *mammary glands*, is itself a specialized type of apocrine gland that is adapted to secreting milk after childbirth (Figure 4-3).

4. **Ceruminous glands** are a specialized gland in the surface of the ear that secretes *cerumen*, a waxy substance that lubricates and protects the ear.

5. **Sebaceous glands,** located in the dermis, secrete an oily substance called **sebum,** which is found at the base of the hair follicles. This substance serves to lubricate and protect the skin. Sebum forms a skin barrier against bacteria and fungi and also softens the surface of the skin.

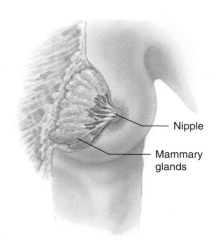

— Nipple

— Mammary glands

FIGURE 4-3 The female breast is a specialized type of apocrine gland.

VOCABULARY REVIEW

In the previous section, you learned terms relating to the integumentary system. Before going on to the exercise section, review the terms below and refer back to the previous section if you have any questions. Pronunciations are provided for certain terms. Sometimes information about where the word came from is included after the term. The etymologies (word histories) are for your information only. You do not need to memorize them.

Term	Definition
adipose [ĂD-ĭ-pōs]	Fatty; relating to fat.
alopecia [ăl-ō-PĒ-shē-ă] Greek *alopekia*, mange	Lack of hair in spots; baldness.
apocrine [ĂP-ō-krĭn] **glands** Greek *apo-krino*, to separate	Glands that appear during and after puberty and secrete sweat, as from the armpits.
ceruminous [sĕ-RŪ-mĭn-ŭs] **glands**	Glands that secrete a waxy substance on the surface of the ear.

Term	Definition
collagen [KŎL-lă-jĕn] Greek *koila*, glue + -gen	Major protein substance that is tough and flexible and that forms connective tissue in the body.
corium [KŌ-rē-ŭm]	See dermis.
cuticle [KYŪ-tĭ-kl]	Thin band of epidermis that surrounds the edge of nails, except at the top.
dermis [DĚR-mĭs]	Layer of skin beneath the epidermis containing blood vessels, nerves, and some glands.
diaphoresis [DĪ-ă-fō-RĒ-sĭs]	Excretion of fluid by the sweat glands; sweating.
eccrine [ĔK-rĭn] **glands** Greek *ek-krino*, to separate	Sweat glands that occur all over the body, except where the apocrine glands occur.
epidermis [ĕp-ĭ-DĚR-mĭs] epi-, upon + dermis, layer of skin	Outer portion of the skin containing several strata.
exocrine [ĔK-sō-krĭn] **glands** exo-, outside + Greek *krino*, to separate	Glands that secrete through ducts toward the outside of the body.
hair follicle [FŎL-ĭ-kl]	Tubelike sac in the dermis out of which the hair shaft develops.
hair root	Portion of the hair beneath the skin surface.
hair shaft	Portion of the hair visible above the skin surface.
hypodermis [hī-pō-DĚR-mĭs] hypo-, under + dermis, layer of skin	Subcutaneous skin layer; layer below the dermis.
integument [ĭn-TĚG-yū-mĕnt] Latin *integumentum*, covering	Skin and all the elements that are contained within and arise from it.
keratin [KĚR-ă-tĭn]	Hard, horny protein that forms nails and hair.
lunula (*pl.*, lunulae) [LŪ-nū-lă (LŪ-nū-lē)] Latin, little moon	Half-moon shaped area at the base of the nail plate.
melanin [MĔL-ă-nĭn]	Pigment produced by melanocytes that determines skin, hair, and eye color.
melanocyte [MĔL-ă-nō-sīt] melano-, black + cyte, cell	Cell in the epidermis that produces melanin.
nail	Thin layer of keratin that covers the distal portion of fingers and toes.
papillary [PĂP-ĭ-lār-ē] **layer**	Thin sublayer of the dermis containing small papillae (nipple-like masses).
pore	Opening or hole, particularly in the skin.
reticular [rĕ-TĬK-yū-lăr] **layer**	Bottom sublayer of the dermis containing reticula (network of structures with connective tissue between).

Term	Definition
sebaceous [sĕ-BĀ-shŭs] **glands**	Glands in the dermis that open to hair follicles and secrete sebum.
sebum [SĒ-bŭm] Latin *sebum*, tallow	Oily substance, usually secreted into the hair follicle.
squamous epithelium [SKWĂ-mŭs ĕp-ĭ-THĒ-lē- ŭm]	Flat, scaly layer of cells that makes up the epidermis.
stratified squamous epithelium	Layers of epithelial cells that make up the strata of epithelium of the epidermis.
stratum (*pl.*, strata) [STRĂT-ŭm (STRĂ-tă)] Latin *stratum*, layer, bed cover	Layer of tissue, especially a layer of the skin.
stratum [KŌR-nē-ŭm] **corneum**	Top sublayer of the epidermis.
stratum germinativum [jĕr-mĭ-NĀT-ĭ-vŭm]	Bottom sublayer of the epidermis.
striae [STRĪ-ē] Latin, plural of *stria*, furrow	Stretch marks made in the collagen fibers of the dermis layer.
subcutaneous [sŭb-kyū-TĀ-nē-ŭs] **layer** sub-, beneath + Latin *cutis*, skin	Bottom layer of the skin containing fatty tissue.
sweat glands	Coiled glands of the skin that secrete perspiration to regulate body temperature and excrete waste products.

CASE STUDY

The Dermatologist's Office

Madeline Charles arrived at the office a few minutes early. She knew that Dr. Lin had a busy morning scheduled, and she wanted to set up before the doctor arrived. As secretary to Dr. Lin, Madeline handles incoming calls, scheduling, billing, new patient information forms, and insurance matters. She reports to James Carlson, the CMA and office manager for this small office. James assists the doctor with patients, oversees the work Madeline does, and helps when Madeline's load is too great. This morning, the first three patients are scheduled at 8:30, 9:00, and 9:30. Madeline looks at the schedule, realizes that one of the patients is new, and gets the folders for the other two. She sets up the clipboard with the forms the new patient will have to complete and attaches the privacy practices statement of the office (a requirement of the HIPAA laws). She had previously asked the new patient to arrive 15 minutes early in order to have time to fill out the necessary forms.

Bob Luis, the first patient, is 48 years old and has a long history of diabetes (a disease of the endocrine system discussed in Chapter 15). He sees Dr. Lin several times a year for treatment of skin irritations that do not seem to heal. Yesterday, Mr. Luis called with a specific problem. He has an extensive rash on his left ankle. It sounded serious enough to warrant an appointment for the next morning. When Mr. Luis arrives, James escorts him to an examination room and helps him prepare for his visit.

Critical Thinking

1. What do we know about Mr. Luis's condition that would warrant an immediate appointment with Dr. Lin?
2. Does a dermatologist treat a disease such as diabetes, or only symptoms related to the integumentary system?

Build Your Medical Vocabulary

3. The dermis is a layer of skin. Using your knowledge of prefixes learned in Chapter 2, put the following words in order according to how close they are to the outside of the body.

   a. hypodermis _____

   b. epidermis _____

   c. dermis _____

4. Name three types of glands, two of which were compound terms even in ancient Greece.

Complete the Diagram

5. Fill in the missing labels on the figure shown here.

   a. _____

   b. _____

   c. _____

   d. _____

   e. _____

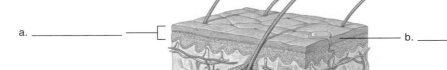

a. _____

b. _____

d. _____

c. _____

e. _____

Fill in the Blanks

Complete the sentences below by filling in the blank(s).

6. The thin layer of skin around the edge of a nail is called a(n) _____.

7. A hair follicle is in the _____ (layer of the skin).

8. The outer layer of skin is the _____.

9. The top sublayer of the dermis is called _____ _____.

10. Small sweat glands found all over the body are called _____ glands.

11. The subcutaneous layer consists of _____ tissue.

12. A pinkish nail is a sign of a(n) _____ nail.

13. The area where keratin and other cells mix with air under the nail is called the _____.

14. Sebaceous glands secrete _____.

15. The female breast is a(n) _____ gland.

Match the Terms

Write the letter of the meaning of the term in the space provided.

16. ____ adipose

17. ____ collagen

18. ____ cuticle

19. ____ dermis

20. ____ epidermis

21. ____ keratin

22. ____ lunula

23. ____ melanin

24. ____ sebum

25. ____ striae

a. layer of skin beneath the epidermis containing blood vessels, nerves, and some glands

b. hard, horny protein that forms nails and hair

c. oily substance, usually secreted into the hair follicle

d. thin band of epidermis that surround the edge of nails, except the top

e. pigment produced by melanocytes that determines skin, hair, and eye color

f. outer portion of the skin containing several strata

g. stretch marks made in the collagen fibers of the dermis layer

h. fatty, relating to fat

i. half-moon shaped area at the base of the nail

j. major protein substance that is tough and flexible and that forms connective tissue in the body

Know Your Glands

Write the letter of the glands that match the description.

26. ____ apocrine glands

27. ____ ceruminous glands

28. ____ eccrine glands

29. ____ exocrine

30. ____ sebaceous glands

31. ____ sweat glands

a. glands that secrete a waxy substance on the surface of the ear

b. glands in the dermis that open to hair follicles and secrete an oily substance

c. glands that secrete through ducts toward the outside of the body

d. glands that appear during and after puberty and secrete sweat

e. sweat glands that occur all over the body, except where apocrine glands occur

f. coiled glands of the skin that secrete perspiration to regulate body temperature and excrete waste products

Combining Forms and Abbreviations

The tables below include combining forms and abbreviations that relate specifically to the integumentary system. Pronunciations are included for the examples.

Combining Form	Meaning	Example
adip(o)	fatty	*adiposis* [ăd-ĭ-PŌ-sĭs], excessive accumulation of body fat
dermat(o)	skin	*dermatitis* [dĕr-mă-TĪ-tĭs], inflammation of the skin

Combining Form	Meaning	Example
derm(o)	skin	*dermabrasion* [dĕr-mă-BRĀ-zhŭn], surgical procedure to remove acne scars and marks, using an abrasive product to remove part of the skin
hidr(o)	sweat, sweat glands	*hidrosis* [hī-DRŌ-sĭs], production and excretion of sweat
ichthy(o)	fish, scaly	*ichthyosis* [ĭk-thē-Ō-sĭs], congenital skin disorder characterized by dryness and peeling
kerat(o)	horny tissue	*keratosis* [kĕr-ă-TŌ-sĭs], skin lesion covered by a horny layer of tissue
lip(o)	fatty	*liposuction* [lĭp-ō-SŬK-shŭn], removal of unwanted fat by suctioning through tubes placed under the skin
melan(o)	black, very dark	*melanoma* [mĕl-ă-NŌ-mă], malignancy arising from cells that form melanin
myc(o)	fungus	*mycosis* [mī-KŌ-sĭs], any condition caused by fungus
onych(o)	nail	*onychotomy* [ŏn-ĭ-KŎT-ō-mē] incision into a nail
pil(o)	hair	*pilocystic* [pī-lō-SĬS-tĭk], relating to a skin cyst with hair
seb(o)	sebum, sebaceous glands	*seborrhea* [sĕb-ō-RĒ-ă], excessive sebum caused by overactivity of the sebaceous glands
steat(o)	fat	*steatitis* [stē-ă-TĪ-tĭs], inflammation of fatty tissue
trich(o)	hair	*trichopathy* [trī-KŎP-ă-thē], disease of the hair
xanth(o)	yellow	*xanthoma* [zăn-THŌ-mă], yellow growth or discoloration of the skin
xer(o)	dry	*xeroderma* [zēr-ō-DĔR-mă], excessive dryness of the skin

Abbreviation	Meaning	Abbreviation	Meaning
bx	biopsy (see surgical terms on page 92)	PUVA	psoralen—ultraviolet A light therapy (used in the treatment of some disorders such as psoriasis)
DLE	discoid lupus erythematosus (see pathological terms on page 85)	SLE	systemic lupus erythematosus (see pathological terms on page 88)
MRSA	A form of staphylococcus aureus that is resistant to a common group of antibiotics that include methicillin, penicillin, and amoxicillin.	VRE	A form of enterococcus that is resistant to most antibiotics
PPD	purified protein derivative (of tuberculin)		

CASE STUDY

Understanding Information

While Dr. Lin is examining his first patient, Bob Luis, the new patient arrives for her 9:00 appointment. Madeline explains which parts of the forms have to be filled out, asks for the patient's insurance card so she can copy it, and completes the file for Dr. Lin before 9:00. Meanwhile, Dr. Lin hands Madeline his notes with a diagnosis for Bob Luis, including a new prescription for treatment of xeroderma. In addition, Dr. Lin gives Mr. Luis samples of a cream to relieve itching.

Critical Thinking

32. Why does the new patient have to fill out forms with questions about family history?
33. Mr. Luis is to be given samples of a prescription cream to try. Can the medical assistant decide which samples to give him?

COMBINING FORMS AND ABBREVIATIONS EXERCISES

Build Your Medical Vocabulary

Build a word for each of the following definitions. Use the combining form vocabulary review in this chapter and the combining forms you have learned earlier.

34. Plastic surgery of the skin: _____
35. Inflammation of the skin and veins: _____
36. Horny growth on the epidermis: _____
37. Fungal eruption on the skin: _____
38. Excess pigment in the skin: _____
39. Fungal infection of the nail: _____
40. Surgical repair of the nail: _____
41. Of the hair follicles and sebaceous glands: _____
42. Pigment-producing cell: _____
43. Examination of the hair: _____
44. Removal of fat by cutting: _____
45. Relating to both fatty and cellular tissue: _____
46. Study of hair: _____
47. Disease of the nail: _____
48. Poison produced by certain fungi: _____
49. Virus that infects fungi: _____
50. Yellow coloration of the skin: _____
51. Condition of extreme dryness: _____
52. Removal or shedding of the horny layer of the epidermis: _____
53. Abnormally darkened skin: _____
54. Lessening of the rate of sweating: _____
55. A doctor who specializes in the diagnosis and treatment of the skin: _____
56. Nail biting: _____
57. Causing the growth of horny tissue or skin and hair: _____
58. The formation of sweat: _____
59. A skin disorder characterized by dry flaking or scaling of the skin: _____
60. The study of fungus: _____
61. Any disease of the skin: _____
62. Hardening of the skin: _____
63. Grafting of skin from one part of the body to another: _____
64. Inflammation of the nail bed: _____
65. Fear of loose hairs on the clothing or elsewhere: _____

66. A tumor of the sebaceous glands:

_____

67. Abnormal sensitivity (of the skin) to light:

_____

68. A rapidly spreading (malignant) skin tumor that arises from a pigment-producing cell in the skin:

_____

69. Another term for *fatty* tissue: _____

Root Out the Meaning

Separate the following terms into word parts; define each word part.

70. trichoma _____

71. xerosis _____

72. mycocide _____

73. xanthoderma _____

74. onychoid _____

75. dermatofibroma _____

76. onychomalacia _____

77. hypodermic _____

78. erythroderma _____

79. pachyderma _____

80. mycogenic _____

81. xeroderma _____

82. trichomycosis _____

83. lipoma _____

84. onychocryptosis _____

Diagnostic, Procedural, and Laboratory Terms

The field of **dermatology** studies, diagnoses, and treats ailments of the skin. The first diagnostic test is usually visual observation of the surface of the skin. Clinical procedures and laboratory tests can result in diagnosis and treatment of specific skin conditions.

Diagnostic Procedures and Tests

Once a visual assessment has been made, the dermatologist determines which procedures and tests will help find the underlying cause of a skin problem. Samples of **exudate** (material that passes out of tissues) or pus may be sent to a laboratory for examination. The laboratory can determine what types of bacteria are present. A scraping may also be taken and placed on a growth medium to be examined for the presence of fungi.

Skin is a reliable place to test for various diseases and allergies. A suspected *allergen*, something that provokes an allergic reaction, is mixed with a substance that can be used in tests. That substance containing the allergen is called an *antigen*. Skin tests are typically performed in one of three ways:

1. The **patch test** calls for placing a suspected antigen on a piece of gauze and applying it to the skin. If a reaction results, the test is considered positive.
2. The **scratch test** (in which a suspected antigen is scratched onto the skin, and redness or swelling within ten minutes indicates a positive reaction).

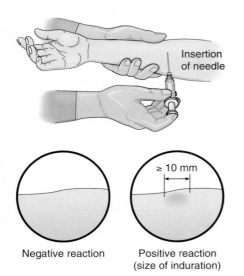

Insertion of needle

Negative reaction

≥ 10 mm

Positive reaction (size of induration)

FIGURE 4-4 A Mantoux test is performed by injecting a small dose of tuberculin intradermally. A positive result is a small raised bump on the skin. No reaction indicates that tuberculosis is not present.

3. The **intradermal test** (in which a suspected antigen is injected between layers of skin). Infectious diseases may also be detected by an intradermal test. Some common intradermal tests are:

   a. The **Mantoux test** for diagnosing tuberculosis. In the Mantoux test, **PPD** (a purified protein derivative of tuberculin) is injected intradermally. Figure 4-4 shows a Mantoux test.

   b. The **tine test** (also called **TB tine**), a screening test for tuberculosis, injects the tuberculin using a tine (an instrument with a number of pointed ends).

   c. The **Schick test** is a test for diphtheria, in which a small amount of toxin is injected into the skin of one arm and a small amount of deactivated toxin is injected into the skin of the other arm for comparison.

> The American Lung Association (www.lungusa.org) has extensive information about tuberculosis.

VOCABULARY REVIEW

In the previous section, you learned terms relating to diagnosis, clinical procedures, and laboratory tests. Before going on to the exercise section, review the terms below and refer to the previous section if you have questions. Pronunciations are provided for certain terms. Sometimes information about where the word came from is included after the term. The etymologies (word histories) are for your information only. You do not need to memorize them.

Term	Definition
dermatology [dĕr-mă-TŎL-ō-jē] dermato-, skin + -logy, study	Medical specialty that deals with diseases of the skin.
exudate [ĔKS-yū-dāt] ex-, out + Latin *sudo*, sweat	Any fluid excreted out of tissue, especially fluid excreted out of an injury to the skin.
intradermal [ĬN-tră-DĔR-măl] **test** intra, within + derm(o)-, skin	Test that injects antigen or protein between layers of skin.
Mantoux [măn-TŪ] **test**	Test for tuberculosis in which a small dose of tuberculin is injected intradermally with a syringe.
patch test	Test for allergic sensitivity in which a small dose of antigen is applied to the skin on a small piece of gauze.
PPD	Purified protein derivative of tuberculin.
Schick [shĭk] **test**	Test for diphtheria.
scratch test	Test for allergic sensitivity in which a small amount of antigen is scratched onto the surface of the skin.
tine [tīn] **test, TB tine**	Screening test for tuberculosis in which a small dose of tuberculin is injected into a series of sites within a small space with a tine (instrument that punctures the surface of the skin).

Testing for Allergic Reactions

Several days ago, Dr. Lin had given a series of scratch tests to a teenager who had allergic skin rashes. The doctor had noted all the places where redness or swelling appeared within ten minutes.

He had also noted the negative reactions, where no changes appeared within thirty minutes. There were also some mild, inconclusive reactions. Dr. Lin reviewed the results of the tests. He asked Madeline to send a report to the patient and to set up a phone appointment to discuss the results. Madeline thought the results looked interesting. She didn't know that people could be allergic to so many things at once. However, Madeline knows she cannot discuss this patient's case with anyone not allowed to see that specific medical record. So, while it may be something interesting to talk to some of her friends about, she will not say anything.

Critical Thinking

85. What does a negative reaction to a scratch test indicate?
86. If the patient avoids the allergens that gave the most positive reactions, what is likely to happen to the rashes?

Diagnostic, Procedural, and Laboratory Terms Exercises

Check Your Knowledge

Circle T for true and F for false.

87. The Mantoux test detects allergies. T F
88. An intradermal test may detect an infectious disease. T F
89. PPD is used in the Mantoux test. T F
90. An intradermal injection usually reaches into the hypodermis. T F
91. Visual observation of the skin is a diagnostic tool. T F

Fill in the Blanks

Complete the sentences below by filling in the blanks.

92. A scraping from the skin is placed on a growth medium to detect the presence of _____.
93. Samples of _____ may be sent to a laboratory for examination.
94. Scratch tests are often used to detect _____.
95. Suspected antigens are injected between layers of skin in a(n) _____ test.

Pathological Terms

At the Skin Cancer Foundation's Web site (www.skincancer.org), you can find out a lot about the different kinds of skin cancers.

The skin is a place where both abnormalities occur and some internal diseases show dermatological symptoms. **Lesions** are areas of tissues that are altered because of a pathological condition. Primary lesions appear on previously normal skin. Secondary lesions are abnormalities that result from changes in primary lesions. **Vascular lesions** are blood vessel lesions that show through the skin. Figure 4-5 shows various types of skin lesions.

Some common primary lesions are areas of discoloration, such as a **macule** (freckle or flat mole) or **patch.** Elevated, solid masses include:

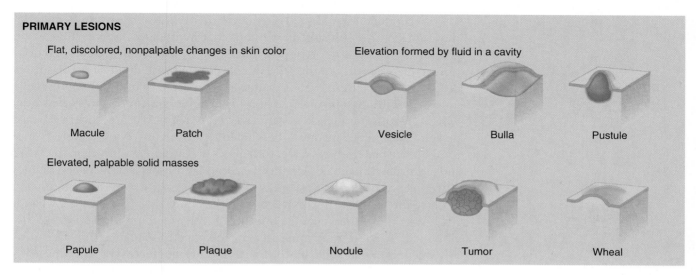

PRIMARY LESIONS

Flat, discolored, nonpalpable changes in skin color

Macule   Patch

Elevation formed by fluid in a cavity

Vesicle   Bulla   Pustule

Elevated, palpable solid masses

Papule   Plaque   Nodule   Tumor   Wheal

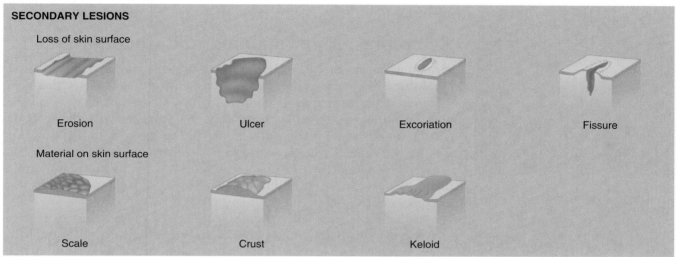

SECONDARY LESIONS

Loss of skin surface

Erosion   Ulcer   Excoriation   Fissure

Material on skin surface

Scale   Crust   Keloid

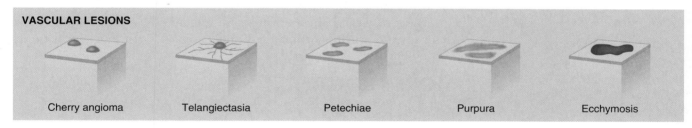

VASCULAR LESIONS

Cherry angioma   Telangiectasia   Petechiae   Purpura   Ecchymosis

FIGURE 4-5 Various types of skin lesions.

papule, a small elevated mass, also called a *pimple;* **plaque,** a small patch on the skin; **nodule,** a large pimple or a small node; **polyp,** any mass that projects upward, either on a slender stalk (**pediculated polyp**) or from a broad base (**sessile polyp**); **tumor,** any swelling or, specifically, any abnormal tissue growth; and **wheal,** a smooth, slightly elevated area, usually associated with allergic itching. A **bulla,** a large blister; a **pustule,** a small elevated mass containing pus; and a **vesicle,** a small mass containing fluid, are all elevated skin pockets filled with fluid. A **cyst** may be solid or filled with fluid or gas. A **pilonidal cyst** contains hairs, and a **sebaceous cyst** contains yellow sebum.

Secondary lesions usually involve either loss of skin surface or material that forms on the skin surface. Lesions that involve loss of skin surface are: **erosion,** a shallow area of the skin worn away by friction or pressure; **excoriation,** a scratched area of the skin, usually covered with dried blood; **fissure,** a deep furrow or crack in the skin surface; and **ulcer,** a wound with loss of tissue and often with inflammation, especially **decubitus ulcers** or **pressure sores,** which are chronic ulcers on skin over bony parts that are under constant pressure, as when someone is bedridden or wheelchair-bound. Lesions that form surface material are: **scale,** thin plates of epithelium formed on the skin's surface; **crust,** dried blood or pus that forms on the skin's surface; and **keloid,** a firm, raised mass of scar tissue. A **cicatrix,** a general word for scar, usually refers to internal scarring (as a lesion on the brain) or growth inside a wound.

Vascular lesions may be a result of disease, aging, or a vascular disturbance. A **cherry angioma** is a dome-shaped vascular lesion that usually occurs on the skin of elderly people. **Telangiectasia** is an area with a permanent dilation of the small blood vessels that usually appears on the skin.

Symptoms, Abnormalities, and Conditions

Symptoms of disease can appear on the skin. For example, **exanthematous viral diseases** are rashes that develop during a viral infection. Other common viral rashes are: **rubeola,** measles with an accompanying rash; **rubella,** disease with a rash caused by the rubella virus (also known as *German measles*); **roseola,** disease with small, rosy patches on the skin, usually caused by a virus; and **varicella,** disease with a rash known as *chicken pox,* caused by the varicella virus. Chicken pox (Figure 4-6) does not usually cause harm (other than possible scarring) in young children. However, young adult males who become infected may become sterile.

Infectious agents, such as staphylococci, may cause **impetigo,** which is a **pyoderma,** or pus-containing, contagious skin disease. At times, staphylococci infections can become deadly, as is the case with flesh-eating bacteria (known as necrotizing fasciitis), a fatal type of staph infection.

Fungi may cause **tinea** or **ringworm** (Figure 4-7), a skin condition that causes intense **pruritus** or itching. **Candidiasis** is a yeast fungus that causes

> The National Skin Centre in Singapore (www.nsc.gov.sg) provides a guide to many skin diseases.

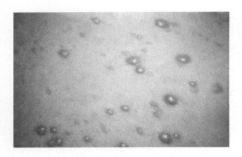

FIGURE 4-6 Pustules typical of chicken pox.

MORE ABOUT . . .

Infections

Necrotizing fasciitis is a rare but very serious infection that involves the skin and soft tissue of the body. The infection is most commonly caused by the bacterial organism *Streptococcus pyogenes.* This bacterial organism, which is a type of Strep A bacteria, is also responsible for strep throat and impetigo infections. It is commonly known as the "skin-eating" bacteria. Sufferers of this infection usually have weakened immune systems, chronic health problems, non-intact skin due to wounds or surgery, certain viral infections such as chickenpox, and/or have been on extended steroid medication use that can lower the body's immune system. The infection develops quickly and requires immediate action and hospitalization. Treatments include care for shock, respiratory problems, and kidney failure. Surgery is required in most cases as is extensive use of antibiotics to kill the bacteria.

common rashes such as diaper rash. Other common fungi are *tinea pedis* or athlete's foot; *tinea capitis*, scalp ringworm; and *tinea barbae*, ringworm of the beard. Some autoimmune diseases, such as **pemphigus,** cause skin blistering.

Skin conditions, particularly skin irritations or **dermatitis,** can reflect systemic allergies or diseases. **Urticaria** or **hives** may arise from many causes, such as a food allergy; itching or pruritus can also be the result of allergies. **Eczema** is an acute form of dermatitis often caused by allergies.

Ecchymosis (plural, **ecchymoses**) is a bluish-purple skin mark that may result from a skin injury that can cause blood to leak out of blood vessels. **Petechiae** are tiny, pinpoint ecchymoses. **Purpura** is a condition with extensive hemorrhages into the skin covering a wide area. Purpura starts out with red areas, which turn purplish, and then brown, in a couple of weeks. **Rosacea** is a vascular disorder that appears as red blotches on the skin, particularly around the nose and cheeks.

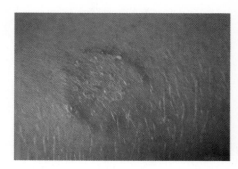

FIGURE 4-7 Skin showing ringworm.

Some diseases, infections, or inflammations cause skin conditions, such as a **furuncle,** a localized, pus-producing infection originating in a hair follicle; a **carbuncle,** a pus-producing infection that starts in subcutaneous tissue and is usually accompanied by fever and an ill feeling; **abscess,** a localized infection usually accompanied by pus and inflammation; and **gangrene,** necrosis (death) of tissue due to loss of blood supply.

Some skin areas lack color, which may be the result of **depigmentation,** partial or complete loss of pigment; **leukoderma,** white patches on the skin; or **vitiligo,** patches with loss of pigment surrounded by patches with extensive pigment. These conditions often indicate a systemic autoimmune disease. A rare congenital condition called **albinism** causes either extensive or total lack of pigmentation. People with albinism often have very white, almost translucent, skin and white hair. A pigmented skin lesion found at birth is a **nevus** (plural, **nevi**) or **birthmark. Chloasma** is a group of fairly large, pigmented facial patches, often associated with pregnancy.

Some viruses cause skin problems. In some cases, these viruses are STDs, or sexually transmitted diseases (such as some types of **herpes** and genital warts). (Sexually transmitted diseases are discussed with the female and male reproductive systems, covered in Chapters 10 and 11.) **Herpes simplex virus Type 1, herpes simplex virus Type 2,** and **herpes zoster** are all viral diseases caused by herpes viruses. Herpes 1, also called **cold sores** or **fever blisters,** usually appears around the mouth. Herpes 2, also known as **genital herpes,** affects the genital area. Herpes zoster or **shingles** is an inflammation that affects the nerves on one side of the body and results in skin blisters. It can be extremely painful. A virus may also cause a **wart** or **verruca.** A **plantar wart** appears on the soles of the feet.

Lupus, a chronic disease with erosion of the skin, may appear in different forms. Two common forms are **DLE** or **discoid lupus erythematosus,** a mild form of lupus that usually causes only superficial eruption of the skin, and **SLE** or **systemic lupus erythematosus,** a chronic inflammation of the collagen in the skin and joints that usually causes inflammation of connective tissue throughout the body and is often accompanied by fever, weakness, arthritis, and other serious symptoms. Inflammation of the dermis and subcutaneous skin layers is called **cellulitis** (Figure 4-8), which can spread infection via the blood to the brain.

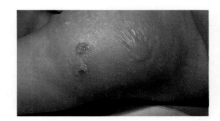

FIGURE 4-8 Cellulitis.

Other skin conditions include **acne** (also called **acne vulgaris**), a skin condition with eruptions on the face and upper back. Acne usually starts around puberty and is often caused by overproduction of sebum. It usually includes several types of skin eruptions, such as **comedones** or **blackheads, whiteheads,** pustules, and nodules.

Scleroderma is a chronic disease with abnormal thickening of the skin caused by the formation of new collagen. **Psoriasis,** a recurrent skin condition with scaly lesions on the trunk, arms, hands, legs, and scalp, is often associated with stress. **Seborrhea,** a condition with excessive production of sebum, is a result of overactivity of the sebaceous glands. *Seborrheic dermatitis* (also called *dandruff*), scaly eruptions on the face or scalp, is due to the overproduction of seborrhea.

Exposure of the skin to heat, chemicals, electricity, radiation, or other irritants may cause a **burn.** Burns are classified by the amount or level of skin involvement.

1. **First-degree burns** are superficial burns of the epidermis without blistering, but with redness and swelling. Sunburn is an example of a first-degree burn. There is mild to moderate pain and the skin is intact but is often swollen and reddened, and it radiates heat. Cold compresses will relieve the pain and reduce the swelling. Various creams may help the healing process. Recovery is usually complete but continual sunburns may be a cause of later skin cancer.
2. **Second-degree burns** involve the epidermis and dermis and involve blistering. The wound is sensitive to touch and very painful.
3. **Third-degree burns** involve complete destruction of the skin, sometimes reaching into the muscle and bone and causing extensive scarring.

Figure 4-9 shows the "rule of 9s," which is used to determine the extent of burning.

The National Psoriasis Foundation (www.psoriasis.org) provides information about new treatments for psoriasis on their Web site.

FIGURE 4-9 Burns are categorized by the extent and depth of burning.

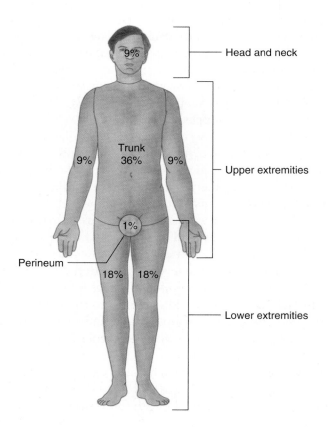

Head and neck

9%

Trunk
36%

9%   9%

Upper extremities

1%

Perineum

18%   18%

Lower extremities

Some skin conditions are caused by insects. **Pediculosis** is an inflammation with lice, often on the head (*pediculosis capitis*) or the genital area (*pediculosis pubis*). **Scabies,** a contagious skin eruption that often occurs between fingers, on other areas of the trunk, or on the male genitalia, is caused by mites.

Inflammations of the nail can be caused by infection, irritation, or fungi. **Onychia** or **onychitis** is a nail inflammation. **Paronychia** is an inflammation in the nail fold, the flap of skin overlapping the edges of the nail. Both of these inflammations often occur spontaneously in debilitated people. They may also result from a slight trauma. A general term for disease of the nails is **onychopathy.**

Some abnormal growths or **neoplasms** are benign. The most common benign neoplasms are a **callus,** a hard, thickened area of skin; a **corn,** hardening or thickening of skin on a toe; **keratosis,** overgrowth of horny tissue on skin (especially **actinic keratosis**), such as overgrowth due to excessive sun exposure; and **leukoplakia,** thickened white patches of epithelium. A growth may be of fibrous tissue: for example, a cicatrix is a growth of fibrous tissue inside a wound that forms a scar.

Some neoplasms are malignant. **Basal cell carcinoma** is cancer of the basal layer of the epidermis; **squamous cell carcinoma** affects the squamous epithelium. **Kaposi's sarcoma** is often associated with AIDS. The incidence of **malignant melanoma** is rapidly increasing. Figure 4-10 shows a benign mole and a malignant melanoma. This increase in malignant melanomas is thought to be due to the depletion of the Earth's ozone layer, which protects the skin from harmful UV rays. Many protective products, such as sunblock or sunscreen, are widely available. One of the odd results of widespread sunscreen use is that skin cancers have increased in people who use them. This is because people who use the screens actually feel that they can stay in the sun for much longer periods. The only effective skin cancer prevention is to avoid exposure to the sun as much as possible.

In most instances, hair loss is hereditary or due to a side effect of medication. However, hair loss can be a pathological condition, as in **alopecia areata,** a condition in which hair falls out in patches.

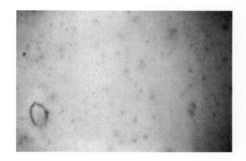

FIGURE 4-10 Scabies.

VOCABULARY REVIEW

In the previous section, you learned terms relating to pathology. Before going on to the exercises, review the terms below and refer to the previous section if you have questions. Pronunciations are provided for certain terms. Sometimes information about where the word came from is included after the term. The etymologies (word histories) are for your information only. You do not need to memorize them.

Term	Definition
abscess [ĂB-sĕs] Latin *abscessus*, a going away	Localized collection of pus and other exudate, usually accompanied by swelling and redness.
acne [ĂK-nē]	Inflammatory eruption of the skin, occurring in or near sebaceous glands on the face, neck, shoulder, or upper back.
acne vulgaris [vŭl-GĀR-ĭs]	*See* acne.
actinic keratosis [ăk-TĬN-ĭk KĔR-ă-tō-sĭs]	Overgrowth of horny skin that forms from over-exposure to sunlight; sunburn.
albinism [ĂL-bĭ-nĭzm] albin(o) + -ism, state	Rare, congenital condition causing either partial or total lack of pigmentation.
alopecia areata [ăl-ō-PĒ-shē-ă ā-rē-Ă-tă]	Loss of hair in patches.
basal cell carcinoma [BĀ-săl sĕl kăr-sĭn-Ō-mă]	Slow-growing cancer of the basal cells of the epidermis, usually a result of sun damage.
birthmark	Lesion (especially a hemangioma) visible at or soon after birth; nevus.
blackhead	*See* comedo.
bulla (*pl.,* bullae) [BŬL-ă (BŬL-ī)]	Bubble-like blister on the surface of the skin.
burn	Damage to the skin caused by exposure to heat, chemicals, electricity, radiation, or other skin irritants.
callus [KĂL-ŭs] Latin	Mass of hard skin that forms as a cover over broken skin on certain areas of the body, especially the feet and hands.
candidiasis [kăn-dĭ-DĪ-ă-sĭs] Candid(a) + -iasis, condition	Yeastlike fungus on the skin, caused by Candida; characterized by pruritus, white exudate, peeling, and easy bleeding; examples are thrush and diaper rash.
carbuncle [KĂR-bŭng-kl]	Infected area of the skin producing pus and usually accompanied by fever.
cellulitis [sĕl-yū-LĪ-tĭs] cellul(ar) + -itis, inflammation	Severe inflammation of the dermis and subcutaneous portions of the skin, usually caused by an infection that enters the skin through an opening, as a wound; characterized by local heat, redness, pain, and swelling.

Term	Definition
cherry angioma [ăn-jē-Ō-mă]	A dome-shaped vascular angioma lesion that usually occurs in the elderly.
chloasma [klō-ĂZ-mă] Greek *chloazo*, to become green	Group of fairly large, pigmented facial patches, often associated with pregnancy.
cicatrix [SĬK-ă-trĭks] Latin	Growth of fibrous tissue inside a wound that forms a scar; also, general term for scar.
cold sore	Eruption around the mouth or lips; herpes simplex virus Type 1.
comedo (*pl.*, comedos, comedones) [KŌM-ē-dō, kō-MĒ-dō (KŌM-ē-dōz, kō-mē-DŌ-nēz)] Latin, a glutton	Open hair follicle filled with bacteria and sebum; common in acne; blackhead.
corn	Growth of hard skin, usually on the toes.
crust	Hard layer, especially one formed by dried pus, as in a scab.
cyst [sĭst] Greek *kystis*, bladder	Abnormal sac containing fluid.
decubitus (*pl.*, decubiti) [dĕ-KYŪ-bĭ-tŭs (dĕ-KYŪ-bĭ-tī)] **ulcer**	Chronic ulcer on skin over bony parts that are under constant pressure; pressure sore.
depigmentation [dē-pĭg-mĕn-TĀ-shŭn] de-, removal + pigmentation	Loss of color of the skin.
dermatitis [dĕr-mă-TĪ-tĭs] dermat-, skin + -itis	Inflammation of the skin.
discoid lupus erythematosus (DLE) [DĬS-kŏyd LŪ-pŭs ĕr-ĭ-THĔM-ă-tō-sŭs]	Mild form of lupus.
ecchymosis (*pl.*, ecchymoses) [ĕk-ĭ-MŌ-sĭs (ĕk-ĭ-MŌ-sēz)] Greek	Purplish skin patch (bruise) caused by broken blood vessels beneath the surface.
eczema [ĔK-sē-mă, ĔG-zē-mă] Greek	Severe inflammatory condition of the skin, usually of unknown cause.
erosion	Wearing away of the surface of the skin, especially when caused by friction.
exanthematous [ĕks-zăn-THĔM-ă-tŭs] **viral disease**	Viral disease that causes a rash on the skin.
excoriation [ĕks-KŌ-rē-Ā-shŭn] Latin *excoriatio*, to skin	Injury to the surface of the skin caused by a scratch, abrasion, or burn, usually accompanied by some oozing.
fever blister	Eruption around the mouth or lips; herpes simplex virus Type 1.
first-degree burn	Least severe burn, causes injury to the surface of the skin without blistering.
fissure [FĬSH-ŭr] Latin	Deep slit in the skin.

Term	Definition
furuncle [FYŪ-rŭng-kl]	Localized skin infection, usually in a hair follicle and containing pus; boil.
gangrene [GĂNG-grēn] Greek *gangraina*, eating sore	Death of an area of skin, usually caused by loss of blood supply to the area.
genital herpes	*See* herpes simplex virus Type 2.
herpes [HĔR-pēz] Greek, shingles	An inflammatory skin disease caused by viruses of the family Herpesviridae.
herpes simplex virus Type 1	Herpes that recurs on the lips and around the area of the mouth, usually during viral illnesses or states of stress.
herpes simplex virus Type 2	Herpes that recurs on the genitalia; can be easily transmitted from one person to another through sexual contact.
herpes zoster [ZŎS-tĕr]	Painful herpes that affects nerve roots; shingles.
hives	*See* urticaria.
impetigo [ĭm-pĕ-TĪ-gō] Latin	A type of pyoderma.
Kaposi's sarcoma [KĂ-pō-sēz săr-KŌ-mă] After Moritz Kaposi (1837–1902), Hungarian dermatologist	Skin cancer associated with AIDS.
keloid [KĒ-lŏyd] Greek *kele*, tumor + *-oid*, like	Thick scarring of the skin that forms after an injury or surgery.
keratosis [kĕr-ă-TŌ-sĭs] kerat(o)-, horny layer + -osis, condition	Lesion on the epidermis containing keratin.
lesion [LĒ-zhŭn]	Wound, damage, or injury to the skin.
leukoderma [lū-kō-DĔR-mă] leuko-, white + -derma, skin	Absence of pigment in the skin or in an area of the skin.
leukoplakia [lū-kō-PLĀ-kē-ă] leuko- + -plakia, plaque	White patch of mucous membrane on the tongue or cheek.
macule [MĂK-yūl]	Small, flat, noticeably colored spot on the skin.
malignant melanoma [mĕl-ă-NŌ-mă]	Virulent skin cancer originating in the melanocytes, usually caused by overexposure to the sun.
neoplasm [NĒ-ō-plăzm] neo-, recent, new + -plasm, formation	Abnormal tissue growth.
nevus (*pl.*, nevi) [NĒ-vŭs (NĒ-vī)]	Birthmark.
nodule [NŎD-yūl]	Small knob of tissue.
onychia, onychitis [ō-NĬK-ē-ă, ŏn-ĭ-KĪ-tĭs] onycho-, nail + -ia, condition; onych(o)- + -itis	Inflammation of the nail.

Term	Definition
onychopathy [ŏn-ĭ-KŎP-ă-thē] onycho- + -pathy, disease	Disease of the nail.
papule [PĂP-yūl]	Small, solid elevation on the skin.
paronychia [păr-ŏ-NĬK-ē-ă] par(a)-, abnormal + Greek *onyx*, nail	Inflammation, with pus, of the fold surrounding the nail plate.
patch	Small area of skin differing in color from the surrounding area; plaque.
pediculated [pĕ-DĬK-yū-lā-tĕd] **polyp**	Polyp that projects upward from a slender stalk.
pediculosis [pĕ-DĬK-yū-LŌ-sĭs] Latin *pediculus*, louse + -osis	Lice infestation.
pemphigus [PĔM-fĭ-gŭs] Greek *pemphix*, blister	Autoimmune disease that causes skin blistering.
petechia (*pl.,* petechiae) [pē-TĒ-kē-ă, pē-TĔK-ē-ă (pē-TĒ-kē-ē)]	A tiny hemorrhage beneath the surface of the skin.
pilonidal [pī-lō-NĬ-dă] **cyst** pilo-, hair + Latin *nidus*, nest	Cyst containing hair, usually found at the lower end of the spinal column.
plantar [PLĂN-tăr] **wart**	Wart on the sole of the foot.
plaque [plăk]	*See* patch.
polyp [PŎL-ĭp]	Bulging mass of tissue that projects outward from the skin surface.
pressure sore	*See* decubitus ulcer.
pruritus [prū-RĪ-tŭs]	Itching.
psoriasis [sō-RĪ-ă-sĭs]	Chronic skin condition accompanied by scaly lesions with extreme pruritus.
purpura [PŬR-pū-ră]	Skin condition with extensive hemorrhages underneath the skin covering a wide area.
pustule [PŬS-tūl]	Small elevation on the skin containing pus.
pyoderma [pī-ō-DĔR-mă] pyo-, pus + -derma, skin	Any inflammation of the skin that produces pus.
ringworm	Fungal infection; tinea.
rosacea [rō-ZĀ-shē-ă]	Vascular disease that causes blotchy, red patches on the skin, particularly on the nose and cheeks.
roseola [rō-ZĒ-ō-lă]	Skin eruption of small, rosy patches, usually caused by a virus.
rubella [rū-BĔL-ă]	Disease that causes a viral skin rash; German measles.
rubeola [rū-BĒ-ō-lă]	Disease that causes a viral skin rash; measles.

Term	Definition
scabies [SKĀ-bēz]	Skin eruption caused by a mite burrowing into the skin.
scale	Small plate of hard skin that falls off.
scleroderma [sklēr-ō-DĔR-mă] sclero-, hardness + -derma, skin	Thickening of the skin caused by an increase in collagen formation.
sebaceous [sĕ-BĀ-shŭs] cyst	Cyst containing yellow sebum.
seborrhea [sĕb-ō-RĒ-ă] sebo-, sebum + -rrhea, flowing	Overproduction of sebum by the sebaceous glands.
second-degree burn	Moderately severe burn that affects the epidermis and dermis; usually involves blistering.
sessile [SĔS-ĭl] polyp	Polyp that projects upward from a broad base.
shingles [SHĬN-glz]	Viral disease affecting peripheral nerves and caused by herpes zoster.
squamous cell carcinoma [SKWĂ-mŭs sĕl kăr-sĭn-NŌ-mă]	Cancer of the squamous epithelium.
systemic lupus erythematosus (SLE)	Most severe form of lupus, involving internal organs.
telangiectasia [tĕl-ĂN-jē-ĕk-TĀ-zhē-ă]	A permanent dilation of the small blood vessels.
third-degree burn	Most severe type of burn; involves complete destruction of an area of skin.
tinea [TĬN-ē-ă]	Fungal infection; ringworm.
tumor [TŪ-mŏr]	Any mass of tissue; swelling.
ulcer [ŬL-sĕr]	Open lesion, usually with superficial loss of tissue.
urticaria [ŬR-tĭ-KĀR-ē-ă]	Group of reddish wheals, usually accompanied by pruritus and often caused by an allergy.
varicella [vār-ĭ-SĔL-ă]	Contagious skin disease, usually occurring during childhood, and often accompanied by the formation of pustules; chicken pox.
vascular [VĂS-kyū-lăr] lesion	Lesion in a blood vessel that shows through the skin.
verruca (pl., verrucae) [vĕ-RŪ-kă (vĕ-RŪ-kē)]	Flesh-colored growth, sometimes caused by a virus; wart.
vesicle [VĔS-ĭ-kl]	Small, raised sac on the skin containing fluid.
vitiligo [vĭt-ĭ-LĪ-gō]	Condition in which white patches appear on otherwise normally pigmented skin.
wart [wōrt]	See verruca.
wheal [hwēl]	Itchy patch of raised skin.
whitehead [WHĪT-hĕd]	Closed comedo that does not contain the dark bacteria present in blackheads.

CASE STUDY

Treating Adolescent Acne

Dr. Lin's new patient, Maria Cardoza, is 17 years old and has a persistent case of acne. She had been treating it with soap and Oxy-10 with limited success in the past couple of years, but recently her condition has worsened and her pediatrician recommended that she see Dr. Lin. After careful examination and removal of some comedones, Dr. Lin prescribed a course of antibiotics and asked Maria to return in three weeks. Dr. Lin put the following notes on Maria's record:

"Mild-to-moderate acne on the face, neck, and upper back. Lesions consist of macules, papules, mild oily comedones, and an occasional nodule, but no cysts or boils. Erythromycin, 400 mg., t.i.d. for 3 months. Recheck in 3 months."

Critical Thinking

96. Dr. Lin recommended that Maria wash her face with soap three times a day. Acne occurs in the sebaceous glands. How will frequent washing help?
97. As Maria gets older, why might her acne improve even without treatment?

PATHOLOGICAL TERMS EXERCISES

Build Your Medical Vocabulary

Put C for correct in the blank next to each word that is spelled correctly. Put the correct spelling next to words that are spelled incorrectly.

98. pemfigus _____

99. varicella _____

100. purpora _____

101. urticaria _____

102. rosola _____

Add the missing suffix to the following terms.

103. Nail inflammation: onych _____

104. Skin condition: dermat _____

105. Black tumor: melan _____

106. Hair disease: tricho _____

107. White skin: leuko _____

Check Your Knowledge

Circle T for true or F for false.

108. Basal cell carcinoma is characterized by blackened areas on the skin. T F

109. All neoplasms are malignant. T F

110. A nevus is a third-degree burn. T F

111. Pruritus can be present in many skin conditions. T F

112. Rubella causes a viral skin rash. T F

113. Tinea barbae is ringworm of the feet. T F

114. Warts may be caused by a virus. T F

115. Seborrhea is abnormal pigmentation. T F

116. The herpes virus is not curable and recurs at various times. T F

117. Food allergies can cause skin eruptions. T F

Fill in the Blanks

118. Most adult hair loss is caused by _____ or _____.

119. Scabies is caused by _____.

120. Herpes simplex virus Type 1 usually occurs around the area of the _____.

121. Herpes simplex virus Type 2 usually occurs on the _____.

122. What percent of the body surface would be considered burned if only the upper extremities
     were involved? _____.

123. If the lower extremities, perineum, and trunk were involved, what percent of the body
     would this be? _____.

124. The head, neck and trunk constitute what percent of the body? _____.

125. The right leg and right arm would be _____% of the body surface.

Choose the Correct Term

Circle the term that best describes the *italicized* description in the sentences below.

126. Patient presented to the office with a *flesh-colored growth, sometimes caused by a virus* (wheal, macule,
     verruca) on his right index finger.

127. A *cyst containing a yellow sebum* is known as a (pilonidal, sebaceous, pustule) cyst.

128. An *area of tissue that is altered because of pathological conditions* is known as a (lesion, erosion, fissure).

129. The physician asked for your assistance in lancing a/an *localized collection of pus and other exudates*
     (callus, abscess, bulla) to alleviate the pressure.

130. This fungus is also known as *athlete's foot.* (tinea capitis, tinea barbae, tinea pedis)

131. A five-year-old boy was brought into the office with a viral infection commonly known as *German measles.*
     The medical term is (roseola, varicella, rubella).

132. The diagnosis was listed as a *chronic skin condition accompanied by scaly lesions* also known as: (psoriasis,
     eczema, excoriation).

133. _____ is a *condition in which white patches appear on otherwise normally pigmented skin.* (leukoderma,
     keratosis, vitiligo)

134. *Urticaria* is another name for (pruritus, hives, pyoderma).

135. A lesion caused by an *overgrowth of horny skin that forms due to overexposure to sunlight; sunburn* is called:
     (actinic keratosis, cellulitis, seborrheic dermatitis)

Matching Conditions and Diseases

Write the letter of the common term next to its medical term equivalent.

136. ____verucca
137. ____urticaria
138. ____ varicella
139. ____herpes zoster
140. ____rubeola
141. ____ tinea
142. ____decubitus ulcer
143. ____nevus
144. ____rubella
145. ____ comedo
146. ____ cicatrix
147. ____ pruritus
148. ____herpes simplex I
149. ____pediculosis

a. blackhead
b. head lice
c. cold sore/fever blister
d. pressure sore
e. shingles
f. hives
g. birthmark
h. itching
i. ringworm
j. German measles
k. measles
l. chickenpox
m. wart
n. scar

Surgical Terms

Skin surgery includes the repair of various conditions. Sutures, stitches, or staples hold skin together while healing takes place. Various types of plastic surgery may involve reconstructing areas of the skin, as after severe burns or radiation. Other types of skin surgery result in the removal of a part of a growth to test for the presence of cancer. Growths are also removed to keep a cancer from spreading.

Plastic surgery is a general term for a variety of surgeries to correct defects resulting from injuries, birth defects, or to enhance someone's idea of how they should look (Figure 4-11). Surgical correction of disfiguring physical defects is also known as *cosmesis*. Plastic surgery may involve the use of **skin grafts.** An **autograft** uses skin from one's own body. An **allograft** or **homograft** uses donor skin from another person. A **heterograft** or **xenograft** uses donor skin from one species to another (such as animal, for example a pig, to human). A *dermatome* is an implement used to remove layers of skin for grafts.

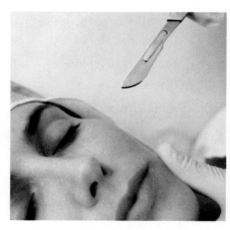

FIGURE 4-11 Some cosmetic surgeries are for minor improvements.

Plastic surgery may also use various methods to remove unwanted growths or scrape tissue or discolorations. **Cryosurgery** involves the removal of tissue by applying cold liquid nitrogen. **Dermabrasion** is the use of brushes and emery papers to remove wrinkles, scars, and tattoos. **Debridement** and **curettage** are the removal of dead tissue from a wound by scraping.

Some surgical procedures of the skin involve the use of electricity or lasers to stop bleeding, remove tissue, or excise tissues for examination. Wounds may be **cauterized** or burned to coagulate an area that is bleeding.

They may be dried with electrical current (**electrodesiccation**). **Fulguration** is the use of electric sparks to destroy tissue.

A **biopsy** is a cutting of tissue for microscopic examination. A *needle biopsy* is the removal of tissue by aspirating it through a needle. A *punch biopsy* is the use of a cylindrical instrument to remove a small piece of tissue. A *shave biopsy* is the removal of a layer of skin using a surgical blade. **Mohs' surgery** is the removal of thin layers of malignant growth until a nonmalignant area is reached.

VOCABULARY REVIEW

In the previous section, you learned terms relating to surgery. Before going on to the exercises, review the terms below and refer to the previous section if you have any questions. Pronunciations are provided for certain terms. Sometimes information about where the word came from is included after the term. The etymologies (word histories) are for your information only. You do not need to memorize them.

Term	Definition
allograft [ĂL-ō-grăft] allo-, other + graft	*See* homograft.
autograft [ĂW-tō-grăft] auto-, self + graft	Skin graft using skin from one's own body.
biopsy [BĪ-ŏp-sē] bi(o)-, life + -opsy, view of	Excision of tissue for microscopic examination.
cauterize [KĂW-tĕr-ĭz]	To apply heat to an area to cause coagulation and stop bleeding.
cryosurgery [KRĪ-ō-SĔR-jĕr-ē] cryo-, cold + surgery	Surgery that removes tissue by freezing it with liquid nitrogen.
curettage [kyū-rĕ-TĂZH]	Removal of tissue from an area, such as a wound, by scraping.
debridement [dā-brēd-MŎN]	Removal of dead tissue from a wound.
dermabrasion [dĕr-mă-BRĀ-zhŭn] derm-, skin + abrasion	Removal of wrinkles, scars, tattoos, and other marks by scraping with brushes or emery papers.
electrodesiccation [ē-LĔK-trō-dĕ-sĭ-KĀ-shŭn]	Drying with electrical current.
fulguration [fŭl-gŭ-RĀ-shŭn]	Destruction of tissue using electric sparks.
heterograft [HĔT-ĕr-ō-grăft] hetero-, other + graft	Skin graft using donor skin from one species to another; xenograft.
homograft [HŌ-mō-grăft] homo-, alike + graft	Skin graft using donor skin from one person to another; allograft.
Mohs' [mōz] **surgery** After Frederic Edward Mohs (1910–1979), U.S. surgeon.	Removal of thin layers of malignant tissue until nonmalignant tissue is found.
plastic surgery	Repair or reconstruction (as of the skin) by means of surgery.
skin graft	Placement of fresh skin over a damaged area.
xenograft [ZĔN-ō-grăft] xeno-, foreign + graft	*See* heterograft.

CASE STUDY

Skin Biopsy

Dr. Lin has hospital hours scheduled for tomorrow morning. He will see two patients in the one-day surgery unit for minor operations. The first patient is to have cryosurgery for removal of several moles. Later, Dr. Lin will take a biopsy from a suspicious-looking skin patch of a patient who was treated earlier for a basal cell carcinoma. The pathology report follows:

The specimen consists of two ellipses of skin, each stated to be from the left upper arm. The larger measures 1.7 × 0.7 cm and has a slightly raised and roughened outer surface. Sections of skin exhibit a dermal nodular lesion consisting of interlacing bundles of elongated cells surrounded by fibrous stroma.

Critical Thinking

150. If the patch turns out to be a malignant melanoma, will that be more serious than the patient's earlier diagnosis?

151. What steps can you take to avoid permanent skin damage?

SURGICAL TERMS EXERCISES

Build Your Medical Vocabulary

Fill in the blanks in the statements that follow.

152. Tattoos can be removed through _____.

153. The repair of various conditions or the changing of one's appearance surgically is called _____ surgery.

154. Cauterizing a wound helps to stop _____.

155. The use of one's own skin to cover a wound is called a/an _____.

156. The use of someone else's skin to cover a wound is called a/an _____ or _____.

Pharmacological Terms

Treatment of skin disorders involves the use of various medications. A wide variety of topical preparations can relieve symptoms and even kill agents that cause disease. Other treatments involve heat, light, and radiation.

Cancer of the skin is sometimes successfully treated by **chemotherapy** and/or **radiation therapy,** most of the time successfully. Chemotherapy uses chemicals to treat the malignant cells systematically. Radiation therapy uses high-energy radiation to bombard malignant cells in order to destroy them.

The sun is beneficial in healing certain skin problems. Some lesions are treated with **ultraviolet light,** which imitates some of the sun's rays. On the other hand, sunlight may also be the cause of many skin problems, such as certain carcinomas.

Antihistamines are medications used to control allergic skin reactions. They do so by blocking the effects of *histamines*, chemicals present in tissues that heighten allergic reactions. Other skin conditions are controlled by different medications. For example, **antibiotics** kill or slow the growth of microorganisms on the skin. **Antiseptics** perform the same function. **Antibacterials** kill or slow the growth of bacteria. **Antifungals** kill or slow the growth of fungal infections. **Parasiticides** destroy insect parasites, such as

TABLE 4-1 Medications Used to Treat Skin Disorders

Drug Class	Purpose	Generic Name	Trade Name
anesthetic	to relieve pain	benzocaine dibucaine lidocaine	Anbesol, Orajel, Solarcaine Nupercainal Lidoderm
antifungal	to slow stop fungi growth	tolnaftate clotrimazole ketoconazole	Absorbine, Desenex, Tinactin Lotrimin Nizoral
antihistamine	to slow, stop, or prevent an allergic reaction	diphenhydramine loratidine fexofenadine	Allerdryl, Benadryl, Caladryl Claritin Allegra
antibacterial	to slow or stop the growth of bacteria	neomycin bacitracin benzoyl peroxide	Myciguent Neosporin Clearisil
antipruritic	to relieve itching	hydrocortisone doxapin	Bactine, Caldecort, Cortaid, Hydrocortone Zonalon
anti-inflammatory (corticosteroid)	to reduce inflammation	triamcinolone betamethasone	Aristocort, Triamolone, Tri-Kort, Kenacort A 10 Diprosone, Betnovate

lice and mites, that cause some skin conditions. **Anti-inflammatory** agents, particularly **corticosteroids,** reduce inflammation, and **antipruritics** control itching. Some skin conditions are painful because of nerve conduction near the skin surface. An **anesthetic** (especially, in the case of surface pain, a **topical anesthetic**) can relieve some of the pain associated with such conditions.

Some skin conditions result in either oversecretion of oils or extreme dryness. **Emollients** are agents that soothe or soften skin by moistening it or adding oils to it. **Astringents** temporarily lessen the formation of oily material on the surface of the skin. These types of agents are often present in over-the-counter products. Other vitamin-based products to control skin aging (often containing Vitamins A and C) are also often available over the counter. **Keratolytics** remove warts and corns from the skin surface. **Alpha-hydroxy acids** are fruit acids added to cosmetics to improve the skin's appearance. Table 4-1 lists drugs commonly used in treating skin conditions.

VOCABULARY REVIEW

In the previous section, you learned terms relating to pharmacology. Before going on to the exercises, review the terms below and refer to the previous section if you have questions. Pronunciations are provided for certain terms. Sometimes information about where the word came from is included after the term. The etymologies (word histories) are for your information only. You do not need to memorize them.

CHAPTER REVIEW

True or False

Circle T for true or F for false. If the answer is false, write the correct answer in the space provided.

178. Another name for a boil is a bulla. T F _____

179. Herpes simplex virus Type 2 is a painful condition that affects the nerve root. T F_____

180. Rosacea is a vascular disease that causes blotchy, red patches on the skin. T F _____

181. A wart that is found on the bottom of the foot is known as a plantar wart. T F _____

182. Any inflammation of the skin that causes pus is called a pachyderma. T F _____

183. A tiny hemorrhage beneath the surface of the skin is called a microdermorrhagia. T F _____

184. A first-degree burn involved complete destruction of an area of skin. T F _____

185. A whitehead and a blackhead are both called comedos; one is open and one is closed. T F _____

186. An overgrowth of scar tissue is known as a keloid. T F _____

187. Secondary lesions result from changes in vascular lesions. T F _____

188. Another name for hair that falls out in patches is alopecia areata. T F _____

189. With the widespread use of sunscreens the incidence of skin cancers has decreased. T F _____

190. Inflammation of the dermis and subcutaneous skin layers is called cellulitis. T F _____

191. DLE is a mild form of lupus that usually causes only superficial eruption of the skin. T F _____

192. The subcutaneous layer is the layer between the dermis and the body's inner organs. T F _____

193. A Mantoux test is given to test for diphtheria. T F _____

194. Dead skin is removed by exfoliation or diaphoresis. T F _____

195. Hair growth, thickness, and curliness are generally determined by heredity. T F _____

196. When collagen fibers stretch they form fissures. T F _____

197. Chloasma are pigmented patches that appear on the face, often associated with pregnancy. T F _____

Pluralizing Terms

Give the plural for form for each of the integumentary terms below. Consult Table 1-2 in Chapter 1 if you need assistance with this exercise.

198. fungus _____

199. abscess _____

200. ecchymosis _____

201. nevus _____

202. bulla _____

203. verruca _____

204. staphylococcus _____

205. comedo _____

DEFINITIONS

Define the following terms and combining forms. Review the chapter before starting, and check your answers by looking in the vocabulary reviews in this chapter. Make sure you know how to pronounce each term. The words in curly brackets are references to the Spanish glossary available online at www.mhhe.com/medterm3e.

TERM

206. abscess [ĂB-sĕs] {absceso}

207. acne [ĂK-nē] {acné}

208. acne vulgaris [vŭl-GĀR-ĭs] {acné vulgar}

209. actinic keratosis [ăk-TĬN-ĭk kĕr-ă-TŌ-sĭs]

210. adip(o)

211. adipose [ĂD-ĭ-pōs] {adiposo}

212. allograft [ĂL-ō-grăft] {aloinjerto}

213. albinism [ĂL-bĭ-nĭzm] {albinismo}

214. alopecia [ăl-ō-PĒ-shē-ă] {alopecia}

215. alopecia areata [ăl-ō-PĒ-shē-ă ā-rē-Ā-tă]

216. alpha-hydroxy [ĂL-fă-hī-DRŎK-sē] acid

217. anesthetic [ăn-ĕs-THĔT-ĭk]

218. antibacterial [ĂN-tē-băk-TĒR-ē-ăl]

219. antibiotic [ĂN-tē-bī-ŎT-ĭk]

220. antifungal [ĂN-tē-FŬNG-ăl]

221. antihistamine [ĂN-tē-HĬS-tă-mēn]

222. anti-inflammatory

223. antipruritic [ĂN-tē-prū-RĬT-ĭk]

224. antiseptic

225. apocrine [ĂP-ō-krĭn] glands

226. astringent [ăs-TRĬN-jĕnt]

227. autograft [ĂW-tō-grăft] {autoinjerto}

228. basal cell carcinoma [BĀ-săl sĕl kăr-sĭn-Ō-mă]

229. biopsy [BĪ-ŏp-sē] {biopsia}

230. birthmark

231. blackhead {punto Negro}

232. bulla (pl., bullae) [BŬL-ă (BŬL-ī)] {bulla}

233. burn {quemadura}

234. callus [KĂL-ŭs] {callo}

235. candidiasis [kăn-dĭ-DĪ-ă-sĭs] {candidiasis}

236. carbuncle [KĂR-bŭng-kl] {carbunco}

237. cauterize [KĂW-tĕr-īz] {cauterizar}

238. cellulitis [sĕl-yū-LĪ-tĭs] {celulitis}

239. ceruminous [sĕ-RŪ-mĭn-ŭs] glands

240. chemotherapy [KĒ-mō-THĀR-ă-pē]

241. cherry angioma [ăn-jē-Ō-mă]

242. chloasma [klō-ĂZ-mă] {cloasma}

243. cicatrix [SĬK-ă-trĭks] {cicatriz}

244. cold sore

245. collagen [KŎL-lă-jĕn] {colágeno}

246. comedo (pl., comedos, comedones) [KŌM-ē-dō, kō-MĒ-dō (KŌM-ē-dōz, kō-mē-DŌ-nĕz)]

247. corium [KŌ-rē-ŭm] {corium}

248. corn {callo}

249. corticosteroid [KŌR-tĭ-kō-STĔR-ŏyd]

250. crust {costar}

251. cryosurgery [KRĪ-ō-SĔR-jer-ē] {criocirugía}

252. curettage [kyū-rĕ-TĂZH]

253. cuticle [KYŪ-tĭ-kl] {cutícula}

254. cyst [sĭst] {quiste}

255. debridement [dā-brēd-MŎN]

256. decubitus (pl., decubiti) [dĕ-KYŪ-bĭ-tŭs (dĕ-KYŪ-bĭ-tī)] ulcer

257. depigmentation [dē-pĭg-mĕn-TĀ-shŭn]

258. dermabrasion [dĕr-mă-BRĀ-zhŭn] {dermabrasión}

259. dermatitis [dĕr-mă-TĪ-tĭs] {dermatitis}

260. dermat(o)

261. dermatology [dĕr-mă-TŎL-ō-jē] {dermatologia}

262. dermis [DĔR-mĭs] {dermis}

263. derm(o)

264. diaphoresis [DĪ-ă-fō-RĒ-sĭs] {diaforesis}

265. discoid lupus erythematosus (DLE) [DĬS-kŏyd LŪ-pŭs ĕr-ĭ-THĔM-ă-tō-sĭs]

266. ecchymosis (pl., ecchymoses) [ĕk-ĭ-MŌ-sĭs (ĕk-ĭ-MŌ-sēz)] {equimosis}

267. eccrine [ĔK-rĭn] glands {glándulas ecrinas}

268. eczema [ĔK-sē-mă, ĔG-zē-mă] {eccema}

269. electrodesiccation [ē-LĔK-trō-dĕ-sĭ-KĀ-shŭn]

270. emollient [ē-MŎL-ē-ĕnt]

271. epidermis [ĕp-ĭ-DĔR-mĭs] {epidermis}

272. erosion {erosion}

273. exanthematous [ĕks-zăn-THĔM-ă-tŭs] viral disease

274. excoriation [ĕks-KŌ-rē-Ā-shŭn] {excoriación}

275. exocrine [ĔK-sō-krĭn] glands

276. exudate [ĔKS-yū-dāt] {exudado}

277. fever blister

278. first-degree burn

279. fissure [FĬSH-ŭr] {fisura}

280. fulguration [fŭl-gū-RĀ-shŭn] {fulguración}

281. furuncle [FYŪ-rŭng-kl] {furúnculo}

282. gangrene [GĂNG-grēn] {gangrena}

283. genital herpes

284. hair follicle [FŎL-ĭ-kl]

285. hair root {raiz del pelo}

286. hair shaft

287. herpes [HĔR-pēz] {herpes}

288. herpes simplex virus Type 1

289. herpes simplex virus Type 2

290. herpes zoster [ZŎS-tĕr]

291. heterograft [HĔT-ĕr-ō-grăft] {heteroinjerto}

292. hidr(o)

293. hives {urticaria}

294. homograft [HŌ-mō-grăft] {homoinjerto}

295. hypodermis [hī-pō-DĔR-mĭs] {hipodermis}

296. ichthy(o)

297. impetigo [ĭm-pĕ-TĪ-gō] {impétigo}

298. integument [ĭn-TĔG-yū-mĕnt] {integumento}

299. intradermal [ĭn-tră-DĔR-măl] {intradérmico}

300. Kaposi's sarcoma [KĂ-pō-sēz săr-KŌ-mă]

301. keloid [KĒ-lŏyd] {queloide}

302. keratin [KĔR-ă-tĭn] {queratina}

303. kerat(o)

304. keratolytic [KĔR-ă-tō-LĬT-ĭk]

305. keratosis [kĕr-ă-TŌ-sĭs] {queratosis}

306. lesion [LĒ-zhŭn] {lesión}

307. leukoderma [lū-kō-DĔR-mă] {leucodermia}

308. leukoplakia [lū-kō-PLĀ-kē-ă] {leucoplaquia}

309. lip(o)

310. lunula (pl., lunulae) [LŪ-nū-lă (LŪ-nū-lē)] {lúnula}

311. macule [MĂK-yūl] {macula}

312. malignant melanoma [mĕl-ă-NŌ-mă]

313. Mantoux [măn-TŪ] test

314. melan(o)

315. melanin [MĔL-ă-nĭn] {melanina}

316. melanocyte [MĔL-ă-nō-sīt] {melanocito}

317. Mohs' [mōz] surgery

318. myc(o)

319. nail {uña}

320. neoplasm [NĒ-ō-plăzm] {neoplasma}

321. nevus (pl., nevi) [NĒ-vŭs (NĒ-vī)] {nevo}

322. nodule [NŎD-yūl] {nódulo}

323. onych(o)

324. onychia, onychitis [ō-NĬK-ē-ă, ŏn-ĭ-KĪ-tĭs] {oniquia}

325. onychopathy [ŏn-ĭ-KŎP-ă-thē] {onicopatia}

326. papillary [PĂP-ĭ-lār-ē] layer

327. papule [PĂP-yūl] {pápula}

328. parasiticide [păr-ă-SĬT-ĭ-sīd]

329. paronychia [păr-ŏ-NĬK-ē-ă] {paroniquia}

330. patch {placa}

331. patch test

332. pediculated [pĕ-DĬK-yū-lā-tĕd] polyp

333. pediculosis [pĕ-DĬK-yū-LŌ-sĭs] {pediculosis}

334. pemphigus [PĔM-fĭ-gŭs] {pénfigo}

335. petechia (pl., petechiae) [pē-TĒ-kē-ă, (pē-TĒ-kē-ē)] {petequia}

336. pil(o)

337. pilonidal [pī-lō-NĪ-dăl] cyst

338. plantar [PLĂN-tăr] wart

339. plaque [plăk] {placa}

340. plastic surgery

341. polyp [PŎL-ĭp] {pólipo}

342. pore {poro}

343. pressure sore

344. pruritus [prū-RĪ-tŭs] {prurita}

345. psoriasis [sō-RĪ-ă-sĭs] {psoriasis}

346. purpura [PŬR-pū-ră] {púrpura}

347. pustule [PŬS-tūl] {pústula}

348. pyoderma [pī-ō-DĔR-mă] {pioderma}

349. radiation therapy
350. reticular [rĕ-TĬK-yū-lăr] layer
351. ringworm {tiña}
352. rosacea [rō-ZĀ-shē-ă] {rosácea}
353. roseola [rō-ZĒ-ō-lă]
354. rubella [rū-BĔL-ă] {rubéola}
355. rubeola [rū-BĒ-ō-lă] {rubéola}
356. scabies [SKĀ-bēz] {sarna}
357. scale {escala}
358. Schick [shĭk] test
359. scleroderma [sklēr-ō-DĔR-mă] {esclerodermia}
360. scratch test
361. sebaceous [sĕ-BĀ-shŭs] cyst
362. sebaceous glands
363. seb(o)
364. seborrhea [sĕb-ō-RĒ-ă] {seborrea}
365. sebum [SĒ-bŭm] {sebo}
366. second-degree burn
367. sessile [SĔS-ĭl] polyp
368. shingles [SHĬN-glz] {culebrilla}

369. skin graft {injerto de la piel}
370. squamous cell carcinoma [SKWĂ-mŭs sĕl kăr-sĭn-NŌ-mă]
371. squamous epithelium [ĕp-ĭ-THĒ-lē-ŭm]
372. steat(o)
373. stratified squamous epithelium
374. stratum (pl., strata) [STRĂT-ŭm (STRĂ-tă)] {estrato}
375. stratum corneum [KŌR-nē-ŭm]
376. stratum germinativum [jĕr-mĭ-NĀT-ĭ-vŭm]
377. striae [STRĪ-ē] {estrías}
378. subcutaneous [sŭb-kyū-TĀ-nē-ŭs] layer
379. sweat glands
380. systemic lupus erythematosus (SLE)
381. telangiectasia [tĕl-ĂN-jē-ĕk-TĀ-zhē-ă]
382. third-degree burn
383. tine [tīn] test, TB tine
384. tinea [TĬN-ē-ă] {tiña}

385. topical anesthetic
386. trich(o)
387. tumor [TŪ-mŏr] {tumor}
388. ulcer [ŬL-sĕr] {úlcera}
389. ultraviolet [ŭl-tră-VĪ-ō-lĕt] light
390. urticaria [ŬR-tĭ-KĀR-ē-ă] {urticaria}
391. varicella [vār-ĭ-SĔL-ă] {varicela}
392. vascular [VĂS-kyū-lăr] lesion
393. verruca (pl., verrucae) [vĕ-RŪ-kă (vĕ-RŪ-kē)] {verruga}
394. vesicle [VĔS-ĭ-kl] {vesícula}
395. vitiligo [vĭt-ĭ-LĪ-gō] {vitiligo}
396. wart [wŏrt] {verruga}
397. wheal [hwēl] {roncha}
398. whitehead [WHĪT-hĕd] {punto blanco}
399. xanth(o)
400. xenograft [ZĔN-ō-grăft] {xenoinjerto}
401. xer(o)

Abbreviations

Write the full meaning of each abbreviation.

ABBREVIATION

402. bx
403. DLE

404. PPD
405. PUVA

406. SLE

Answers to Chapter Exercises

1. He is a diabetic and has a stubborn skin rash, which may become infected.
2. symptoms
3. a. 3; b. 1; c. 2
4. apocrine, eccrine, and exocrine
5. a. epidermis
   b. stratum corneum
   c. hair follicle
   d. sebaceous gland
   e. subcutaneous layer (hypodermis)
6. cuticle
7. dermis
8. epidermis
9. papillary layer
10. eccrine
11. adipose
12. healthy
13. lunula
14. sebum
15. apocrine
16. h
17. j
18. d
19. a
20. f
21. b
22. I
23. e
24. c
25. g
26. d
27. a
28. e
29. c
30. b
31. f
32. Family history can give clues to hereditary disorders.
33. No, only a medical doctor may prescribe prescription medication, whether in sample form or not.
34. dermatoplasty
35. dermophlebitis
36. keratoderma
37. mycodermatitis
38. melanoderma
39. onychomycosis
40. onychoplasty
41. pilosebaceous

42. melanocyte
43. trichoscopy
44. lipotomy
45. adipocellular
46. trichology
47. onychopathy
48. mycotoxin
49. mycovirus
50. xanthoderma
51. xerosis
52. keratolysis
53. melanoderma
54. hidromeiosis dermatologist
56. onychophagia
57. keratogenic
58. hidropoiesis
59. icthyosis
60. mycology
61. dermatopathy
62. dermatosclerosis
63. dermatoautoplasty
64. onychitis or onychia
65. trichophobia
66. steatoma
67. photosensitivity
68. melanocarcinoma
69. adipose
70. tricho-, hair + -oma, tumor
71. xer(o)-, dry + -osis, condition
72. myco-, fungus + -cide, killing
73. xantho-, yellow + -derma, skin
74. onych(o)-, nail + -oid, resembling
75. dermat(o), skin + fibr(o), fibrous tissue + -oma, tumor
76. onych(o), nail + -malacia, softening
77. hypo-, under + derm(o)-, skin + -ic, pertaining to
78. erythr(o)-, red + -derma, skin
79. pachy-, thick + -derma, skin
80. myc(o), fungus + -genic, producing
81. xer(o), dry + -derma, skin
82. trich(o)-, hair + myc(o)-, fungus + -osis, condition
83. lip(o)-, fatty + -oma, tumor
84. onycho-, nail + crypt(o), hidden + -osis, condition
85. Patient does not have allergies to the allergens being tested.

86. The rashes would subside or even disappear.
87. F
88. T
89. T
90. F
91. T
92. fungi
93. exudate or pus
94. allergies
95. intradermal
96. Washing helps to remove excess sebum from the skin.
97. Hormonal changes that occur as one ages affect the occurrence of acne.
98. pemphigus
99. C
100. purpura
101. C
102. roseola
103. -itis
104. -osis
105. -oma
106. -pathy
107. -derma
108. F
109. F
110. F
111. T
112. T
113. F
114. T
115. F
116. T
117. T
118. heredity, medication
119. mites
120. mouth
121. genitalia
122. 18%
123. 73%
124. 45%
125. 27%
126. verruca
127. sebaceous
128. lesion
129. abscess
130. tinea pedis
131. rubella
132. psoriasis
133. vitiligo

134. hives
135. actinic keratosis
136. m
137. f
138. l
139. e
140. k
141. i
142. d
143. g
144. j
145. a
146. n
147. h
148. c
149. b
150. yes
151. Avoid baking in the sun; use protectant lotions; wear a hat outside.
152. dermabrasion
153. plastic
154. bleeding
155. autograft
156. allograft, homograft
157. the woman
158. allergic rash
159. anti-, against
160. anti-, against
161. chemo-, chemistry

162. fungi-, fungus/-cide, killing
163. myco-, fungus/-cide, killing
164. kerato-, horny tissue/-lysis, destruction of
165. F
166. T
167. T
168. F
169. T
170. f; to relieve itching
171. a; to reduce inflammation
172. d; to slow or stop the growth of fungi
173. b; to slow or stop the growth of bacteria
174. e; to slow, stop, or prevent an allergic reaction
175. c; to relieve pain
176. Inflammation of the dermis and subcutaneous skin layers. Yes, infection can spread via bloodstream.
177. The infection will not be destroyed and may recur.
178. F; furuncle
179. F; herpes zoster
180. T
181. T
182. F; pyoderma

183. F; petechia
184. F; third-degree
185. T
186. T
187. F; changes in primary lesions
188. T
189. F; increased—because people think that they can stay in the sun for much longer periods
190. T
191. T
192. T
193. F; detects presence of TB
194. F; exfoliation and desquamation.
195. T
196. Fstriae
197. T
198. fungi
199. abscesses
200. ecchymoses
201. nevi
202. bullae
203. verrucae
204. staphylococci
205. comedo or comedones
206–406. Answers are available in the vocabulary reviews in this chapter.

The Musculoskeletal System

After studying this chapter, you will be able to:

5.1 Name the parts of the musculoskeletal system and discuss the function of each part

5.2 Define combining forms used in building words that relate to the musculoskeletal system

5.3 Identify the meaning of related abbreviations

5.4 Name the common diagnoses, laboratory tests, and clinical procedures used in treating disorders of the musculoskeletal system

5.5 List and define the major pathological conditions of the musculoskeletal system

5.6 Define surgical terms related to the musculoskeletal system

5.7 List common pharmacological agents used in treating disorders of the musculoskeletal system

Structure and Function

The **musculoskeletal system** forms the framework that holds the body together, enables it to move, and protects and supports all the internal organs. This system includes **bones, joints,** and **muscles.** Figure 5-1 shows the musculoskeletal system.

Bones are made of **osseous tissue** and include a rich network of blood vessels and nerves. The cells of bone, called **osteocytes,** are part of a dense network of connective tissue. The cells themselves are surrounded by calcium salts. During fetal development, bones are softer and flexible and are composed of **cartilage** until the hardening process begins.

Bone-forming cells are called **osteoblasts.** As bone tissue develops, some of it dies and is reabsorbed by **osteoclasts** (also called **bone phagocytes**). The reabsorption of dead bone cells prevents the bone from becoming overly thick and heavy. Later, if a bone breaks, osteoblasts will add new mineral matter to repair the break and the osteoclasts will remove any bone debris, thereby smoothing over the break. The hardening process and development of the osteocytes is called **ossification.** This process is largely dependent on **calcium, phosphorus,** and **vitamin D.**

The **skeleton** of the body is made up of bones and joints. A mature adult has 206 bones that work together with joints and muscles to move the various parts of the body. The *axial* portion of the skeleton includes the trunk and head. The *appendicular* portion of the skeleton includes the limbs.

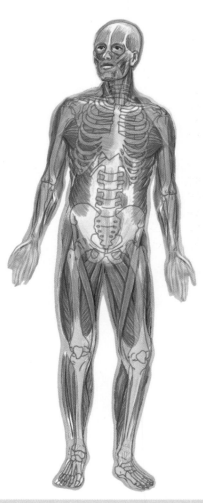

Calcium is important for the formation of bones. It is recommended that you pay attention to your daily calcium intake throughout your life, since lack of calcium is a factor in certain diseases, such as osteoporosis. To find out about the recommended levels, go to the National Osteoporosis Foundation's Web site (www.nof.org) and click on prevention.

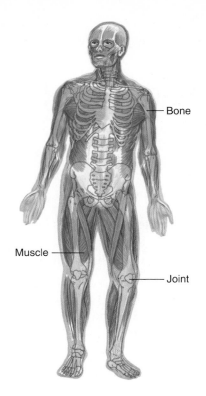

Bone

Muscle

Joint

FIGURE 5-1 Muscles and bones hold the body together, enable it to move, and protect and support the internal organs.

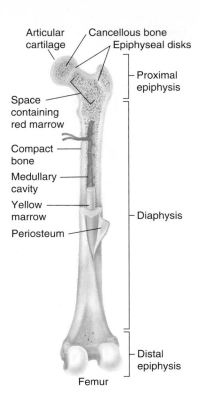

Articular cartilage

Cancellous bone
Epiphyseal disks

Proximal epiphysis

Space containing red marrow

Compact bone

Medullary cavity

Yellow marrow

Periosteum

Diaphysis

Distal epiphysis

Femur

FIGURE 5-2 Parts of a long bone. The legs and arms are made up of long bones.

Bones

There are many types of bones. The five most common categories include:

1. The **long bones** form the extremities of the body. The legs and arms include this type of bone. The longest portion of a long bone is called the shaft. The outer portion is **compact bone,** solid bone that does not bend easily. Compact bone is where oxygen and nutrients are brought from the bloodstream to the bone. This shaft is also called the **diaphysis** or place where bone growth occurs first.

   Each end of the shaft has an area shaped to connect to other bones by means of ligaments and muscle. These ends are called the *proximal epiphysis* and the *distal epiphysis*. As long bones grow, the **metaphysis,** the space between the diaphysis and the two epiphyses, develops. The **epiphyseal plate** is cartilaginous tissue that is replaced during growth years, but eventually calcifies and disappears when growth has stopped. The epiphysis is covered by **articular cartilage,** a thin, flexible substance that provides protection at movable points.

   Inside the compact bone is **cancellous bone** (which has a latticelike structure and is also called **spongy bone**) that covers the **medullary cavity.** The medullary contains yellow bone marrow or red bone marrow. Spongy bone is also in the epiphyses. The medullary cavity has a lining called the **endosteum.** The outside of the bone is covered by a fibrous membrane called the **periosteum.** Figure 5-2 shows the parts of long bones.

2. **Short bones** are the small, cube-shaped bones of the wrists, ankles, and toes. Short bones consist of an outer layer of compact bone with an inner layer of cancellous bone.
3. **Flat bones** generally have large, somewhat flat surfaces that cover organs or that provide a surface for large areas of muscle. The shoulder blades, pelvis, and skull include flat bones.
4. **Irregular bones** are specialized bones with specific shapes. The bones of the ears, vertebrae, and face are irregular bones.
5. **Sesamoid bones** are bones formed in a tendon near joints. The patella (kneecap) is a sesamoid bone. Sesamoid bones are also found in the hands and feet.

Commonly, bones have various extensions and depressions that serve as sites for attaching muscles and tendons. Bone extensions are enlargements usually at the ends of bones. Muscles, tendons, and other bones are attached at these extensions. The seven different kinds of bone extensions are:

1. The **bone head,** the end of a bone, often rounded, that attaches to other bones or connective material and is covered with cartilage.
2. The **crest,** a bony ridge.
3. The **process,** any bony projection to which muscles and tendons attach.
4. The **tubercle,** a slight elevation on a bone's surface where muscles or ligaments are attached.
5. The **trochanter,** a bony extension near the upper end of the femur where muscle is attached.
6. A **tuberosity,** a large elevation on the surface of a bone for the attachments of muscles or tendons.
7. A **condyle,** a rounded surface protrusion at the end of a bone, usually where (covered with cartilage) it articulates with another bone. The *epiondyle* projects from the condyle.

Figure 5-3 shows some of the extensions on a long bone.

Depressions in bone also allow bones to attach to each other. In addition, they are the passageways for blood vessels and nerves throughout the body. The most common types of depressions in bone are:

1. A **fossa,** a shallow pit in bone
2. A **foramen,** an opening through bone for blood vessels and nerves.
3. A **fissure,** a deep cleft in bone
4. A **sulcus,** a groove or furrow on the surface of a bone
5. A **sinus,** a hollow space or cavity in a bone.

Figure 5-4 shows the types of bone depressions.

Marrow is soft connective tissue and serves important functions in the production of blood cells. *Red bone marrow* can be found in the cancellous bone of the epiphysis and in flat bones. In infants and young children, all bone marrow is red, allowing much opportunity for red blood cells to develop. As people age, most of the red bone marrow decreases and is replaced by *yellow bone marrow.* Yellow bone marrow is found in most other adult bones and is made up of connective tissue filled with fat.

Bones of the Head

Cranial bones form the skull, which protects the brain and the structures inside the skull. The skull or cranial bones join at points called **sutures.**

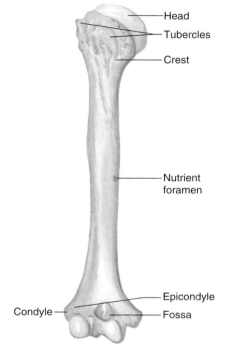

FIGURE 5-3 Bone extensions on a long bone.

Bone marrow can be transplanted from one person to another to help in curing certain diseases. To find out more about bone marrow donation, go to the Bone Marrow Foundation's Web site (www.bonemarrow.org).

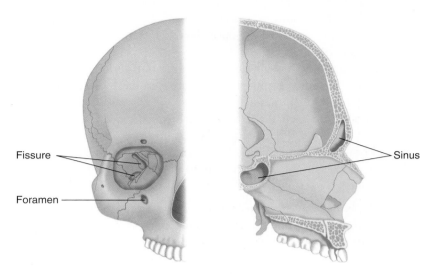

Fissure

Foramen

Sinus

FIGURE 5-4 Types of bone depressions.

The skull of a newborn is not completely joined and has soft spots, called **fontanelles.**

The skull contains the **frontal bone** (the forehead and roof of the eye sockets), the **ethmoid bone** (the nasal cavity and the orbits of the eyes), the **parietal bone** (top and upper parts of the sides of the skull), and the **temporal bone** (lower part of the skull and the lower sides, including the openings for the ears). The **temporomandibular joint (TMJ)** is the connection point for the temporal bone and the mandible (lower jawbone). A round extension behind the temporal bone is the **mastoid process.** It sits behind the ear. The **styloid process** is a peg-shaped protrusion from a bone, as the one that extends down from the temporal bone. The back and base of the skull are covered by the **occipital bone.** An opening in the occipital bone, the **foramen magnum,** is the structure through which the spinal cord passes. The skull bones are held together by the **sphenoid bone,** which joins the frontal, occipital, and ethmoid bones and forms the base of the cranium. The pituitary gland sits in the **sella turcica,** a depression in the sphenoid bone.

The skull has sinuses, specific cavities that reduce its weight. The **frontal sinuses** are above the eyes. The **sphenoid sinus** is above and behind the nose. The **ethmoid sinuses** are a group of small sinuses on both sides of the nasal cavities, between each eye and the sphenoid sinus. The **maxillary sinuses** are on either side of the **nasal cavity** below the eyes. Figure 5-5 shows the bones of the skull and the location of the sinuses.

The head also has facial bones, each with a specific function:

1. **Nasal bones** form the bridge of the nose.
2. **Lacrimal bones** hold the lacrimal gland and the canals for the tear ducts.
3. The **mandibular bone** or **mandible** is the lower jawbone and contains the sockets for the lower teeth. The mandible is the only movable bone in the face.
4. **Maxillary bones** form the upper jawbone and contain the sockets for the upper teeth.
5. The **vomer** is a flat bone that joins with the ethmoid bone to form the nasal septum.
6. **Zygomatic bones** form the prominent shape of the cheek.

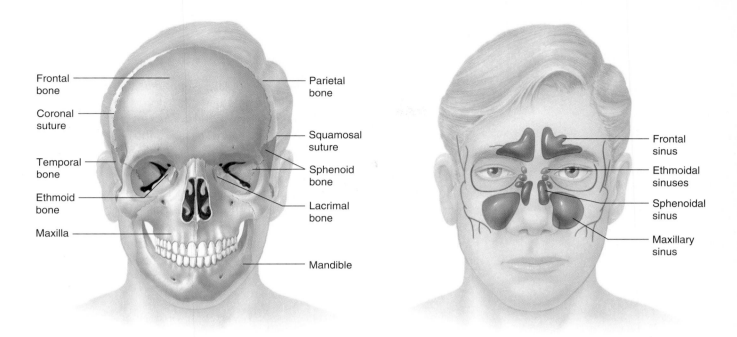

FIGURE 5-5   The bones of the skull and the sinus cavities.

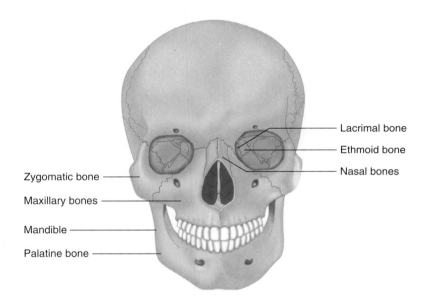

FIGURE 5-6   The bones of the face.

7. The **palatine bone** sits behind the maxillary bones and helps to form
the nasal cavity and the hard palate.

Figure 5-6 shows the bones of the face.

Spinal Column

The **spinal column** (also called the **vertebral column**) consists of five sets of
vertebrae. Each vertebra is a bone segment with a thick, **cartilaginous disk**
(also called **intervertebral disk** or **disk**) that separates the vertebrae. In the
middle of the disk is a fibrous mass called the **nucleus pulposus.** The disks

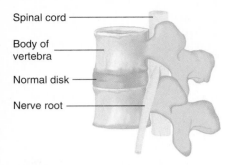

Spinal cord

Body of
vertebra

Normal disk

Nerve root

FIGURE 5-7   Details of two vertebrae.

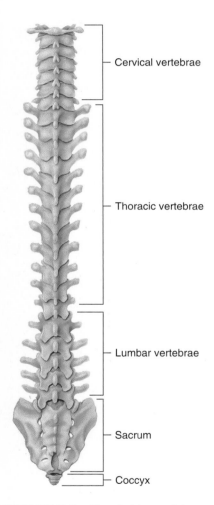

Cervical vertebrae

Thoracic vertebrae

Lumbar vertebrae

Sacrum

Coccyx

FIGURE 5-8   The divisions of the
spinal column.

cushion the vertebrae and help in movement and flexibility of the spinal column. The space between the **vertebral body** and the back of the vertebra is called the **neural canal.** This is the space through which the spinal cord passes. At the back of the vertebra, the **spinous process, transverse process,** and **lamina** form the posterior side of the spinal column. Figure 5-7 shows two vertebrae.

The five divisions of vertebrae are:

1. The **cervical vertebrae,** the seven vertebrae of the neck bone, which include the first vertebra (T1, first thoracic vertebra), called the **atlas,** and the second vertebra (T2, second thoracic vertebra), called the **axis.**
2. The **thoracic vertebrae** (also called the **dorsal vertebrae**), the twelve vertebrae that connect to the ribs.
3. The **lumbar vertebrae,** the five bones of the middle back.
4. The **sacrum,** the curved bone of the lower back, consisting of five separate bones at birth that fuse together in early childhood.
5. The **coccyx,** the tailbone, formed from four bones fused together.

Figure 5-8 shows the divisions of the spinal column.

Bones of the Chest

At the top of the **thorax** (chest cavity) are the **clavicle** (anterior collar bone) and **scapula** (posterior shoulder bone). The scapula joins with the clavicle at a point called the **acromion.** There are two weight-transferring sections of bones. The upper is the group formed by the clavicle and scapula, which transfers the weight of the upper body to distribute it evenly to the spine. Any additional weight carried by one arm, such as a person holding a child, will be distributed evenly to the spine. The second weight-transferring transverse section is formed by the pelvic girdle (see Bones of the Pelvis below).

Next is the **sternum** (breastbone), which extends down the middle of the chest. Extending out from the sternum are the twelve pairs of **ribs.** The first seven pairs of ribs, the **true ribs,** are joined both to the vertebral column and to the sternum by costal cartilage. The next three pairs of ribs, called *false ribs*, attach to the vertebral column but not to the sternum. Instead, they join the seventh rib. The last two ribs, which are also called false ribs, are known as *floating ribs* because they do not attach to the sternum anteriorly. Figure 5-9 on page 111 shows the ribs of the chest.

Bones of the Pelvis

Below the thoracic cavity is the pelvic area. The **pelvic girdle** is a large bone that forms the hips and supports the trunk of the body. It is composed of

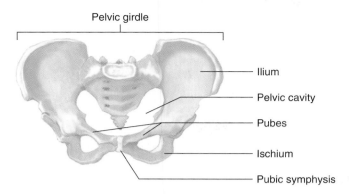

FIGURE 5-10   Bones of the pelvis.

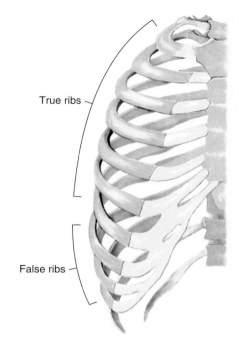

FIGURE 5-9   Ribs of the chest.

three fused bones, including the **ilium, ischium,** and **pubes** (the anteroinferior portion of the hip bone). It is also the point of attachment for the legs. This is the second weight-transferring transverse section of bone. The pelvic girdle easily transfers weight of the body from one leg to the other during running, walking, or any movement.

Inside the pelvic girdle is the **pelvic cavity.** In the pelvic cavity are located the female reproductive organs, the sigmoid colon, the bladder, and the rectum. The area where the two pubic bones join is called the **pubic symphysis.** Figure 5-10 shows the bones of the **pelvis.**

Bones of the Extremities

The upper arm bone, the **humerus,** attaches to the scapula and clavicle. The two lower arm bones are the **ulna,** which has a bony protrusion called the **olecranon (elbow),** and the **radius,** which attaches to the eight **carpal bones** of the wrist (**carpus**). The **metacarpals** are the five bones of the palm that radiate out to the finger bones, the **phalanges.** Each **phalanx** (except for the thumbs and great toes) has a *distal* (furthest from the body), *middle,* and *proximal* (nearest to the body) segment. Figure 5-11 shows the bones of the arm and hand.

The hip bone has a cup-shaped depression or socket called the **acetabulum** into which the **femur** (thigh bone) fits. The femur is the longest bone in the body. It meets the two bones of the lower leg, the **tibia** (also called the **shin**) and **fibula,** at the kneecap or **patella.** The tibia and fibula have bony protrusions near the foot called the **malleoli** (singular, **malleolus**). The protrusion of the tibia is called the *medial malleolus.* The protrusion of the fibula is called the *lateral malleolus.* The malleoli and the **tarsal bones** (seven small bones of the **tarsus** or instep) form the **ankle.** The largest tarsal is the **calcaneus (heel).** The **metatarsals** connect to the phalanges of the toes. Figure 5-12 shows the bones of the lower extremities.

Joints

Joints are also called **articulations,** points where bones connect. The movement at a particular joint varies depending on the body's needs. **Diarthroses** are joints that move freely, such as the knee joint. **Amphiarthroses** are cartilaginous joints that move slightly, such as the joints between vertebrae.

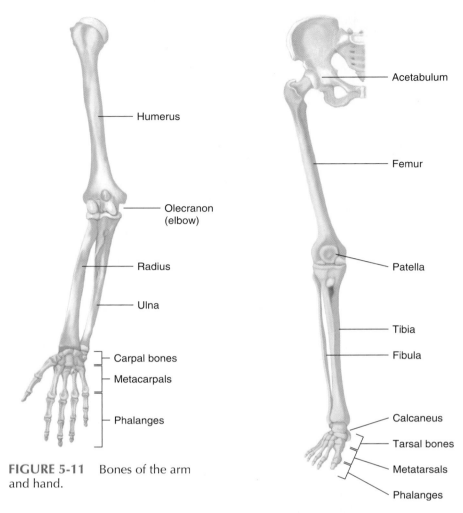

Humerus

Olecranon
(elbow)

Radius

Ulna

Carpal bones

Metacarpals

Phalanges

FIGURE 5-11   Bones of the arm
and hand.

Acetabulum

Femur

Patella

Tibia

Fibula

Calcaneus

Tarsal bones

Metatarsals

Phalanges

FIGURE 5-12   Bones of the leg
and foot.

Synarthroses do not move; examples are the fibrous joints between the skull bones. **Symphyses** are cartilaginous joints that unite two bones firmly; an example is the pubic symphysis.

Joints are also described by the type of movement they allow. Ball-and-socket joints (the hip and shoulder joints for example) are set up like a ball sitting in a socket. A hinge joint (the elbow or knee, for example) moves as though swinging like a hinge. The joints and muscles allow the parts of the body to move in specific ways.

Bones are connected to other bones with **ligaments,** bands of fibrous tissue. **Tendons** are bands of fibrous tissue that connect muscles to bone. Movement takes place at the joints using the muscles, ligaments, and tendons. **Synovial joints** are covered with a **synovial membrane,** which secretes **synovial fluid,** a joint lubricant, and which helps the joint move easily. The hip joint is an example of a synovial joint. Some spaces between tendons and joints have a **bursa,** a sac lined with a synovial membrane. Bursae help the movement of hands and feet. Figure 5-13 shows the three types of joints and the parts of a joint.

MORE ABOUT . . .

Body Movement

Bones, joints, and muscles allow parts of the body to move in certain directions. To determine if movement can be done correctly, medical practitioners in a variety of fields look at the range of motion of the parts of the body. Also, position of the body involves placement in certain positions.

- *Flexion*—the bending of a limb.
- *Extension*—the straightening of a limb.
- *Rotation*—the circular movement of a part, such as the neck.
- *Abduction*—movement away from the body.
- *Adduction*—movement toward the body.
- *Supination*—a turning up, as of the hand.
- *Pronation*—a turning down, as of the hand.
- *Dorsiflexion*—a bending up, as of the ankle.
- *Plantar flexion*—a bending down, as of the ankle.

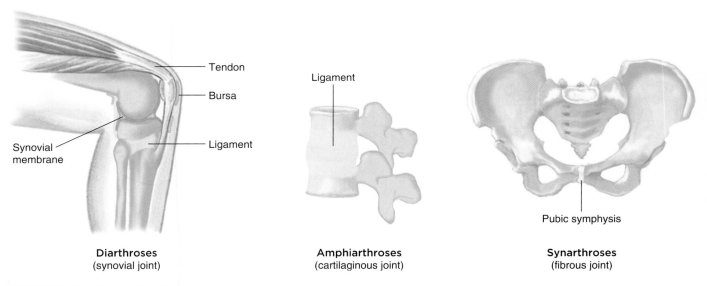

Diarthroses
(synovial joint)

Amphiarthroses
(cartilaginous joint)

Synarthroses
(fibrous joint)

FIGURE 5-13   Types of and parts of a joint.

Muscles

Muscles contract and extend to provide body movement. The **voluntary (striated) muscles** can be contracted at will. These muscles are called *skeletal muscles*, as they are responsible for the movement of all skeletal bones, including facial bones, such as the mandible. The **involuntary (smooth or visceral) muscles** control movement that is not controlled by will, such as respiration, urination, and digestion. Involuntary muscles move the internal organs and systems, such as the digestive system and the blood. **Cardiac muscle,** which controls the contractions of the heart, is the only involuntary muscle that is also striated.

MORE ABOUT . . .

Muscles

Normal muscles contract and extend during routine movement and exercise. In unusual circumstances, muscles can *atrophy* (waste away). This can happen from a number of diseases that affect muscles and movement or from lack of use, as in a sedentary lifestyle. People who are paralyzed and find it difficult to get help moving muscles generally have areas where muscle atrophies. On the other hand, overuse of muscles can cause *hyperplasia,* an abnormal increase in muscle cells.

Building muscle by exercising is generally a healthy thing to do. However, some athletes take dangerous shortcuts to building muscle. They take *anabolic steroids* or supplements containing products similar to anabolic steroids that build muscle quickly. Unfortunately, these products can have devastating health and emotional consequences, sometimes even fatal ones. Also, athletes who take these illegal substances often have an unfair advantage in competition over those who don't. These substances are outlawed in most competitive sports.

For more information about steroid abuse, go to the National Institute on Drug Abuse's Web site on steroid abuse (www.steroidabuse.org).

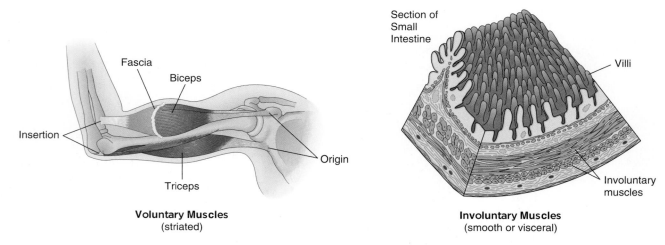

Voluntary Muscles
(striated)

Involuntary Muscles
(smooth or visceral)

FIGURE 5-14 Types and parts of muscle.

Most muscles are covered by **fascia,** a band of connective tissue that supports and covers the muscle. Muscles attach to a stationary bone at a point called the **origin.** They attach to a movable bone at a point called the **insertion.** During movement, the muscle contracts and extends and the moveable bone moves in a specific direction. Different muscles have different functions. For example, the deltoid muscles are used to extend the arms, the biceps of the arm flex the forearms, and the masticatory muscles close and open the jaw for chewing. Figure 5-14 shows the various types of muscle.

VOCABULARY REVIEW

In the previous section, you learned terms relating to the musculoskeletal system. Before going on to the exercises, review the terms below and refer to the previous chapters if you have any questions. Pronunciations are provided for certain terms. Sometimes information about where the word came from is included after the term. These etymologies (word histories) are for your information only. You do not need to memorize them.

Term	Definition
acetabulum [ăs-ĕ-TĂB-yū-lŭm]	Cup-shaped depression in the hip bone into which the top of the femur fits.
acromion [ă-KRŌ-mē-oñ]	Part of the scapula that connects to the clavicle.
amphiarthrosis *(pl.,* **amphiarthoses)** [ĂM-fĭ-ăr-THRŌ-sĭs (ĂM-fĭ-ăr-THRŌ-sĕs)] Greek *amphi-*, both + *arthrosis*, joint	Cartilaginous joint having some movement at the union of two bones.
ankle [ĂNG-kl]	Hinged area between the lower leg bones and the bones of the foot.
articular [ăr-TĬK-yū-lăr] **cartilage**	Cartilage at a joint.
articulation [ăr-tĭk-yū-LĀ-shŭn]	Point at which two bones join together to allow movement.
atlas [ĂT-lăs]	First cervical vertebra.
axis [ĂK-sĭs]	Second cervical vertebra.
bone	Hard connective tissue that forms the skeleton of the body.
bone head	Upper, rounded end of a bone.
bone phagocyte [FĂG-ō-sīt]	Bone cell that ingests dead bone and bone debris.
bursa *(pl.,* **bursae)** [BŬR-să(BŬR-sē)]	Sac lined with a synovial membrane that fills the spaces between tendons and joints.
calcaneus [kăl-KĀ-nē-ŭs]	Heel bone.
calcium [KĂL-sē-ŭm]	Mineral important in the formation of bone.
cancellous [KĂN-sĕ-lŭs] **bone**	Spongy bone with a latticelike structure.
cardiac [KĂR-dē-ăk] **muscle**	Striated involuntary muscle of the heart.
carpus, carpal [KĂR-pŭs, KĂR-păl] **bone**	Wrist; wrist bone.
cartilage [KĂR-tĭ-lăj]	Flexible connective tissue found in joints, fetal skeleton, and the lining of various parts of the body.
cartilaginous [kăr-tĭ-LĂJ-ĭ-nŭs] **disk**	Thick, circular mass of cartilage between the vertebrae of the spinal column.
cervical [SĔR-vĭ-kl] **vertebrae**	Seven vertebrae of the spinal column located in the neck.
clavicle [KLĂV-ĭ-kl]	Curved bone of the shoulder that joins to the scapula; collar bone.

Term	Definition
coccyx [KŎK-sĭks]	Small bone consisting of four fused vertebrae at the end of the spinal column; tailbone.
compact bone	Hard bone with a tightly woven structure.
condyle [KŎN-dīl]	Rounded surface at the end of a bone.
crest	Bony ridge.
diaphysis [dī-ĂF-ĭ-sĭs] Greek, a growing between	Long middle section of a long bone; shaft.
diarthroses (*sing.*, diarthrosis) [dī-ăr-THRŌ-sēz (dī-ăr-THRŌ-sĭs] Greek, articulations	Freely movable joints.
disk [dĭsk] Latin *discus*	*See* cartilaginous disk.
dorsal vertebrae	Thoracic vertebrae.
elbow [ĔL-bō]	Joint between the upper arm and the forearm.
endosteum [ĕn-DŎS-tē-ŭm] end(o)-, within + Greek *osteon*, bone	Lining of the medullary cavity.
epiphyseal [ĕp-ĭ-FĬZ-ē-ăl] plate	Cartilaginous tissue that is replaced during growth years, but eventually calcifies and disappears when growth stops.
ethmoid [ĔTH-mŏyd] bone	Irregular bone of the face attached to the sphenoid bone.
ethmoid sinuses	Sinuses on both sides of the nasal cavities between each eye and the sphenoid sinus.
fascia (*pl.*, fasciae) [FĂSH-ē-ă (FĂSH-ē-ē)]	Sheet of fibrous tissue that encloses muscles.
femur [FĒ-mūr]	Long bone of the thigh.
fibula [FĬB-yū-lă]	Smallest long bone of the lower leg.
fissure [FĬSH-ŭr]	Deep furrow or slit.
flat bones	Thin, flattened bones that cover certain areas, as of the skull.
fontanelle [FŎN-tă-nĕl]	Soft, membranous section on top of an infant's skull.
foramen [fō-RĀ-mĕn]	Opening or perforation through a bone.
foramen magnum [MĂG-nŭm]	Opening in the occipital bone through which the spinal cord passes.
fossa (*pl.*, fossae) [FŎS-ă (FŎS-ē)]	Depression, as in a bone.
frontal [FRŬN-tăl] bone	Large bone of the skull that forms the top of the head and forehead.
frontal sinuses	Sinuses above the eyes.

CASE STUDY

Seeing a Specialist

Mary Edgarton was referred to Dr. Alana Wolf, a rheumatologist, by her internist. Mary's five-month bout of joint pain, swelling, and stiffness had not shown improvement. Dr. Wolf gave her a full musculoskeletal examination to check for swelling, abnormalities, and her ability to move her joints. Even though Mary remains a fairly active person, her movement in certain joints is now limited. She shows a moderate loss of grip strength.

In checking earlier for a number of systemic diseases, Mary's internist felt that Mary's problems were the result of some disease of her musculoskeletal system. Many of the laboratory tests that were forwarded to Dr. Wolf showed normal levels.

Critical Thinking

1. What lubricates the joints, allowing movement?
2. Exercise is usually recommended to alleviate musculoskeletal problems. Is it possible to exercise both involuntary and voluntary muscles?

STRUCTURE AND FUNCTION EXERCISES

Check Your Knowledge

Fill in the blanks.

3. The extremities of the body include mostly _____ bones.

4. A mature adult has a total of _____ bones.

5. Soft connective tissue with high nutrient content in the center of some bones is called _____.

6. An infant's skull generally has soft spots known as _____.

7. Disks in the spinal column have a soft, fibrous mass in the middle called the _____ _____.

8. The scapula and the clavicle join at a point called the _____.

9. Ribs that attach to both the vertebral column and the sternum are called _____ _____.

10. Another name for kneecap is _____.

11. The largest tarsal is called the _____ or heel.

12. The only muscle that is both striated and involuntary is the _____ muscle.

13. The first two cervical vertebrae are known as the _____ and the _____.

14. The longest bone in the body is the _____.

15. Bones are connected to bones by _____.

16. Muscles connect to bones by _____.

17. The _____ is the connection point for the temporal bone and the mandible (lower jawbone).

18. Joints are also called _____, points where bones connect.

19. Joints are described by the type of _____ they allow.

Circle T for true or F for false.

20. Compact bone is another name for cancellous bone. T F

21. Yellow bone marrow is found in adults. T F

22. The mandible is the upper jawbone. T F
23. The twelve vertebrae that connect to the ribs are the dorsal vertebrae. T F

Match the Movement

Put the letter of the correct movement in the space provided.

24. _____ extension

25. _____ rotation

26. _____ abduction

27. _____ adduction

28. _____ supination

29. _____ pronation

30. _____ flexion

31. _____ dorsiflexion

32. _____ plantar flexion

a. a bending down, as of the ankle

b. movement toward the body

c. the straightening of a limb

d. a bending up, as of the ankle

e. the bending of a limb

f. the circular movement of a part, such as the neck

g. movement away from the body

h. a turning up as of the hand

i. a turning down, as of the hand

Match the Terms

Put the letter of the correct definition in the space provided.

33. _____ articulation

34. _____ atlas

35. _____ axis

36. _____ carpal bone

37. _____ clavicle

38. _____ coccyx

39. _____ olecranon

40. _____ origin

41. _____ insertion

42. _____ sternum

43. _____ tarsal bones

a. bony prominence of the elbow

b. point at which muscles attach to stationary bone

c. wrist, wrist bone

d. tailbone

e. first cervical vertebrae

f. second cervical vertebra

g. collar bone

h. bones of the instep (arch) of the foot

i. point at which two bones join together

j. point at which muscle attaches to moveable bone

k. breast bone

Combining Forms and Abbreviations

The lists below include combining forms and abbreviations that relate specifically to the musculoskeletal system. Pronunciations are provided for the examples.

Combining Form	Meaning	Example
acetabul(o)	acetabulum	*acetabulectomy* [ĂS-ĕ-tăb-yū-LĔK-tō-mē], excision of the acetabulum
acromi(o)	end point of the scapula	*acromioscapular* [ă-KRŌ-mē-ō-SKĂP-yū-lăr], relating to the acromion and the body of the scapula
ankyl(o)	bent, crooked	*ankylosis* [ĂNG-kĭ-LŌ-sĭs], fixation of a joint in a bent position, usually resulting from a disease
arthr(o)	joint	*arthrogram* [ĂR-thrō-grăm], x-ray of a joint
brachi(o)	arm	*brachiocephalic* [BRĀ-kē-ō-sĕ-FĂL-ĭk], relating to both the arm and head
burs(o)	bursa	*bursitis* [bŭr-SĪ-tĭs], inflammation of a bursa
calcane(o)	heel	*calcaneodynia* [kăl-KĀ-nē-ō-DĬN-ē-ă], heel pain
calci(o)	calcium	*calciokinesis* [KĂL-sē-ō-kĭ-NĒ-sĭs], mobilization of stored calcium in the body
carp(o)	wrist	*carpopedal* [KĂR-pō-PĔD-ăl], relating to the wrist and foot
cephal(o)	head	*cephalomegaly* [SĔF-ă-lō-MĔG-ă-lē], abnormally large head
cervic(o)	neck	*cervicodynia* [SĔR-vĭ-kō-DĬN-ē-ă], neck pain
chondr(o)	cartilage	*chondroplasty* [KŎN-drō-plăs-tē], surgical repair of cartilage
condyl(o)	knob, knuckle	*condylectomy* [kŏn-dĭ-LĔK-tō-mē], excision of a condyle
cost(o)	rib	*costiform* [KŎS-tĭ-fŏrm], rib-shaped
crani(o)	skull	*craniotomy* [krā-nē-ŎT-ō-mē], incision into the skull
dactyl(o)	fingers, toes	*dactylitis* [dăk-tĭ-LĪ-tĭs], inflammation of the finger(s) or toe(s)
fasci(o)	fascia	*fasciotomy* [făsh-ē-ŎT-ō-mē], incision through a fascia
femor(o)	femur	*femorocele* [FĔM-ō-rō-sēl], hernia in the femur
fibr(o)	fiber	*fibroma* [fī-BRŌ-mă], benign tumor in fibrous tissue

Combining Form	Meaning	Example
humer(o)	humerus	*humeroscapular* [HYŪ-měr-ō-SKĂP-yū-lăr], relating to both the humerus and the scapula
ili(o)	ilium	*iliofemoral* [ĬL-ē-ō-FĔM-ō-răl], relating to the ilium and the femur
ischi(o)	ischium	*ischiodynia* [ĬS-kē-ō-DĬN-ē-ă], pain in the ischium
kyph(o)	hump; bent	*kyphoscoliosis* [KĪ-fō-skō-lē-Ō-sĭs], kyphosis and scoliosis combined
lamin(o)	lamina	*laminectomy* [LĂM-ĭ-NĔK-tō-mē], removal of part of one or more of the thick cartilaginous disks between the vertebrae
leiomy(o)	smooth muscle	*leiomyosarcoma* [LĪ-ō-MĪ-ō-săr-KŌ-mă], malignant tumor of smooth muscle
lumb(o)	lumbar	*lumboabdominal* [LŬM-bō-ăb-DŎM-ĭ-năl], relating to the lumbar and abdominal regions
maxill(o)	upper jaw	*maxillofacial* [măk-SĬL-ō-FĀ-shăl], pertaining to the jaws and face
metacarp(o)	metacarpal	*metacarpectomy* [MĔT-ă-kăr-PĔK-tō-mē], excision of a metacarpal
my(o)	muscle	*myocardium* [mī-ō-KĂR-dē-ŭm], cardiac muscle in the middle layer of the heart
myel(o)	spinal cord; bone marrow	*myelocyst* [MĪ-ĕ-lō-sĭst], cyst that develops in bone marrow
oste(o)	bone	*osteoarthritis* [ŎS-tē-ō-ăr-THRĪ-tĭs], arthritis characterized by erosion of cartilage and bone and joint pain
patell(o)	knee	*patellectomy* [PĂT-ĕ-LĔK-tō-mē], excision of the patella
ped(i), ped(o)	foot	*pedometer* [pĕ-DŎM-ĕ-tĕr], instrument for measuring walking distance
pelv(i)	pelvis	*pelviscope* [PĔL-vĭ-skōp], instrument for viewing the pelvic cavity
phalang(o)	finger or toe bone	*phalangectomy* [făl-ăn-JĔK-tō-mē], removal of a finger or toe
pod(o)	foot	*podalgia* [pō-DĂL-jē-ă], foot pain

Combining Form	Meaning	Example
pub(o)	pubis	*puborectal* [PYŪ-bō-RĔK-tăl], relating to the pubis and the rectum
rachi(o)	spine	*rachiometer* [rā-kē-ŎM-ĕ-tĕr], instrument for measuring spine curvature
radi(o)	forearm bone	*radiomuscular* [RĀ-dē-ō-MŬS-kyū-lăr], relating to the radius and nearby muscles
rhabd(o)	rod-shaped	*rhabdosphincter* [RĂB-dō-SFĬNGK-tĕr], striated muscular sphincter
rhabdomy(o)	striated muscle	*rhabdomyolysis* [RĂB-dō-mī-ŎL-ĭ-sĭs], acute disease that includes destruction of skeletal muscle
scapul(o)	scapula	*scapulodynia* [SKĂP-yū-lō-DĬN-ē-ă], scapula pain
scoli(o)	curved	*scoliokyphosis* [SKŌ-lē-ō-kī-FŌ-sĭs], lateral and posterior curvature of the spine
spondyl(o)	vertebra	*spondylitis* [spŏn-dĭ-LĪ-tĭs], inflammation of a vertebra
stern(o)	sternum	*sternodynia* [stĕr-nō-DĬN-ē-ă], sternum pain
synov(o)	synovial membrane	*synovitis* [sĭn-ō-VĪ-tĭs], inflammation of a synovial joint
tars(o)	tarsus	*tarsomegaly* [tăr-sō-MĔG-ă-lē], congenital abnormality with overgrowth of a tarsal bone
ten(o), tend(o), tendin(o)	tendon	*tenodynia* [tĕn-ō-DĬN-ē-ă], tendon pain; *tendoplasty* [TĔN-dō-plăs-tē], surgical repair of a tendon; *tendinitis* [tĕn-dĭ-NĪ-tĭs], tendon inflammation
thorac(o)	thorax	*thoracoabdominal* [THŌR-ă-kō-ăb-DŎM-ĭ-năl], relating to the thorax and the abdomen
tibi(o)	tibia	*tibiotarsal* [tĭb-ē-ō-TĂR-săl], relating to the tarsal and tibia bones
uln(o)	ulna	*ulnocarpal* [ŬL-nō-KĂR-păl], relating to the ulna and the wrist
vertebr(o)	vertebra	*vertebroarterial* [VĔR-tĕ-brō-ăr-TĒR-ē-ăl], relating to a vertebral artery or to a vertebra and an artery

ABBREVIATION	MEANING	ABBREVIATION	MEANING
A-K	above the knee (amputation)	L	left
ASIS	anterior superior iliac spine	L_1, L_2, etc.	first lumbar vertebra, second lumbar vertebra, etc.
B	bilateral	MCP	metacarpophalangeal
B-K	below the knee (amputation)	NSAID	nonsteroidal anti-inflammatory drug
C_1, C_2, etc.	first cervical vertebra, second cervical vertebra, etc.	OA	osteoarthritis
Ca	calcium	P	phosphorus
CTS	carpal tunnel syndrome	PIP	proximal interphalangeal joints
D_1, D_2, etc.	first dorsal vertebra, second dorsal vertebra, etc. (now referred to as first thoracic vertebra, second thoracic vertebra, etc.)	PSIS	posterior superior iliac spine
		R	right
DJD	degenerative joint disease	RA	rheumatoid arthritis
DTR	deep tendon reflex	ROM	range of motion
EMG	electromyogram	T_1, T_2, etc.	first thoracic vertebra, second thoracic vertebra, etc.
Fx	fracture		
IM	intramuscularly	TMJ	temporomandibular joint

COMBINING FORMS AND ABBREVIATIONS EXERCISES

Build Your Medical Vocabulary

Complete the words using combining forms listed in this chapter.

44. Joint pain: _____ dynia

45. Plastic surgery of the skull: _____ plasty

46. Of the upper jaw and its teeth: _____ dental

47. Relating to the large area of the hip bone and the tibia: _____ tibial

48. Operation on the instep of the foot: _____ tomy

49. Relating to the head and chest: cephalo _____

50. Production of fibrous tissue: _____ plasia

51. Inflammation of the foot: _____ itis

52. Instrument for measuring spine curvature: _____ meter

53. Incision through the sternum: _____ tomy

CASE STUDY

Checking Medication

Dr. Wolf's next patient, Laura Spinoza, is in for a follow-up visit for fibromyalgia, a disease that causes chronic muscle pain. In addition, Laura has tested positive for CTS (carpal tunnel syndrome). The patient suffers from depression, for which she is currently being treated. Laura has had earlier reactions to some of the medications meant to relieve the symptoms of fibromyalgia. She is receiving new prescriptions for the fibromyalgia as well as directions for an exercise program. Dr. Wolf sent a follow-up letter to Laura's primary care physician after her visit.

Critical Thinking

54. Dr. Wolf gets referrals from general practitioners and internists. As a specialist in rheumatology, most of her cases involve diseases of the musculoskeletal system. Refer to the letter from Dr. Wolf and use the combining forms list to provide definitions of two diseases given as examples.

55. Laura has a physical condition in addition to fibromyalgia. What is it? Give both the abbreviation and the full spelling.

Alana Wolf, M.D.
285 Riverview Road
Belle Harbor, MI 09999

March 12, 20XX

Dr. Robert Johnson
16 Tyler Court
Newtown, MI 09990

Dear Dr. Johnson

I saw Laura Spinoza on March the 7th for evaluation of her fibromyalgia. I reviewed her history with her and discussed her treatment for depression. The history suggests that there has not been any new development of an inflammatory rheumatic disease process within the last two years. She does have right thumb-carpal pain, which represents some osteoarthritis. Headaches are frequent but she is receiving no specific therapy. Her sleep pattern remains disturbed at times.

Her height was 62 inches, her weight was 170 lbs, while her BP was 162/100 in the right arm in the reclining position. Pelvic and rectal examinations were not done. The abdominal examination revealed some mild tenderness in the right lower quadrant without other abnormalities. The musculoskeletal examination revealed rotation and flexion to the left with no other cervical abnormalities. The remainder of the musculo-skeletal examination revealed hypermobility in the elbow and knees and slight bony osteoarthritic enlargement of the thumb-carpal joint. Slight deformity was noted in the right knee with mild patellar-femoral crepitus. Severe bilateral pas planus was present, with the right foot more involved than the left, and ankle vagus deformity with mild bony osteoarthritic enlargement of both 1st MTP joints.

Hope these thoughts are helpful. I want to thank you for the consultation. If I can be of future service with her or other rheumatic-problem patients, please do not hesitate to contact me.

Alana Wolf, MD

Alana Wolf, M.D.

Find the Word Parts

Give the term that fits the definition given below. Each term must contain at least one of the combining forms given in the previous section. You may refer to the Appendix of combining forms at the back of the book.

56. Joint pain _____ .

57. Removal of a bursa _____ .

58. Inflammation of cartilage _____ .

59. Removal of a vertebra _____ .

60. Bone-forming cell _____ .

61. Abnormal bone hardening _____ .

62. Plastic surgery on the neck _____ .

63. Inflammation of the spinal cord _____ .

64. Foot spasm _____ .

65. Of the ulna and the carpus _____ .

Find the misspelled word part. Write the corrected word part in the space with its definition.

66. sinovotomy _____

67. myellogram _____

68. arthrodunia _____

69. ostiomyelitis _____

70. takiometer _____

Know the Word Parts

Write the meaning of the following word parts in the space provided. As additional practice, use your dictionary to find at least two words for each word part listed below. Learn the meanings of each word you find.

71. arthr(o) _____

72. ankyl(o) _____

73. brachi(o) _____

74. calcane(o) _____

75. cephal(o) _____

76. cervic(o) _____

77. chondr(o) _____

78. cost(o) _____

79. crani(o) _____

80. fasci(o) _____

81. kyph(o) _____

82. my(o) _____

83. myel(o) _____

84. oste(o) _____

85. patell(o) _____

86. rachi(o) _____

87. scoli(o) _____

Diagnostic, Procedural, and Laboratory Terms

The musculoskeletal system is often the site of pain caused by conditions in the system itself or by symptoms of other systemic conditions. Specialists in the musculoskeletal system include **orthopedists** or **orthopedic surgeons,** physicians who treat disorders of the musculoskeletal system; **osteopaths,** physicians who combine manipulative procedures with conventional treatment; **rheumatologists,** physicians who treat disorders of the joints, specifically, and of the musculoskeletal system generally; **podiatrists,** medical specialists who treat disorders of the foot; and **chiropractors,** health care professionals who manipulate the spine to treat certain ailments.

Diagnosing bone and muscle ailments often involves taking x-rays (Figure 5-15), scans, or radiographs or performing internal examinations to determine if an abnormality is present. **Arthrography** is the examination of joints using radiography. **Arthroscopy** is the examination of a joint internally using a lighted instrument capable of direct viewing, cutting, irrigation, obtaining biopsy material, and more, through a small incision. **Diskography** is the examination of disks by injecting a contrast medium and using radiography. Computed tomography (CT) scans (Figure 5-16) can reveal joint, bone, or connective tissue disease. **Myelography** is the use of radiography of the spinal cord to identify spinal cord conditions. An **electromyogram** is a graphic image of the electrical activity of muscles. Magnetic resonance imaging (MRI) may be used to detect disorders of the musculoskeletal system, especially of soft tissue (see Figure 5-17). A **bone scan** is used to detect tumors.

Physicians examine bones and joints externally, often using small rubber mallets to provoke responses. **Tinel's sign** is a "pins and needles" sensation felt when an injured nerve site is tapped. The sign indicates a partial lesion in a nerve and is a common test for carpel tunnel syndrome.

Laboratory tests measure the levels of substances found in some musculoskeletal disorders. Rheumatoid arthritis may be confirmed by a **rheumatoid factor test.** High levels of **serum creatine phosphokinase (CPK)** appear in some disorders such as a skeletal injury. The measurement of **serum calcium** and **serum phosphorus** in the blood indicates the body's incorporation of those substances in the bones. **Uric acid tests** can detect gout.

Tests for range of motion (ROM) in certain joints can indicate movement or joint disorders. A **goniometer** is used to measure motion in the joints (Figure 5-18). A **densitometer** uses light and x-ray images to measure bone density for osteoporosis, a disease with bone fractures that is most common in post-menopausal women.

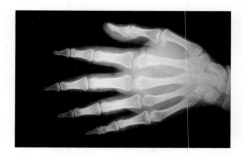
FIGURE 5-15 An x-ray of the hand showing arthritis in most of the joints

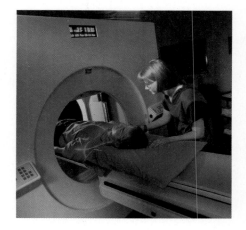
FIGURE 5-16 CT scans are valuable diagnostic tools.

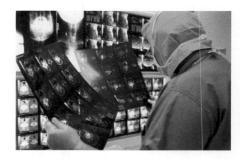
FIGURE 5-17 A radiologist examining MRI scans to see if there are any abnormalities.

The National Osteoporosis Foundation (www.nof.org) gives tips on prevention.

FIGURE 5-18 A goniometer is used to measure the range of motion of a joint.

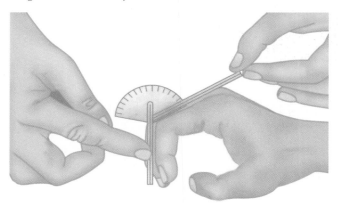

VOCABULARY REVIEW

In the previous section, you learned terms relating to diagnosis, clinical procedures, and laboratory tests. Before going on to the exercises, review the terms below and refer to the previous section if you have any questions. Pronunciations are provided for certain terms. Sometimes information about where the word came from is included after the term. These etymologies (word histories) are for your information only. You do not need to memorize them.

Term	Definition
arthrography [ăr-THRŎG-ră-fē] arthro-, joint + -graphy, process of recording	Radiography of a joint.
arthroscopy [ăr-THRŎS-kō-pē] arthro-, joint + -scopy, a viewing with an instrument	Examination with an instrument that explores the interior of a joint.
bone scan	Radiographic or nuclear medicine image of a bone.
chiropractor [kī-rō-PRĂK-tōr] chiro-, hand + Greek praktikos, efficient	Health care professional who works to align the spinal column so as to treat certain ailments.
densitometer [děn-sĭ-TŎM-ě-těr]	Device that measures bone density using light and x-rays.
diskography [dĭs-KŎG-ră-fē]	Radiographic image of an intervertebral disk by injection of a contrast medium into the center of the disk.
electromyogram [ē-lěk-trō-MĪ-ō-grăm] electro-, electrical + myo-, muscle + -gram, recording	A graphic image of muscular action using electrical currents.
goniometer [gō-nē-ŎM-ě-těr] Greek gonia, angle + -meter, measuring device	Instrument that measures angles or range of motion in a joint.
myelography [MĪ-ě-LŎG-ră-fē] myelo-, spinal cord + -graphy, process of recording	Radiographic imaging of the spinal cord.
orthopedist [ōr-thō-PĒ-dĭst], **orthopedic** [ōr-thō-PĒD-ĭk] **surgeon** ortho-, straight + Greek pais (paid-), child	Physician who examines, diagnoses, and treats disorders of the musculoskeletal system.
osteopath [ŎS-tē-ō-păth] osteo-, bone + -path(y), disease	Physician who combines manipulative treatment with conventional therapeutic measures.
podiatrist [pō-DĪ-ă-trĭst]	Medical specialist who examines, diagnoses, and treats disorders of the foot.
rheumatoid factor test	Test used to detect rheumatoid arthritis.
rheumatologist [rū-mă-TŎL-ō-jĭst]	Physician who examines, diagnoses, and treats disorders of the joints and musculoskeletal system.
serum calcium [SĒR-ŭm KĂL-sĭ-ŭm]	Test for calcium in the blood.

Term	Definition
serum creatine phosphokinase [KRĒ-ă-tēn fŏs-fō-KĪ-nās]	Enzyme active in muscle contraction; usually phosphokinase is elevated after a myocardial infarction and in the presence of other degenerative muscle diseases.
serum phosphorus [FŎS-fōr-ŭs]	Test for phosphorus in the blood.
Tinel's [tĭ-NĔLZ] **sign**	"Pins and needles" sensation felt when an injured nerve site is tapped.
uric [YŪR-ĭk] **acid test**	Test for acid content in urine; elevated levels may indicate gout.

CASE STUDY

Preventing Disease

Louella Jones (age 48) visited her gynecologist, Dr. Phillips, for her annual examination. During the past year, Louella had stopped menstruating. She had some symptoms of menopause, but they did not bother her tremendously. Louella is tall and very thin. Dr. Phillips sent her for a bone density test. The densitometer measured the density of Louella's bones and found that there was a slight increase in her bones' porosity from three years ago. Dr. Phillips suggested hormone replacement therapy and a program of weight-bearing exercises.

However, Louella wanted more information about the treatment's potential impact on her condition before beginning therapy.

Critical Thinking

88. Why are bone density measurements important in the diagnosis?

89. Louella wanted more information before taking medication and starting an exercise program. What kind of information might she be given?

DIAGNOSTIC, PROCEDURAL, AND LABORATORY TERMS EXERCISES

Test Your Knowledge

Answer the following questions.

90. Tests for calcium and phosphorus are given to determine blood levels of these minerals. What significance do these minerals have for the musculoskeletal system? _____

_____

_____

_____

91. Is it likely that a chiropractor would order a uric acid test? Why or why not? _____

_____

_____

92. Would a bone scan be likely to show bone cancer? _____

93. How is an osteopath like a chiropractor? _____

_____

94. What might a goniometer show about a muscle's action? _____

_____

True or False

For each of the following statements, circle T for true or F for false.

95. A diskography is used to check bone density. T F

96. An electromyogram uses a contrast medium to check for range of motion in a joint. T F

97. A chiropractor can perform surgery. T F

98. A rheumatologist examines, diagnoses, and treats disorders of the joints and musculoskeletal system. T F

99. A podiatrist is a medical specialist who examines, diagnoses, and treats disorders of the foot. T F

Check Your Spelling

For each of the following terms, place a C if the spelling is correct. If it is not, write the correct spelling in the space provided.

100. chiropractor _____

101. densitiometer _____

102. electromelogram _____

103. rhuematoid _____

104. goniometer _____

105. orthepodist _____

106. Tenil's sign _____

Pathological Terms

Musculoskeletal disorders arise from congenital conditions, injury, degenerative disease, or other systemic disorders. Birth defects, such as **spina bifida,** affect the development of the spinal cord. Injuries to the spinal cord may produce paralysis. In some situations, surgery on the fetus while it is in utero can alleviate some of the effects of spina bifida. In such surgery, the abnormal spinal cord opening is repaired.

A **herniated disk,** in which the center of the disk is compressed and presses on nerves in the neural canal, can lead to **sciatica,** pain radiating down the leg from the lower back. Some diseases, such as **rickets,** which causes deformities in the legs, may result from a vitamin D deficiency.

Foot deformities may occur in or involve the ankle joint. **Talipes calcaneus** is a deformity of the heel due to weakened calf muscles; **talipes valgus** is *eversion* (a turning outward) of the foot; and **talipes varus** is *inversion* (a turning inward) of the foot. A **calcar** or **spur** is a bony projection growing out of a bone.

Fractures are breaks or cracks in bones (see Figure 5-19). There are many different types of fractures:

- A **closed fracture** is a break with no open wound.
- An **open (compound) fracture** is a break with an open wound.
- A **simple (hairline** or **closed) fracture** does not move any part of the bone out of place.
- A **complex fracture** is a separation of part of the bone and usually requires surgery for repair.
- A **greenstick fracture** is an incomplete break of a soft (usually, a child's) bone.
- An **incomplete fracture** is a break that does not go entirely through any type of bone.
- A **comminuted fracture** is a break in which the bone is fragmented or shattered.
- A **Colles' fracture** is a break of the distal part of the radius.
- A **complicated fracture** involves extensive soft tissue injury.
- An **impacted fracture** occurs when a fragment from one part of a fracture is driven into the tissue of another part.
- A **pathological fracture** occurs at the site of bone already damaged by disease.
- A **compression fracture** is a break in one or more vertebrae caused by a compressing or squeezing of the space between the vertebrae. Compression fractures often result from loss of bone density as in osteoporosis.

There are many other types of fractures; for example, an *avulsion fracture* is one caused by the pulling of a ligament and an *intracapsular fracture* is one within the capsule of a joint.

Figure 5-20 shows various types of fractures.

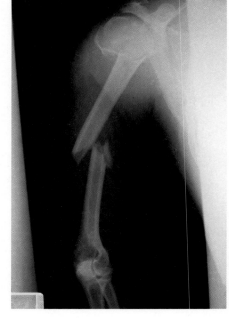

FIGURE 5-19 An x-ray of a complex fracture.

The National Library of Medicine has an online encyclopedia where you can learn more about almost any medical subject. Go to their Medline encyclopedia (www.nlm.nih.gov/medlineplus) and search for fractures to learn more about types and treatments for fractures.

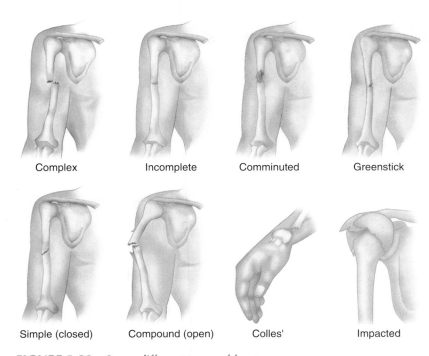

Complex   Incomplete   Comminuted   Greenstick

Simple (closed)   Compound (open)   Colles'   Impacted

FIGURE 5-20 Some different types of fractures.

MORE ABOUT . . .

Fractures

Some types of fractures are possible indicators of child abuse. This is particularly true of *spiral fractures,* fractures caused by twisting an extremity until the bone breaks. This type of fracture is usually investigated as to its cause in a child. Also, if a child's x-rays show a number of old fractures, child abuse may be suspected. Unfortunately, there are some diseases that cause continual bone fracturing and, as a result, some people have been falsely accused of child abuse in such cases.

FIGURE 5-21 The damage caused to the spine by osteoporosis.

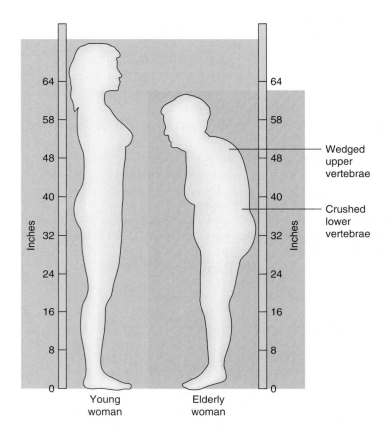

Injury or trauma to a ligament may cause a **sprain.** Overuse or improper use of a muscle may cause a **strain.** Overworking a joint may cause **tendinitis (tendonitis),** an inflammation of a tendon. **Dislocation** may result from an injury or from a strenuous, sudden movement. A **subluxation** is a partial dislocation. Bones may lose their density (**osteoporosis**). Figure 5-21 shows the damage caused by osteoporosis. **Contracture,** extreme resistance to stretching of a muscle, usually results from diseases of the muscle fibers or from an injury.

Pain in the musculoskeletal system may appear in the bones (**ostealgia, osteodynia**), muscles (**myalgia, myodynia**), or joints (**arthralgia**). Stiffness of the joints (**ankylosis**) may be an indicator of several diseases. **Spastic** muscles have abnormal contractions (**spasms**) in diseases such as multiple sclerosis. An abnormal increase in muscle size is **hyper-trophy. Flaccid** muscles are flabby in tone. **Hypotonia** is abnormally reduced muscle tension, and **rigor** (also called **rigidity**) is abnormal muscle stiffness as seen in lockjaw. **Dystonia** is abnormal tone (tension) in a muscle. A painfully long muscle contraction is **tetany.** Shaking (**tremors**) appears in a number of diseases such as Parkinson's Disease. Some muscles **atrophy** (shrink) as a result of disuse or specific diseases such as **muscular dystrophy,** a progressive, degenerative disorder affecting skeletal muscles. A muscle inflammation is **myositis.**

Some bone tissue dies (**bony necrosis, sequestrum**), often as a result of loss of blood supply. Abnormal bone growths may be capped with cartilage, as in **exostosis.** The bursa may become inflamed, causing **bursitis.** Inflammation of the bursa in the big toe causes a **bunion.** The epiphyses may also become inflamed, causing **epiphysitis.**

A common inflammation of the joints is **arthritis** (Figure 5-22). Arthritis is a name for many different joint diseases, such as **osteoarthritis** or **degenerative arthritis** (arthritis characterized by erosion of joint cartilage), **rheumatoid arthritis** (a systemic disease affecting connective tissue), and **gouty arthritis** or **gout** (a disease characterized by joint pain, as in **podagra,** pain in the big toe). Certain types of arthritis may cause **crepitation** (also called **crepitus**), noise made when affected surfaces rub together. Infections in the bone may cause **osteomyelitis.**

Cartilage may soften (**chondromalacia**) or become fragmented, as in a herniated disk. Disks may also slip or become misaligned with other vertebrae (**spondylolisthesis**) or become stiff (**spondylosis**). Various tumors may develop in the muscle, bone, bone marrow, and joints. **Myeloma, myoma, leiomyoma, leiomyosarcoma, rhabdomyoma, rhabdomyosarcoma, osteoma,** and **osteosarcoma** are types of musculoskeletal tumors.

Some abnormal posture conditions (**spinal curvature, kyphosis, lordosis,** and **scoliosis**) may cause pain (see Figure 5-23). Pain may even be felt in limbs that have been paralyzed or amputated. **Phantom limb** or **phantom pain** afflicts many who are paralyzed or are missing a limb. Repetitive motion of the hand may cause **carpal tunnel syndrome,** which is signaled by pain and paresthesia (numbness or tingling) of the hand. Chiropractors treat some spinal conditions by manipulation. **Physical therapy** is movement therapy to restore use of damaged areas of the body.

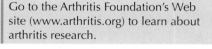
Go to the Arthritis Foundation's Web site (www.arthritis.org) to learn about arthritis research.

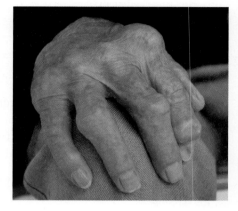

FIGURE 5-22   An arthritic hand.

Carpal tunnel syndrome usually requires some rest period. For people who work on computers this may be difficult. There are alternative devices, such as the hands-free mouse (it uses head motion) available at www.ctsplace.com.

FIGURE 5-23   The three types of spinal curvature.

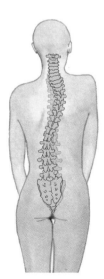 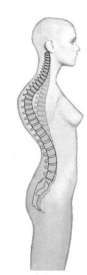 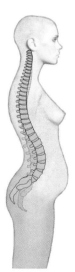

Scoliosis   Kyphosis ("hunchback")   Lordosis ("swayback")

MORE ABOUT . . .

Cartilage

The replacement of damaged or lost cartilage is now possible. The procedure is to remove some of a patient's cartilage through a small incision, grow more cartilage in the laboratory using the patient's own cells, and inject them back into the small incision.

MORE ABOUT . . .

What Fractures Can Tell Us

Fractures can be caused by many types of injuries or diseases. Osteoporosis in older people may result in hip fractures which, in many cases, are thought to precede the actual fall. A twisting fracture may result from a twisting injury in a sports game. A comminuted fracture may result from the impact of a car crash. The type of fracture often gives clues as to how the initial injury occurred.

VOCABULARY REVIEW

In the previous section, you learned terms relating to pathology. Before going on to the exercises, review the terms below and refer to the previous section if you have any questions. Pronunciations are provided for certain terms. Sometimes information about where the word came from is included after the term. These etymologies (word histories) are for your information only. You do not need to memorize them.

Term	Definition
ankylosis [ĂNG-kĭ-LŌ-sĭs]	Stiffening of a joint, especially as a result of disease.
arthralgia [ăr-THĂL-jē-ă] arthro-, joint + -algia, pain	Severe joint pain.
arthritis [ăr-THRĪ-tĭs] Greek, from arthro-, joint + -itis, inflammation	Any of various conditions involving joint inflammation.
atrophy [ĂT-rō-fē] Greek *atrophia*, without nourishment	Wasting away of tissue, organs, and cells, usually as a result of disease or loss of blood supply.
bony necrosis [nĕ-KRŌ-sĭs]	Death of portions of bone.
bunion [BŬN-yŭn]	An inflamed bursa at the foot joint, between the big toe and the first metatarsal bone.
bursitis [bŭr-SĪ-tĭs] burs(a) + -itis, inflammation	Inflammation of a bursa.
calcar [KĂL-kăr]	Spur.
carpal [KĂR-păl] **tunnel syndrome**	Pain and paresthesia in the hand due to repetitive motion injury of the median nerve.
chondromalacia [KŎN-drō-mă-LĀ-shē-ă] chondro-, cartilage + malacia, softening	Softening of cartilage.
closed fracture	Fracture with no open skin wound.
Colles' [kōlz] **fracture**	Fracture of the lower end of the radius.
comminuted [KŎM-ĭ-nū-tĕd] **fracture**	Fracture with shattered bones.

Term	Definition
complex fracture	Fracture with part of the bone displaced.
complicated fracture	Fracture involving extensive soft tissue injury.
compound fracture	Fracture with an open skin wound; open fracture.
compression fracture	Fracture of one or more vertebrae caused by compressing of the space between the vertebrae.
contracture [kŏn-TRĂK-chūr]	Extreme resistance to the stretching of a muscle.
crepitation, crepitus [krĕp-ĭ-TĀ-shŭn, KRĔP-ĭ-tŭs]	Noise made by rubbing together of bones.
degenerative arthritis	Arthritis with erosion of the cartilage.
dislocation	Movement of a joint out of its normal position as a result of an injury or sudden, strenuous movement.
dystonia [dĭs-TŌ-nē-ă]	Abnormal tone in tissues.
epiphysitis [ĕ-pĭf-ĭ-SĪ-tĭs]	Inflammation of the epiphysis.
exostosis [ĕks-ŏs-TŌ-sĭs] ex-, out of + ost(eo)-, bone + -osis, condition	Abnormal bone growth capped with cartilage.
flaccid [FLĂK-sĭd]	Without tone; relaxed.
fracture [FRĂK-chŭr]	A break, especially in a bone.
gouty arthritis, gout [GŎWT-ē, gŏwt]	Inflammation of the joints, present in gout; usually caused by uric acid crystals.
greenstick fracture	Fracture with twisting or bending of the bone but no breaking; usually occurs in children.
hairline fracture	Fracture with no bone separation or fragmentation.
herniated [HĔR-nē-ā-tĕd] **disk**	Protrusion of an intervertebral disk into the neural canal.
hypertrophy [hī-PĔR-trō-fē] hyper-, excessive + -trophy, growth	Abnormal increase as in muscle size.
hypotonia [HĪ-pō-TŌ-nē-ă] hypo-, subnormal + Greek *tonos*, tone	Abnormally reduced muscle tension.
impacted fracture	Fracture in which a fragment from one part of the fracture is driven into the tissue of another part.
incomplete fracture	Fracture that does not go entirely through a bone.
kyphosis [kī-FŌ-sĭs]	Abnormal posterior spine curvature.
leiomyoma [LĪ-ō-mī-Ō-mă] leio-, smooth + my(o)-, muscle + -oma, tumor	Benign tumor of smooth muscle.
leiomyosarcoma [LĪ-ō-MĪ-ō-săr-KŌ-mă] leio-, smooth + myo-, muscle + sarcoma	Malignant tumor of smooth muscle.

Term	Definition
lordosis [lōr-DŌ-sĭs]	Abnormal anterior spine curvature resulting in a sway back.
muscular dystrophy [MŬS-kyū-lăr DĬS-trō-fē]	Progressive degenerative disorder affecting the musculoskeletal system and, later, other organs.
myalgia [mī-ĂL-jē-ă] my(o)-, muscle + -algia, pain	Muscle pain.
myeloma [mī-ĕ-LŌ-mă] myel(o)-, bone marrow + -oma, tumor	Bone marrow tumor.
myodynia [MĪ-ō-DĬN-ē-ă] myo-, muscle + -dynia, pain	Muscle pain.
myoma [mī-Ō-mă] my(o)-, muscle + -oma, tumor	Benign muscle tumor.
myositis [mī-ō-SĪ-tĭs] myo-, muscle + -itis, inflammation	Inflammation of a muscle.
open fracture	Fracture with an open skin wound; compound fracture.
ostealgia [ŏs-tē-ĂL-jē-ă] oste(o)-, bone + -algia, pain	Bone pain.
osteoarthritis [ŎS-tē-ō-ăr-THRĪ-tĭs] osteo-, bone + arthritis	Arthritis with loss of cartilage.
osteodynia [ŏs-tē-ō-DĬN-ē-ă] osteo-, bone + -dynia, pain	Bone pain.
osteoma [ŏs-tē-Ō-mă] osteo-, bone + -oma, tumor	Benign bone tumor, usually on the skull or mandible.
osteomyelitis [ŎS-tē-ō-mī-ĕ-LĪ-tĭs] osteo-, bone + myel(o)-, bone marrow + -itis, inflammation	Inflammation of the bone marrow and surrounding bone.
osteoporosis [ŎS-tē-ō-pō-RŌ-sĭs] osteo-, bone + por(e) + -osis, condition	Degenerative thinning of bone.
osteosarcoma [ŎS-tē-ō-săr-KŌ-mă] osteo-, bone + sarcoma	Malignant tumor of bone.
pathological fracture	Fracture occurring at the site of already damaged bone.
phantom limb; phantom pain	Pain felt in a paralyzed or amputated limb.
physical therapy	Movement therapy to restore use of damaged areas of the body.
podagra [pō-DĂG-ră]	Pain in the big toe, often associated with gout.
rhabdomyoma [RĂB-dō-mī-Ō-mă] rhadbdo-, rod-shaped + my(o)-, muscle + -oma, tumor	Benign tumor in striated muscle.

Term	Definition
rhabdomyosarcoma [RĂB-dō-mĭ-ō-săr-KŌ-mă] rhabdo-, rod-shaped + myo-, muscle + sarcoma	Malignant tumor in striated muscle.
rheumatoid [RŪ-mă-tŏyd] **arthritis**	Autoimmune disorder affecting connective tissue.
rickets [RĬK-ĕts]	Disease of the skeletal system, usually caused by vitamin D deficiency.
rigidity	Stiffness.
rigor [RĬG-ōr]	Stiffening.
sciatica [sī-ĂT-ĭ-kă]	Pain in the lower back, usually radiating down the leg, from a herniated disk or other injury or condition.
scoliosis [skō-lē-Ō-sĭs]	Abnormal lateral curvature of the spinal column.
sequestrum [sē-KWĔS-trŭm]	Piece of dead tissue or bone separated from the surrounding area.
simple fracture	Fracture with no open skin wound.
spasm [spăzm]	Sudden, involuntary muscle contraction.
spastic [SPĂS-tĭk]	Tending to have spasms.
spina bifida [SPĪ-nă BĬF-ĭ-dă]	Congenital defect with deformity of the spinal column.
spinal curvature	Abnormal curvature of the spine.
spondylolisthesis [SPŎN-dĭ-lō-lĭs-THĒ-sĭs] spondyl(o)-, vertebrae + Greek *olisthesis*, slipping	Degenerative condition in which one vertebra misaligns with the one below it; slipped disk.
spondylolysis [spŏn-dĭ-LŌL-ĭ-sĭs] spondylo-, vertebrae + -lysis, destruction of	Degenerative condition of the moving part of a vertebra.
sprain [sprān]	Injury to a joint without dislocation or fracture. (can involve a ligament). This is worse than a strain and often takes longer to heal than does a fracture and can be more painful.
spur [spŭr]	Bony projection growing out of a bone; calcar.
strain [strān]	Injury to a muscle as a result of improper use or overuse.
subluxation [sŭb-lŭk-SĀ-shŭn]	Partial dislocation, as between joint surfaces.
talipes calcaneus [TĂL-ĭ-pēz kăl-KĀ-nē-ŭs]	Deformity of the heel resulting from weakened calf muscles.
talipes valgus [VĂL-gŭs]	Foot deformity characterized by eversion of the foot.
talipes varus [VĀ-rŭs]	Foot deformity characterized by inversion of the foot.
tendinitis, tendonitis [tĕn-dĭn-ĪT-ĭs]	Inflammation of a tendon.
tetany [TĔT-ă-nē]	Painfully long muscle contraction.
tremor [TRĔM-ōr]	Abnormal, repetitive muscle contractions.

Making a Referral

Dr. Millet, a chiropractor, sees many patients for back pain. His treatments consist primarily of spinal manipulation, heat, and nutritional and exercise counseling. He currently sees a group of patients, mainly middle-aged men, who complain of sciatica. He has been able to relieve the pain for about 50 percent of them. The others seem to have more persistent pain. Dr. Millet is not allowed to prescribe medications because he is not a licensed medical doctor. He refers some of his patients to Dr. Wolf, a specialist, who believes that Dr. Millet provides a valuable service.

Critical Thinking

107. Chiropractic is one way for some people to manage pain. Why might spinal manipulation help?

108. If spinal manipulation does not work, why should the patient see a medical specialist?

PATHOLOGICAL TERMS EXERCISES

Build Your Medical Vocabulary

Match the word roots on the left with the proper definition on the right.

109. ____ myo-	a.	bone
110. ____ myelo-	b.	hand
111. ____ rhabdo-	c.	rod-shaped
112. ____ osteo-	d.	joint
113. ____ arthro-	e.	bone marrow
114. ____ chiro-	f.	muscle

Know the Word Parts

Match the following terms with the letter that gives the best definition.

115. ____ myeloma	a.	malignant tumor of smooth muscle
116. ____ myoma	b.	benign tumor in striated muscle
117. ____ leiomyoma	c.	benign tumor of smooth muscle
118. ____ leiomyosarcoma	d.	benign muscle tumor
119. ____ rhabdomyoma	e.	malignant bone tumor
120. ____ rhabdomyosarcoma	f.	bone marrow tumor
121. ____ osteoma	g.	malignant tumor in striated muscle
122. ____ osteosarcoma	h.	benign tumor, usually on the skull or mandible

Check Your Knowledge

Complete the sentences below by filling in the blanks.

123. A patient with painful joints and bulges around the knuckles probably has _____.

124. Fractures that are most likely to occur in young children are called _____ fractures.

125. Osteoporosis is usually a disease found in _____ women.

126. Playing tennis too vigorously may cause _____ of the elbow.

127. Underworked muscles may become _____.

128. A muscle tumor is a(n) _____.

129. A slipped disk is called _____.

130. A compound fracture is a break accompanied by a(n) _____ wound.

131. Arthritis is a general term for a number of _____ diseases.

132. Paralysis may be caused by an injury to the _____.

133. A break in soft bone is a(n) _____ fracture.

134. A strain is a(n) _____ of the muscle, while a(n) _____ is a torn or damaged ligament or damaged muscle due to trauma or injury.

135. An injury or a strenuous, sudden movement of a joint may result in _____.

136. A partial dislocation is called a(n) _____.

137. Pain in the muscle is called _____ or _____.

138. Pain in the bone is called _____.

139. Pain in the joints is called _____.

140. The suffix–desis means fixation or fusion, so the fixing of a joint so it does not move it is called _____ desis.

141. Hypertrophy is an increase in muscle _____, while hypertonia is an increase in muscle _____.

142. Abnormal muscle tone is called _____.

143. An infection in the bone is _____.

144. Repetitive motion of the hand may cause _____.

Know the Fractures

Write the letter of the correct fracture description in the space provided.

145. ____ closed fracture

146. ____ open fracture

147. ____ simple fracture

148. ____ greenstick fracture

149. ____ comminuted fracture

150. ____ impacted fracture

151. ____ pathological fracture

152. ____ compression fracture

a. break with shattered bones

b. break that does not move the bone out of place

c. break with no open wound

d. break with an open wound

e. incomplete break of a soft bone

f. break in a vertebrae caused by compression

g. fragment from one part of the bone driven into the tissue of another part

h. break in bone due to disease (bone may be already diseased in that area)

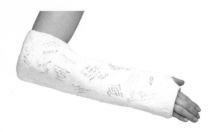

FIGURE 5-24 A cast is an external fixation device.

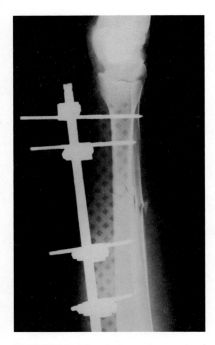

FIGURE 5-25 Surgery is required to place internal fixation devices.

Historically, before the advent of antibiotics, limb amputations were often necessary due to infections or wounds that would have no way to heal. Now, amputations are much rarer. New techniques of bone repair and infection control make it more likely that they can be avoided.

Surgical Terms

Orthopedic surgery may involve repair, grafting, replacement, excision, or reconstruction of parts of the musculoskeletal system. Surgeons also make incisions to take biopsies. Almost any major part of the musculoskeletal system can now be surgically replaced. In some situations (as with loss of circulation in diabetes, cancer of a limb, or severe infection), **amputation** may be necessary. **Prosthetic devices** now routinely replace knees and hips, as when injury or degenerative disease has worn down joints. **Bone grafting** can be used to repair a defect. An **orthosis** or **orthotic** may be used to provide support and prevent movement during treatment.

Fractures are treated by **casting, splinting,** surgical manipulation, or placement in **traction.** Casts and splints are considered **external fixation devices**—devices that surround a fractured body part to hold the bones in place while healing (see Figure 5-24). They may be used in combination with an **internal fixation device,** such as a pin placed internally to hold bones together (see Figure 5-25). Pins for internal fixation are usually metal or hard plastic. A pin may be placed permanently or it may be removed after the bone has healed. **Reduction** is the return of a part to its normal position. An *open reduction* is done surgically to repair either fractured or dislocated bones; a *closed reduction* is external manipulation used for dislocated bones, such as a shoulder bone. In some surgeries, artificial bone is now being used. Some products in development may actually replace injured or diseased bone and allow for new bone growth while gradually dissolving as it is not needed.

Osteoplasty is repair of a bone. **Osteoclasis** is the breaking of bone for the purpose of repairing it (as when a fracture has not healed properly). **Osteotomy** is an incision into a bone. **Tenotomy** is the cutting into a tendon to repair a muscle. **Myoplasty** is muscle repair. **Arthroplasty** is joint repair. **Arthrocentesis** is a puncture into a joint. A **synovectomy** is the removal of part or all of the synovial membrane of a joint. **Arthrodesis** and **spondylosyndesis** are two types of fusion. A **bursectomy** is the removal of an affected bursa. A **bunionectomy** is the removal of a bunion. This operation it usually performed on the *great toe*. Other types of toe repair may correct such things as *hammer toe*, where one or more toes are permanently flexed to one side. Some musculoskeletal surgery is done by arthroscopy. **Laminectomy** or removal of part of a spinal disk may alleviate the pain of a herniated disk.

VOCABULARY REVIEW

In the previous section, you learned terms relating to surgery. Before going on to the exercises, review the terms below and refer to the previous section if you have questions. Pronunciations are provided for certain terms. Sometimes information about where the word came from is included after the term. These etymologies (word histories) are for your information only. You do not need to memorize them.

Term	Definition
amputation [ĂM-pyū-TĀ-shŭn]	Cutting off of a limb or part of a limb.
arthrocentesis [ĂR-thrō-sĕn-TĒ-sĭs] arthro-, joint + Greek *kentesis*, puncture	Removal of fluid from a joint with use of a puncture needle.
arthrodesis [ăr-thrō-DĒ-sĭs] arthro-, + Greek *desis*, a binding	Surgical fusion of a joint to stiffen it.
arthroplasty [ĂR-thrō-plăs-tē] arthro- + -plasty, repair	Surgical replacement or repair of a joint.
bone grafting	Transplantation of bone from one site to another.
bunionectomy [bŭn-yŭn-ĔK-tō-mē] bunion + -ectomy, removal	Removal of a bunion.
bursectomy [bŭr-SĔK-tō-mĕ] burs(a) + -ectomy, removal	Removal of a bursa.
casting	Forming of a cast in a mold; placing of fiberglass or plaster over a body part to prevent its movement.
external fixation device	Device applied externally to hold a limb in place.
internal fixation device	Device, such as a pin, inserted in bone to hold it in place.
laminectomy [LĂM-ĭ-NĔK-tō-mē] lamin(a) + -ectomy, removal	Removal of part of an intervertebral disk.
myoplasty [MĪ-ō-plăs-tē] myo-, muscle + -plasty, repair	Surgical repair of muscle tissue.
orthosis, orthotic [ōr-THŌ-sĭs, ōr-THŎT-ĭk]	External appliance used to immobilize or assist the movement of the spine or limbs.
osteoclasis [ŎS-tē-ŎK-lā-sĭs] osteo-, bone + -clasis, breaking	Breaking of a bone in order to repair or reposition it.
osteoplasty [ŎS-tē-ō-plăs-tē] osteo-, bone + -plasty, repair	Surgical replacement or repair of bone.
osteotomy [ŏs-tē-ŎT-ō-mē] osteo-, bone + -tomy, cutting	Cutting of bone.
prosthetic [prŏs-THĔT-ĭk] **device**	Artificial device used as a substitute for a missing or diseased body part.
reduction	Return of a part to its normal position.
splinting	Applying a splint to immobilize a body part.
spondylosyndesis [SPŎN-dĭ-lō-sĭn-DĒ-sĭs] spondylo-, vertebrae + Greek *syndesis*, a binding together	Fusion of two or more spinal vertebrae.
synovectomy [sĭn-ō-VĔK-tō-mē] synovi(o)-, synovial fluid + -ectomy, removal	Removal of part or all of a joint's synovial membrane.
tenotomy [tĕ-NŎT-ō-mē] teno-, tendon + -tomy, cutting	Surgical cutting of a tendon.
traction [TRĂK-shŭn]	Dragging or pulling or straightening of something, as a limb, by attachment of elastic or other devices.

CASE STUDY

Musculoskeletal Injury

John Positano, a track star at a large university, suffered a knee injury during a meet. The team physician prescribed rest and medication first, to be followed by a gradual program of physical therapy. John missed about six weeks of meets and seemed fine until the end of the season, when a particularly strenuous run in which he twisted his knee left him writhing in pain. It was the same knee on which fluid had accumulated during the previous week. X-rays showed no fractures. Later, after examination by a specialist, arthroscopic surgery was recommended. John had to go through another rehabilitative program (rest, medication, and physical therapy) after the surgery.

Critical Thinking

153. A program of physical therapy was prescribed for John. Which one of his tests was most important in determining whether or not he could exercise?

154. Is physical therapy always appropriate for a musculoskeletal injury?

SURGICAL TERMS EXERCISES

Build Your Medical Vocabulary

Form two surgical words for each of the following word roots by adding suffixes learned in Chapter 2.

155. osteo- _____

156. arthro-_____

157. myo- _____

158. spondylo- _____

Find a Match

Match the terms in the second column to the terms in the first.

159. _____ amputation   **a.** replacement device

160. _____ prosthesis   **b.** molding

161. _____ orthosis, orthotic   **c.** muscle repair

162. _____ traction   **d.** bone cutting

163. _____ casting   **e.** limb removal

164. _____ splinting   **f.** bone repair

165. _____ myoplasty   **g.** external supporting or immobilizing device

166. _____ osteoplasty   **h.** wrapping to immobilize

167. _____ osteotomy   **i.** pulling to straighten

168. _____ arthroplasty   **j.** joint repair

Understanding Surgical Procedures

Explain the following surgical terms in simple words.

169. reduction (of a bone) _____

170. synovectomy _____

171. arthrodesis _____

172. bunionectomy _____

173. laminectomy _____

174. orthotic _____

175. arthrocentesis _____

Pharmacological Terms

Most medications for treatment of the musculoskeletal system treat symptoms, not causes. Pain medications, such as **analgesics, narcotics, anti-inflammatories (corticosteroids), muscle relaxants,** and **nonsteroidal anti-inflammatory drugs (NSAIDs),** all relieve or relax the area of pain either by numbing the area or by reducing the inflammation. Table 5-1 shows some common medications.

TABLE 5-1 Some Medications for the Musculoskeletal System

Drug Class	Purpose	Generic	Trade Name
analgesic	to relieve pain	aspirin acetaminophen (NSAIDs are also analgesics.)	Bayer, Excedrin, and various Tylenol and various
anti-inflammatory (corticosteroids)	to reduce inflammation	prednisone (Aspirin and NSAIDs also reduce inflammation.)	Deltasone, Orasone, Cortan
muscle relaxant	to relieve stiffness	carisoprodol cyclobenzaprine methocarbamol	Soma Flexeril Delaxin, Robaxin
NSAIDs	to reduce inflammation	ibuprofen naproxen ketorolac, tromethamine nabutemone	Advil, Motrin, Nuprin Naproxyn Toradol (IV) Relafen

VOCABULARY REVIEW

In the previous section, you learned terms relating to pharmacology. Before going on to the exercises, review the terms below and refer to the previous section if you have questions. Pronunciations are provided for certain terms.

Sometimes information about where the word came from is included after the term. These etymologies (word histories) are for your information only. You do not need to memorize them.

Term	Definition
analgesic [ăn-ăl-JĒ-zĭk]	Agent that relieves pain.
anti-inflammatory (corticosteroid)	Agent that reduces inflammation.
muscle relaxant	Agent that relieves muscle stiffness.
narcotic	Agent that relieves pain by affecting the body in ways that are similar to opium.
nonsteroidal [nŏn-STĔR-ŏy-dăl] anti-inflammatory drug (NSAID)	Agent that reduces inflammation without the use of steroids.

CASE STUDY

Treating the Symptoms

In her follow-up letter on Laura Spinoza's visit, Dr. Wolf listed a number of medications to treat the symptoms of fibromyalgia. Part of the difficulty in treating musculoskeletal disorders is that many of the diseases are degenerative, and damage cannot be reversed. Some of these diseases, such as muscular dystrophy, currently have no cure. Many forms of arthritis are degenerative and, short of replacing joints, cannot be improved significantly. Alleviating the pain is the only available course of treatment in many instances.

Critical Thinking

176. Narcotics can be addictive. The long-term use of steroids can cause other health problems. What does Dr. Wolf prescribe to avoid these two problems?

177. Many athletes use anabolic steroids illegally for strength and endurance building. (Corticosteroids are not used for this purpose.) Anabolic-steroid use can cause heart damage and many other serious health problems. What are some ways to increase strength and endurance without the use of dangerous drugs?

PHARMACOLOGICAL TERMS EXERCISES

Fill in the Blank

Choose one or more of the following terms to fill in each blank. Each term may be used more than once.

analgesic   anti-inflammatory   antibiotic

178. Treatment for bursitis _____.

179. Treatment for myalgia _____.

180. Treatment for bone infection _____.

181. Treatment for arthritis _____.

182. Treatment for arthralgia _____.

CHALLENGE SECTION

The notes of Janet Azrah's examination give the results of all observations and tests. The treatment protocol is described.

Critical Thinking

183. The notes in this section indicate a probable diagnosis of rheumatoid arthritis. Was the musculoskeletal examination normal?

184. Why might a physician perform a general examination on a patient who only shows symptoms related to the musculoskeletal system?

TERMINOLOGY IN ACTION

After an x-ray given in the emergency room, Ellen was told that she would need to be seen by the orthopedist on call. The notes in her chart are as follows:

> X-RAY: X-ray of the right wrist reveals distal radial fracture with about 20 degrees dorsal angulation and displaced about 30% from normal position. There is no ulnar fracture. Right knee x-ray shows a fracture of the patella with no displacement of the fragments.

From the notes, describe what she has fractured and what you think the treatment will be.

USING THE INTERNET

Osteoporosis can be a serious affliction of late adulthood. Visit the National Osteoporosis Foundation's Web site (http://www.nof.org). From what you read at the site, what can you do to prevent osteoporosis as you age?

CHAPTER REVIEW

The material that follows is to help you review all the material in this chapter.

Explain the Terms

Write out the following sentences in lay terms.

185. The pt had a Fx of L1 _____

186. The ROM was decreased in the right shoulder due to myalgia _____

187. The pt was placed on an NSAID due to OA _____

188. The pt has CTS, it is B _____

189. The pt has severe RA, which has caused arthrodynia and hypertonic muscles in the R leg _____

190. On review of the medical history, the pt has TMJ, CTS, has had a Fx of the R wrist, has some DJD _____

191. On examination it was found the DTR of the R leg was decreased. The ROM was also decreased on the R side of the body. The muscles in the R leg were flaccid and hypotonic _____

Know the Medical Terms

Rewrite the following sentences to include proper medical terminology and abbreviations.

192. The patient came in today for a test that uses electricity to check muscle activity _____

_____

193. The pt will have a below the knee amputation on his right leg due to severe frostbite _____

_____

194. The child's break needs to be set _____

_____

True or False

For each of the following statements, circle T for true or F for false.

195. The clavicle is the posterior shoulder bone. T F

196. The femur is the upper arm bone. T F

197. The tibia is a flat bone on the front of the leg. T F

198. The sternum is also known as the breastbone. T F

199. The coccyx is also known as the tailbone. T F

200. The cervical vertebrae attach to ribs. T F

201. The false ribs do not attach to the sternum. T F

202. A tight muscle could be considered hypotonic. T F

203. A massage therapist would help someone with subluxations. T F

204. A chiropractor works only on the spine. T F

205. The radius is a bone in the leg. T F

206. The patella is another name for kneecap. T F

207. A fracture is considered a break in the continuity of the bone. T F

208. There are many types of fractures. T F

209. A fracture always goes completely through the bone. T F

DEFINITIONS

Define the following terms and combining forms. Review the chapter before starting. Make sure you know how to pronounce each term as you define it. The blue words in curly brackets are references to the Spanish glossary the student Web site (www.mhhe.com/medterm3e).

WORD

210. acetabul(o)

211. acetabulum [ăs-ĕ-TĂB-yū-lŭm] {acetábulo}

212. acromi(o)

213. acromion [ă-KRŌ-mē-ōn] {acromion}

214. amphiarthrosis [ĂM-fĭ-ăr-THRŌ-sĭs] {anfiartrosis}

215. amputation [ĂM-pyū-TĀ-shŭn] {amputación}

216. analgesic [ăn-ăl-JĒ-zĭk]

217. ankle [ĂNG-kl] {tobillo}

218. ankyl(o)

219. ankylosis [ĂNG-kĭ-LŌ-sĭs] {anquilosis}

220. anti-inflammatory

221. arthr(o)

222. arthralgia [ăr-THRĂL-jē-ă] {artralgia}

223. arthritis [ăr-THRĬ-tĭs] {artritis}

224. arthrocentesis [ĂR-thrō-sĕn-TĒ-sĭs] {artrocentesis}

225. arthrodesis [ăr-thrō-DĒ-sĭs]

226. arthrography [ăr-THRŎG-ră-fē]

227. arthroplasty [ĂR-thrō-plăs-tē]

228. arthroscopy [ăr-THRŌS-kŏ-pē]

229. articular [ăr-TĬK-yū-lăr] cartilage

230. articulation [ăr-tĭk-yū-LĀ-shŭn] {articulación}

231. atlas [ĂT-lăs] {atlas}

232. atrophy [ĂT-rō-fē] {atrofia}

233. axis [ĂK-sĭs] {axis}

234. bone {hueso}

235. bone grafting

236. bone head

237. bone phagocyte [FĂG-ō-sīt]

238. bone scan

239. bony necrosis [nĕ-KRŌ-sĭs]

240. brachi(o)

241. bunion [BŬN-yŭn] {bunio}

242. bunionectomy [bŭn-yŭn-ĔK-tō-mē] {bunionectomía}

243. burs(o)

244. bursa (*pl.*, bursae) [BŬR-să (BŬR-sē)] {bursa}

245. bursectomy [bŭr-SĔK-tō-mē] {bursectomía}

246. bursitis [bŭr-SĪ-tĭs] {bursitis}

247. calcane(o)

248. calcaneus [kăl-KĀ-nē-ŭs] {calcáneo}

249. calcar [KĂL-kăr] {calcar}

250. calci(o)

251. calcium [KĂL-sē-ŭm] {calcio}

252. cancellous [KĂN-sĕ-lŭs] {canceloso} bone

253. cardiac [KĂR-dē-ăk] muscle

254. carp(o)

255. carpal [KĂR-păl] tunnel syndrome

256. carpus [KĂR-pŭs], carpal bone

257. cartilage [KĂR-tĭ-lăj] {cartílago}

258. cartilaginous [kăr-tĭ-LĂJ-ĭ-nŭs] disk

259. casting {colado}

260. cephal(o)

261. cervic(o)

262. cervical [SĔR-vĭ-kăl] vertebrae

263. chiropractor [kī-rō-PRĂK-tĕr] {quiropráctico}

264. chondr(o)

265. chondromalacia [KŎN-drō-mă-LĀ-shē-ă] {condromalacia}

266. clavicle [KLĂV-ĭ-kl] {clavicula}

267. closed fracture

268. coccyx [KŎK-sĭks] {cóccix}

269. Colles' [kōlz] fracture

270. comminuted [KŎM-ĭ-nū-tĕd] fracture

271. compact bone

272. complex fracture

273. complicated fracture

274. compound fracture

275. compression fracture

276. condyl(o)

277. condyle [KŎN-dīl]

278. contracture [kŏn-TRĂK-chŭr]

279. corticosteroid

280. cost(o)

281. crani(o)

282. crepitation [krĕ-pĭ-TĀ-shŭn], crepitus [KRĔP-ĭ-tŭs]

283. crest {cresta}

284. dactyl(o)

285. degenerative arthritis

286. densitometer [děn-sǐ-TŎM-ě-těr]
287. diaphysis [dī-ĂF-ǐ-sǐs] {diáfisis}
288. diarthroses [dī-ǎr-THRŌ-sēz]
289. disk [dǐsk] {disco}
290. diskography [dǐs-KŎG-ră-fē] {discografía}
291. dislocation {dislocación}
292. dorsal vertebrae
293. dystonia [dǐs-TŌ-nē-ǎ] {distonia}
294. elbow [ĚL-bō] {codo}
295. electromyogram [ē-lěk-trō-MĪ-ō-grăm] {electromiógrafo}
296. endosteum [ěn-DŎS-tē-ŭm] {endostio}
297. epiphyseal [ěp-ǐ-FĬZ-ē-ǎl] plate
298. epiphysitis [ě-pǐf-ǐ-SĪ-tǐs] {epifisitis}
299. ethmoid [ĚTH-mǒyd] bone
300. ethmoid sinuses
301. exostosis [ěks-ŏs-TŌ-sǐs] {exostosis}
302. external fixation device
303. fasci(o)
304. fascia (pl., fasciae [FĂSH-ē-ǎ (FĂSH-ē-ē)] {fascia}
305. femor(o)
306. femur [FĒ-mūr] {fémur}
307. fibr(o)
308. fibula [FĬB-yū-lǎ] {peroné}
309. fissure [FĬSH-ŭr] {fisura}
310. flaccid [FLĂK-sǐd] {fláccido}
311. flat bones
312. fontanelle [FŎN-tǎ-něl] {fontanela}
313. foramen [fō-RĀ-měn] {agujero}
314. foramen magnum [MĂG-nŭm]
315. fossa (pl., fossae) [FŎS-ǎ (FŎS-ē)] {fosa}
316. fracture [FRĂK-chŭr] {fractura}
317. frontal [FRŬN-tǎl] bone

318. frontal sinuses
319. goniometer [gō-nē-ŎM-ě-těr] {goniómetro}
320. gouty arthritis, gout [GŎWT-ē, gŏwt]
321. greenstick fracture
322. hairline fracture
323. heel [hēl] {talon}
324. herniated [HĔR-nē-ā-těd] disk
325. humer(o)
326. humerus [HYŪ-měr-ŭs] {húmero}
327. hypertrophy [hī-PĔR-trō-fē]
328. hypotonia [HĪ-pō-TŌ-nē-ǎ]
329. ili(o)
330. ilium [ĬL-ē-ŭm] {ilium}
331. impacted fracture
332. incomplete fracture
333. insertion {inserción}
334. internal fixation device
335. intervertebral [ǐn-těr-VĔR-tě-brǎl] disk
336. involuntary muscle
337. irregular bones
338. ischi(o)
339. ischium [ĬS-kē-ŭm] {isquión}
340. joint [jǒynt] {empalme}
341. kyph(o)
342. kyphosis [kī-FŌ-sǐs] {cifosis}
343. lacrimal [LĂK-rǐ-mǎl] bone
344. lamin(o)
345. lamina (pl., laminae) [LĂM-ǐ-nǎ(LĂM-ǐ-nē)] {lamina}
346. laminectomy [LĂM-ǐ-NĔK-tō-mē]
347. leiomy(o)
348. leiomyoma [LĪ-ō-mī-Ō-mǎ]
349. leiomyosarcoma [LĪ-ō-MĪ-ō-sǎr-KŌmǎ]
350. ligament [LĬG-ǎ-měnt] {ligamento}
351. long bone
352. lordosis [lōr-DŌ-sǐs] {lordosis}

353. lumb(o)
354. lumbar [LŬM-bǎr] vertebrae
355. malleolus (pl., malleoli) [mǎ-LĒ-ō-lŭs (mǎ-LĒ-ō-lī)]
356. mandible [MĂN-dǐ-bl] {mandíbula}
357. mandibular [măn-DĬB-yū-lǎr]
358. marrow [MĂR-ō] {médula}
359. mastoid [MĂS-tǒyd] process
360. maxill(o)
361. maxillary [MĂK-sǐ-lār-ē] bone
362. maxillary sinus
363. medullary [MĔD-ū-lār-ē] cavity
364. metacarp(o)
365. metacarpal [MĔT-ǎ-KĂR-pǎl] {metacarpiano}
366. metaphysis [mě-TĂF-ǐ-sǐs] {metáfisis}
367. metatarsal [MĔT-ǎ-tǎr-sǎl] bones
368. muscle [MŬS-ěl] {músculo}
369. muscle relaxant
370. muscular dystrophy [MŬS-kyū-lǎr DĬS-trō-fē] {distrofia muscular}
371. musculoskeletal [MŬS-kyū-lō-SKĔL-ě-tǎl] {musculoesquelético} system
372. my(o)
373. myalgia [mī-ĂL-jē-ǎ] {mialgia}
374. myel(o)
375. myelography [MĪ-ě-LŎG-ră-fē] {mielografia}
376. myeloma [mī-ě-LŌ-mǎ] {mieloma}
377. myodynia [MĪ-ō-DĬN-ē-ǎ] {miodinia}
378. myoma [mī-Ō-mǎ] {mioma}
379. myoplasty [MĪ-ō-plǎs-tē]
380. myositis [mī-ō-SĪ-tǐs] {miositis}
381. narcotic
382. nasal bones

383. nasal cavity

384. neural [NŪR-ăl] canal

385. nonsteroidal [nŏn-STĔR-ŏy-dăl] anti-inflammatory drug (NSAID)

386. nucleus pulposus [NŪ-klē-ŭs pŭl-PŌ-sŭs]

387. occipital [ŏk-SĬP-ĭ-tăl] bone

388. olecranon [ō-LĔK-ră-nŏn] {olecranon}

389. open fracture

390. origin {origen}

391. orthopedist [ōr-thō-PĒ-dĭst], orthopedic [ōr-thō-PĒ-dĭk] {ortopedista} surgeon

392. orthosis [ōr-THŌ-sĭs], orthotic [ōr-THŎT-ĭk] {ortosis, ortótica}

393. osseus [ŎS-ē-ŭs] tissue

394. ossification [ŎS-ĭ-fĭ-KĀ-shŭn] {ossificación}

395. oste(o)

396. ostealgia [ŏs-tĕ-ĂL-jē-ă] {ostealgia}

397. osteoarthritis [ŎS-tē-ō-ăr-THRĪ-tĭs] {osteoartritis}

398. osteoblast [ŎS-tē-ō-blăst] {osteoblasto}

399. osteoclasis [ŎS-tē-ŎK-lā-sĭs] {osteoclasia}

400. osteoclast [ŎS-tē-ō-klăst] {osteoclasto}

401. osteocyte [ŎS-tē-ō-sīt] {osteocito}

402. osteodynia [ŏs-tē-ō-DĬN-ē-ă] {osteodinia}

403. osteoma [ŏs-tē-Ō-mă] {osteoma}

404. osteomyelitis [ŎS-tē-ō-mī-ĕ-LĪ-tĭs] {osteomielitis}

405. osteopath [ŎS-tē-ō-păth] {osteópata}

406. osteoplasty [ŎS-tē-ō-plăs-tē] {osteoplastia}

407. osteoporosis [ŎS-tē-ō-pō-RŌ-sĭs] {osteoporosis}

408. osteosarcoma [ŎS-tē-ō-săr-KŌ-mă] {osteosarcoma}

409. osteotomy [ŏs-tē-ŎT-ō-mē] {osteotomía}

410. palatine [PĂL-ă-tīn] bone

411. parietal [pă-RĪ-ĕ-tăl] bone

412. patell(o)

413. patella [pă-TĔL-ă] {rótula}

414. pathological fracture

415. ped(i), ped(o)

416. pelv(i)

417. pelvic [PĔL-vĭk] cavity

418. pelvic girdle

419. pelvis [PĔL-vĭs] {pelvis}

420. periosteum [pĕr-ē-ŎS-tē-ŭm] {periostio}

421. phalang(o)

422. phalanges (sing., phalanx) [fă-LĂN-jēz (FĂ-lăngks)] {falangeo}

423. phantom limb; phantom pain

424. phosphorus [FŎS-fōr-ŭs] {fósforo}

425. physical therapy

426. pod(o)

427. podagra [pō-DĂG-ră] {podagra}

428. podiatrist [pō-DĪ-ă-trĭst] {podiatra}

429. process [PRŌS-sĕs, PRŌS-ĕs]

430. prosthetic [prŏs-THĔT-ĭk] device

431. pub(o)

432. pubes [PYŪ-bĭs] {pubis}

433. pubic symphysis [PYŪ-bĭk SĬM-fĭ-sĭs]

434. rachi(o)

435. radi(o)

436. radius [RĀ-dē-ŭs] {radio}

437. reduction {reducción}

438. rhabd(o)

439. rhabdomy(o)

440. rhabdomyoma [RĂB-dō-mī-Ō-mă] {rabdomioma}

441. rhabdomyosarcoma [RĂB-dō-mī-ō-săr-KŌ-mă] {rabdomiosarcoma}

442. rheumatoid arthritis

443. rheumatoid factor test

444. rheumatologist [rū-mă-TŎL-ō-jĭst] {reumatólogo}

445. rib {costilla}

446. rickets [RĬK-ĕts] {raquitismo}

447. rigidity {rigidez}

448. rigor [RĬG-ōr] {rigor}

449. sacrum [SĀ-krŭm] {sacro}

450. scapul(o)

451. scapula [SKĂP-yū-lă] {escápula}

452. sciatica [sī-ĂT-ĭ-kă] {ciática}

453. scoli(o)

454. scoliosis [skō-lē-Ō-sĭs] {escolisis}

455. sella turcica [SĔL-ă-TŬR-sĭ-kă] {silla turcica}

456. sequestrum [sĕ-KWĔS-trŭm] {secuestro}

457. serum calcium

458. serum creatine phosphokinase [SĒR-ŭm KRĒ-ă-tēn fŏs-fō-KĪ-nās]

459. serum phosphorus

460. sesamoid [SĔS-ă-mŏyd] bone

461. shin [shĭn] {espinilla}

462. short bones

463. simple fracture

464. sinus [SĪ-nŭs] {seno}

465. skeleton [SKĔL-ĕ-tŏn] {esqueleto}

466. smooth muscle

467. spasm [spăzm] {espasmo}

468. spastic [SPĂS-tĭk] {espástico}

469. sphenoid [SFĒ-nŏyd] bone

470. sphenoid sinus

471. spina bifida [SPĪ-nă BĬF-ĭ-dă] {espina bífido}

472. spinal column

473. spinal curvature
474. spinous [SPĪ-nŭs] process
475. splinting {ferulización}
476. spondyl(o)
477. spondylolisthesis [SPŎN-dĭ-lō-lĭs-THĒ-sĭs] {espondilolistesis}
478. spondylolysis [spŏn-dĭ-LŎL-ĭ-sĭs] {espodilolisis}
479. spondylosyndesis [SPON-di-lō-sin-DĒ-sĭs] {espondilosindesis}
480. spongy bone
481. sprain [sprān]
482. spur [spŭr]
483. stern(o)
484. sternum [STĔR-nŭm] {esternón}
485. strain [strān] {distender}
486. striated [strī-ĀT-ĕd] muscle
487. styloid [STĪ-lŏyd] process
488. subluxation [sŭb-lŭk-SĀ-shŭn] {subluxación}
489. sulcus (pl., sulci) [SŬL-kŭs, [SŬL-sī] {surco}
490. suture [SŪ-chūr] {sutura}
491. symphysis [SĬM-fĭ-sĭs] {sinfisis}
492. synarthrosis [SĬN-ăr-THRŌ-sĭs] {sinartrosis}
493. synov(o)

494. synovectomy [sĭn-ō-VĔK-tō-mē] {sinovectomi}
495. synovial [sĭ-NŌ-vē-ăl] fluid
496. synovial joint
497. synovial membrane
498. talipes calcaneus [TĂL-ĭ-pēz kăl-KĀ-nē-ŭs]
499. talipes valgus [TĂL-ĭ-pēz VĂL-gŭs]
500. talipes varus [TĂL-ĭ-pēz VĀ-rŭs]
501. tars(o)
502. tarsus, tarsal [TĂR-sŭs, TĂR-săl] bones
503. temporal [TĔM-pō-RĂL] bone
504. temporomandibular [TĔM-pō-rō-măn-DĬB-yū-lăr] joint
505. ten(o), tend(o), tendin(o)
506. tendinitis, tendonitis {tendonitis}
507. tendon [TĔN-dŏn] {tendon}
508. tenotomy [tĕ-NŎT-ō-mē] {tenotomía}
509. tetany [TĔT-ă-nē] {tetania}
510. thorac(o)
511. thoracic [thō-RĂS-ĭk] vertebrae
512. thorax [THŌ-răks] {tórax}
513. tibi(o)

514. tibia [TĬB-ē-ă] {tibia}
515. Tinel's [tĭ-NĔLZ] sign
516. traction [TRĂK-shŭn] {tracción}
517. transverse process
518. tremor [TRĔM-ōr] {temblor}
519. trochanter [trō-KĂN-těr] {trocánter}
520. true ribs
521. tubercle [TŪ-běr-kl] {tubérculo}
522. tuberosity [TŪ-běr-ŏs-ĭ-tē] {tuberosidad}
523. uln(o)
524. ulna [ŬL-nă] {ulna}
525. uric [YŪR-ĭk] acid test
526. vertebr(o)
527. vertebra (pl., vertebrae) [VĔR-tĕ-bră (VĔR-tĕ-brē)] {vertebra}
528. vertebral [věr-TĔ-brăl, VĔR-tĕ-brăl] body
529. vertebral column
530. visceral [VĬS-ĕr-ăl] muscle
531. vitamin D
532. voluntary muscle
533. vomer [VŌ-měr] {vómer}
534. zygomatic [ZĪ-gō-MĂT-ĭk] bone

Abbreviations

Write out the full meaning of each abbreviation.

535. A-K
536. ASIS
537. B-K
538. C_1, C_2, etc.
539. Ca
540. CTS
541. D_1, D_2, etc.
542. DJD

543. DTR
544. EMG
545. Fx
546. IM
547. L
548. L_1, L_2, etc.
549. MCP
550. NSAID

551. OA
552. P
553. PIP
554. PSISRRA
555. ROM
556. T_1, T_2, etc.
557. TMJ

Answers to Chapter Exercises

1. Synovial fluid lubricates joints.
2. Yes, exercise can increase breathing and heart rate which can exercise certain involuntary muscles. Voluntary muscles may be exercised at will.
3. long
4. 206
5. marrow
6. fontanelles
7. nucleus pulposus
8. acromion
9. true ribs
10. patella
11. calcaneus
12. cardiac
13. atlas, axis
14. femur
15. ligaments
16. tendons
17. TMJ (temporal mandibular joint)
18. articulations
19. movement
20. F
21. T
22. F
23. T
24. c
25. f
26. b
27. g
28. h
29. i
30. e
31. d
32. a
33. i
34. e
35. f
36. c
37. g
38. d
39. a
40. b
41. j
42. k
43. h
44. arthro
45. cranio
46. maxillo
47. ilio
48. tarso
49. thoracic

50. fibro
51. pod
52. rachio
53. sterno
54. fibromyalgia, pain in the fibrous tissue of muscles; osteoarthritis, arthritis of the bone
55. CTS, carpel tunnel syndrome
56. arthralgia, arthrodynia
57. bursectomy
58. chondritis
59. spondylectomy
60. osteoblast
61. osteosclerosis
62. cervicoplasty
63. myelitis
64. podospasm
65. ulnocarpal
66. synovo-, synovial fluid; synovial membrane
67. myelo-, spinal cord; bone marrow
68. -dynia, pain
69. osteo-, bone
70. rachio-, spine
71. joint: (sample dictionary answers); arthroplasty, arthroscopy, arthrodynia, arthritis, arthrostomy
72. bent
73. arm
74. heel
75. head
76. neck
77. cartilage
78. rib
79. skull
80. fascia
81. hump
82. muscle
83. spinal cord; bone marrow
84. bone
85. knee
86. spine
87. curved
88. Porous bone can result in breakage.
89. alternative treatment plans, side effects, potential benefits, potential risks, and the negative effect of not taking the medicine
90. These elements are crucial to bone formation.

91. No. Chiropractors are concerned with spinal manipulation.
92. Yes, the picture of the bone should show abnormalities.
93. Both believe in spinal manipulation.
94. A goniometer can measure range of motion of a joint.
95. f
96. f
97. f
98. t
99. t
100. C
101. densitometer
102. electromyelogram
103. rheumatoid
104. C
105. orthopedist
106. Tinel's sign
107. It may help ease pain by loosening and realigning.
108. Because the pain may be due to a condition other than back misalignment.
109. f
110. e
111. c
112. a
113. d
114. b
115. f
116. d
117. c
118. a
119. b
120. g
121. h
122. e
123. arthritis
124. greenstick
125. older
126. tendinitis (tendonitis)
127. flaccid
128. myoma
129. spondylolisthesis
130. open
131. joint
132. spinal cord
133. greenstick
134. overstretching; sprain
135. dislocation
136. subluxation

137. myalgia; myodynia
138. osteodynia or ostealgia
139. arthralgia
140. arthrodesis
141. size; tension
142. dystonia
143. osteomyelitis
144. carpel tunnel syndrome
145. c
146. d
147. b
148. e
149. a
150. g
151. h
152. f
153. The x-rays showed no fractures; therefore, no area needed to be held in place for a long period of time to allow the bone to heal.
154. No, not if there are certain kinds of fractures that must heal before movement is attempted. Answers to 155–158 may vary. Sample answers are shown below.
155. osteotomy, osteoplasty, osteoclasis
156. arthroplasty, arthrotomy
157. myotomy, myoplasty
158. spondylotomy, spondylectomy
159. e
160. a
161. g
162. i
163. b
164. h
165. c
166. f
167. d
168. j

169. The putting of a bone back in its place.
170. The removal of synovial fluid
171. Surgical fusion or fixation of a joint.
172. The removal of a bunion
173. The removal of a vertebra
174. A device to immobilize the foot
175. Puncture to remove fluid from a joint
176. She suggests no narcotics, since the patient has fairly continuous pain episodes, and she suggests switching to nonsteroidal compounds.
177. diet, weight-bearing exercises, cardiovascular exercise, aerobics
178. anti-inflammatory
179. analgesic
180. anti-inflammatory, antibiotic
181. anti-inflammatory
182. analgesic
183. no
184. to eliminate possible diseases (such as multiple sclerosis) that might mimic symptoms of musculoskeletal diseases
185. The patient had a fracture of the first lumbar verterbra.
186. The range of motion was decreased in the right shoulder due to muscle pain.
187. The patient was given a nonsteroidal anti-inflammatory drug due to osteoarthritis.
188. The patient has carpel tunnel syndrome on both sides.
189. The patient has severe rheumatoid arthritis, which has caused joint paint and overly tense muscles in the right leg.

190. A review of the patient's medical history shows problems with her temperomandibular joint and carpal tunnel syndrome and has had a fracture of the right wrist with has some degenerative joint disease.
191. On examination it was the found the deep tendon reflex of the left leg was decreased. The range of motion was also decreased on the left side of the body. The muscles in the left leg were limp and weak with little muscle tone.
192. The pt came in today for an EMG.
193. The pt will have a B-K amputation on his R leg due to severe frostbite.
194. The greenstick fracture needs casting.
195. F
196. F
197. T
198. T
199. T
200. F
201. T
202. F
203. F
204. F
205. F
206. T
207. T
208. T
209. F
210–557. Answers are available in the vocabulary reviews in this chapter.

The Cardiovascular System

After studying this chapter, you will be able to:

6.1 Name the parts of the cardiovascular system and discuss the function of each part

6.2 Define combining forms used in building words that relate to the cardiovascular system

6.3 Identify the meaning of related abbreviations

6.4 Name the common diagnoses, clinical procedures, and laboratory tests used in treating disorders of the cardiovascular system

6.5 List and define the major pathological conditions of the cardiovascular system

6.6 Explain the meaning of surgical terms related to the cardiovascular system

6.7 Recognize common pharmacological agents used in treating disorders of the cardiovascular system

Structure and Function

The **cardiovascular** system is the body's delivery service. Figure 6-1 on the next page shows the routes of blood circulation throughout the cardiovascular system. The **heart** pumps **blood** through the **blood vessels** to all the cells of the body. The average adult heart is about 5 inches long and 3.5 inches wide and weighs anywhere from 7 ounces to almost 14 ounces, depending on an individual's size and gender.

The heart wall consists of a double-layered protective sac and two additional layers:

1. The protective sac is the **pericardium.** The pericardium covers the *pericardial cavity* which is filled with *pericardial fluid*, a lubricant for the membranes of the heart. The pericardium itself consists of the *visceral pericardium* (the inner layer) which is also called the **epicardium** and is attached to the heart wall and the *parietal pericardium* (the outer portion of the pericardium).
2. The second layer is the **myocardium,** a thick layer of muscular tissue.
3. The inner layer, the **endocardium,** forms a membranous lining for the chambers and valves of the heart.

The heart is divided into right and left sides. Each side of the heart pumps blood to a specific area of the body. The right side of the heart pumps oxygen-poor blood from the body to the lungs. The left side of the heart pumps oxygen-rich blood from the lungs to all other areas of the body, where

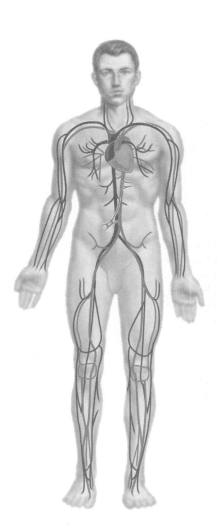

Remember epi- means upon or on and endo- means within. It is easy to remember that the epicardium is on the heart wall and the endocardium is the lining within the heart.

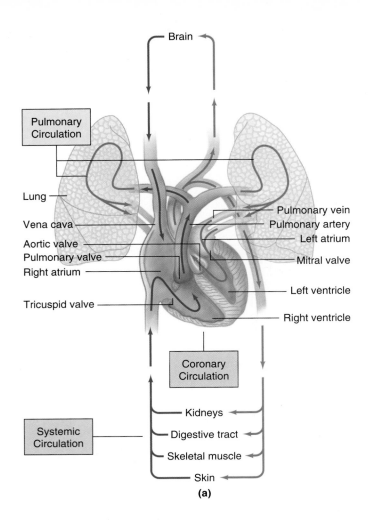

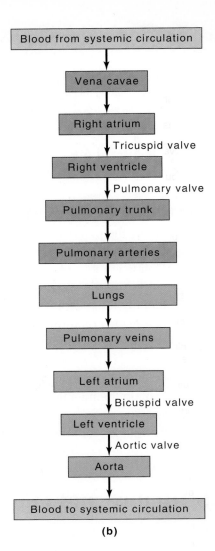

FIGURE 6-1 The heart pumps blood throughout the cardiovascular system via the blood vessels, arteries, and veins. **(a)**. The flow chart **(b)** Shows the path of deoxygenated blood in blue and oxygenated blood in red.

it will deliver nutrients and oxygen. Each side of the heart has two chambers. The **right atrium** and **right ventricle** on the right side are separated from the **left atrium** and **left ventricle** on the left side by a muscular partition called a **septum** (plural, **septa**). The part of the septum between the two **atria** (plural of **atrium**) is called the *interatrial septum;* the part between the two **ventricles** is called the *interventricular septum.*

Blood flows through the chambers of the heart in only one direction, with the flow regulated by one-way **valves.** The blood is pumped throughout the body through the system of **arteries** and **veins.** Arteries carry blood away from the heart. Veins carry blood toward the heart. The arteries carry oxygenated blood, except in pulmonary circulation. The veins carry deoxygenated blood, except in pulmonary circulation. Arteries have a lining called the **endothelium,** which secretes enzymes and other substances into the blood. The space within the arteries through which blood flows is called the **lumen.**

The valves of the heart also control the blood flow through the heart. The two **atrioventricular valves** (located between the atria and the ventricles)—the **tricuspid valve** and the **bicuspid valve** (also called the **mitral**

Superior vena cava

Pulmonary valve

Aortic valve

Right pulmonary artery

Right pulmonary veins

Right atrium

Interatrial septum

Opening of coronary sinus

Tricuspid valve

Chordae tendineae

Inferior vena cava

Right ventricle

Aorta

Left pulmonary artery

Pulmonary trunk

Left pulmonary veins

Left atrium

Bicuspid (mitral) valve

Purkinje fibers

Left ventricle

Interventricular septum

Visceral pericardium

Parietal pericardium

Oxygenated blood

Deoxygenated blood

valve)—control the flow of blood within the heart. The two **semilunar valves**—the **pulmonary valve** and the **aortic valve**—prevent the backflow of blood into the heart. The tricuspid valve has three cusps (flaps) that open and close to allow blood to flow from the right atrium into the right ventricle. The two cusps of the bicuspid valve are said to resemble a bishop's miter (hat), so this valve is commonly known as the mitral valve. The bicuspid valve controls blood flow on the left side of the heart, from the atrium to the ventricle. Figure 6-2 shows the heart and the structures leading to and from it.

The Vessels of the Cardiovascular System

Arteries and veins are the vessels that carry blood to and from the heart and lungs and to and from the heart and the rest of the body. This circulation of blood is the essential function of the cardiovascular system, which includes *coronary circulation*, the circulation of blood within the heart; *pulmonary circulation*, the flow of blood between the heart and lungs; and *systemic circulation*, the flow of blood between the heart and the cells of the body.

Coronary Circulation

The **coronary arteries,** which branch off the **aorta** (the body's largest artery and the artery through which blood exits the heart), supply blood to the heart muscle. The aortic semilunar valves control this flow of blood. The heart needs more oxygen than any other organ except the brain. The amount

The Web site www.heartinfo.org has heart animations that illustrate different parts of the heart and how they are affected by disease and surgery.

FIGURE 6-3 Coronary circulation is the circulation of blood within the heart **(a)**. The flowchart **(b)** gives an overview of this type of circulation.

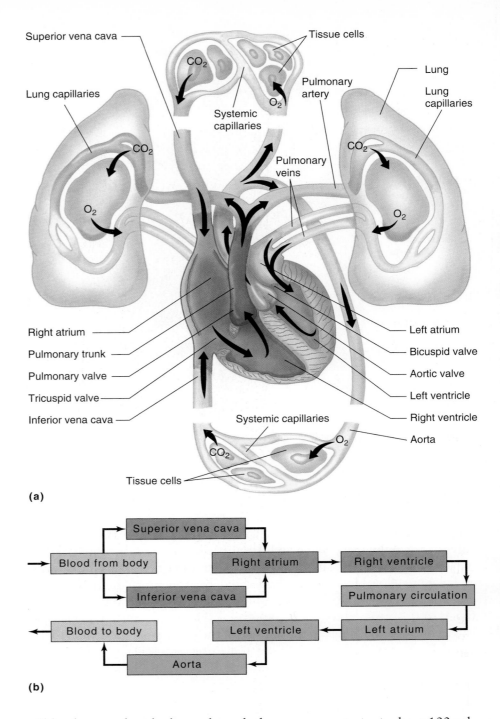

(a)

(b)

of blood pumped to the heart through the coronary arteries is about 100 gallons per day. The atrioventricular valves control the circulation of blood within the heart, between the atria and the ventricles. Figure 6-3 diagrams coronary circulation.

Pulmonary Circulation

The **pulmonary arteries** carry blood that is low in oxygen (*deoxygenated blood*) from the right ventricle of the heart to the lungs to get oxygen. Blood that is rich in oxygen (oxygenated blood) flows from the lungs to the left atrium of the heart through the **pulmonary veins.** Figure 6-4 on p. 160 traces the circulation of blood from the heart to the lungs and back.

The average adult has about 5-6 liters of blood in the body.

MORE ABOUT . . .

The Heart

The heart is the body's main pump, sending blood, oxygen, and nutrients to sustain all parts of the body. The heart is surprisingly small for such a large body function—only the size of an average adult fist. Although the heart has two sides, its shape is not symmetrical.

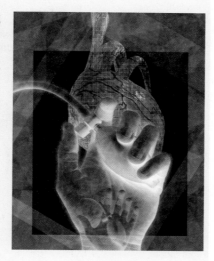

Systemic Circulation

The heart pumps blood through the arteries to the cells of the body. The blood moves in a surge caused by the muscular contraction of the heart. This surge is called the **pulse.** The blood that goes from the heart to the cells of the body (except the lungs) is oxygenated.

Specialized arteries (branching off the aorta) carry the oxygen-rich blood to different areas of the body. For example, the **carotid artery** supplies the head and neck; the **femoral artery** supplies the thigh; and the **popliteal artery** supplies the back of the knee. The arteries divide into smaller vessels called **arterioles,** which then divide into even smaller vessels called **capillaries.** The capillaries are the transfer station of the delivery system. The thin-walled capillaries allow the essential nutrients to leave the capillary through its single-celled walls via *osmosis*, the movement from a greater concentration to a lesser concentration through a membrane. The capillaries provide the cells they serve with essential nutrients and, in turn, remove waste products (including **carbon dioxide, CO_2**) from the cells, sending it to the **venules,** which are small branches of veins that then dump into the veins.

The veins take the deoxygenated blood back to the heart. An example of specialized veins are the **saphenous veins,** which remove oxygen-poor blood from the legs. Veins move the blood by gravity, skeletal muscle contractions, and respiratory activity. The veins contain small one-way valves that prevent the blood from flowing backward. The blood from the upper part of the body (above the diaphragm) is collected and carried to the heart through a large vein called the **superior vena cava.** The blood from the lower part of the body (below the diaphragm) goes to the other large vein called the **inferior vena cava** and then to the heart. Both of these large veins, the **venae cavae** (plural of **vena cava**), bring the blood to the right atrium of the heart. Figure 6-5 shows the major pathways in the systemic circulation.

Blood pressure   Blood pressure measures the force of the blood surging against the walls of the arteries. Each heartbeat consists of two parts. The first is the contraction, called **systole,** and the second is the relaxation, the

Although interpretation of pulse rates is controversial, most health practitioners agree that normal pulse rates for adults at rest range from 60 to 100 beats per minute. Children's pulse rates vary depending on age, size, level of activity, and so on. If a heart beats 70 times a minute, pumping 70 ml of blood into the aorta each time; 70 ml × 70 equals 4900 ml or almost 5 liters of blood every 60 seconds. This volume of blood is called the *cardiac output*. The volume of blood ejected from the ventricles during each heartbeat is called the *stroke volume*.

FIGURE 6-4 Pulmonary circulation is the circulation of blood between the hearts and lungs **(a)**. The flowchart **(b)** is a diagram of the blood flow in this type of circulation.

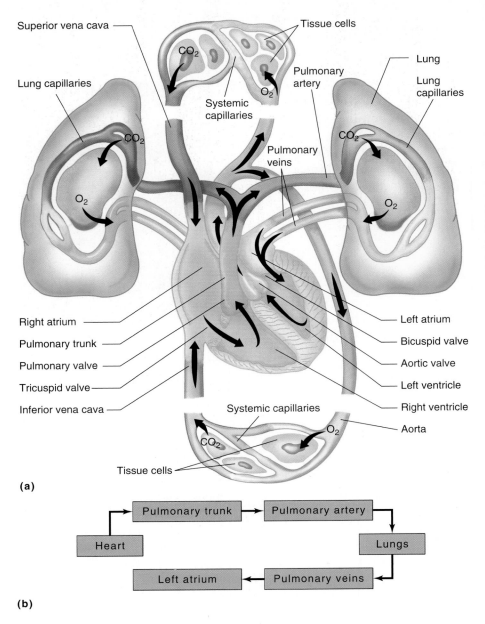

Superior vena cava

Tissue cells

CO_2

O_2

Lung capillaries

Systemic capillaries

CO_2

O_2

Lung

Lung capillaries

Pulmonary artery

Pulmonary veins

CO_2

O_2

Right atrium

Pulmonary trunk

Pulmonary valve

Tricuspid valve

Inferior vena cava

Left atrium

Bicuspid valve

Aortic valve

Left ventricle

Right ventricle

Aorta

Systemic capillaries

CO_2

O_2

Tissue cells

(a)

```
        ┌→ Pulmonary trunk → Pulmonary artery ─┐
        │                                        ↓
     Heart                                     Lungs
                                                 │
        Left atrium ← Pulmonary veins ←──────────┘
```

(b)

If a stethoscope is placed on the anterior chest wall, two distinct sounds can be heard that are often described as *lub dup.* The first or *lub* sound is caused when the atrioventricular valves slam tightly shut as the ventricles contract pushing blood out of the heart to the lungs and cells of the body. The second or *dup* sound is caused by the shutting of the semilunar valves as the ventricles relax and rest from the contraction in anticipation of the next contraction. Each complete heartbeat is referred to as the *cardiac cycle* and includes the contraction (systole) and relaxation (diastole) of atria and ventricles. If the heart was beating at a rate of 72 beats per minute (bpm), each cycle would take about 0.8 seconds to complete.

diastole. **Blood pressure** is the measurement of the systolic pressure followed by the diastolic pressure. Normal blood pressure for an adult is 120/80. The number 120 represents the pressure within the walls of an artery during systole; the number 80 represents the pressure within the arterial wall during diastole. Pulse pressure represents the difference between the distolic and systolic readings. In blood pressure of 120/80, the pulse pressure is 40, which represents the strength of the left ventricle pumping blood to the body.

Conduction system The heart has the unique ability to control its own rhythm. This electrical ability is called the **conduction system,** which is contained in special heart tissue called *conductive tissue* in the right atrium. This region is called the **sinoatrial (SA) node** and is known as the heart's **pacemaker** because its electrical impulse causes the regular contractions that result in a regular heartbeat or pulse. The contractions take place in the myocardium, which cycles through **polarization** (resting state) to **depolarization** (contracting state) to **repolarization** (recharging from contracting to resting) in the heartbeat. The electrical current from the SA node

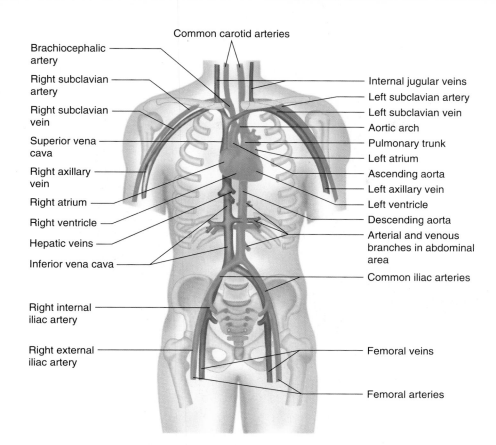

Common carotid arteries

Brachiocephalic artery

Right subclavian artery

Right subclavian vein

Superior vena cava

Right axillary vein

Right atrium

Right ventricle

Hepatic veins

Inferior vena cava

Right internal iliac artery

Right external iliac artery

Internal jugular veins

Left subclavian artery

Left subclavian vein

Aortic arch

Pulmonary trunk

Left atrium

Ascending aorta

Left axillary vein

Left ventricle

Descending aorta

Arterial and venous branches in abdominal area

Common iliac arteries

Femoral veins

Femoral arteries

FIGURE 6-5 Systemic circulation is the flow of blood between the heart and the cells of the entire body. In addition to arteries and veins, smaller blood vessels branch off to connect with cellular material. Specific arteries and veins are named for the area of the body that they serve. The brachiocephalic artery serves the arms and head, the subclavian arteries and veins serve the area beneath the shoulder or collar bone, the iliac arteries and veins serve the small intestines, the hepatic vessels serve the liver, and the jugular veins serve the throat and neck.

causes fibers in the atria to contract. This current then passes to a portion of the interatrial septum called the **atrioventricular (AV) node,** which sends the charge to a group of specialized muscle fibers called the **atrioventricular bundle,** also called the **bundle of His.** The bundle of His divides into left and right bundle branches and causes the ventricles to contract, forcing blood away from the heart during systole. At the end of these branches are the *Purkinje fibers*, specialized fibers that conduct the change.

Heart rate can vary depending on a person's health, physical activity, or emotions at any one time. The repeated beating of the heart takes place in the **cardiac cycle,** during which the heart contracts and relaxes as it circulates blood. Normal heart rhythm is called **sinus rhythm.**

The National Heart, Lung, and Blood Institute's Web site (www.nhlbi.nih.gov) can be searched for good information about blood pressure.

Fetal Circulation

The circulatory system of the fetus bypasses pulmonary circulation, because a fetus's lungs do not function until after birth and because the fetus gets oxygen and nutrients through the umbilical cord, which contains arteries and a vein. Fetal blood is transported back and forth to the placenta, where deoxygenated blood is oxygenated and returned to the fetus. Three structures are important to fetal circulation (Figure 6-6). The **ductus venosus** is the connection from the umbilical vein to the fetus's inferior vena cava, through which oxygenated blood is delivered to the fetal heart, bypassing the fetal liver. Deoxygenated blood flows from the fetal heart through the **ductus arteriosus** and back through the umbilical cord to the placenta. The septum between the atria of the fetal heart has a small opening called the **foramen ovale,** which allows blood to flow from the right atrium intro the left atrium. After birth, this opening closes. Chapter 17 discusses fetal development.

FIGURE 6-6 Fetal blood moves back and forth between the placenta and the growing fetus. The diagram shows the flow of oxygenated and deoxygenated blood from the fetus's heart through its nonfunctioning lungs to the umbilicus to the placenta. Structures unique to the fetus that change after birth are the foramen ovale and the ductus venosus.

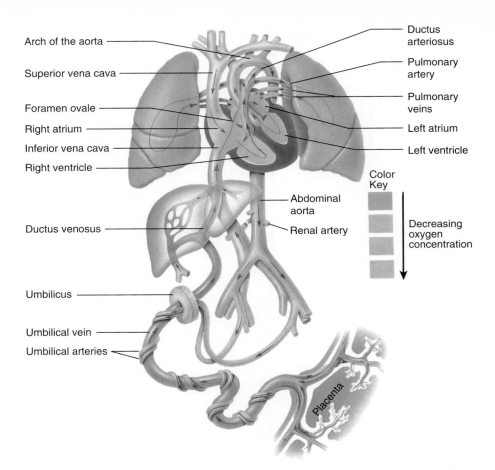

Arch of the aorta
Superior vena cava
Foramen ovale
Right atrium
Inferior vena cava
Right ventricle
Ductus venosus
Umbilicus
Umbilical vein
Umbilical arteries
Ductus arteriosus
Pulmonary artery
Pulmonary veins
Left atrium
Left ventricle
Abdominal aorta
Renal artery
Placenta

Color Key
Decreasing oxygen concentration

MORE ABOUT . . .

Controlling High Blood Pressure

High blood pressure is a dangerous condition with virtually no symptoms felt by the patient. At almost every doctor visit, blood pressure is measured, usually with a sphygmomanometer. Blood pressure measurements are characterized as normal, low, or high. Blood pressure may gradually increase with age or may decrease with consistent athletic training. The generally regarded normal arterial blood pressure for an adult is 120/80 or 120 mm Hg systolic pressure (as the ventricles contract) and 80 mm Hg diastolic pressure (as the ventricles relax). High blood pressure is sometimes the result of heredity or lifestyle factors. Overeating leading to overweight, smoking, lack of exercise, and stress are lifestyle factors that affect blood pressure. For consistently high systolic pressures, most doctors recommend lifestyle changes along with medication.

The American Heart Association (www.amheart.org) categorizes blood pressure as follows:

Blood Pressure Category	Systolic (mm Hg)		Diastolic (mm Hg)
Normal	less than 120	and	less than 80
Prehypertension (considered hypertension in some high-risk cases)	120–139	or	80–89
High			
Stage 1	140–159	or	90–99
Stage 2	160 or higher	or	100 or higher

Your doctor should evaluate unusually low readings.

VOCABULARY REVIEW

In the previous section, you learned terms relating to the cardiovascular system. Before going on to the exercises, review the terms below and refer to the previous section if you have any questions. Pronunciations are provided for certain terms. Sometimes information about where the word came from is included after the term. The etymologies (word histories) are for your information only. You do not need to memorize them.

Term	Definition
aorta [ā-ŌR-tă] Greek *aorte*	Largest artery of the body; vessel through which oxygenated blood exits the heart.
aortic [ā-ŌR-tĭk] **valve**	Valve between the aorta and the left ventricle.
arteriole [ăr-TĒ-rē-ōl] arteri-, artery + -ole, small	A tiny artery connecting to a capillary.
artery [ĂR-tĕr-ē] Latin and Greek *arteria*	A thick-walled blood vessel that, in systemic circulation, carries oxygenated blood away from the heart.
atrioventricular [Ā-trē-ō-vĕn-TRĬK-yū-lăr] **bundle** atrio-, atrium + ventricular	Bundle of fibers in the interventricular septum that transfers charges in the heart's conduction system; also called bundle of His.
atrioventricular (AV) node	Specialized part of the interatrial septum that sends a charge to the bundle of His.
atrioventricular valve	One of two valves that control blood flow between the atria and ventricles.
atrium (*pl.,* atria) [Ā-trē-ŭm (Ā-trē-ă)]	Either of the two upper chambers of the heart.
bicuspid [bī-KŬS-pĭd] **valve** bi-, two + cuspid, having one cusp	Atrioventricular valve on the left side of the heart.
blood [blŭd] Old English *blod*	Essential fluid made up of plasma and other elements that circulates throughout the body; delivers nutrients to and removes waste from the body's cells.
blood pressure	Measure of the force of blood surging against the walls of the arteries.
blood vessel	Any of the tubular passageways in the cardiovascular system through which blood travels.
bundle of His [hĭz, hĭs] After Wilhelm His (1863–1934), German Physician	*See* atrioventricular bundle.
capillary [KĂP-ĭ-lār-ē]	The smallest blood vessel that forms the exchange point between the arterial and venous vessels.
carbon dioxide (CO_2)	Waste material transported in the venous blood.
cardiac cycle	Repeated contraction and relaxation of the heart as it circulates blood within itself and pumps it out to the rest of the body or the lungs.

Term	Definition
cardiovascular [KĂR-dē-ō-VĂS-kyū-lĕr]	Relating to or affecting the heart and blood vessels.
carotid [kă-RŎT-ĭd] **artery**	Artery that transports oxygenated blood to the head and neck.
conduction system	Part of the heart containing specialized tissue that sends electrical charges through heart fibers, causing the heart to contract and relax at regular intervals.
coronary [KŌR-ō-nār-ē] **artery** Latin *coronarius* from *corona*, crown	Blood vessel that supplies oxygen-rich blood to the heart.
depolarization [dē-pō-lă-rĭ-ZĀ-shŭn] de-, away from + polarization	Contracting state of the myocardial tissue in the heart's conduction system.
diastole [dī-ĂS-tō-lē] Greek, *dilation*	Relaxation phase of a heartbeat.
ductus arteriosus [DŬK-tŭs ăr-tēr-ē-Ō-sŭs]	Structure in the fetal circulatory system through which blood flows to bypass the fetus's nonfunctioning lungs.
ductus venosus [vĕn-Ō-sŭs]	Structure in the fetal circulatory system through which blood flows to bypass the fetal liver.
endocardium [ĕn-dō-KĂR-dē-ŭm] endo-, within + Greek *kardia*, heart	Membranous lining of the chambers and valves of the heart; the innermost layer of heart tissue.
endothelium [ĕn-dō-THĒ-lē-ŭm] endo- + Greek *thele*, nipple	Lining of the arteries that secretes substances into the blood.
epicardium [ĕp-ĭ-KĂR-dē-ŭm] epi-, upon + Greek *kardia*, heart	Outermost layer of heart tissue.
femoral [FĔM-ŏ-răl, FĒ-mŏ-răl] **artery**	An artery that supplies blood to the thigh.
foramen ovale [fō-RĀ-mĕn ō-VĂ-lē]	Opening in the septum of the fetal heart that closes at birth.
heart [hărt] Old English *heorte*	Muscular organ that receives blood from the veins and sends it into the arteries.
inferior vena cava [VĒ-nă KĂ-vă, KĀ-vă]	Large vein that draws blood from the lower part of the body to the right atrium.
left atrium	Upper left heart chamber.
left ventricle	Lower left heart chamber.
lumen [LŪ-mĕn]	Channel inside an artery through which blood flows.
mitral [MĪ-trăl] **valve**	*See* bicuspid valve.
myocardium [mī-ō-KĂR-dē-ŭm] myo-, muscle + Greek *kardia*, heart	Muscular layer of heart tissue between the epicardium and the endocardium.

Term	Definition
pacemaker	Term for the sinoatrial (SA) node; also, an artificial device that regulates heart rhythm.
pericardium [pĕr-ĭ-KĂR-dē-ŭm] peri-, around + Greek *kardia*, heart	Protective covering of the heart.
polarization [pō-lăr-ĭ-ZĀ-shŭn]	Resting state of the myocardial tissue in the conduction system of the heart.
popliteal [pŏp-LĬT-ē-ăl] **artery**	An artery that supplies blood to the cells of the area behind the knee.
pulmonary [PŬL-mō-nār-ē] **artery**	One of two arteries that carry blood that is low in oxygen from the heart to the lungs.
pulmonary valve	Valve that controls the blood flow between the right ventricle and the pulmonary arteries.
pulmonary vein	One of four veins that bring oxygenated blood from the lungs to the left atrium.
pulse [pŭls]	Rhythmic expansion and contraction of a blood vessel, usually an artery.
repolarization [rē-pō-lăr-ĭ-ZĀ-shŭn] re, again + polarization	Recharging state; transition from contraction to resting that occurs in the conduction system of the heart.
right atrium	Upper right chamber of the heart.
right ventricle	Lower right chamber of the heart.
saphenous [să-FĒ-nŭs] **vein**	Any of a group of veins that transport deoxygenated blood from the legs.
semilunar [sĕm-ē-LŪ-năr] **valve** semi-, half + Latin *luna*, moon	One of the two valves that prevent the backflow of blood flowing out of the heart into the aorta and the pulmonary artery.
septum (*pl.,* septa) [SĔP-tŭm (SĔP-tă)]	Partition between the left and right chambers of the heart.
sinoatrial [sī-nō-Ā-trē-ăl] **(SA) node**	Region of the right atrium containing specialized tissue that sends electrical impulses to the heart muscle, causing it to contract.
sinus rhythm	Normal heart rhythm.
superior vena cava	Large vein that transports blood collected from the upper part of the body to the heart.
systole [SĬS-tō-lē]	Contraction phase of the heartbeat.
tricuspid [trī-KŬS-pĭd] **valve** tri-, three + cuspid, having one cusp	Atrioventricular valve on the right side of the heart.
valve [vălv]	Any of various structures that slow or prevent fluid from flowing backward or forward.

Term	Definition
vein [vān]	Any of various blood vessels carrying deoxygenated blood toward the heart, except the pulmonary vein.
vena cava (*pl.*, **venae cavae**) [VĒ-nă KĂ-vă, KĀ-vă (VĒ-nē KĂ-vē, KĀ-vē)]	*See* superior vena cava and inferior vena cava.
ventricle [VĔN-trĭ-kl]	Either of the two lower chambers of the heart.
venule [VĔN-yūl, VĒ-nŭl]	A tiny vein connecting to a capillary.

CASE STUDY

A Cardiovascular Emergency

On a hot summer afternoon, Joseph Davino entered the emergency room at Stone General Hospital with severe shortness of breath (SOB). Dr. Mary Woodard was the cardiologist on call that day. She immediately started examining Mr. Davino and made a preliminary diagnosis based upon the physical assessment and the patient's history. She learned that Mr. Davino is 44 years old, is a smoker, is overweight, and has a sedentary lifestyle.

Mr. Davino's past medical history shows that he has a high cholesterol level, has a history of angina, and takes medication to control high blood pressure. The physical exam shows normal temperature and a blood pressure of 190/100. Dr. Woodard orders an ECG and a cardiac panel.

Critical Thinking

1. Shortness of breath may indicate cardiovascular disease. What lifestyle factors put Mr. Davino at risk?
2. Was Mr. Davino's blood pressure normal?

STRUCTURE AND FUNCTION EXERCISES

Finish the Picture

Complete the labeling of the parts of the heart on the diagram on page 167.

3. Describe the function of each lettered part from the diagram in the space below.

a. _____

b. _____

c. _____

d. _____

e. _____

f. _____

g. _____

h. _____

i. _____

j. _____

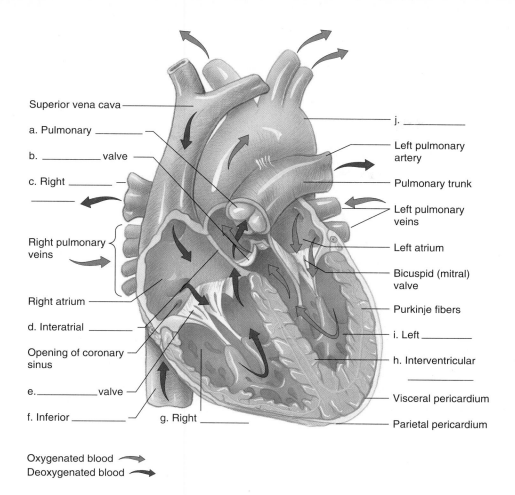

Superior vena cava
a. Pulmonary _____
b. _____ valve
c. Right _____
_____
Right pulmonary veins
Right atrium
d. Interatrial _____
Opening of coronary sinus
e. _____ valve
f. Inferior _____
g. Right _____

j. _____
Left pulmonary artery
Pulmonary trunk
Left pulmonary veins
Left atrium
Bicuspid (mitral) valve
Purkinje fibers
i. Left _____
h. Interventricular _____
Visceral pericardium
Parietal pericardium

Oxygenated blood
Deoxygenated blood

Spell It Correctly

For each of the following words, write C if the spelling is correct. If it is not, write the correct spelling.

4. atriaventricular _____

5. capillairy _____

6. ductus arteriosus _____

7. Purkine fibers _____

8. myocardium _____

9. arteryole _____

10. bundle of His _____

11. popliteal _____

12. sistole _____

Test Your Knowledge

Complete the sentences below by filling in the blanks.

13. A vessel that carries oxygenated blood is a(n) _____.

14. Deoxygenated blood flows through the _____.

15. The innermost layer of heart tissue is called the _____.

16. The two atrioventricular valves control the flow of blood between the _____ and the _____.

17. Carbon dioxide is carried back to the heart via the _____.

18. Three lifestyle factors that may result in high blood pressure are _____, _____, and _____.

19. The fetal circulatory system does not include _____ circulation.

20. The lining of the arteries that secretes substances into the blood is called the _____.

21. Pulmonary circulation is the flow of blood between the _____ and _____.

22. The head and neck receive oxygen-rich blood via the _____.

23. Fill in the missing part in the following sequence: pulmonary arteries → _____ → pulmonary veins.

Combining Forms and Abbreviations

The lists below include combining forms and abbreviations that relate specifically to the cardiovascular system. Pronunciations are provided for the examples.

COMBINING FORM	MEANING	EXAMPLE
angi(o)	blood vessel	*angiogram* [ĂN-jē-ō-grăm], image of a blood vessel
aort(o)	aorta	*aortitis* [ā-ōr-TĪ-tĭs], inflammation of the aorta
arteri(o), arter(o)	artery	*arteriosclerosis* [ăr-TĒR-ē-ō-sklĕr-Ō-sĭs], hardening of the arteries
ather(o)	fatty matter	*atherosclerosis* [ĂTH-ĕr-ō-sklĕr-Ō-sĭs], hardening of the arteries with irregular plaque deposits
atri(o)	atrium	*atrioventricular* [Ā-trē-ō-vĕn-TRĬK-yū-lăr], relating to the atria and ventricles of the heart
cardi(o)	heart	*cardiomyopathy* [KĂR-dē-ō-mī-ŎP-ă-thē], disease of the heart muscle
hemangi(o)	blood vessel	*hemangioma* [hĕ-MĂN-jē-ō-mă], abnormal mass of blood vessels
pericardi(o)	pericardium	*pericarditis* [PĔR-ĭ-kăr-DĪ-tĭs], inflammation of the pericardium
phleb(o)	vein	*phlebitis* [flĕ-BĪ-tĭs], inflammation of a vein
sphygm(o)	pulse	*sphygmomanometer* [SFĬG-mō-mă-NŎM-ĕ-tĕr], instrument for measuring blood pressure
thromb(o)	blood clot	*thrombocytosis* [THRŎM-bō-sī-TŌ-sĭs], abnormal increase in blood platelets in the blood

COMBINING FORM	MEANING	EXAMPLE
vas(o)	blood vessel	*vasodepressor* [VĀ-sō-dē-PRĔS-ŏr], agent that lowers blood pressure by relaxing blood vessels
ven(o)	vein	*venography* [vē-NŎG-ră-fē], radiographic imaging of a vein

ABBREVIATION	MEANING	ABBREVIATION	MEANING
AcG	accelerator globulin	ECHO	echocardiogram
AF	atrial fibrillation	ETT	exercise tolerance test
AMI	acute myocardial infarction	GOT	glutamic oxaloacetic transaminase
AS	aortic stenosis		
ASCVD	arteriosclerotic cardiovascular disease	HDL	high-density lipoprotein
		HR	heart rate
ASD	atrial septal defect	LDH	lactate dehydrogenase
ASHD	arteriosclerotic heart disease	LDL	low-density lipoprotein
AV	atrioventricular	LV	left ventricle
BP	blood pressure bpm beats per minute	LVH	left ventricular hypertrophy
		MI	mitral insufficiency; myocardial infarction
CABG	coronary artery bypass graft		
CAD	coronary artery disease	MR	mitral regurgitation
cath	catheter	MS	mitral stenosis
CCU	coronary care unit	MUGA	multiple-gated acquisition scan
CHD	coronary heart disease	MVP	mitral valve prolapse
CHF	congestive heart failure	PAC	premature atrial contraction
CO	cardiac output	PTCA	percutaneous transluminal coronary angioplasty
CPK	creatine phosphokinase		
CPR	cardiopulmonary resuscitation	PVC	premature ventricular contraction
CVA	cerebrovascular accident	SA	sinoatrial
CVD	cardiovascular disease	SV	stroke volume
DIC	disseminated intravascular coagulation	TC	total cholesterol
		tPA, TPA	tissue plasminogen activator
DSA	digital subtraction angiography	VLDL	very low-density lipoprotein
DVT	deep venous thrombosis	VSD	ventricular septal defect
ECG, EKG	electrocardiogram	VT	ventricular tachycardia

Build Your Medical Vocabulary

Build a word for each of the following definitions. Use the combining forms in this chapter as well as in Chapters 1, 2, and 3.

24. Disease of the heart muscle _____

25. Inflammation of the membrane surrounding the heart _____

26. X-ray of a vein _____

27. Inflammation of a vein _____

28. Operation for reconstruction of an artery _____

29. A disease involving both nerves and blood vessels _____

30. Tending to act on the blood vessels _____

31. Of cardiac origin _____

32. Enlargement of the heart _____

33. Inflammation of the artery with a thrombus _____

Use the following combining forms and the suffixes and prefixes you learned in Chapters 1, 2, and 3 to fill in the missing word parts: atrio-, arterio-, phlebo-, thrombo-, veno-

34. _____ itis, inflammation of a vein

35. _____ ectomy, surgical removal of a thrombus

36. _____ plasty, vein repair

37. _____ megaly, enlargement of the atrium

38. _____ graph, radiograph of veins

Give the term that fits each definition. Each term must contain at least one of the combining forms shown in the previous section. You may also refer to Chapters 1, 2, and 3.

39. Enlargement of the heart _____

40. Relating to the heart and lungs _____

41. Establishing an opening into the pericardium _____

42. Inflammation of the endocardium _____

43. Repair of a vein _____

44. Paralysis of a blood vessel _____

45. Suturing of a blood vessel _____

Check Your Knowledge

Complete the sentences below by filling in the blanks.

46. An inflammation of a vein is _____.

47. Atherosclerosis is hardening of the _____.

48. A venogram is an x-ray of a(n) _____.

49. An abbreviation for a term meaning heart attack is _____.

50. CABG is a surgical procedure that bypasses a blocked _____.

Reading the Record

The nurse on duty the night of Mr. Davino's admittance observed that his blood pressure dropped gradually from 190/100 to 160/90. The nurse, Joan Aquino, marked each change of blood pressure on his record. In addition to blood pressure, she also took Mr. Davino's temperature and pulse every two hours. All his measurements seemed to show improvement, except that Mr. Davino was running a slight fever. However, Joan did not like Mr. Davino's appearance. His skin had a gray pallor and he seemed very disoriented. Dr. Mirkhan, the cardiologist on call that night, spoke with Nurse Aquino and looked over the results of the tests ordered earlier. The doctor also made the notes shown on the record.

Critical Thinking

51. Nurse Aquino made very specific comments to Dr. Mirkhan about her observations of Mr. Davino's appearance. What are the two items that Nurse Aquino noticed?
52. Referring to Mr. Davino's chart below, how long did Mr. Davino's temperature remain slightly elevated?

MEDICAL RECORD	PROGRESS NOTES
DATE 8/15/XX	3:30 pm Chest clear to auscultation bilaterally with mild crackles; Heart rate and rhythm regular; no
	audible murmur; no rubs; ECG, blood gases, and SED rate were ordered. Recommended transfer to
	CCU.—A. Mirkhan, M.D.
8/15/XX	4 pm BP 190/100; temp 100.4°; no urine in catheter bag.—J. Aquino, R.N.
8/15/XX	5 pm BP 182/95; temp 100.5°; still no urine in catheter bag; if no urine by 8 pm, notify Dr. Mirkhan.—
	J.Aquino, R.N.
8/15/XX	6 pm BP 176/97; temp 100.6°; catheter bag empty.—J. Aquino, R.N.
8/15/XX	7 pm Catheter bag empty.—J. Aquino, R.N.
8/15/XX	8 pm BP 168/94; temp 100.7°; catheter bag empty; paged Dr. Mirkhan.—J. Aquino, R.N.
8/15/XX	9 pm BP 162/96; temp 100.8°; start IV; ECG; blood gases.—A. Mirkhan, M.D.
8/15/XX	10 pm Catheter bag contains 50 ml of urine; patient resting comfortably.—J. Aquino, R.N.
8/15/XX	11 pm Catheter bag contains about 200 ml of urine; patient still sleeping.—J. Aquino, R.N.
8/15/XX	12 pm Woke patient; BP 160/90; temp 100.2°; 300 ml of urine.—J. Aquino, R.N.

PATIENT'S IDENTIFICATION (For typed or written entries give: Name—last, first, middle; grade; rank; hospital or medical facility)	REGISTER NO.	WARD NO. 4B

Matching

Match the following combining forms used in cardiovascular terms with the correct meanings. Some answers may be used more than once or not at all.

53. _____ angi(o)
54. _____ arteri(o)
55. _____ ather(o)
56. _____ aden(o)
57. _____ aort(o)

a. aorta
b. vein
c. blood
d. vessel
e. electric

58. _____ cardi(o)   f. artery

59. _____ ech(o)   g. heart

60. _____ electr(o)   h. thick, yellowish fatty plaque

61. _____ hem(o)   i. gland

62. _____ phleb(o)   j. sound

Match the following combining forms used in cardiovascular terms with the correct meanings. Some answers may be used more than once or not at all.

63. _____ atri(o)   a. heat

64. _____ hemangi(o)   b. vein

65. _____ pericardi(o)   c. blood vessel

66. _____ sphygm(o)   d. deficiency, blockage

67. _____ thromb(o)   e. sound

68. _____ vas(o)   f. pericardium

69. _____ son(o)   g. blood clot

70. _____ valv(o)   h. atrium

71. _____ isch(o)   i. pulse

72. _____ therm(o)   j. valve

Define these abbreviations used on Mr. Davino's record.

73. ECG _____   76. BP _____

74. CCU _____   77. ECHO _____

75. MI _____

Diagnostic, Procedural, and Laboratory Terms

Treatment of cardiovascular disease requires a precise understanding of the structure and function of the heart and of the parts of the body that affect the heart's functioning. Doctors order many types of diagnostic tests based on their observations of a patient. They may order clinical procedures whose results will indicate certain specific conditions or they may order laboratory tests to find disease-causing factors or evidence of a specific disease. Sometimes, test results are used to rule out conditions, in which case, physicians look for other causes of disease.

Diagnostic Procedures and Tests

Doctors who specialize in the diagnosis and treatment of cardiovascular disease (*cardiology*) are called *cardiologists*. Cardiologists usually see patients who already have some type of cardiovascular problem or indication of disease. In addition, cardiac surgeons are specialists who perform heart surgery.

The cardiologist often starts an examination with **auscultation** (listening to sounds within the body through a stethoscope). Some abnormal sounds a physician may hear are a *murmur*, a *bruit*, or a *gallop*. Each sound is a clue to the patient's condition. A **sphygmomanometer** is then usually used to measure blood pressure.

One common diagnostic test is a **stress test** (Figure 6-7) or *exercise tolerance test* (*ETT*). Patients are asked to exercise on a treadmill while technicians take certain measurements, such as heart rate and respiration. A stress test may be used to diagnose coronary artery disease or it may give a risk factor for heart attack.

Another common test is **electrocardiography,** which produces an *electrocardiogram* (**ECG, EKG**), which measures the amount of electricity flowing through the heart by means of electrodes placed on the patient's skin at specific points surrounding the heart. Figure 6-8 illustrates the printout that results from an electrocardiogram. Figure 6-9 illustrates some of the abnormalities that may show up on ECGs. A **Holter monitor** is a portable type of electrocardiograph or instrument that performs an electrocardiogram over a 24-hour period.

Various diagnostic procedures can be performed by producing some type of image. Taking x-rays after a dye has been injected is called **angiocardiography** (x-ray of the heart and its large blood vessels), **angiography** (x-ray of the heart's large blood vessels), **arteriography** (x-ray of a specific artery), **aortography** (x-ray of the aorta), or **venography** or **phlebography** (x-ray of a specific vein). The tests are called an *angiocardiogram, angiogram, arteriogram, aortogram,* or *venogram* or *phlebogram.* A **ventriculogram** is an x-ray showing the ventricles. Ventriculograms measure *stroke volume* (**SV**),

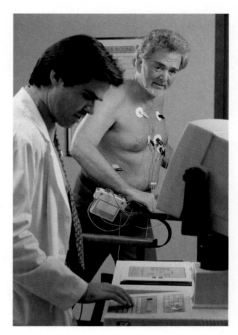

FIGURE 6-7 A stress test includes monitoring of heart function.

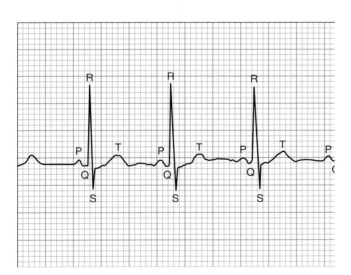

FIGURE 6-8 A normal ECG. The waves of electrical changes in the heart are mapped as P, QRS, and T waves. The P wave is the first electrical impulse through the atria, the QRS complex is the point at which the ventricles contract, and the T wave represents relaxation of the ventricles.

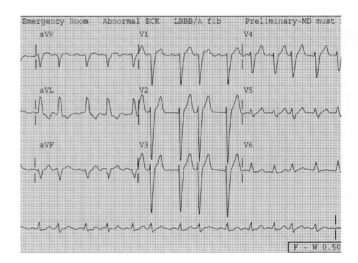

FIGURE 6-9 An abnormal ECG taken in the emergency room. Note the irregularities compared to Figure 6-8. These irregularities show atrial fibrillation and a blockage. In atrial fibrillation, the heart's rhythm is irregular, chaotic, and out of sync, with as many as 350 beats per minute. It results from the atria discharging blood simultaneously. If not treated with medication, it can result in heart failure. Heart blockage represents a delay in the heart's conduction system.

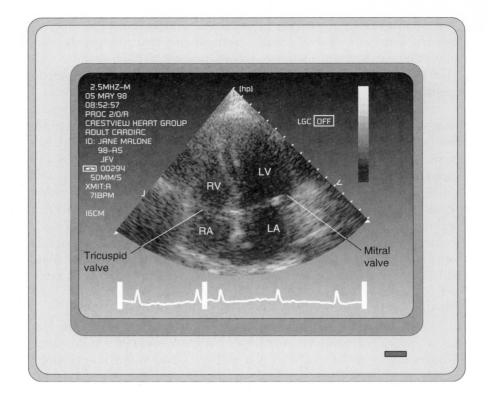

FIGURE 6-10 An echocardiogram is a test that shows the structure and movement of the heart.

the amount of blood going out of a ventricle in one contraction; *cardiac output* (**CO**), the amount of blood ejected from a ventricle every minute; and the **ejection fraction,** the percentage of volume of the contents of the left ventricle ejected with each contraction. Another x-ray test, **digital subtraction angiography (DSA)**, requires two angiograms with different contrast material to compare the results of the two tests in a computer.

Ultrasound tests, or *ultrasonography* or **sonography,** produce images by measuring the echoes of sound waves against various structures. **Doppler ultrasound** measures blood flow in certain blood vessels. **Echocardiography** records sound waves to show the structure and movement of the heart. The test itself is called an *echocardiogram*. Figure 6-10 shows an echocardiogram.

Radioactive substances that are injected into the patient can provide information in a **cardiac scan,** a test that measures movement of areas of the heart, or in *nuclear medicine imaging*. **Positron emission tomography (PET) scans** are one form of nuclear imaging. A PET scan of the heart produces three-dimensional images of the heart's blood flow and other functional processes. Another form of nuclear imaging is **multiple-gated acquisition (MUGA) angiography.** A MUGA scan is a noninvasive method that provides a movielike image of the beating heart. It allows for evaluation of the function of ventricles.

Magnetic resonance imaging (MRI) uses magnetic waves to produce images. A **cardiac MRI** uses radio waves to provide images of the heart while beating and provides a detailed image of the heart and shows any lesions in the large blood vessels of the heart.

Cardiac catheterization is used to sample the blood in the chambers of the heart to determine the oxygen content and blood pressure in the chambers. Cardiac output can also be checked. This procedure involves passing a small plastic catheter into the heart through a vein or artery. A vein is used for right-sided catheterization while an artery is used for a left-sided approach into the heart. The veins and arteries of the legs and arms are most commonly used.

Laboratory Tests

Laboratory tests are crucial for determining what may be happening to a patient or for evaluating risk factors for heart disease. Drug therapy, clinical procedures, and lifestyle changes may all be recommended largely on the basis of laboratory test results. All laboratory tests have a range of normal values (also called *reference ranges*—see the Appendix section on laboratory values). Some of these ranges change as new studies are done and views of what constitutes a healthy value (such as for cholesterol readings) is revised. Laboratory tests may fall outside of normal ranges due to a variety of reasons, age, gender, dietary habits, problems with collection, and so on. Results are viewed as one part of an entire exam in focusing on a diagnosis.

The flow of blood in the arteries is affected by the amount of **cholesterol** and **triglycerides** (fatty substances or *lipids*) contained in the blood. Lipids are carried through the blood by *lipoproteins*. *Low-density lipoproteins* (**LDL**) and *very low-density lipoproteins* (**VLDL**) cause cholesterol to form blockages in the arteries and are referred to as "bad" cholesterol. *High-density lipoproteins* (**HDL,** referred to as "good" cholesterol) actually remove lipids from the arteries and help protect people from the formation of blockages or fatty deposits, called *plaque*. One factor that increases LDL and VLDL is a diet high in *saturated fats* (animal fats and some vegetable fats that tend to be solid). The processing of some shortenings or margarines produces *transfats* (man-made fats), which are thought to cause particular risk for heart disease and cancer. *Polyunsaturated fats* (certain vegetable oils such as safflower or olive) do not raise LDL or VLDL. Laboratory tests performed on blood samples determine the levels of lipoproteins in the blood.

Adult cholesterol readings below 200 are considered to pose little risk for coronary artery disease (this number is controversial and varies as new studies are performed). The importance of cholesterol testing is evidenced by the fact that the chance of heart disease is reduced by 2 to 3 percent for each percentage point reduction in the cholesterol level. A **lipid profile** (a series of laboratory tests performed on a blood sample) gives the lipid, triglyceride, glucose, and other values that help in evaluating a patient's risk factors. Figure 6-11 is an example of a patient's lipid profile.

A laboratory test that can be used to diagnose a myocardial infarction earlier than most other laboratory tests measures the levels of *troponin T* and *troponin I*, proteins found in the heart. As levels of the two rise, it usually indicates the early states of an acute myocardial infarction. If only one level rises,

	RESULTS		
TEST	OUT OF RANGE	WITHIN RANGE	REFERENCE RANGE/UNITS
HDL	36 mg/dL		>40 mg/dL
LDL	192 mg/dL		<130mg/dL
Triglycerides	204 mg/dL		40–199 mg/dL
Cholesterol	208 mg/dL		120–199mg/dL

Laboratory Report
Emhar Diagnostics
Three Riverview Drive
Wesley, OH 66666
(800) 999–0000

PATIENT NAME _Mary Helfer_
PATIENT ID _777-888-6666_
DATE RECEIVED _06/14/XXXX_
DATE REPORTED _06/15/XXXX_

FIGURE 6-11 This lipid profile reveals the need to cut cholesterol in the patient's diet.

MORE ABOUT . . .

Cholesterol

Cholesterol is just one of the risk factors for heart disease but it is one that can be changed by lifestyle and/or medication. That is why many researchers focus on cholesterol levels and ratios. It is generally thought that low LDL levels and high HDL levels are healthier.

To learn more about cardiac enzyme tests, visit the information site of the BBC (www.bbc.co.uk/health/talking/tests/blood_cardiac_enzymes.shtml).

it can indicate a number of conditions not related to the heart, such as kidney failure or muscle trauma. A fairly new test for the evaluation of heart disease is the IMA (ischemia modified albumin). It is used with troponin and ECG to rule out acute coronary syndrome (ACS) patients with chest pain. Tests for C-reactive protein indicate levels of inflammation which is considered an accurate predictor of cardiovascular disease.

Another important laboratory test of blood is the **cardiac enzyme test** or **study** (also called a **serum enzyme test**), which measures the levels of enzymes released into the blood by damaged heart muscle during a myocardial infarction. The three enzymes that help evaluate the condition of the patient are **GOT** (*glutamic oxaloacetic transaminase*), **CPK** (*creatine phosphokinase*), and **LDH** (*lactate dehydrogenase*). The enzymes may indicate the degree of injury to the heart or the seriousness of an attack. Research to find markers for heart disease is ongoing. For example, brain natriuretic peptide (a hormone found in the body) levels have been found to be higher in patients with congestive heart failure. Looking for such markers in laboratory tests may be a reliable predictor of future disease.

VOCABULARY REVIEW

In the previous section, you learned terms relating to diagnosis, clinical procedures, and laboratory tests. Before going on to the exercises, review the terms below and refer to the previous section if you have questions. Pronunciations are provided for certain terms. Sometimes information about where the word came from is included after the term. The etymologies (word histories) are for your information only. You do not need to memorize them.

Term	Definition
angiocardiography [ăn-jē-ō-kăr-dē-ŎG-ră-fē] angio-, vessel + cardio-, heart + -graphy, a recording	Viewing of the heart and its major blood vessels by x-ray after injection of a contrast medium.
angiography [ăn-jē-ŎG-ră-fē] angio- + -graphy	Viewing of the heart's major blood vessels by x-ray after injection of a contrast medium.
aortography [ā-ōr-TŎG-ră-fē] aorto-, aorta + -graphy	Viewing of the aorta by x-ray after injection of a contrast medium.
arteriography [ăr-tēr-ē-ŎG-ră-fē] arterio-, artery + -graphy	Viewing of a specific artery by x-ray after injection of a contrast medium.
auscultation [ăws-kŭl-TĀ-shŭn]	Process of listening to body sounds via a stethoscope.
cardiac catheterization [kăth-ĕ-tĕr-ĭ-ZĀ-shŭn]	Process of passing a thin catheter through an artery or vein to the heart to take blood samples, inject a contrast medium, or measure various pressures.
cardiac enzyme tests/studies	Blood tests for determining levels of enzymes during a myocardial infarction; serum enzyme tests.
cardiac MRI	Viewing of the heart by magnetic resonance imaging.
cardiac scan	Process of viewing the heart muscle at work by scanning the heart of a patient into whom a radioactive substance has been injected.

Term	Definition
cholesterol [kō-LĔS-tĕr-ōl]	Fatty substance present in animal fats; cholesterol circulates in the bloodstream, sometimes causing arterial plaque to form.
digital subtraction angiography	Use of two angiograms done with different dyes to provide a comparison between the results.
Doppler [DŎP-lĕr] **ultrasound** After Christian Doppler (1803–1853), Austrian physicist	Ultrasound test of blood flow in certain blood vessels.
echocardiography [ĕk-ō-kăr-dē-ŎG-ră-fē] echo-, sound + cardio- + -graphy	Use of sound waves to produce images showing the structure and motion of the heart.
ejection fraction	Percentage of the volume of the contents of the left ventricle ejected with each contraction.
electrocardiography [ē-lĕk-trō-kăr-dē-ŎG-ră-fē] electro-, electrical + cardio- + -graphy	Use of the electrocardiograph in diagnosis.
Holter [HŌL-tĕr] **monitor** After Norman Holter (1914–1983), U.S. biophysicist	Portable device that provides a 24-hour electrocardiogram.
lipid profile [LĬP-ĭd] Greek *lipos*, fat	Laboratory test that provides the levels of lipids, triglycerides, and other substances in the blood.
multiple-gated acquisition (MUGA) angiography	Radioactive scan showing heart function.
phlebography [flĕ-BŎG-ră-fē] phlebo-, vein + -graphy	Viewing of a vein by x-ray after injection of a contrast medium.
positron emission tomography [tō-MŎG-ră-fē] **(PET) scan**	Type of nuclear image that measures movement of areas of the heart.
serum enzyme tests	Laboratory tests performed to detect enzymes present during or after a myocardial infarction; cardiac enzyme studies.
sonography [sō-NŎG-ră-fē] Latin *sonus*, sound + -graphy	Production of images based on the echoes of sound waves against structures.
sphygmomanometer [SFĬG-mō-mă-NŎM-ĕ-tĕr] sphygmo-, pulse + Greek *manos*, thin + -meter	Device for measuring blood pressure.
stress test	Test that measures heart rate, blood pressure, and other body functions while the patient is exercising on a treadmill.
triglyceride [trī-GLĬS-ĕr-īd] tri-, three + glyceride	Fatty substance; lipid.
venography [vē-NŎG-ră-fē] veno-, vein + -graphy	Viewing of a vein by x-ray after injection of a contrast medium.
ventriculogram [vĕn-TRĬK-yū-lō-grăm] ventricle + -gram, a recording	X-ray of a ventricle taken after injection of a contrast medium.

CASE STUDY

Diagnosing the Problem

Dr. Woodard, the admitting physician, had made notations on the patient's chart, but her shift ended before the results of the tests she had ordered were in. The doctor on call that night was Dr. Mirkhan, a cardiologist. He agreed with Nurse Aquino that the patient's pallor and disorientation warranted further tests. First, Dr. Mirkhan reviewed the ECG that Dr. Woodard had ordered. It showed a sinus rhythm with Q waves in 2 AVF and a mild ST elevation in V2 and V3. Dr. Mirkhan ordered some more laboratory tests to help in his diagnosis of

Mr. Davino's current condition. He made the additions to Mr. Davino's record. He also made some notes for Mr. Davino's personal physician.

Critical Thinking

78. From the notations added to the chart, is his cholesterol still high?

79. Which of his laboratory tests shows an abnormal level that can often be corrected by dietary changes?

MEDICAL RECORD	PROGRESS NOTES
DATE 8/15/XX	3:30 pm Have reviewed nursing notes. Chest clear to auscultation bilaterally with mild crackles; Heart rate and rhythm regular; no audible murmur; no rubs; ECG, blood gases, and SED rate were ordered. Recommend transfer to CCU.—A. Mirkhan, M.D.
8/15/XX	9 pm BP 162/96; temp 100.8°; start IV; ECG, blood gases.—A. Mirkhan, M.D.
8/16/XX	2 am ECG—sinus rhythm with Q waves in 2 AVF; mild ST elevation in V2 and V3; cholesterol 296; SED rate 15 mm/1 hr.—A. Mirkhan, M.D.

PATIENT'S IDENTIFICATION (For typed or written entries give: Name—last, first, middle; grade; rank; hospital or medical facility)	REGISTER NO.	WARD NO. 4B
Davino, Joseph A. 000-77-9999	**PROGRESS NOTES** STANDARD FORM 509	

DIAGNOSTIC, PROCEDURAL, AND LABORATORY TERMS EXERCISES

Apply What You Learn

Dr. Mirkhan also works in private practice. Patients' notes from his practice that follow give you an idea of the types of clinical problems he treats.

80. What is Marvin's diagnosis? _____

81. List five laboratory tests Dr. Mirkhan reviewed on 9/7/xx.

_____

_____

_____

_____

_____

Patient name _Angela O'Toole_	Age _57_	Current Diagnosis _angina_

DATE/TIME	
9/7/XX 9:30	_Exercise thallium test with no post-exercise changes; continue current medication._

Patient name _Marvin Hochstadter_	Age _64_	Current Diagnosis _arteriosclerosis_

DATE/TIME	
9/7/XX 10:15	_Two-year post angioplasty; SOB; cardiac pain; schedule cardiac catheterization._

Patient name _Lou Lawisky_	Age _49_	Current Diagnosis _unstable angina_

DATE/TIME	
9/7/XX 1:20	_Negative stress cardiolite scan to 12 MET; peak heart rate of 153/min with no ischemia or infarction; epigastric burning, no angina; recommend Tagamet to control reflux._

Patient name _Marlena Castelli_	Age _68_	Current Diagnosis _R/O MI_

DATE/TIME	
9/7/XX 2:30	_Neck and jaw discomfort; two previous MIs (last 1/23/XX); PTCA 2/6/XX; BP 126/84, pulse 88, heart: Apical impulse discrete. S1 and S2 are regular in rate and intensity. There is an S4 gallop, no S3 gallop, no cardiac murmur. Laboratory: Sodium 142, potassium 3.7, CO_2 29, chloride 103, creatinine 1.1, BUN 13, cholesterol 293, triglycerides 28; HDL 35; LDL 156; CPK 133._

Pathological Terms

Cardiovascular disease (**CVD**) can have many causes and can take many forms. Some diseases are caused by heredity or a congenital anomaly, whereas others may be caused by other pathology or by lifestyle factors (**risk factors**), such as poor diet, smoking, and lack of exercise.

> Almost one-third of all deaths in Western countries are attributed to heart disease.

Heart Rhythm

The rhythm of the heart maintains the blood flow through and in and out of the heart. Abnormal rhythms are called **arrhythmias** or dysrhthymias. Figure 6-12 shows a patient with an arrhythmia being treated with an auto-mated external defibrillator (AED). Heart rates may be too slow (**brady-cardia**), too fast (**tachycardia**), or irregular (also called **atrial fibrillation, fibrillation,** or **dysrhythmia**). Ventricular fibrillation is considered lethal and must be treated immediately. A **flutter** is a rapid but regular heartbeat. The heart rate may be regular, but the sound of the heartbeat may be abnor-mal (**bruit,** heard on auscultation of the carotid artery, or **murmur,** a soft humming sound), which may indicate valve leakage. A new murmur heard during a heart attack may indicate a rupture of the heart muscle, which is life-threatening and an urgent surgical emergency. Other sounds indicate

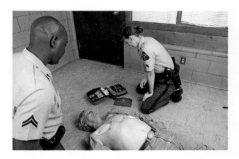

FIGURE 6-12 An automated external defibrillator (AED) is used for patients with a sudden arrhythmia.

specific problems; for example, a **rub** (a frictional sound) usually indicates a pericardial murmur, and a **gallop** (a triple heart sound) usually indicates serious heart disease. Some pulsations of the heart (**palpitations**) can be felt by the patient as thumping in the chest. An **atrioventricular block** or **heart block** is caused by a blocking of impulses from the AV node. The electrical impulses of the heart control contractions. Irregularities in the heart's contractions, such as **premature atrial contractions** (**PACs**) or **premature ventricular contractions** (**PVCs**), can cause palpitations.

Blood Pressure

Abnormalities in blood pressure (**hypertensive heart disease**) can damage the heart as well as other body systems. If the blood pressure is too high (**hypertension** or **high blood pressure**) or too low (**hypotension** or **low blood pressure**), the blood vessels do not have the proper pressure of blood flowing through them. **Essential hypertension** is high blood pressure that is *idiopathic* or without any known cause. **Secondary hypertension** has a known cause, such as a high-salt diet, renal disease, adrenal gland disease, and so on. Hypertension is the most common cardiovascular disease. Hypotension often results from another disease process or trauma (as in shock). Hypotension may lead to fainting or becoming unconscious. Extremely low hypotension may lead to death.

Diseases of the Blood Vessels

Blood vessels can become damaged, diseased, or even destroyed, as when **plaque,** buildup of fatty material, is deposited on the wall of an artery. An **atheroma** is plaque specifically on the wall of an artery, which can build up to cause **atherosclerosis.** An **embolus** is a mass traveling through the bloodstream causing a blockage in the vessel. A **thrombus** is a stationary blood clot, usually formed from elements of the blood. Figure 6-13 shows the difference between an embolus and a thrombus. **Thrombophlebitis** is an inflammation of a vein with a thrombus. **Thrombosis** is the presence of a thrombus in a blood vessel. **Deep vein thrombosis (DVT)** forms in a deep vein or in a vein within a structure rather than one on the surface of a structure. **Thrombotic occlusion** is the occlusion or closing of a vessel caused by a thrombus. Any blockage in a blood vessel can lead to *ischemia*, or insufficient blood flow.

Blood vessels can have a **constriction,** or narrowing, due to contraction. An **occlusion** is the closing off of a blood vessel due to a blockage. A weakness in an artery wall can cause a ballooning or **aneurysm,** which can fatally rupture. Loss of elasticity or hardening of the arteries (**arteriosclerosis**) can lessen blood flow. Inadequate blood supply, particularly to the blood vessels in the legs, causes **claudication,** limping. **Intermittent claudication,** irregular attacks of claudication, is helped by resting.

Peripheral vascular disease is a general term for vascular disease in the lower extremities. A sudden drop in the supply of blood to a vessel (an **infarction**) can cause an area of dead tissue, or **necrosis** (an **infarct**). The general term for lack of flow through a blood vessel is **perfusion deficit.** An area of blood insufficiency in the body is called **ischemia.** Insufficiently oxygenated areas of the body may develop **cyanosis,** a bluish or purplish discoloration of the skin caused by deficient oxygenation of the blood.

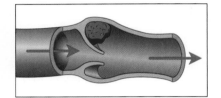

A thrombus.

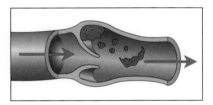

An embolus.

FIGURE 6-13 A thrombus is a stationary blood clot, while an embolus is a traveling mass of material that blocks a blood vessel.

Veins sometimes become twisted or enlarged (**varicose veins**). **Hemorrhoids** are varicose veins in the anal region. An inflammation of a vein is called **phlebitis** (which most often occurs in the lower legs). An inflammation of an artery is called **arteritis.** Minute hemorrhages in the blood vessels in the skin are called **petechiae.**

Numbness or pain in the fingers caused by arterial spasms is called **Raynaud's phenomenon.** Raynaud's phenomenon may be an indicator of some serious connective tissue or autoimmune diseases. Most often, it is a reaction to cold or to emotional stress. Once a "trigger" starts the phenomenon, three color changes usually take place. First, the finger(s) turn absolutely white when the blood flow is blocked by the spasm; second, the finger becomes cyanotic from the slow return of blood to the site; and third, as blood fills the finger, a darker red color appears. Treatment of Raynaud's not linked to another disease is usually as simple as wearing gloves when removing items from the freezer and when going out in cold weather. *Buerger's Disease* is an inflammation of the peripheral arteries and veins in the arms and legs with clot formations. Symptoms of Buerger's include intense pain in the affected area that is exacerbated or aggravated by exercise and relieved by rest. The primary cause of Buerger's is long-term smoking of tobacco that results in clot formation in the vessels until the entire vessel is destroyed and circulation to that area is seriously compromised.

> There are three basic forms of aneurysms; **saccular** which is a bulge in one arterial wall that involves all three of the vessel layers; **fusiform** which has both walls in the same area ballooning outward; and **dissecting** where the arterial wall splits allowing blood to enter into the vessel and blood within the artery to flow in both directions.

Coronary Artery Disease

Coronary artery disease (CAD) refers to any condition that reduces the nourishment the heart receives from the blood flowing through the arteries of the heart. Such diseases include **aortic stenosis** or narrowing of the aorta. **Coarctation of the aorta** is also an abnormal narrowing of the aorta. **Stenosis** is any narrowing of a blood vessel. **Pulmonary artery stenosis** slows the flow of blood to the lungs. **Angina** or **angina pectoris** (sometimes referred to as cardiac pain) can result from lack of oxygen to the heart muscle. Angina is usually categorized in degrees from class I to class IV. A person with class I angina (able to withstand prolonged exertion) will have no limits to normal activity. Severe angina (class IV) requires strict limitations on any activity except rest.

General Heart and Lung Diseases

When the heart suffers an attack that causes insufficient blood flow to the heart or ischemia, one is said to have a *coronary* or *heart attack.* These are informal terms for a **myocardial infarction (MI)** or *acute myocardial infarction (AMI)*, a disruption in the heart's activity usually caused by blockage (a clot or plaque) of blood flow to a coronary artery. Myocardial infarctions are often classified by the location of the area to which blood flow is restricted; for example, an anterior myocardial infarction is one in which the anterior wall of the heart is affected, and a posterior one involves the heart's posterior wall.

Cardiac arrest or **asystole** is a sudden stopping of the heart. Such an attack can be fatal or, with treatment, can be a warning to make medical and lifestyle changes to ward off a further attack. Approximately 1.5 million people suffer heart attacks annually. One-third of these people do not survive. Before age 50, men are much more likely to suffer heart attacks than are women, who are thought to be protected by their production of estrogen before menopause. After menopause, the risk for women is approximately the same as for men. In March 2008, in a major announcement, the American Heart Association (AHA) issued an advisory statement regarding revisions in how CPR was to be performed on a patient suffering cardiac arrest. Called "Hands-Only CPR," the directive included the recommendation that lay persons or bystanders should perform CPR using hands-only chest compressions without attempting to give the patient mouth-to-mouth breaths or rescue breaths. Hands-only CPR calls for immediate activation of 911 and then uninterrupted chest presses at a rate of approximately 100 per minute until paramedics take over or an automated external defibrillator (AED) is available to restore a normal or sustainable heart rhythm. Although not recommended for children or infants, experts hope bystanders will now be more willing to help if they see someone suddenly collapse. Hands-only CPR is simpler and easier to remember and removes a big barrier for people skittish about the mouth-to-mouth breathing.

Some diseases of the heart are specific inflammations, such as **endocarditis, myocarditis, pericarditis,** or **bacterial endocarditis.** Other conditions of the heart have to do with fluid accumulation. **Congestive heart failure** occurs when the heart is unable to pump the necessary amount of blood. People suffering from congestive heart failure usually experience shortness of breath, edema, enlarged organs and veins, and irregular breathing patterns. **Pulmonary edema** or accumulation of fluid in the lungs can result from this failure. Fluid accumulation in the pericardial sac causes **cardiac tamponade.**

An **intracardiac tumor** is a tumor in a heart chamber. **Cardiomyopathy** is disease of the heart muscle.

Valve Conditions

The heart valves control the flow of blood into, through, and out of the heart. Valve irregularities affecting the flow of blood can be serious. **Aortic regurgitation** or **reflux** is a backward flow of blood through the aortic valve. An abnormal narrowing of the opening of the mitral valve (**mitral stenosis**) affects the opening and closing of the valve. **Mitral insufficiency** or **reflux** is a backward flow of blood through the mitral valve. Similarly, **mitral valve prolapse** is a backward flow of blood, but it is due to the abnormal protrusion of one or both of the mitral cusps into the left atrium. **Tricuspid stenosis** is an abnormal narrowing of the opening of the tricuspid valve.

MORE ABOUT . . .

Familiar Terms for Heart Disease

Cardiovascular disease is a common ailment all Americans today. Many familiar terms are used by lay people to describe common cardiovascular diseases and procedures. A myocardial infarction may be called a *coronary* or a *heart attack.* Arteriosclerosis is often referred to as *hardening of the arteries.* Congestive heart failure may be called *heart failure. Vein stripping* is a common term for removal of veins for transplanting elsewhere or for treating varicosities.

Sometimes, infections or inflammation may cause valve damage. **Valvulitis** is the general term for a heart valve inflammation. **Rheumatic heart disease** is damage to the heart, usually to the valves, caused by an untreated streptococcal infection. Some infections can cause a clot on a heart valve or opening (**vegetation**).

Congenital Heart Conditions

Congenital heart disease results from a condition present at birth. Some common conditions are **patent ductus arteriosus,** a disease in which a small duct remains open at birth; **septal defect,** an abnormal opening in the septum between the atria or ventricles; and **tetralogy of Fallot,** actually a combination of four congenital heart abnormalities (ventricular septal defect, pulmonary stenosis, incorrect position of the aorta, and right ventricular hypertrophy) that appear together.

VOCABULARY REVIEW

In the previous section, you learned terms relating to pathology. Before going on to the exercises, review the terms below and refer to the previous section if you have questions. Pronunciations are provided for certain terms. Sometimes information about where the word came from is included after the term. The etymologies (word histories) are for your information only. You do not need to memorize them.

Term	Definition
aneurysm [ĂN-yū-rĭzm] Greek *aneurysma*, dilation	Ballooning of the artery wall caused by weakness in the wall.
angina [ĂN-jĭ-nă, ăn-JĪ-nă] Latin, sore throat	Angina pectoris.
angina pectoris [PĔK-tōr-ĭs, pĕk-TŌR-ĭs] Latin, sore throat of the chest	Chest pain, usually caused by a lowered oxygen or blood supply to the heart.
aortic regurgitation [rē-GŬR-jĭ-TĀ-shŭn] or **reflux** [RĒ-flŭks]	Backward flow or leakage of blood through a faulty aortic valve.
aortic stenosis [stĕ-NŌ-sĭs]	Narrowing of the aorta.
arrhythmia [ā-RĬTH-mē-ă] a-, without + Greek *rhythmos*, rhythm	Irregularity in the rhythm of the heartbeat.
arteriosclerosis [ăr-TĒR-ē-ō-sklĕr-Ō-sĭs] arterio-, artery + sclerosis	Hardening of the arteries.
arteritis [ăr-tĕr-Ī-tĭs] arter-, artery + -itis, inflammation	Inflammation of an artery or arteries.
asystole [ā-SĬS-tō-lē] a- + Greek *systole*, a contracting	Cardiac arrest.
atheroma [ăth-ĕr-Ō-mă] ather-, fatty matter + oma, tumor	A fatty deposit (plaque) in the wall of an artery.

Term	Definition
atherosclerosis [ĂTH-ĕr-ō-sklĕr-ō-sĭs] athero-, fatty matter + sclerosis	Hardening of the arteries caused by the buildup of atheromas.
atrial fibrillation [fĭ-brĭ-LĀ-shŭn]	An irregular, usually rapid, heartbeat caused by overstimulation of the AV node.
atrioventricular block atrio-, atrium + ventricle	Heart block; partial or complete blockage of the electrical impulses from the atrioventricular node to the ventricles.
bacterial endocarditis	Bacterial inflammation of the inner lining of the heart.
bradycardia [brād-ē-KĂR-dē-ă] brady-, slow + Greek *kardia*, heart	Heart rate of fewer than 60 beats per minute.
bruit [brū-Ē] French, noise	Sound or murmur, especially an abnormal heart sound heard on auscultation, especially of the carotid artery.
cardiac arrest	Sudden stopping of the heart; also called asystole.
cardiac tamponade [tăm-pō-NĀD]	Compression of the heart caused by fluid accumulation in the pericardial sac.
cardiomyopathy [KĂR-dē-ō-mī-ŎP-ă-thē] cardio-, heart + myo-, muscle + -pathy, disease	Disease of the heart muscle.
claudication [klăw-dĭ-KĀ-shŭn] Latin *claudicatio*, limping	Limping caused by inadequate blood supply during activity; usually subsides during rest.
coarctation [kō-ărk-TĀ-shŭn] **of the aorta** Latin *coarcto*, to press together	Abnormal narrowing of the aorta.
congenital [kŏn-JĔN-Ĭ-tăl] **heart disease**	Heart disease (usually a type of malformation) that exists at birth.
congestive [kŏn-JĔS-tĭv] **heart failure**	Inability of the heart to pump enough blood out during the cardiac cycle; collection of fluid in the lungs results.
constriction [kŏn-STRĬK-shŭn]	Compression or narrowing caused by contraction, as of a vessel.
coronary artery disease	Condition that reduces the flow of blood and nutrients through the arteries of the heart.
cyanosis [sī-ă-NŌ-sĭs] Greek, dark blue color	Bluish or purplish coloration, as of the skin, caused by inadequate oxygenation of the blood.
deep vein thrombosis [thrŏm-BŌ-sĭs]	Formation of a thrombus (clot) in a deep vein, such as a femoral vein.
dysrhythmia [dĭs-RĬTH-mē-ă] dys-, difficult + Greek *rhythmos*, rhythm	Abnormal heart rhythm.
embolus [ĔM-bō-lŭs] Greek *embolos*, plug	Mass of foreign material blocking a vessel.

Term	Definition
endocarditis [ĔN-dō-kăr-DĪ-tĭs] endo-, within + card-, heart + -itis, inflammation	Inflammation of the endocardium, especially an inflammation caused by a bacterial (for example, staphylococci) or fungal agent.
essential hypertension	High blood pressure without any known cause.
fibrillation [fĭ-brĭ-LĀ-shŭn] Latin *fibrilla*, little fiber	Random, chaotic, irregular heart rhythm.
flutter	Regular but very rapid heartbeat.
gallop	Triple sound of a heartbeat, usually indicative of serious heart disease.
heart block	*See* atrioventricular block.
hemorrhoids [HĔM-ō-rŏydz] Greek *haima*, blood + *rhoia*, flow	Varicose condition of veins in the anal region.
high blood pressure	*See* hypertension.
hypertension [HĪ-pĕr-TĔN-shŭn] hyper-, excessive + tension	Chronic condition with blood pressure greater than 140/90.
hypertensive heart disease	Heart disease caused, or worsened, by high blood pressure.
hypotension [HĪ-pō-TĔN-shŭn] hypo-, below normal + tension	Chronic condition with blood pressure below normal.
infarct [ĬN-fărkt] Latin *infarcto*, to stuff into	Area of necrosis caused by a sudden drop in the supply of arterial or venous blood.
infarction [ĭn-FĂRK-shŭn]	Sudden drop in the supply of arterial or venous blood, often due to an embolus or thrombus.
intermittent claudication	Attacks of limping, particularly in the legs, due to ischemia of the muscles.
intracardiac [ĭn-tră-KĂR-dē-ăk] **tumor** intra-, within + cardiac	A tumor within one of the heart chambers.
ischemia [ĭs-KĒ-mē-ă] From Greek *ischo*, to keep back + *haima*, blood	Localized blood insufficiency caused by an obstruction.
low blood pressure	*See* hypotension.
mitral [MĪ-trăl] **insufficiency** or **reflux**	Backward flow of blood due to a damaged mitral valve.
mitral stenosis	Abnormal narrowing at the opening of the mitral valve.
mitral valve prolapse	Backward flow of blood into the left atrium due to protrusion of one or both mitral cusps into the left atrium during contractions.
murmur	Soft heart humming sound heard between normal beats.

Term	Definition
myocardial infarction myocardi(um) + -al, pertaining to	Sudden drop in the supply of blood to an area of the heart muscle, usually due to a blockage in a coronary artery.
myocarditis [MĪ-ō-kăr-DĪ-tĭs] myocard(ium) + -itis	Inflammation of the myocardium.
necrosis [nĕ-KRŌ-sĭs] Greek *nekrosis*, death	Death of tissue or an organ or part due to irreversible damage; usually a result of oxygen deprivation.
occlusion [ŏ-KLŪ-zhŭn] From Latin *ob-*, against + *claudo*, to close	The closing of a blood vessel.
palpitations [păl-pĭ-TĀ-shŭnz] Latin *palpito*, to throb	Uncomfortable pulsations of the heart felt as a thumping in the chest.
patent ductus arteriosus [PĂ-tĕnt DŬK-tŭs ăr-tēr-ē-Ō-sĭs]	A condition at birth in which the ductus arteriosus, a small duct between the aorta and the pulmonary artery, remains abnormally open.
perfusion deficit	Lack of flow through a blood vessel, usually caused by an occlusion.
pericarditis [PĔR-ĭ-kăr-DĪ-tĭs] pericard(ium) + -itis	Inflammation of the pericardium.
peripheral vascular disease	Vascular disease in the lower extremities, usually due to blockages in the arteries of the groin or legs.
petechiae (*sing.*, petechia) [pĕ-TĒ-kē-ē, pĕ-TĔK-ē-ē, (pĕ-TĒ-kē-ă, pĕ-TĔK-ē-ă)] Italian *petecchie*	Minute hemorrhages in the skin.
phlebitis [flĕ-BĪ-tĭs] phleb-, vein + -itis	Inflammation of a vein.
plaque [plăk] French, plate	Buildup of solid material, such as a fatty deposit, on the lining of an artery.
premature atrial contractions (PACs)	Atrial contractions that occur before the normal impulse; can be the cause of palpitations.
premature ventricular contractions (PVCs)	Ventricular contractions that occur before the normal impulse; can be the cause of palpitations.
pulmonary artery stenosis	Narrowing of the pulmonary artery, preventing the lungs from receiving enough blood from the heart to oxygenate.
pulmonary edema	Abnormal accumulation of fluid in the lungs.
Raynaud's phenomenon [rā-NŌZ] After Maurice Raynaud (1834–1881), French physician	Spasm in the arteries of the fingers causing numbness or pain.

Term	Definition
rheumatic heart disease Greek *rheumatikos*, subject to flux, the discharge of fluids	Heart valve and/or muscle damage caused by an untreated streptococcal infection.
risk factor	Any of various factors considered to increase the probability that a disease will occur; for example, high blood pressure and smoking are considered risk factors for heart disease.
rub	Frictional sound heard between heartbeats, usually indicating a pericardial murmur.
secondary hypertension	Hypertension having a known cause, such as kidney disease.
septal defect	Congenital abnormality consisting of an opening in the septum between the atria or ventricles.
stenosis [stĕ-NŌ-sĭs]	Narrowing, particularly of blood vessels or of the cardiac valves.
tachycardia [TĂK-ĭ-KĂR-dē-ă] tachy-, fast + Greek *kardia*, heart	Heart rate greater than 100 beats per minute.
tetralogy of Fallot [fă-LŌ] After Étienne-Louis A. Fallot (1850–1911), French physician	Set of four congenital heart abnormalities appearing together that cause deoxygenated blood to enter the systemic circulation: ventricular septal defect, pulmonary stenosis, incorrect position of the aorta, and right ventricular hypertrophy.
thrombophlebitis [THRŎM-bō-flĕ-BĪ-tĭs] thrombo-, thrombus + phleb- + -itis	Inflammation of a vein with a thrombus.
thrombosis [thrŏm-BŌ-sĭs] Greek, a clotting	Presence of a thrombus in a blood vessel.
thrombotic [thrŏm-BŎT-ĭk] **occlusion**	Narrowing caused by a thrombus.
thrombus [THRŎM-bŭs] Latin, clot	Stationary blood clot in the cardiovascular system, usually formed from matter found in the blood.
tricuspid stenosis	Abnormal narrowing of the opening of the tricuspid valve.
valvulitis [văl-vyū-LĪ-tĭs] New Latin *valvula*, value + -itis	Inflammation of a heart valve.
varicose [VĂR-ĭ-kōs] **vein** Latin *varix*, dilated vein	Dilated, enlarged, or twisted vein, usually on the leg.
vegetation [vĕj-ĕ-TĀ-shŭn]	Clot on a heart valve or opening, usually caused by infection.

Applying Medical Technology to Reimbursement

Mr. Davino had a follow-up visit in Dr. Mirkhan's office. The doctor's billing clerk received the records and notes for Mr. Davino. Mr. Davino's insurance company will pay the claim once the doctor's office submits it for payment. A section of the claim is shown below

Critical Thinking

82. On the claim, what is the procedure code for the service provided to Mr. Davino?

83. On the claim, what is the code for Mr. Davino's diagnosis?

24. A DATE(S) OF SERVICE From MM DD YY — To MM DD YY	B Place of Service	C Type of Service	D PROCEDURES, SERVICES, OR SUPPLIES (Explain Unusual Circumstances) CPT/HCPCS MODIFIER	E DIAGNOSIS CODE	F $ CHARGES	G DAYS OR UNITS	H EPSDT Family Plan	I EMG	J COB	K RESERVED FOR LOCAL USE
1 08 15 XXXX			82803	1	74 00	1				
2										
3										
4										
5										
6										

25. FEDERAL TAX I.D. NUMBER SSN EIN	26. PATIENT'S ACCOUNT NO.	27. ACCEPT ASSIGNMENT? (For govt. claims, see back)	28. TOTAL CHARGE	29. AMOUNT PAID	30. BALANCE DUE
12-34-56789 [X] [ ]	000-77-9999	[X] YES [ ] NO	$ 74 00	$	$ 74 00

PHYSICIAN OR SUPPLIER INFORMATION

PATHOLOGICAL TERMS EXERCISES

Make an Educated Guess

For each of the following four situations, insert the likely age of the patient from the following age ranges. Use each range only once.

A. 0–2

B. 11–18

C. 40–55

D. 67–90

84. A patient going into surgery for a septal defect _____

85. Arteriosclerosis with pulmonary edema _____

86. Cardiac arrest of an athlete during a stressful game _____

87. Hypertension due to stress _____

Check Your Knowledge

Complete the sentences below by filling in the blanks.

88. Heart rhythms may be dangerously fast (called _____) or dangerously slow (called _____).

89. Atrial fibrillation is another name for _____ or _____, irregular rhythm.

90. An embolus travels in the blood while a(n) _____ is stationary.

91. An abnormal sound heard on auscultation is called a(n) _____.

92. An abnormal heartbeat with a soft humming sound is called a(n) _____.

93. The most common cardiovascular disease is _____.

94. Smoking, poor diet, and lack of exercise are _____ _____ for heart disease.

95. A heart attack is also called a(n) _____ _____.

Surgical Terms

Cardiovascular surgery usually involves opening up or repairing blood vessels or valves; removal, repair, or replacement of diseased portions of blood vessels; or bypass of blocked areas. The goal of most cardiovascular surgery is to improve blood flow, thereby allowing proper oxygenation and nourishment of all the cells of the body. Many types of heart surgery are now *minimally invasive procedures*. Most heart operations require opening up the chest to access the heart. However, devices such as lasers, robotic devices, and miniature surgical instruments now allow surgeons to perform certain procedures through a "keyhole," a small opening in the chest.

A balloon catheter is used in **balloon catheter dilation** (also called **percutaneous transluminal coronary angioplasty** or **PTCA**) to open the passageway inside a blood vessel so that blood can flow freely (see Figure 6-14).

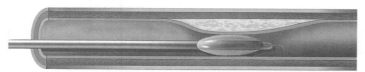

Narrowed artery with balloon catheter positioned.

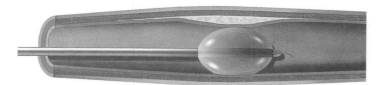

Inflated balloon presses against arterial wall.

FIGURE 6-14 Balloon catheter dilation.

MORE ABOUT . . .

Surgical Devices

New surgical devices are being developed all the time. The Da Vinci System is a robotic device that uses a tiny camera with multiple lenses inserted into the patient's chest, providing a three-dimensional image of the heart. The surgeon, at a nearby computer workstation, watches through a viewer to see inside the chest as a pair of joysticks control two robotic arms. The arms hold specially designed surgical instruments that mimic the actual movement of the surgeon's hands on the joysticks. This allows for minimal incision into the patient.

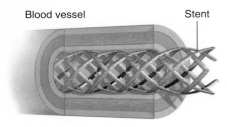

FIGURE 6-15 Drug-eluting stent.

A **balloon valvuloplasty** involves the use of a balloon catheter to open narrowed cardiac valve openings. Similarly, **angioplasty** or **coronary angioplasty** is the opening of a blood vessel using a balloon catheter. *Cardiac catheterization* uses a catheter threaded through an artery or vein into the heart to observe blood flow. It is the most common type of operation performed in the United States; over 1 million operations are performed annually. **Angioscopy** uses a fiberoptic catheter to view the interior of a blood vessel. Surgery that involves the use of cardiac catheterization is called **endovascular surgery.** During surgery, a **stent** or an **intravascular stent** may be inserted to hold a blood vessel passageway open. Many stents are now *drug-eluting* stents (Figure 6-15), meaning that they include slowly released medication that helps to maintain the open passageways. Such procedures also help to break up blockages.

Sometimes it becomes necessary to create a detour or a **bypass** around blockages. **Coronary bypass surgery** or **CABG** (coronary artery bypass graft) is performed to attach the vessel to be used for the bypass. A **graft,** particularly of a blood vessel from another part of the body, can be used to bypass an arterial blockage. Saphenous (leg) veins or mammary (chest) arteries are two types of vessels used for this procedure. The number of arteries that are bypassed determines whether a CABG is a triple (three arteries bypassed) bypass, a quadruple (four) bypass, and so on. **Fontan's operation** creates a bypass from the right atrium to the main pulmonary artery. Sometimes it is necessary to divert blood flow from the heart during surgery. This procedure, **cardiopulmonary bypass** (also called *extracorporeal circulation*), circulates the blood through a heart-lung machine and back into systemic circulation.

Surgical removal and replacement of the entire heart is called a **heart transplant. Valve replacement** is the removal and replacement of a heart valve. Surgical removal of a thrombus is a **thrombectomy;** of an embolus, an **embolectomy;** of an atheroma, an **atherectomy;** and of hemorrhoids, a **hemorrhoidectomy.** An **endarterectomy** removes the diseased lining of an artery, while an **arteriotomy** is an incision into an artery, as to remove a clot. A **valvotomy** is the incision into a cardiac valve to remove an obstruction. **Venipuncture** is a small puncture for the purpose of drawing blood (**phlebotomy**). Figure 6-16 shows a phlebotomist preparing to draw blood from a patient.

Some surgeries are for the purpose of reconstruction or repair—a **valvuloplasty** is done to reconstruct a cardiac valve. Other surgical procedures, such as **anastomosis,** are performed to connect blood vessels and to implant devices, such as *pacemakers*, that help regulate body functions. Pacemakers are small computers that provide electrical stimulation to regulate the heart rate. They can be attached temporarily (usually with a small box worn outside the body and a sensor attached to the outside of the chest) or permanently (the lead is surgically inserted into a blood vessel leading to the heart).

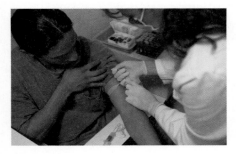

FIGURE 6-16 Phlebotomists must follow standard precautions when drawing blood.

VOCABULARY REVIEW

In the previous section, you learned terms relating to surgery. Before going on to the exercises, review the terms below and refer to the previous section if you have questions. Pronunciations are provided for certain terms. Sometimes information about where the word came from is included after the term. The etymologies (word histories) are for your information only. You do not need to memorize them.

Term	Definition
anastomosis [ă-năs-tō-MŌ-sĭs] Greek, to furnish with a mouth	Surgical connection of two blood vessels to allow blood flow between them.
angioplasty [ĂN-jē-ō-plăs-tē] angio-, vessel + -plasty, repair	Opening of a blocked blood vessel, as by balloon dilation.
angioscopy [ăn-jē-ŎS-kō-pē] angio- + -scopy, viewing	Viewing of the interior of a blood vessel using a fiberoptic catheter inserted or threaded into the vessel.
arteriotomy [ăr-tēr-ē-ŎT-ō-mē] arterio-, artery + -tomy, cutting	Surgical incision into an artery, especially to remove a clot.
atherectomy [ăth-ĕ-RĔK-tō-mē] ather-, fatty matter + -ectomy, removal	Surgical removal of an atheroma.
balloon catheter dilation	Insertion of a balloon catheter into a blood vessel to open the passage so blood can flow freely.
balloon valvuloplasty [VĂL-vyū-lō-PLĂS-tē]	Procedure that uses a balloon catheter to open narrowed orifices in cardiac valves.
bypass	A structure (usually a vein graft) that creates a new passage for blood to flow from one artery to another artery or part of an artery; used to create a detour around blockages in arteries.
cardiopulmonary [KĂR-dē-ō-PŬL-mŏ-nēr-ē] **bypass**	Procedure used during surgery to divert blood flow to and from the heart through a heart-lung machine and back into circulation.
coronary angioplasty	*See* angioplasty.
coronary bypass surgery	*See* bypass.
embolectomy [ĕm-bō-LĔK-tō-mē] embol(us) + -ectomy	Surgical removal of an embolus.
endarterectomy [ĕnd-ăr-tēr-ĔK-tō-mē] end-, within + arter-, artery + -ectomy	Surgical removal of the diseased portion of the lining of an artery.
endovascular [ĕn-dō-VĂS-kyū-lăr] **surgery** endo-, within + vascular	Any of various procedures performed during cardiac catheterization, such as angioscopy and atherectomy.
Fontan's [FŎN-tănz] **operation** After François Fontan (1929–), French surgeon	Surgical procedure that creates a bypass from the right atrium to the main pulmonary artery; Fontan's procedure.
graft	Any tissue or organ implanted to replace or mend damaged areas.
heart transplant	Implantation of the heart of a person who has just died into a person whose diseased heart cannot sustain life.
hemorrhoidectomy [HĔM-ō-rŏy-DĔK-tō-mē] hemorrhoid + -ectomy;	Surgical removal of hemorrhoids.

Term	Definition
intravascular stent intra-, within + vascular	Stent placed within a blood vessel to allow blood to flow freely.
percutaneous transluminal [pĕr-kyū-TĀ-nē-ŭs trăns-LŪ-mĭn-ăl] **coronary angioplasty**	*See* balloon catheter dilation.
phlebotomy [flĕ-BŎT-ō-mē] phlebo-, vein + -tomy	Drawing blood from a vein via a small incision.
stent [stĕnt]	Surgically implanted device used to hold something (as a blood vessel) open.
thrombectomy [thrŏm-BĔK-tō-mē] thromb-, thrombus + -ectomy	Surgical removal of a thrombus.
valve replacement	Surgical replacement of a coronary valve.
valvotomy [văl-VŎT-ō-mē] valve + -tomy	Incision into a cardiac valve to remove an obstruction.
valvuloplasty [VĂL-vyū-lō-PLĂS-tē] New Latin *valvula*, valve + -plasty	Surgical reconstruction of a cardiac valve.
venipuncture [VĔN-ĭ-pŭnk-chŭr, VĒ-nĭ-PŬNK-chŭr] veni-, vein + puncture	Small puncture into a vein, usually to draw blood or inject a solution.

CASE STUDY

Surgery Helps

Mr. Davino's progress is poor after three days in the hospital. After determining that his heart has extensive blockages, the doctors decide to perform a CABG on him. Mr. Davino has a smooth postoperative recovery. He is told that he must make some lifestyle changes and will have to attend a cardiac rehabilitation center as an outpatient.

Critical Thinking

96. What are some of the lifestyle changes the staff at the cardiac rehabilitation center will probably recommend?
97. Evaluate your own general cardiovascular health based on your lifestyle. What changes should you make to prevent heart disease?

SURGICAL TERMS EXERCISES

Check Your Knowledge

Define the following terms.

98. Anastomosis is _____

99. Valvuloplasty is _____

100. Valvotomy is _____

101. Embolectomy is _____

102. Angioplasty is _____

Spell It Correctly

Check the spelling of the following terms. If the term is spelled correctly, put "C" in the blank. If not, put the correct spelling.

103. thromboctomy _____

104. atherectomy _____

105. arteritomy _____

106. angiascopy _____

107. hemorrhoidectomy _____

108. valvitomy _____

109. veinipuncture _____

110. valvuloplasty _____

111. coronery _____

Pharmacological Terms

Drug therapy for the cardiovascular system generally treats the following conditions: angina, heart attack, high blood pressure, high cholesterol, congestive heart failure, rhythm disorders, and vascular problems. Many of the pharmacological agents treat several problems at once. Table 6-1 lists some of the medications commonly used to treat the cardiovascular system. These are just a sample of the many cardiovascular medications available. To find about more details about heart medications, go to www.americanheart.org and search medications.

TABLE 6-1 Medications for the Cardiovascular System

Drug Class	Purpose	Generic Name	Trade Name
coronary vasodilators	dilate veins, arteries, and coronary arteries; used to treat angina, myocardial infarction, congestive heart failure	nitroglycerin	Nitrocot, Nitrong, Deponit, Nitro-Dur, Nitro-Bid, Transderm-Nitro, and many others
beta blockers	reduce contraction strength of heart muscle; lower blood pressure; slow heartbeat	propanolol metroprolol atenolol bisoprolol	Inderal Lopressor Tenormin Zabeta
calcium channel blockers	inhibit ability of calcium ions to enter heart muscle and blood vessel muscle cells; reduce heart rate; lower squeezing strength of heart contraction; lower blood pressure; dilate coronary arteries to enhance blood flow; normalize some fast or irregular heartbeats	verapamil nifedipine diltiazem nicardipine amlodipine bepridil felodipine	Calan, Isoptin, Verelan Procardia, Adalat Cardizem, Dilacor XR Cardene Noravsc, Istin Vascor Plendil, Hydac
thrombolytics	dissolve blood clots	urokinase tissue-type plasminogen activator (tPA, TPA)	Abbokinase Activase

(continued)

TABLE 6-1 (continued)

Drug Class	Purpose	Generic Name	Trade Name
bile acid sequestrants	lipid-lowering medications that bind to bile acids and require more body cholesterol to create other bile acids; more cholesterol used up and hence lowered	cholestyramine colestipol colesevalam	Prevalite, Questran, Cholybar Colestid Welchol
lipid-lowering medications	reduce triglycerides and cholesterol (but mechanisms not totally understood)	atorvastatin lovastatin pravastatin simvastatin	Lipitor Mevacor Pravachol Zocor
centrally acting hypertensive agents, antihypertensive	decrease blood pressure by affecting brain control centers	methyldopa guanfacine guanabenz	Aldomet Tenex Wytensin
direct-acting vasodilators	lower blood pressure by relaxing walls of blood vessels	hydralazine minoxidil	Apresoline Loniten
peripherally acting hypertensive agents	lower blood pressure by affecting nerves involved in blood pressure regulation	guanadrel guanethidine mecamylamine prazosin rauwolfia alkaloids	Hylorel Ismelin Inversine Minipres Harmonyl, Raudixin,
ACE inhibitors	ease heart pumping and lower blood pressure by dilating arteries	lisinopril enalapril quinapril	Zestril, Prinivil Vasotec, Renitec Accupril
angiotensin II receptor blockers	block the action of angiotensin II, a chemical that causes blood vessels to narrow. The blood vessels then dilate and blood pressure is lowered.	lasartan valsarartan irbesartan	Cozaar Diovin Avapro
diuretics	promote removal of water by kidneys to lower blood pressure and relieve edema	furosemide hydrochlorothiazide spironolactone bumetanide	Lasix Esidrix, Hydrodiuril Aldactone Bumex
combination diuretics		hydrochlorothiazide plus triamterene	Maxzide
inotropic agents	increase amount of blood the heart is able to pump by increasing squeezing strength of heart muscle	digitalis milrinone digoxin digitoxin dopamine	Primacor Lanoxin, Lanoxicap Crystodigin Intropin
antiarrhythmics	alter the electrical flow through the heart's conduction system thereby regulating fast or irregular heartbeats	quinidine procainamide disopyramide mexiletine	Cardioquin, Quinagulte, Quinidex, Quinora Procan SR, Pronestyl Norpace, Norpace CR Mexitil

TABLE 6-1 (continued)

Drug Class	Purpose	Generic Name	Trade Name
anticoagulants, anticlotting	reduce proteins involved in blood clotting so clots cannot form as readily	warfarin enoxaparin dicumarol heparin	Coumadin Lovenox
antiplatelet medications	reduce ability of blood platelets to clot	aspirin dipyridamole clopidogrel	(numerous) Persantine Plavix
hemorrheologic agents	decrease viscosity of blood; used to treat claudication	pentoxifylline cukistazik	Trental Pletal

Antianginals relieve the pain and prevent attacks of angina. Three categories of drugs—**nitrates, beta blockers,** and **calcium channel blockers**—are used as antianginals. Figure 6-17 illustrates how antianginals can be administered. **Thrombolytics** are used to dissolve blood clots in heart-attack victims. **Tissue-type plasminogen activator (tPA or TPA)** is an agent used to prevent the formation of a thrombus. Nitrates and beta blockers are used to treat myocardial infarctions.

High blood pressure may require treatment with one drug or a combination of drugs. Such drugs are called **antihypertensives.** Beta blockers and calcium channel blockers are used along with a number of agents that affect the control centers in the brain that regulate blood pressure. **Vasodilators** relax the walls of the blood vessels. Other treatments for high blood pressure include **diuretics,** to relieve edema (swelling) and increase kidney function; **angiotensin converting enzyme (ACE) inhibitors,** which dilate arteries thus making it easier for blood to flow out of the heart; and agents that affect the nerves of the body. Congestive heart failure is treated with ACE inhibitors, diuretics, and **cardiotonics,** which increase myocardial contractions. In certain situations, **vasoconstrictors** may be needed to narrow blood vessels.

Rhythm disorders are treated with a number of medications(some are called **antiarrhythmics**) that normalize heart rate by affecting the nervous system that controls the heart rate. Beta blockers and calcium channel blockers may also be used for rhythm disorders.

Cholesterol is a substance the body needs in certain quantities. Excesses of certain kinds of cholesterol such as LDL can cause fatty deposits or plaque to form on blood vessels. **Lipid-lowering** drugs work in various ways (some of which are not understood) to help the body excrete unwanted cholesterol. Blood clotting in vessels can cause dangerous blockages. The most common type of lipid-lowering drugs are **statins.** The widespread use of statins is thought to be helping reduce the incidence of coronary artery disease. **Anticoagulants,** anticlotting and *antiplatelet* medications (such as **heparin**) inhibit the ability of the blood to clot. Other medications used for vascular problems may include drugs that decrease the thickness of the blood, or drugs that increase the amount of blood the heart is able to pump.

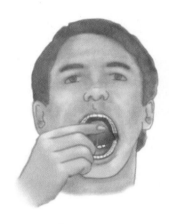
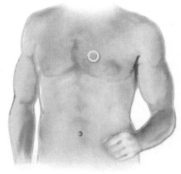

FIGURE 6-17 The most common antianginal is nitroglycerin, which is administered sublingually under the tongue or via a patch on the skin.

VOCABULARY REVIEW

In the previous section, you learned terms relating to pharmacology. Before going on to the exercises, review the terms below and refer to the previous section if you have questions. Pronunciations are provided for certain terms. Sometimes information about where the word came from is included after the term. The etymologies (word histories) are for your information only. You do not need to memorize them.

Agent	Purpose
angiotensin converting enzyme (ACE) inhibitor [ăn-jē-ō-TĔN-sĭn] angio-, vessel + (hyper)tension	Medication used for heart failure and other cardiovascular problems; acts by dilating arteries to lower blood pressure and makes heart pump easier.
antianginal [ăn-tē-ĂN-jĭ-năl] anti-, against + angina	Agent used to relieve or prevent attacks of angina.
antiarrhythmic [ăn-tē-ā-RĬTH-mĭ] anti- + arrhythmic	Agent used to help normalize cardiac rhythm.
anticlotting anti- + clotting	*See* anticoagulant.
anticoagulant anti- + coagulant	Agent that prevents the formation of dangerous clots
antihypertensive anti- + hypertensive	Agent that helps control high blood pressure.
beta [BĀ-tă] **blocker**	Agent that lowers blood pressure by reducing contraction strength of the heart muscle; slows heartbeat.
calcium channel blocker	Medication that lessens the ability of calcium ions to enter heart and blood vessel muscle cells; used to lower blood pressure and normalize some arrhythmias.
cardiotonic [KĂR-dē-ō-TŎN-ĭk] cardio-, heart + Greek *tonos*, tension	Medication for congestive heart failure; increases the force of contractions of the myocardium.
diuretic [dī-yū-RĔT-ĭk] di-, throughout + Greek *uresis*, urine	Medication that promotes the excretion of urine.
heparin [HĔP-ă-rĭn] From Greek *hepar*, liver	Anticoagulant present in the body; also, synthetic version administered to prevent clotting.
lipid-lowering	Helpful in lowering cholesterol levels.
nitrate [NĪ-trāt]	Any of several medications that dilate the veins, arteries, or coronary arteries; used to control angina.
statins [STĀ-tĭnz]	A class of lipid-lowering agents that are the most frequently used today.
thrombolytic [thrŏm-bō-LĬT-ĭk] thrombo-, thrombus + -lytic, destroying destroying	Agent that dissolves a thrombus.
tissue-type plasminogen [plăz-MĬN-ō-jĕn] **activator (tPA, TPA)**	Agent that prevents a thrombus from forming.
vasoconstrictor [VĀ-sō-kŏn-STRĬK-tŏr] vaso-, vessel + constrictor	Agent that narrows the blood vessels.
vasodilator [VĀ-sō-dī-LĀ-tŏr] vaso- + dilator	Agent that dilates or widens the blood vessels.

The Long-Term Treatment

As part of Mr. Davino's long-term rehabilitation, medication has been prescribed, as shown on the prescription forms given to him upon his release.

Critical Thinking

112. For what condition is Mr. Davino's medication in prescriptin form (a) most likely being prescribed?

113. Prescription form (b) prescribes a medication for what other condition?

a

Dr. Andar Mirkhan
16 Courtyard Lane • Andover, Ohio 66666

PATIENT'S NAME _Joseph Davino_ AGE _44_

ADDRESS _____

CITY _Wesley_____ DATE _9/1/XX_

℞

      Questran 4g ac TID
      _#90_

DEA NO. 54321x
LICENSE NO. 12345y   _Andar Mirkhan, M.D._
               SIGNATURE

b

Dr. Andar Mirkhan
16 Courtyard Lane • Andover, Ohio 66666

PATIENT'S NAME _Joseph Davino_ AGE _44_

ADDRESS _____

CITY _Wesley_____ DATE _9/1/XX_

℞

      Lasix 80 mg q12h
      _#60_

DEA NO. 54321x
LICENSE NO. 12345y   _Andar Mirkhan, M.D._
               SIGNATURE

PHARMACOLOGICAL TERMS EXERCISES

Reverse Diagnosis

Using Table 6-1, describe the condition for which each combination of medications is probably being prescribed.

114. metroprolol, Vasotec, and Bumex _____

115. Coumadin, aspirin, and pentoxifylline _____

116. nitroglycerin, Avapro, and furosmide _____

Check Your Knowledge

From Table 6-1, name at least one medication used to treat each of the following conditions.

117. hypertension _____

118. water retention _____

119. arrhythmia _____

120. high cholesterol _____

121. clotting _____

122. arterial plaque _____

123. angina _____

124. congestive heart failure _____

Matching

Match the following cardiovascular pharmacological classifications with their correct definitions.

125. _____ diuretics

126. _____ ACE inhibitors

127. _____ calcium channel blockers

a. reduce ability of blood platelets to clot

b. decrease viscosity of blood

c. dissolve blood clots

128. _____ vasodilators
129. _____ beta blockers
130. _____ antiplatelet medication
131. _____ anticoagulants
132. _____ hemorrheologic agents
133. _____ antiarrhyhmics
134. _____ thrombolytics

d. ease heart pumping, lower blood pressure

e. alter electrical flow through the heart

f. increase urine production, relieve edema

g. reduce contraction of heart, slow heartbeat

h. dilate veins and arteries, used to treat angina

i. reduce blood clotting

j. reduce heart rate, lower squeezing strength of heart contraction, lower blood pressure by inhibiting calcium from entering heart muscle

Match the following medications with their correct pharmacological classification. Some answers may be used more than once and some not at all.

135. _____ Coumadin
136. _____ aspirin
137. _____ procainamide
138. _____ nitroglycerin
139. _____ verapamil
140. _____ Lipitor
141. _____ Accupril
142. _____ Lasix
143. _____ Inderal
144. _____ digitalis

a. anticoagulant

b. inotropic agent

c. antiarrhythmic

d. lipid-lowering medication

e. diuretic

f. beta blocker

g. antiplatelet medication

h. coronary vasodilator

i. calcium channel blocker

j. ACE inhibitor

CHALLENGE SECTION

The cardiologists on the hospital staff have a weekly meeting to review cases. Dr. Woodard and Dr. Mirkhan have discussed the admission of Mr. Davino to the CCU and have reported on his progress. Another interesting case is a 50-year-old woman who presented with no symptoms except chest pain when she was admitted for possible coronary disease. After she was stabilized in the emergency room, the cardiologist on call examined her closely. The patient was found to have very few risk factors (nonsmoker, normal weight, normal BP). However, upon discussions with her, they found she has a high-stress job and a moderate-to-poor diet. The notes on the woman's record are shown here.

Referring physician: Margaret Lao, M.D.

Examination: Resting pulse was 78 beats per minute. The blood pressure was 126/80 mm/Hg. Lungs clear. Soft systolic ejection murmur along left sternal border.

ECG: Patient's resting, modified 12-lead ECG had no resting abnormalities.

Patient was given a stress electrocardiogram one month ago. Her doctor noted no exercise-associated arrythmias and found mild-to-moderate hypokinesis of inferior and posterior segments. Her improved contractility with exercise suggested adequate myocardial perfusion.

Critical Thinking

From the cardiologist's notes, describe the patient's condition.

_____

_____

_____

_____

TERMINOLOGY IN ACTION

Shown below is a medical chart entry in SOAP format for a 61-year-old male. What is his diagnosis and what are some ways it could be treated in addition to the prescribed medication?

Patient Name: Donald Arelio   March 29, 2XXX

S: Mr. Arelio is a 61-year-old male who has a problem with nosebleeds. No history of nose trauma. Hemorrhage occurs spontaneously approximately once a week for a couple of months often followed by a period of no nosebleeds for several weeks. The bleeding often starts at rest and sometimes upon exertion. He has been able to stop them with pressure up until the last week. He has no other bleeding problems and is not currently taking any medication.

O: BP 180/71; pulse 80; height 69"; weight 235 lb. No active bleeding at this time, but there is a small clot over the anterior midseptum.

A: 1. Hypertension

   2. Recurrent epistaxis

P: Patient was given Procardia sublingually with blood pressure dropping to 140/70. Patient was instructed in treatment of nosebleeds. Schedule for a recheck of blood pressure in 5 days. IF nosebleeds continue, he may need a referral.

USING THE INTERNET

If you search the World Wide Web for the American Heart Association (http://www.amhrt.org), you will find many discussions of all aspects of heart disease.

Use the Internet to find and list at least three inherited (genetic) risk factors and at least three acquired risk factors for heart disease.

List at least three things you can do personally to prevent heart disease.

What are three heart attack warning signs listed on the American Heart Association's Web site?

CHAPTER REVIEW

The material that follows is to help you review all the material in this chapter.

Building Cardiovascular Terms

Using word parts you have learned in this chapter and earlier chapters, build the correct medical term for each of the following definitions.

145. Hardening of fatty plaque on the arterial wall: _____

146. Inflammation of the inner layer of the heart: _____

147. Abnormally slow heart rate: _____

148. Narrowed blood vessels: _____

149. Disease of the heart muscle: _____

150. A blood clot: _____

151. Narrowing of the aorta: _____

152. Mass of blood in the tissues: _____

153. Abnormally enlarged heart: _____

154. Viewing the aorta by x-ray with contrast: _____

155. Using sound waves to produce images of the heart (structure and motion): _____

156. An electrical tracing of the heart conduction system: _____

157. Deficiency of blood flow: _____

158. Unusually rapid, fast heart rate: _____

159. Hardening of the arteries: _____

160. Study of the heart: _____

161. Abnormally low body temperature: _____

162. Study of blood: _____

163. Dissolving of a blood clot: _____

164. Study of veins: _____

165. Originating in the heart: _____

166. Formation of blood cells: _____

167. Pertaining to the heart: _____

168. Instrument used to record the electrical activity of the heart: _____

169. Radiographic imaging of a blood vessel: _____

170. Process of recording the electrical activity of the heart: _____

171. Incision into a vein: _____

172. Excision of fatty plaque: _____

173. Inflammation of the sac surrounding the heart: _____

Know the Meaning

For each of the following definitions, write the correct term in the space provided.

174. Connect arterioles with venules: _____

175. Carry oxygen-rich blood away from the heart: _____

176. The body's smallest veins: _____

177. Vessels that carries blood back to the heart: _____

178. Outermost layer of the heart muscle: _____

179. The body's largest, most pressurized vessel: _____

180. Vessel that delivers oxygen-poor blood to the heart from the upper portion of the body: _____

181. Tube-like vessels that supply blood to the entire body: _____

182. Controls blood flow between left atrium and left ventricle: _____

183. Vessels that return oxygen-rich blood from the lungs to the heart: _____

184. Inner opening of a vessel that the blood flows through: _____

185. Structure in the fetal circulatory system that allows the blood to bypass the undeveloped lungs: _____

186. Organ of muscle that receives blood from the veins and returns it to the body through the arteries: _____

187. Innermost layer of the heart muscle: _____

188. Opening in the septum of the fetal heart that closes soon after birth: _____

189. Upper right chamber of the heart: _____

190. Separates the right and left halves of the heart: _____

191. Vessel that supplies the heart with oxygen-rich blood: _____

True or False

Circle T for true or F for false.

192. The term *atrioventricular* relates to the atria and the ventricles of the heart. T F

193. *Thrombocytosis* is an abnormal decrease in the number of platelets in the blood. T F

194. An image of a blood vessel is called an *angiography*. T F

195. A patient with an abnormally large heart is diagnosed with *cardiopathy*. T F

196. *Arteriography* is the x-ray of an artery after the injection of a contrast medium. T F

197. A normal heart rhythm is called *normal sinus rhythm*. T F

198. The amount of blood pushed out of the ventricles with each contraction is measured as the *ejection fraction*. T F

199. Laboratory blood tests performed to determine whether a patient has experienced a myocardial infarction are called *serum enzyme tests*. T F

200. A test that measures the blood pressure, heart rate, and other functions while the patient is exercising on a treadmill is called an *echocardiogram*. T F

201. A portable device that is used to perform a 24-hour electrocardiogram is a *Holter monitor*. T F

Matching

Match the following heart rhythms with their correct descriptions.

202. _____ unusually fast heart beat above 100 bpm

203. _____ a regular but very rapid heartbeat
more than 250 bpm

204. _____ a normal, regular heart beat

205. _____ slow but regular heartbeat below 60 bpm

206. _____ chaotic, irregular, life-threatening rhythm

207. _____ rapid, triple beat of the heart

208. _____ the heart has completely stopped beating

209. _____ sudden drop in blood supply to the heart,
usually due to a blockage in a coronary artery

a. normal sinus

b. bradycardiae

c. fibrillation

d. flutter

e. tachycardia

f. asystole

g. myocardial infarction

h. gallop

Match the following cardiac terms with their correct definitions. Some answers may be used twice and some not at all.

210. _____ ductus arteriosus

211. _____ aorta

212. _____ myocardium

213. _____ aortic valve

214. _____ septum

215. _____ systole

216. _____ pulmonary valve

a. contraction

b. muscular tissue

c. semilunar valve

d. thrombocytes

e. fetal circulation

f. partition

g. largest artery

Remembering Suffixes

Write the suffix (used in cardiovascular terms) belonging to the following definitions.

217. pertaining to _____

218. hardening _____

219. removal _____

220. abnormal decrease _____

221. pain _____

222. disease _____

223. cell _____

224. destroying _____

225. condition, state of _____

226. sound _____

227. condition of cells _____

228. relating to blood _____

229. inflammation _____

230. enlargement _____

231. surgical repair _____

Remembering Prefixes

Write the prefix (used in cardiovascular terms) belonging to the following definitions.

232. blood clot _____
233. half _____
234. reflected sound _____
235. slow _____
236. surround _____
237. rapid, fast _____
238. inner _____
239. below normal _____
240. muscle _____
241. small _____
242. before _____
243. against _____
244. two _____
245. above normal _____
246. many _____
247. after _____
248. large _____
249. within _____
250. three _____
251. more than one _____

DEFINITIONS

Define the following terms and combining forms. Review the chapter before starting. Make sure you know how to pronounce each term as you define it. The blue words in curly brackets are references to the Spanish glossary available online at www.mhhe.com/medterm3e.

TERM

252. anastomosis [ă-năs-tō-MŌ-sĭs] {anastomosis}
253. aneurysm [ĂN-yū-rĭzm] {aneurisma}
254. angina [ĂN-jĭ-nă, ăn-JĪ-nă] {angina}
255. angina pectoris [PĔK-tōr-ĭs, pĕk-TŌR-ĭs] {angina de pecho}
256. angi(o)
257. angiocardiography [ăn-jē-ō-kăr-dē-ŎG-ră-fē]

258. angiography [ăn-jē-ŎG-ră-fē]
259. angioplasty [ĂN-jē-ō-plăs-tē] {angioplastia}
260. angioscopy [ăn-jē-ŎS-kō-pē] {angioscopia}
261. angiotensin [ăn-jē-ō-TĔN-sĭn] converting enzyme (ACE) inhibitor
262. antianginal [ăn-tē-ĂN-jĭ-năl]
263. antiarrhythmic [ăn-tē-ā-RĬTH-mĭk]

264. anticlotting
265. anticoagulant
266. antihypertensive
267. aorta [ā-ŌR-tă] {aorta}
268. aort(o)
269. aortic regurgitation [ā-ŌR-tĭk rē-GŬR-jĭ-TĀ-shŭn] or reflux [RĒ-flŭks]
270. aortic stenosis [stĕ-NŌ-sĭs]
271. aortic valve

272. aortography [ā-ōr-TŎG-ră-fē]

273. arrhythmia [ā-RĬTH-mē-ă] {arritmia}

274. arteri(o), arter(o)

275. arteriography [ăr-tēr-ē-ŎG-ră-fē]

276. arteriole [ăr-TĒ-rē-ōl] {arteriola}

277. arteriosclerosis [ăr-TĒR-ē-ō-sklĕr-Ō-sĭs] {arteriosclerosis}

278. arteriotomy [ăr-tēr-ē-ŎT-ō-mē]

279. arteritis [ăr-tēr-Ī-tĭs] {arteritis}

280. artery [ĂR-tēr-ē] {arteria}

281. asystole [ā-SĬS-tō-lē] {asistolia}

282. ather(o)

283. atherectomy [ăth-ĕ-RĔK-tō-mē]

284. atheroma [ăth-ĕr-Ō-mă] {ateroma}

285. atherosclerosis [ĂTH-ĕr-ō-sklĕr-ō-sĭs] {arteriosclerosis}

286. atri(o)

287. atrial fibrillation [Ā-trē-ăl fĭ-brĭ-LĀ-shŭn]

288. atrioventricular [Ā-trē-ō-vĕn-TRĬK-yū-lăr] block

289. atrioventricular bundle

290. atrioventricular node (AV node)

291. atrioventricular valve

292. atrium (pl., atria) [Ā-trē-ŭm (Ā-trē-ă)] {atrium}

293. auscultation [ăws-kŭl-TĀ-shŭn] {auscultación}

294. bacterial endocarditis

295. balloon catheter dilation

296. balloon valvuloplasty [VĂL-vyū-lō-PLĂS-tē]

297. beta [BĀ-tă] blocker

298. bicuspid [bī-KŬS-pĭd] valve

299. blood [blŭd] {sangre}

300. blood pressure

301. blood vessel

302. bradycardia [brăd-ē-KĂR-dē-ă] {bradicardia}

303. bruit [brū-Ē] {ruido}

304. bundle of His [hĭz, hĭs]

305. bypass

306. calcium channel blocker

307. capillary [KĂP-ĭ-lār-ē] {capilar}

308. carbon dioxide {dióxido de carbono}

309. cardi(o)

310. cardiac arrest

311. cardiac catheterization [kăth-ĕ-tĕr-ĭ-ZĀ-shŭn]

312. cardiac cycle

313. cardiac enzyme studies

314. cardiac MRI

315. cardiac scan

316. cardiac tamponade [tăm-pō-NĀD]

317. cardiomyopathy [KĂR-dē-ō-mī-ŎP-ă-thē] {cardiomiopatía}

318. cardiopulmonary [KĂR-dē-ō-PŬL-mŏ-nār-ē] bypass

319. cardiotonic [KĂR-dē-ō-TŎN-ĭk]

320. cardiovascular [KĂR-dē-ō-VĂS-kyū-lăr]

321. carotid [kă-RŎT-ĭd] artery

322. cholesterol [kō-LĔS-tĕr-ōl] {colesterol}

323. claudication [klăw-dĭ-KĀ-shŭn] {claudicación}

324. coarctation [kō-ărk-TĀ-shŭn] of the aorta

325. conduction system

326. congenital heart disease

327. congestive heart failure

328. constriction [kŏn-STRĬK-shŭn] {constricción}

329. coronary angioplasty

330. coronary [KŌR-ō-nār-ē] artery

331. coronary artery disease

332. coronary bypass surgery

333. cyanosis [sī-ă-NŌ-sĭs] {cianosis}

334. deep vein thrombosis [thrŏm-BŌ-sĭs]

335. depolarization [dē-pō-lă-rĭ-ZĀ-shŭn] {despolarización}

336. diastole [dī-ĂS-tō-lē] {diástole}

337. digital subtraction angiography

338. diuretic [dī-yū-RĔT-ĭk]

339. Doppler [DŎP-lĕr] ultrasound

340. ductus arteriosus [DŬK-tŭs ăr-tēr-ē-Ō-sŭs]

341. ductus venosus [vĕn-Ō-sĭs]

342. dysrhythmia [dĭs-RĬTH-mē-ă] {disritmia}

343. echocardiography [ĕk-ō-kăr-dē-ŎG-ră-fē] {ecocardiografía}

344. ejection fraction

345. electrocardiography [ē-lĕk-trō-kăr-dē-ŎG-ră-fē]

346. embolectomy [ĕm-bō-LĔK-tō-mē]

347. embolus [ĔM-bō-lŭs] {émbolo}

348. endarterectomy [ĕnd-ăr-tĕr-ĔK-tō-mē]

349. endocarditis [ĔN-dō-kăr-DĪ-tĭs] {endocarditis}

350. endocardium [ĕn-dō-KĂR-dē-ŭm] {endocardio}

351. endothelium [ĕn-dō-THĒ-lē-ŭm] {endotelio}

352. endovascular surgery

353. epicardium [ĕp-ĭ-KĂR-dē-ŭm] {epicardio}

354. essential hypertension

355. femoral [FĔM-ŏ-răl, FĒ-mŏ-răl] artery

356. fibrillation [fĭ-brĭ-LĀ-shŭn] {fibrilación}

357. flutter {aleteo}

358. Fontan's [FŎN-tănz] operation

359. foramen ovale [fō-RĀ-měn ō-VĂ-lē]

360. gallop {galope}

361. graft

362. heart [hărt] {corazón}

363. heart block

364. heart transplant

365. hemangi(o)

366. hemorrhoidectomy [HĔM-ō-rŏy-DĔK-tō-mē] {hemorroidectomía}

367. hemorrhoids [HĔM-ō-rŏydz] {hemorroides}

368. heparin [HĔP-ă-rĭn] {heparina}

369. high blood pressure {presión arterial alta}

370. Holter [HŌL-těr] monitor

371. hypertension [HĪ-pěr-TĔN-shŭn] {hipertensión}

372. hypertensive heart disease

373. hypotension [HĪ-pō-TĔN-shŭn] {hipotensión}

374. infarct [ĬN-fărkt] {infarto}

375. infarction [ĭn-FĂRK-shŭn] {infarto}

376. inferior vena cava [VĒ-nă KĂ-vă, KĀ-vă]

377. intermittent claudication

378. intracardiac [ĭn-tră-KĂR-dē-ăk] tumor

379. intravascular stent

380. ischemia [ĭs-KĒ-mē-ă] {isquemia}

381. left atrium

382. left ventricle

383. lipid-lowering

384. lipid [LĬP-ĭd] profile

385. low blood pressure {presión arterial baja}

386. lumen [LŪ-měn] {lumen}

387. mitral [MĪ-trăl] insufficiency or reflux

388. mitral stenosis

389. mitral [MĪ-trăl] valve

390. mitral valve prolapse

391. multiple-gated acquisition (MUGA) angiography

392. murmur {soplo}

393. myocardial infarction

394. myocarditis [MĪ-ō-kăr-DĪ-tĭs] {miocarditis}

395. myocardium [mī-ō-KĂR-dē-ŭm] {miocardio}

396. necrosis [ně-KRŌ-sĭs] {necrosis}

397. nitrate [NĪ-trāt]

398. occlusion [ŏ-KLŪ-zhŭn] {oclusión}

399. pacemaker {marcapaso}

400. palpitations [păl-pĭ-TĀ-shŭnz] {palpitaciones}

401. patent ductus arteriosus [PĂ-těnt DŬK-tŭs ăr-tēr-ē-Ō-sĭs]

402. percutaneous transluminal [pěr-kyū-TĀ-nē-ŭs trăns-LŪ-mĭn-ăl] coronary angioplasty

403. perfusion deficit

404. pericardi(o)

405. pericarditis [PĔR-ĭ-kăr-DĪ-tĭs] {pericarditis}

406. pericardium [pěr-ĭ-KĂR-dē-ŭm] {pericardio}

407. peripheral vascular disease

408. petechiae (sing., petechia) [pě-TĒ-kē-ē, pě-TĔK-ē-ē (pě-TĒ-kē-ă, pě-TĔK-ē-ă)] {petequia}

409. phleb(o)

410. phlebitis [flě-BĪ-tĭs] {flebitis}

411. phlebography [flě-BŎG-ră-fē] {flebografía}

412. phlebotomy [flě-BŎT-ō-mē] {flebotomía}

413. plaque [plăk] {placa}

414. polarization [pō-lăr-ĭ-ZĀ-shŭn] {polarización}

415. popliteal [pŏp-LĬT-ē-ăl] artery

416. positron emission tomography [tō-MŎG-ră-fē] (PET) scan

417. premature atrial contractions (PACs)

418. premature ventricular contractions (PVCs)

419. pulmonary [PŬL-mō-nār-ē] artery {arteria pulmonar}

420. pulmonary artery stenosis

421. pulmonary edema

422. pulmonary valve

423. pulmonary vein

424. pulse [pŭls] {pulso}

425. Raynaud's [rā-NŌZ] phenomenon

426. repolarization [rē-pō-lăr-ĭ-ZĀ-shŭn] {repolarización}

427. rheumatic heart disease

428. right atrium

429. right ventricle

430. risk factor

431. rub {roce}

432. saphenous [să-FĒ-nŭs] vein

433. secondary hypertension

434. semilunar [sěm-ē-LŪ-năr] valve

435. septal defect

436. septum (pl., septa) [SĔP-tŭm (SĔP-tă)] {tabique}

437. serum enzyme tests

438. sinoatrial [sī-nō-Ā-trē-ăl] node (SA node)

439. sinus rhythm

440. sonography [sō-NŎG-ră-fē] {sonografía}

441. sphygm(o)

442. sphygmomanometer [SFĬG-mō-mă-NŎM-ě-těr] {esfigmomanómetro}

443. statins [STĀ-tĭ-nz]

444. stenosis [stě-NŌ-sĭs] {estenosis}

445. stent [stěnt]

446. stress test

447. superior vena cava

448. systole [SĬS-tō-lē] {sístole}

449. tachycardia [TĂK-ĭ-KĂR-dē-ă] {taquicardia}

450. tetralogy of Fallot [fă-LŌ]

451. thromb(o)

452. thrombectomy [thrŏm-BĔK-tō-mē] {trombectomia}

453. thrombolytic [thrŏm-bō-LĬT-ĭk]

454. thrombophlebitis [THRŎM-bō-flĕ-BĪ-tĭs] {tromboflebitis}

455. thrombosis [thrŏm-BŌ-sĭs] {trombosis}

456. thrombotic [thrŏm-BŎT-ĭk] occlusion

457. thrombus [THRŎM-bŭs] {trombo}

458. tissue-type plasminogen [plăz-MĬN-ō-jĕn] activator (tPA, TPA)

459. tricuspid [trī-KŬS-pĭd] stenosis

460. tricuspid valve

461. triglyceride [trī-GLĬS-ĕr-īd] {triglicérido}

462. valve [vălv] {válvula}

463. valve replacement

464. valvotomy [văl-VŎT-ō-mē]

465. valvulitis [văl-vyū-LĪ-tĭs] {valvulitis}

466. valvuloplasty [VĂL-vyū-lō-PLĂS-tē] {valvuloplastia}

467. varicose [VĂR-ĭ-kōs] vein

468. vas(o)

469. vasoconstrictor [VĂ-sō-kŏn-STRĬK-tŏr]

470. vasodilator [VĂ-sō-dĭ-LĀ-tŏr]

471. vegetation [vĕj-ĕ-TĀ-shŭn] {vegetación}

472. vein [vān] {vena}

473. vena cava (pl., venae cavae) [VĒ-nă KĂ-vă, KĀ-vă (VĒ-nē KĂ-vĕ, KĀ-vĕ)]

474. ven(o)

475. venipuncture [VĔN-ĭ-pŭnk-chŭr, VĒ-nĭ-PŬNK-chŭr] {venipuntura}

476. venography [vē-NŎG-ră-fē] {venografía}

477. ventricle [VĔN-trĭ-kl] {ventrículo}

478. ventriculogram [vĕn-TRĬK-yū-lō-grăm]

479. venule [VĔN-yūl, VĒ-nŭl] {vénula}

Abbreviations

Write out the full meaning of each abbreviation.

480. AcG

481. AF

482. AS

483. ASCVD

484. ASD

485. ASHD

486. AV

487. BP

488. CABG

489. CAD

490. zcath

491. CCU

492. CHD

493. CHF

494. CO

495. CPK

496. CPR

497. CVA

498. CVD

499. DSA

500. DVT

501. ECG, EKG

502. ECHO

503. ETT

504. GOT

505. HDL

506. LDH

507. LDL

508. LV

509. LVH

510. MI

511. MR

512. MS

513. MUGA

514. MVP

515. PAC

516. PTCA

517. PVC

518. SA

519. SV

520. tPA, TPA

521. VLDL

522. VSD

523. VT

Answers to Chapter Exercises

1. overweight, sedentary, smoker
2. no
3. a. pulmonary valve—controls blood flow between the right ventricle and the pulmonary arteries
   b. aortic valve—controls blood flow between the aorta and the left ventricle
   c. right pulmonary artery—one of two arteries that carry blood that is low in oxygen from the heart to the lungs
   d. interatrial septum—partition separating the two atria
   e. tricuspid valve—atrioventricular valve on the right side of the heart
   f. inferior vena cava—large vein that draws blood from the lower part of the body to the right atrium
   g. right ventricle—one of the heart's four chambers
   h. interventricular septum—part of the septum between two ventricles
   i. left ventricle—one of the heart's four chambers
   j. aorta—artery through which blood exits the heart
4. atrioventricular
5. capillary
6. C
7. Purkinje fibers
8. C
9. arteriole
10. C
11. C
12. systole
13. artery
14. veins
15. endocardium
16. atria and ventricles
17. blood
18. poor diet, smoking, and lack of exercise
19. pulmonary
20. endothelium
21. heart and lungs
22. carotid artery
23. lungs
24. cardiomyopathy
25. pericarditis
26. venogram
27. phlebitis
28. arterioplasty
29. vasoneuropathy
30. vasotropic
31. cardiogenic
32. cardiomegaly
33. thromboarteritis
34. phlebitis
35. thrombectomy
36. phleboplasty, venoplasty
37. atriomegaly
38. phlebograph, venograph
39. cardiomegaly
40. cardiopulmonary
41. pericardiostomy
42. endocarditis
43. phleboplasty, venoplasty
44. vasoparalysis
45. angiorrhaphy
46. phlebitis
47. arteries
48. vein
49. MI
50. artery
51. Skin color and disorientation
52. 8 hours
53. d
54. f
55. h
56. I
57. a
58. g
59. I
60. e
61. c
62. b
63. h
64. c
65. f
66. i
67. g
68. c
69. e
70. j
71. d
72. a
73. ECG–electrocardiogram
74. CCU–coronary care unit
75. MI—myocardial infarction
76. BP—blood pressure
77. ECHO—echocardiogram
78. yes
79. cholesterol
80. arteriosclerosis
81. exercise thallium test, sodium, potassium, CO2, chloride, creatinine, BUN, cholesterol, trigliycerides, HDL, LDL, CPK,
82. 82803
83. 414.0
84. A
85. D
86. B
87. C
88. tachycardia, bradycardia
89. arrhythmia, dysrhythmia
90. thrombus
91. bruit
92. murmur
93. hypertension
94. risk factors
95. myocardial infarction
96. dietary changes, quit smoking, exercise program, stress reduction
97. depends on individual, but maintaining a healthy lifestyle will help prevent heart disease
98. surgical connection of two blood vessels
99. repair of a cardiac valve
100. incision into a cardiac valve to remove an obstruction
101. surgical removal of an embolus
102. opening of a blocked blood vessel, as by balloon dilation
103. thrombectomy
104. C
105. arteriotomy
106. angioscopy
107. C
108. valvotomy
109. venipuncture
110. C
111. coronary
112. high cholesterol
113. high blood pressure
114. high blood pressure
115. clotting in blood vessels; anticoagulants
116. myocardial infarction

117. Inderal
118. Lasix
119. Cardioquin
120. Lipitor
121. Coumadin
122. Abbokinase
123. nitroglycerin
124. Dilatrate
125. f
126. d
127. j
128. h
129. g
130. a
131. i
132. b
133. e
134. c
135. a
136. g
137. c
138. h
139. i
140. d
141. j
142. e
143. f
144. b
145. arteriosclerosis
146. endocarditis
147. bradycardia
148. angiostenosis
149. cardiomyopathy
150. thrombus
151. aortic stenosis
152. hematoma
153. cardiomegaly
154. aortogram
155. echocardiogram
156. electrocardiogram
157. ischemia158. tachycardia
159. atherosclerosis
160. cardiology
161. hypothermia
162. hematology
163. thrombolysis

164. phlebology
165. cardiogenesis
166. hematopoiesis
167. cardiac
168. electrocardiograph
169. angiography
170. electrocardiography
171. phlebotomy
172. atherectomy
173. pericarditis
174. capillaries
175. arteries
176. venules
177. veins
178. pericardium
179. aorta
180. superior vena cava
181. blood vessels
182. mitral valve
183. pulmonary veins
184. lumen
185. ductus arteriosus
186. heart
187. endocardium
188. foramen ovale
189. right atrium
190. septum
191. coronary artery
192. T
193. F
194. F
195. F
196. T
197. T
198. T
199. T
200. F
201. T
202. e
203. d
204. a
205. b
206. c
207. h
208. f
209. g

210. e
211. g
212. b
213. c
214. f
215. a
216. c
217. -ac
218. -sclerosis
219. -pheresis
220. -penia
221. -odynia, -algia
222. -pathy
223. -cyte
224. -lysis
225. -osis
226. -phonia
227. -cytosis
228. -emic
229. -it is
230. -megaly
231. -plasty
232. thrombo-
233. semi-
234. echo-
235. brady-
236. peri-
237. tachy-
238. endo-
239. hypo-
240. myo-
241. micro-
242. pre-
243. anti-
244. bi-
245. hyper-
246. multi-
247. post-
248. macro-
249. intra-
250. tri-
251. poly-
252–523. Answers are available in the vocabulary reviews in this chapter.

The Respiratory System

After studying this chapter, you will be able to:

7.1 Name the parts of the respiratory system and discuss the function of each part

7.2 Define combining forms used in building words that relate to the respiratory system and its parts

7.3 Identify the meaning of related abbreviations

7.4 Name the common diagnoses, clinical procedures, and laboratory tests used in treating disorders of the respiratory system

7.5 List and define the major pathological conditions of the respiratory system

7.6 Explain the meaning of surgical terms related to the respiratory system

7.7 Recognize common pharmacological agents used in treating disorders of the respiratory system

▶ OTORHINOLARYNGOLOGY
▶ PULMONOLOGY

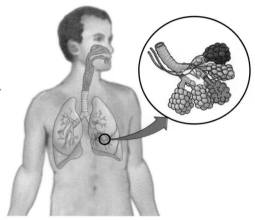

Structure and Function

The **respiratory system** is the body's breathing, or *respiration*, system. It involves the exchange of oxygen and waste gases between the atmosphere and the body and its cells. **External respiration,** breathing or exchanging air between the body and the outside environment is accomplished within the structures of the respiratory system. In external respiration, air from the atmosphere is inhaled and, later, carbon dioxide is exhaled.

Another type of respiration, **internal respiration,** the bringing of oxygen to the cells and removing carbon dioxide from them, happens in the circulation of the blood throughout the body. The carbon dioxide is removed from the body during exhalation.

The respiratory system includes the **lungs,** the **respiratory tract** (passageways through which air moves in and out of the lungs), and the muscles that move air into and out of the lungs (Figures 7-1a and 7-1b). In the upper part of the trachea is the larynx, where most of the sound used in speech and singing is produced.

The Respiratory Tract

The respiratory tract is also known as the *airway*, the route through which air enters the lungs and the route via which air exits the body. **Inspiration** (breathing in or **inhalation**) brings air from the outside environment into the **nose** or mouth. The nose has three functions: to warm, filter,

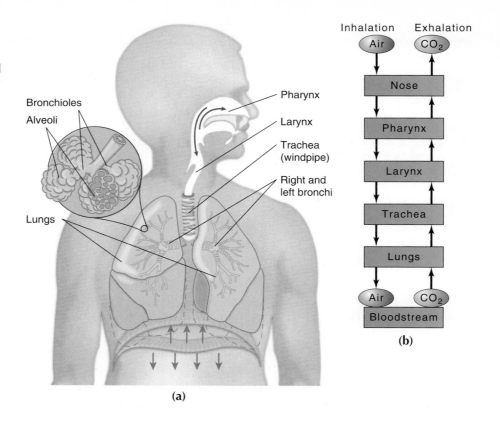

FIGURE 7-1 **(a)** The respiratory system performs the process of inhaling air and exhaling carbon dioxide. **(b)** The diagram shows the pathways of inhaled air (containing oxygen) and exhaled air (containing carbon dioxide).

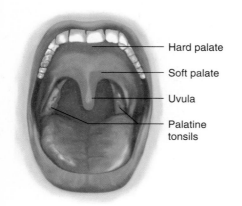

FIGURE 7-2 The inside of the mouth.

and moisten the air. The **nostrils** (also called **external nares**) are the two external openings at the base of the external portion of the nose. The external nose is supported by the nasal bones and is divided into two halves by the **nasal septum,** a strip of cartilage. After air enters the nose, it passes into the **nasal cavity** and the **paranasal sinuses,** where it is warmed by blood in the mucous membranes that line these areas. **Cilia** (hairs) in the nasal cavity filter out foreign bodies.

The air next reaches the **pharynx (throat),** which is a passageway for both air and food. The pharynx is divided into three sections. The **nasopharynx** lies above the **soft palate,** which is a flexible muscular sheet that separates the nasopharynx from the rest of the pharynx. The nasopharynx contains the **pharyngeal tonsils,** more commonly known as the **adenoids,** which aid in the body's immune defense.

The next division of the pharynx is the **oropharynx,** the back portion of the mouth. It contains the **palatine tonsils,** lymphatic tissue that works as part of the immune system. The oropharynx is part of the mechanism of the mouth that triggers swallowing. Figure 7-2 shows the inside of the mouth.

The bottom and third section of the pharynx is the **laryngopharynx** (also called the **hypopharynx**). It is at this point that the respiratory tract divides into the *esophagus*, the passageway for food, and the **larynx** or **voice box,** through which air passes to the **trachea** or **windpipe.**

Food is prevented from going into the larynx by the **epiglottis,** a movable flap of cartilage that covers the opening to the larynx (called the **glottis**) every time one swallows. Food then passes only into the esophagus. Occasionally, a person may swallow and inhale at the same time, allowing some food to be pulled (or *aspirated*) into the larynx. Usually, a strong cough forces out the food, but sometimes the food particle blocks the airway, and the food

MORE ABOUT . . .

Aspiration

Occasionally, food or saliva can be aspirated by inhaling, laughing, or talking with food, gum, or fluid in the mouth. An unconscious person who is lying on his or her back may aspirate some saliva or possibly blood as in a trauma. The body's automatic response to aspiration is violent coughing or choking in an attempt to expel the material. If total obstruction occurs, then the abdominal thrust maneuver (also known as the Heimlich maneuver) must be used.

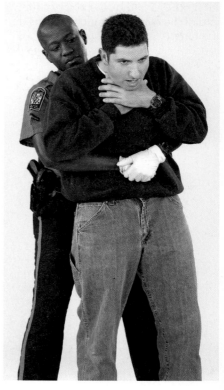

FIGURE 7-3 The abdominal thrust is used to save choking victims.

must be dislodged with help from another person in a technique called the abdominal thrust maneuver (Figure 7-3). This technique is also called the *Heimlich maneuver.* It has saved many people from choking to death.

Air goes into the larynx, which serves both as a passageway to the trachea and as the area where the sounds of speech and singing are produced. The larynx contains **vocal cords,** strips of epithelial tissue that vibrate when muscular tension is applied (Figure 7-4). The size and thickness of the cords determine the pitch of sound. The male's thicker and longer vocal cords produce a lower pitch than do the shorter and thinner vocal cords of most women. Children's voices tend to be higher in pitch because of the smaller size of their vocal cords. Sound volume is regulated by the amount of air that passes over the vocal cords. The larynx is supported by various cartilaginous structures, one of which consists of two disks joined at an angle to form the **thyroid cartilage** or **Adam's apple** (larger in males than in females).

The **trachea** is a tube that connects the larynx to the right and left **bronchi** (plural of **bronchus**), tubular branches into which the larynx divides. The trachea is a cartilaginous and membranous tube. It contains about twenty horseshoe-shaped structures that provide support so that it will not collapse similar to the way a vacuum cleaner hose acts during use. The point at which the trachea divides is called the **mediastinum,** a general term for a median area, especially one with a **septum** or cartilaginous division. The median portion of the thoracic cavity, which contains the heart, esophagus, trachea, and thymus gland, is called the mediastinum. Both bronchi contain cartilage and mucous glands and are the passageways through which air

At the Heimlich Institute's Web site (www.heimlichinstitute.org), you can learn more about saving people and even pets who have something blocking their airway.

The Science Museum of Minnesota (www.smm.org/sound/activity/ssl14.htm) has a simple experiment to show you how vocal cords work as well as a video of vocal cords in action.

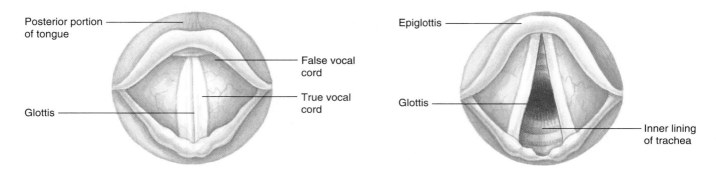

FIGURE 7-4 Vocal cords are the primary instruments of sound. The drawing on the left shows the position of the vocal cords when the voice is high in pitch and the picture on the right illustrates the vocal cords when the voice is low in pitch.

FIGURE 7-5 The alveoli are at the end of the terminal bronchioles inside the lungs.

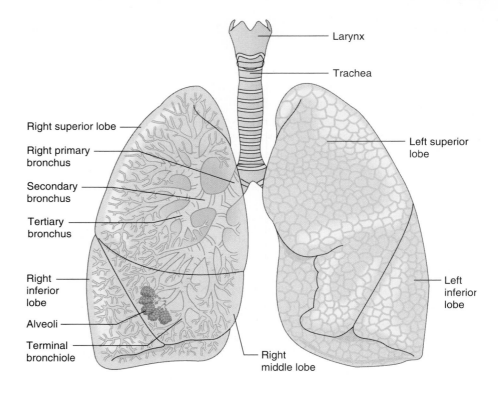

Larynx

Trachea

Right superior lobe

Right primary bronchus

Secondary bronchus

Tertiary bronchus

Right inferior lobe

Alveoli

Terminal bronchiole

Left superior lobe

Left inferior lobe

Right middle lobe

enters the right and left lungs. Air that is pushed out of the lungs travels up through the respiratory tract during **expiration** (breathing out or **exhalation**), where air is expelled into the environment.

The bronchi further divide into many smaller branches called **bronchioles.** Inside the lungs, the structures resemble tree branches, with smaller parts branching off. At the end of each bronchiole is a cluster of air sacs. Each air sac is called an **alveolus** (plural, **alveoli**). There are about 300 million alveoli in the lungs. The one-celled, thin-walled alveoli are surrounded by capillaries, with which they exchange gases. Figure 7-5 shows the alveoli inside of the lungs.

The Structure of the Lungs

The lungs take up most of the thoracic cavity (or **thorax**), reaching from the collarbone to the diaphragm. The outside of the lungs is a moist, double layer of membrane called the **pleura** (plural, **pleurae**). The outer layer, the **parietal pleura,** lines the thoracic cavity, the inside of the ribs. The inner layer, the **visceral pleura,** covers the surface of the lungs. The space between the two pleura is called the **pleural cavity.** This space is filled with fluid. This pleural fluid prevents contact between the lungs and the ribs to avoid the inflammation that would be caused by friction.

Each lung has an **apex,** or topmost section; a middle area called the **hilum** or **hilus;** and a lower section called the **base.** The hilum is the area where the bronchi, blood vessels, and nerves enter the lungs. The right, larger lung is divided into three lobes—a **superior lobe,** a **middle lobe,** and an **inferior lobe.** The left lung is divided into two lobes—a superior lobe and an inferior lobe (Figure 7-5). Humans can function with one or more lobes removed or even an entire lung removed, as is necessary in some cases of lung cancer.

MORE ABOUT . . .

Lung Capacity

Normal inspiration brings about 500 milliliters of air into the lungs. Normal expiration expels about the same amount from the lungs. Forced inspiration brings extra air (even up to six times the normal amount) into the lungs. Forced expiration can expel up to three times the normal amount of air from the lungs.

Some quantity of air always remains in the lungs so that newly inhaled air mixes with the remaining air. This helps to maintain the proper concentrations of oxygen and carbon dioxide in the lungs.

Breathing is the inhalation of oxygen into the lungs. Oxygen is then exchanged from the alveoli into the capillaries of the bloodstream and carbon dioxide is returned from the capillaries into the alveoli. Oxygen is then delivered to the body's other cells. This process is called internal respiration. This type of respiration is affected by how well the cardiovascular system supplies oxygenated blood. Carbon dioxide is expelled back up through the respiratory tract during expiration.

Muscles for Breathing

Inhalation and exhalation is accomplished by changing the capacity of the thoracic cavity. During inhalation, the thoracic cavity expands and the lungs fill with air. During exhalation, the cavity shrinks and the lungs expel air. Muscular contractions enlarge the volume of the thoracic cavity during inspiration and decrease the volume when they relax during expiration. The major muscles that contract are the **diaphragm** and the **intercostal muscles** (the muscles between the ribs). The diaphragm lowers itself when it contracts, allowing more space in the thoracic cavity, and the intercostal muscles pull the ribs upward and outward when they contract, also enlarging the thoracic cavity.

VOCABULARY REVIEW

In the previous section, you learned terms relating to the respiratory system. Before going on to the exercises, review the terms below and refer to the previous section if you have any questions. Pronunciations are provided for certain terms. Sometimes information about where the word came from is included after the term. The etymologies (word histories) are for your information only. You do not need to memorize them.

Term	Definition
Adam's apple	Thyroid cartilage, supportive structure of the larynx; larger in males than in females.
adenoids [ĂD-ĕ-nŏydz] Greek *aden*, gland + *eidos*, resembling	Collection of lymphoid tissue in the nasopharynx; pharyngeal tonsils.
alveolus (*pl.,* alveoli) [ăl-VĒ-ō-lŭs (ăl-VĒ-ō-lī)] Latin, little sac	Air sac at the end of each bronchiole.

Term	Definition
apex [Ā-pĕks] Latin, summit	Topmost section of the lung.
base [bās] Latin *basis*, bottom	Bottom section of the lung.
bronchiole [BRŎNG-ē-ōl] bronchi-, bronchus + -ole, small	Fine subdivision of the bronchi made of smooth muscle and elastic fibers.
bronchus (*pl.*, bronchi) [BRŎNG-kŭs (BRŎNG-kī)] Latin, windpipe	One of the two airways from the trachea to the lungs.
cilia [SĬL-ē-ă] Latin, plural of *cilium*, hair	Hairlike extensions of a cell's surface that usually provide some protection by sweeping foreign particles away.
diaphragm [DĪ-ă-frăm] Greek *diaphragma*, from *dia-*, through + *phrassein*, to enclose	Membranous muscle between the abdominal and thoracic cavities that contracts and relaxes during the respiratory cycle.
epiglottis [ĔP-ĭ-GLŎT-ĭs] Greek, from *epi-*, on + *glottis*, mouth of the windpipe	Cartilaginous flap that covers the larynx during swallowing to prevent food from entering the airway.
exhalation [ĕks-hă-LĀ-shŭn] Latin *exhalo*, to breathe out	Breathing out.
expiration [ĕks-pĭ-RĀ-shŭn] Latin *expiro*, to breathe out	Exhalation.
external nares [NĀR-ēz]	*See* nostrils.
external respiration	Exchange of air between the body and the outside environment.
glottis [GLŎT-ĭs]	Part of the larynx consisting of the vocal folds of mucous membrane and muscle.
hilum (*also* hilus) [HĪ-lŭm (HĪ-lŭs)] Latin, small bit	Midsection of the lung where the nerves and vessels enter and exit.
hypopharynx [HĪ-pō-FĂR-ĭngks] hypo-, below + pharynx	Laryngopharynx.
inferior lobe [ĭn-FĒ-rē-ōr lōb]	Bottom lobe of the lung.
inhalation [ĭn-hă-LĀ-shŭn] Latin *inhalo*, to breathe in	Breathing in.
inspiration [ĭn-spĭ-RĀ-shŭn] Latin *inspiro*, to breath in	Inhalation.
intercostal muscles [ĭn-tĕr-KŎS-tăl MŬS-ĕlz] inter-, between + Latin *costa*, rib	Muscles between the ribs.
internal respiration	Exchange of oxygen and carbon dioxide between the cells.
laryngopharynx [lă-RĬNG-gō-făr-ĭngks] laryngo-, larynx + pharynx	Part of the pharynx below and behind the larynx.

Term	Definition
larynx [LĂR-ĭngks] Greek, larynx	Organ of voice production in the respiratory tract, between the pharynx and the trachea; voice box.
lung [lŭng] Old English *lungen*	One of two organs of respiration (left lung and right lung) in the thoracic cavity, where oxygenation of blood takes place.
mediastinum [MĒ-dē-ăs-TĪ-nŭm]	Median portion of the thoracic cavity; septum between two areas of an organ or cavity.
middle lobe	Middle section of the right lung.
nasal cavity [NĀ-zăl KĂV-ĭ-tē]	Opening in the external nose where air enters the body.
nasal septum [SĔP-tŭm]	Cartilaginous division of the external nose.
nasopharynx [NĀ-zō-FĂR-ĭngks] naso-, nose + pharynx	Portion of the throat above the soft palate.
nose [nōz] Old English *nosu*	External structure supported by nasal bones and containing nasal cavity.
nostrils [NŎS-trĭlz]	External openings at the base of the nose; also called external nares.
oropharynx [ŌR-ō-FĂR-ĭngks] oro-, mouth + pharynx	Back portion of the mouth, a division of the pharynx.
palatine tonsils [PĂL-ă-tīn TŎN-sĭlz] Latin *palatinus*, pertaining to the palate	Lymphatic tissue that works as part of the immune system.
paranasal sinuses [păr-ă-NĀ-săl SĪ-nŭs-ĕz] para-, beside + nasal	Area of the nasal cavity where external air is warmed by blood in the mucous membrane lining.
parietal pleura [pă-RĪ-ĕ-tăl PLŪR-ă]	Outer layer of the pleura.
pharyngeal tonsils [fă-RĬN-jē-ăl TŎN-sĭlz]	Adenoids.
pharynx [FĂR-ĭngks] Greek, pharynx	Passageway at back of mouth for air and food; throat.
pleura (*pl.,* **pleurae**) [PLŪR-ă (PLŪR-ē)] Greek, rib	Double layer of membrane making up the outside of the lungs.
pleural cavity [PLŪR-ăl KĂV-ĭ-tē]	Space between the two pleura.
respiratory [RĔS-pĭ-ră-tōr-ē, rĕ-SPĪR-ă-tōr-ē] **system**	The body's system for breathing.
respiratory tract	Passageways through which air moves into and out of the lungs.
septum [SĔP-tŭm]	Cartilaginous division, as in the nose or mediastinum.
soft palate [sŏft PĂL-ăt]	Flexible muscular sheet that separates the nasopharynx from the rest of the pharynx.
superior lobe	Topmost lobe of each lung.

Term	Definition
thorax [THŌ-răks] Greek, breastplate	Chest cavity.
throat [thrōt]	*See* pharynx.
thyroid cartilage [THĪ-rŏyd KĂR-tĭ-lĭj]	*See* Adam's apple.
trachea [TRĀ-kē-ă]	Airway from the larynx into the bronchi; windpipe.
visceral pleura [VĬS-ĕr-ăl PLŪR-ă]	Inner layer of the pleura.
vocal cords	Strips of epithelial tissue that vibrate and play a major role in the production of sound.
voice box	*See* larynx.
windpipe	*See* trachea.

CASE STUDY

Breathing Emergencies

The emergency department at Midvale Central Hospital often sees patients who complain of breathing problems. The physicians on duty are trained to listen to sounds with a stethoscope to determine the immediate needs of the patient. Many of the patients at Midvale are elderly. Respiratory problems are the number-one reason for seeking emergency help.

Critical Thinking

1. How might an elderly person's weakened muscles affect respiration?

2. Midvale is a retirement community in the South. About six times a year, the state department of environmental protection issues pollution or smog warnings, with suggestions that children, the elderly, and those with chronic illnesses stay indoors, preferably with air conditioning. Polluted air diminishes what gas necessary for respiration?

STRUCTURE AND FUNCTION EXERCISES

Complete the Picture

3. Label the parts of the respiratory system on the following diagram.

   a. _____

   b. _____

   c. _____

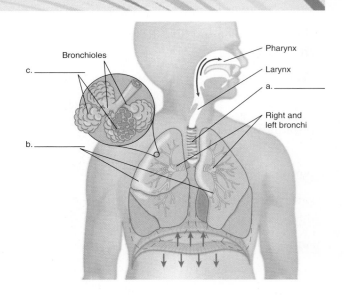

Bronchioles

c. _____

b. _____

Pharynx

Larynx

a. _____

Right and left bronchi

Check Your Knowledge

Complete the sentences below by filling in the blanks.

4. Exchanging air between the body and the outside environment is called _____ _____.

5. Foreign bodies entering the respiratory tract are filtered through _____.

6. The nose is divided into two halves by the _____ _____.

7. Food is prevented from going into the larynx by the _____.

8. A simple technique that has saved many people from death is the _____ _____ _____.

9. At the end of each bronchiole is a small cluster of _____ _____ called _____.

10. The right lung has _____ lobes.

11. The left lung has _____ lobes.

12. A muscle that lowers itself to allow more space when one is breathing in is called a(n) _____.

13. The muscles between the ribs that also aid in breathing are called _____ muscles.

Circle T for true or F for false.

14. The respiratory tract is the major area involved in internal respiration. T F

15. The throat is a passageway for both air and food. T F

16. The pharynx contains the vocal cords. T F

17. Each bronchus enters one lung. T F

18. The pleura are moist layers of membrane surrounding the lungs. T F

19. Humans must have both lungs to live. T F

20. Only the right lung has a middle lobe. T F

21. The hilum is the topmost portion of the lung. T F

22. The larynx is another name for the windpipe. T F

23. The soft palate is at the bottom of the mouth. T F

Spell It Correctly

Write the correct spelling in the blank to the right of any misspelled words. If the word is already correctly spelled, write C.

24. nasopharyngx _____

25. trachae _____

26. resperation _____

27. alveoli _____

28. diagphram _____

29. epiglottus _____

30. pharinx _____

31. mediastinum _____

32. tonsills _____

33. bronchis _____

Know the Respiratory System

Match the respiratory term with its meaning.

34. _____ cilia

35. _____ diaphragm

36. _____ epiglottis

37. _____ exhalation

a. exchange of oxygen and carbon dioxide between the cells.

b. inspiration, breathing in

c. expiration, breathing out

d. chest cavity

38. ____ external nares

39. ____ inhalation

40. ____ internal respiration

41. ____ pharynx

42. ____ larynx

43. ____ thorax

44. ____ external respiration

e. throat

f. hairlike extension of a cells surface

g. muscle between the abdominal and thoracic cavity

h. voicebox

i. nostrils

j. exchange of air between the body and the outside environment.

k. flap that covers the larynx during swallowing.

Combining Forms and Abbreviations

The lists below include combining forms and abbreviations that relate specifically to the respiratory system. Pronunciations are provided for the examples. Some of the abbreviations will be discussed later in the chapter.

COMBINING FORM	MEANING	EXAMPLE
adenoid(o)	adenoid, gland	*adenoidectomy* [ĂD-ĕ-nŏy-DĔK-tō-mē], operation for removal of adenoid growths
alveol(o)	alveolus	*alveolitis* [ĂL-vē-ō-LĪ-tĭs], inflammation of the alveoli
bronch(o), bronchi(o)	bronchus	*bronchitis* [brŏng-KĪ-tĭs], inflammation of the lining of the bronchial tubes
bronchiol(o)	bronchiole	*bronchiolitis* [brŏng-kē-ō-LĪ-tĭs], inflammation of the bronchioles
capn(o)	carbon dioxide	*capnogram* [KĂP-nō-grăm], a continuous recording of the carbon dioxide in expired air
epiglott(o)	epiglottis	*epiglottitis* [ĔP-ĭ-GLŎT-ĭ-tĭs], inflammation of the epiglottis
laryng(o)	larynx	*laryngoscope* [lă-RĬNG-gō-skōp], device used to examine the larynx through the mouth
lob(o)	lobe of the lung	*lobectomy* [lō-BĔK-tō-mē], removal of a lobe
mediastin(o)	mediastinum	*mediastinitis* [MĒ-dē-ăs-tĭ-NĪ-tĭs], inflammation of the tissue of the mediastinum
nas(o)	nose	*nasogastric* [nā-zō-GĂS-tĭk], of the nasal passages and the stomach
or(o)	mouth	*oropharynx* [ŌR-ō-FĂR-ĭngks], the part of the pharynx that lies behind the mouth
ox(o), oxi-, oxy	oxygen	*oximeter* [ŏk-SĬM-ĕ-tĕr], instrument for measuring oxygen saturation of blood
pharyng(o)	pharynx	*pharyngitis* [făr-ĭn-JĪ-tĭs], inflammation in the pharynx

Combining Form	Meaning	Example
phon(o)	voice, sound	*phonometer* [fō-NŎM-ĕ-tĕr], instrument for measuring sounds
phren(o)	diaphragm	*phrenitis* [frĕn-Ī-tĭs], inflammation in the diaphragm
pleur(o)	pleura	*pleuritis* [plū-RĪ-tĭs], inflammation of the pleura
pneum(o), pneumon(o)	air, lung	*pneumolith* [NŪ-mō-lĭth], calculus in the lungs; *pneumonitis* [nū-mō-NĪ-tĭs], inflammation of the lungs
rhin(o)	nose	*rhinitis* [rī-NĪ-tĭs], inflammation of the nose
spir(o)	breathing	*spirometer* [spī-RŎM-ĕ-tĕr], instrument used to measure respiratory gases
steth(o)	chest	*stethoscope* [STĔTH-ō-skōp], instrument for listening to sounds in the chest
thorac(o)	thorax, chest	*thoracotomy* [thōr-ă-KŎT-ō-mē], incision into the chest wall
tonsill(o)	tonsils	*tonsillectomy* [TŎN-sĭ-LĔK-tō-mē], removal of one entire tonsil or of both tonsils
trache(o)	trachea	*tracheoscopy* [trā-kē-ŎS-kō-pē], inspection of the interior of the trachea

Abbreviation	Meaning	Abbreviation	Meaning
ABG	arterial blood gases, a diagnostic test	DPT	diphtheria, pertussis, tetanus (combined vaccination)
AFB	acid-fast bacillus (causes tuberculosis)	ENT	ear, nose, and throat
A&P	auscultation and percussion	ET tube	endotracheal intubation tube
AP	anteroposterior	FEF	forced expiratory flow
ARD	acute respiratory disease	FEV	forced expiratory volume
ARDS	adult respiratory distress syndrome	FVC	forced vital capacity
ARF	acute respiratory failure	HBOT	hyperbaric oxygen therapy
BS	breath sounds	IMV	intermittent mandatory ventilation
COLD	chronic obstructive lung disease	IPPB	intermittent positive pressure breathing
COPD	chronic obstructive pulmonary disease	IRDS	infant respiratory distress syndrome
CPR	cardiopulmonary resuscitation	IRV	inspiratory reserve volume

ABBREVIATION	MEANING	ABBREVIATION	MEANING
CTA	clear to auscultation	LLL	left lower lobe [of the lungs]
CXR	chest x-ray	LUL	left upper lobe [of the lungs]
DOE	dyspnea on exertion	MBC	maximal breathing capacity
MDI	metered dose inhaler	SARS	severe acute respiratory syndrome
PA	posteroanterior	SIDS	sudden infant death syndrome
PCP	pneumocystis carinii pneumonia (a type of pneumonia to which AIDS patients are susceptible)	SOB	shortness of breath
PEEP	positive end expiratory pressure	T&A	tonsillectomy and adenoidectomy
PFT	pulmonary function tests	TB	tuberculosis
PND	paroxysmal nocturnal dyspnea; postnasal drip	TLC	total lung capacity
RD	respiratory disease	TPR	temperature, pulse, and respiration
RDS	respiratory distress syndrome	URI	upper respiratory infection
RLL	right lower lobe [of the lungs]	VC	vital capacity
RUL	right upper lobe [of the lungs]	V/Q scan	ventilation/perfusion scan

CASE STUDY

Coping with COPD

The emergency room nurse admitted Mr. DiGiorno, a patient from a nursing home. He was having difficulty breathing and complained of chest pains. The nurse checked his record and found that he has been positive for COPD for five years. This patient has had four hospital admissions in the last six months. He is overweight, smokes, and is sedentary. He takes medications for his COPD.

Critical Thinking

45. What is COPD? What lifestyle factors might play a role in Mr. DiGiorno's disease?
46. Mr. DiGiorno's chest pains may indicate cardiovascular disease. How might this affect internal respiration?

COMBINING FORMS AND ABBREVIATIONS EXERCISES

Build Your Medical Vocabulary

Complete the words by putting a combining form in the blank.

47. Removal of the adenoids: _____ ectomy.
48. Surgical puncture of the thoracic cavity: _____ centesis.
49. Opening into the trachea: _____ otomy.
50. Inflammation of the tonsils: _____ itis.
51. Inflammation of the pericardium and surrounding mediastinal tissue: _____ pericarditis.

52. Suture of the lung: _____rrhaphy.

53. Relating to the nose and mouth: _____nasal.

54. Inflammation of the pharynx: _____itis.

55. Disease of the vocal cords affecting speech: _____pathy.

56. Record of carbon dioxide in expired air: _____gram.

57. Bronchial inflammation: _____itis.

58. Inflammation of tissue surrounding the bronchi: peri_____itis.

59. Relating to the pericardium and pleural cavity: pericardio _____.

60. Incision into a lobe: _____otomy.

61. Measurement of oxygen in blood: _____metry.

62. Compound of oxygen and a chloride: _____chloride.

63. Swelling in the bronchial area: _____edema.

64. Destruction of an alveolus: _____clasia.

65. Chest pain: _____algia.

66. Incision into the sinus: _____tomy.

Match the Root

Match the respiratory combining forms in the list on the right with the definitions in the list on the left.

67. _____ pain arising in air sacs in the lungs   **a.** broncho

68. _____ instrument to study vocal folds   **b.** capno

69. _____ record of heart sounds   **c.** lob

70. _____ nasal obstruction   **d.** alveol(o)

71. _____ contraction of the bronchus   **e.** pharyngo

72. _____ abnormally dilated windpipe   **f.** laryngo

73. _____ repair of the pharynx   **g.** phono

74. _____ fissure of the chest wall   **h.** thoraco

75. _____ inflammation of a lobe   **i.** rhino

76. _____ instrument for graphing carbon dioxide   **j.** tracheo

Know the Abbreviation

Give the abbreviation for each of the following.

77. Left lower lobe(of the lung) _____

78. Left upper lobe(of the lung) _____

79. acute respiratory disease _____

80. auscultation and percussion _____

81. metered dose inhaler _____

82. severe acute respiratory syndrome _____

83. shortness of breath _____

84. sudden infant death syndrome _____

85. Upper respiratory infection _____

Give the meaning for the following abbreviations.

86. ARF _____

87. BS _____

88. COLD _____

89. CPR _____

90. CXR _____

91. ABG _____

92. DPT _____

93. ENT _____

94. HBOT _____

95. RD _____

96. RDS _____

97. T & A _____

98. TB _____

99. TPR _____

Finding the Meaning

For each of the following terms, guess at the meaning by looking at the word parts. If you need help, consult your allied health dictionary. Then give the meaning of each word part.

100. laryngotracheobronchitis _____

101. tracheotomy _____

102. tracheostomy _____

103. rhinitis _____

104. hypoxia _____

105. otorhinolaryngologist _____

106. bronchostenosis _____

107. pleurocentesis _____

108. alveolitis _____

109. bronchomalacia _____

110. sinusitis _____

Diagnostic, Procedural, and Laboratory Terms

Disorders of the respiratory system can be diagnosed in several ways. First, a physician usually listens to the lungs with a stethoscope, a process called **auscultation** (Figure 7-6). Next, the respiratory rate is determined by counting the number of respirations per minute. One inhalation and one exhalation equal a single respiration. Adult respirations normally range from 15 to 20 per minute. The physician may use **percussion,** tapping over the lung area, to see if the lungs are clear (a hollow sound) or filled with fluid (a dull sound). Sputum can be observed for its color. Pus in sputum usually causes a greenish or yellowish color and indicates infection. Blood in the sputum may indicate tuberculosis.

Pulmonary function tests measure the mechanics of breathing. Breathing may be tested by a **peak flow meter.** Asthmatics often use this type of measuring device to check breathing capacity; they can then take medicine if an attack seems imminent. A **spirometer** is a pulmonary function testing machine that measures the lungs' volume and capacity (*spirometry*). This machine measures the *forced vital capacity* (FVC), or highest breathing capacity, of the lungs when the patient takes the deepest breath possible. Other breathing measurements such as *forced expiratory volume* (FEV) show capacity at different parts of the respiration cycle.

Tuberculosis is a disease that usually affects the respiratory system. Tests for tuberculosis were discussed in Chapter 4, The Integumentary System, because reactions on the surface of the skin indicate a positive result for a tuberculosis test.

Visual images of the chest and parts of the respiratory system play an important role in diagnosing respiratory ailments. Chest x-rays, MRIs, and lung scans can detect abnormalities, such as masses and restricted blood flow within the lungs. A **bronchography** provides a radiological picture of the trachea and bronchi. A thoracic CT scan shows a cross-sectional view of the chest that can reveal tissue masses. A *pulmonary angiography* is an x-ray of the blood vessels of the lungs taken after dye is injected into a blood vessel. A *lung scan* or *V/Q perfusion scan* is a recording of radioactive material, injected or inhaled, to show air flow and blood supply in the lungs.

Parts of the respiratory system can also be observed by *endoscopy*, insertion of an **endoscope** (a viewing tube) into a body cavity. A **bronchoscope** is used for *bronchoscopy*, which is performed to examine airways or retrieve specimens, such as fluid retrieved in **bronchial alveolar lavage** or material for biopsy that is retrieved by **bronchial brushing** (a brush inserted through the bronchoscope). In **nasopharyngoscopy,** a flexible endoscope is used to examine nasal passages and the pharynx. **Laryngoscopy** is the procedure for examining the mouth and larynx, and **mediastinoscopy** for examining the mediastinum area and all the organs within it. Such diagnostic testing can reveal structural abnormalities, tumors, and irritations.

Laboratory Tests

Throat cultures are commonly used to diagnose streptococcal infections. A swab is passed over a portion of the throat, and the swab is then put in contact with a culture. If a strep infection is present, the culture will show certain bacteria. A **sputum sample** or **culture** may be taken and cultured to identify any disease-causing organisms. **Arterial blood gases (ABGs)** measure the levels of pressure of oxygen (O_2) and carbon dioxide (CO_2) in arterial blood. These measurements help diagnose heart and lung functions. A **sweat test** measures the amount of salt in sweat and is used to confirm cystic fibrosis.

Auscultation is from a Latin verb, *ausculto,* to listen to.

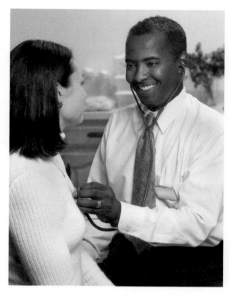

FIGURE 7-6 Auscultation is a part of a normal examination.

The FDA has a food safety site at one of its Web sites (http://vm.cfsan.fda.gov) where you can learn more about infections.

MORE ABOUT...

Streptococcal Infections

Throat cultures are commonly given to children with sore throats. The presence of a streptococcal infection is usually treated with antibiotics because the presence of such an infection can cause health problems (such as heart and kidney damage) if left unchecked.

VOCABULARY REVIEW

In the previous section, you learned terms relating to diagnosis, clinical procedures, and laboratory tests. Before going on to the exercises, review the terms below and refer to the previous section if you have any questions. Pronunciations are provided for certain terms. Sometimes information about where the word came from is included after the term. The etymologies (word histories) are for your information only. You do not need to memorize them.

Term	Definition
arterial [ăr-TĒR-ē-ăl] **blood gases**	Laboratory test that measures the levels of oxygen and carbon dioxide in arterial blood.
auscultation [ăws-kŭl-TĀ-shŭn]	Listening to internal sounds with a stethoscope.
bronchial alveolar lavage [BRŎNG-kē-ăl ăl-VĒ-ō-lăr lă-VĂZH]	Retrieval of fluid for examination through a bronchoscope.
bronchial brushing	Retrieval of material for biopsy by insertion of a brush through a bronchoscope.
bronchography [brŏng-KŎG-ră-fē] broncho-, bronchus + -graphy, a recording	Radiological picture of the trachea and bronchi.
bronchoscope [BRŎNG-kō-skōp] broncho- + -scope, device for viewing	Device used to examine airways.
endoscope [ĔN-dō-skōp] endo-, within + -scope	Tube used to view a body cavity.
laryngoscopy [LĂR-ing-GŎS-kō-pē] laryngo-, larynx + -scopy, a viewing	Visual examination of the mouth and larynx using an endoscope.
mediastinoscopy [MĒ-dē-ăs-tĭ-NŌS-kō-pē] mediastino-, mediastinum + -scopy	Visual examination of the mediastinum and all the organs within it using an endoscope.
nasopharyngoscopy [NĀ-zō-fă-rĭng-GŎS-kō-pē] naso-, nose + pharyngo-, pharynx + -scopy	Examination of the nasal passages and the pharynx using an endoscope.
peak flow meter	Device for measuring breathing capacity.
percussion [pĕr-KŬSH-ŭn]	Tapping on the surface of the body to see if lungs are clear.
pulmonary function tests	Tests that measure the mechanics of breathing.

Term	Definition
spirometer [spī-RŎM-ĕ-tĕr] spiro-, breathing + -meter	Testing machine that measures the lungs' volume and capacity.
sputum [SPŪ-tŭm] sample or culture	Culture of material that is expectorated (or brought back up as mucus).
sweat test	Test for cystic fibrosis that measures the amount of salt in sweat.
throat culture	Test for streptococcal or other infections in which a swab taken on the surface of the throat is placed in a culture to see if certain bacteria grow.

CASE STUDY

Laboratory Testing

Mr. DiGiorno was admitted to Midvale Hospital from the emergency room. His radiological/laboratory data read as follows:

A chest x-ray showed a pneumonic infiltrate in the left lower lobe with some parapneumonic effusion. Follow-up chest x-rays showed progression of infiltrate and then slight clearing. Serial ECGs (ECGs given one after another in succession) showed the development of T-wave inversions anterolaterally compatible with ischemia or a pericardial process. The WBC was 10,000; HCT, 37; platelets, 425,000; PT and PTT were normal. Blood gases showed a pH of 7.43, PCO_2 37, PO_2 71. Sputum culture could not be obtained.

Critical Thinking

111. Why do you think blood gas tests were ordered for Mr. DiGiorno?
112. What part of his blood was measured at 10,000?

DIAGNOSTIC, PROCEDURAL, AND LABORATORY TERMS EXERCISES

Check Your Knowledge

Complete the sentences below by filling in the blanks.

113. The mechanics of breathing are measured by _____ _____ tests.

114. A test that can confirm the presence of cystic fibrosis is called a(n) _____ _____.

115. A tube for viewing a body cavity is called a(n) _____.

116. The highest breathing capacity is called the _____ _____ capacity.

117. A stethoscope is necessary for _____, listening to the lungs.

118. Streptococcal infections can be detected in a _____ _____.

119. Tapping the skin over the lung area to check whether the lungs are clear is called _____.

120. Asthmatics often use a _____ _____ _____ to check breathing capacity.

121. Disease-causing organisms in sputum can be identified in a(n) _____ _____.

122. A device that measures the lung volume and capacity is called a(n) _____.

Root Out the Meaning

Add the appropriate combining form from the list in this chapter.

123. _____scopy means viewing of the pharynx.

124. _____gram means a measure of carbon dioxide in expired air.

125. _____ectomy means removal of the larynx.

126. _____itis means inflammation of a lobe.

127. _____plegia means paralysis of the larynx.

Pathological Terms

The respiratory system is the site for many inflammations, disorders, and infections. This system must contend with foreign material coming into the body from outside, as well as internal problems that may affect any of its parts. Each of its parts may become inflamed. Table 7-1 shows various respiratory inflammations, their symptoms, and some treatments.

Normal breathing (**eupnea**) may become affected by diseases or conditions and change to one of the following breathing difficulties:

- **Bradypnea,** slow breathing
- **Tachypnea,** fast breathing
- **Hypopnea,** shallow breathing
- **Hyperpnea,** abnormally deep breathing
- **Dyspnea,** difficult breathing
- **Apnea,** absence of breathing
- **Orthopnea,** difficulty in breathing, especially while lying down. Physicians determine the degree of orthopnea by the number of pillows required to allow the patient to breathe easily (i.e., two-pillow orthopnea).

Other irregular breathing patterns may indicate various conditions. **Cheyne-Stokes respiration,** for example, is an irregular breathing pattern with a period of apnea followed by deep, labored breathing that becomes shallow, then apneic. Irregular sounds usually indicate specific disorders—**crackles** or **rales** are popping sounds heard in lung collapse and other conditions, such as congestive heart failure and pneumonia. **Wheezes** or **rhonchi** occur during attacks of asthma or emphysema; **stridor** is a high-pitched crowing sound; and **dysphonia** is hoarseness, often associated with laryngitis. **Singultus** or hiccuping (hiccoughing), spasmodic contractions of the diaphragm, can become uncomfortable if not stopped. **Hyperventilation,** excessive breathing in and out, may be caused by anxiety or overexertion. **Hypoventilation,** abnormally low movement of air in and out of the lungs, may cause excessive buildup of carbon dioxide in the lungs, or **hypercapnia. Hypoxemia** is a deficient amount of oxygen in the blood, and **hypoxia** is a deficient amount of oxygen in tissue.

Upper respiratory infection is a term that covers an infection of some or all of the upper respiratory tract. Other disorders of the tract include **croup,** acute respiratory syndrome in children and infants, **diphtheria,** acute infection of the throat and upper respiratory tract caused by Corynebacterium

TABLE 7-1 Respiratory Inflammations

Inflammation	Symptoms	Treatment
adenoiditis, inflammation of the adenoids	swelling, redness	medication; sometimes surgical removal
bronchitis, inflammation of the bronchi	fever, coughing, expectoration	medications, rest
chronic bronchitis, bronchitis that recurs chronically; may be caused by allergies, infections, and pollution	same as for bronchitis	same as for bronchitis
epiglottitis, inflammation of the epiglottis; also known as *supraglottitis*	drooling, distress, and dysphagia; may lead to upper airway obstruction; can be a result of infection or trauma	medication
laryngitis, inflammation of the larynx	sore throat, hoarseness, cough, and dysphagia	medication, treatment or avoidance when caused by allergies, rest
laryngotracheobronchitis	sore throat, cough, hoarseness, dysphagia; may also be cause of croup	same as laryngitis
nasopharyngitis, inflammation of the nose and pharynx	runny nose, discomfort	medication
pansinusitis, inflammation of all the sinuses	may be purulent (pus-producing) or nonpurulent; runny nose, discomfort	medication
pharyngitis (sore throat), inflammation of the pharynx	fever, throat pain, dryness	medication, rest
pleuritis or **pleurisy,** inflammation of the pleura	dry cough, localized chest pain	medication, rest
pneumonitis, inflammation of the lung	fever, dyspnea, coughing	medication, rest, removal from environmental cause if appropriate
rhinitis, inflammation of the nose	runny nose, dryness	medication, removal of any allergic cause
sinusitis, inflammation of the sinuses	same as pansinusitis	same as pansinusitis
tonsillitis, inflammation of the tonsils	swelling, chills, fever, throat pain	medication; in some chronic or severe cases, surgical removal
tracheitis, inflammation of the trachea	a sore, burning sensation when breathing	rest, medication, if severe

diphtheriae bacteria, as well as **SARS (severe acute respiratory distress),** a contagious disease, sometimes fatal, caused by a coronavirus.

Nosebleed or **epistaxis** results from a trauma to, or a spontaneous rupture of, blood vessels in the nose; **rhinorrhea** is nasal discharge usually caused by an inflammation or infection; and **whooping cough** or **pertussis** is a severe infection of the pharynx, larynx, and trachea caused by the Bordetella pertussis bacteria. Diphtheria and pertussis have virtually disappeared in the United States since the regular administration of DPT (diphtheria, pertussis, tetanus) vaccines to most infants. However, pertussis has begun to make a comeback as some children are not receiving that part of the vaccine.

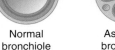

Normal bronchiole | Asthmatic bronchiole, showing constriction

FIGURE 7-7 Asthma causes a narrowing of the bronchi.

The American Academy of Allergy, Asthma, and Immunology (www.aaaai.org) has up-to-date information about asthma. Also, AANMA (Allergy and Asthma Network: Mothers of Asthmatics) provides helpful guidance about living with asthma.

Learn about the risks of lung cancer by going to the Web site www.lungcancer.org.

The Centers for Diseases Control has a Division of Tuberculosis Elimation that maintains a Web site (www.cdc.gov/nchstp/tb/) with information about control of this disease.

Chronic obstructive pulmonary disease (COPD) is a term for any disease with chronic obstruction of the bronchial tubes and lungs. Chronic bronchitis and emphysema are two COPD disease processes. In addition to bronchitis, the bronchial tubes can be the site of **asthma,** a condition of bronchial airway obstruction (Figure 7-7) causing an irritable airway prone to spasm; this spasm is called *bronchospasm.* The underlying cause is allergic inflammation of lung tissue. Asthma can be very serious and is even fatal in rare cases. However, it is usually controllable with the use of inhalers, called *bronchodilators,* and steroids. **Paroxysmal** (sudden spasmodic) movement can occur in asthma as well as in other respiratory conditions.

Hemoptysis is a lung or bronchial hemorrhage that results in the spitting of blood. **Cystic fibrosis,** chronic airway obstruction caused by disease of the exocrine glands, also affects the bronchial tubes. The predominant characteristic of cystic fibrosis is the secretion of abnormally thick mucus in various places in the body, causing chronic bronchitis, emphysema, and recurrent pneumonia, along with other ailments.

Carcinomas, frequently caused by smoking, can also be found in the respiratory system. Lung cancer is one of the leading causes of death in the United States but advances are being made in early detection and treatment.

Some disorders in newborns, such as *hyaline membrane disease* or *respiratory distress syndrome (RDS),* occur most frequently in premature babies and are often the result of underdeveloped lungs. *Adult respiratory distress syndrome (ARDS)* may have a number of causes, especially injury to the lung.

Lung disorders may occur in the alveoli: for example, **atelectasis,** a collapsed lung or part of a lung; **emphysema,** hyperinflation of the air sacs often caused by smoking; and **pneumonia,** acute infection of the alveoli. Pneumonia is a term for a number of infections. Such infections typically affect bedridden and frail people whose internal respiration is compromised. Table 7-2 details several types of pneumonia.

Tuberculosis is a highly infectious disease caused by rod-shaped bacteria **(bacilli),** which invade the lungs and cause small swellings and inflammation. Many forms of tuberculosis have become drug resistant. Tuberculosis is spread though airborne particles from someone with active disease. It usually settles in the lungs but can settle in other areas of the body. A **pulmonary abscess** is a large collection of pus in the lungs, and **pulmonary edema** is a buildup of fluid in the air sacs and bronchioles, usually caused by failure of the heart to pump enough blood to and from the lungs.

TABLE 7-2 Some Types of Pneumonia

Type of Pneumonia	Location	Cause
bacterial pneumonia	lungs	usually streptococcus bacteria
bronchial pneumonia, bronchopneumonia	walls of the smaller bronchial tubes	may be postoperative or from tuberculosis
chronic pneumonia	lungs	any recurrent inflammation or infection
double pneumonia	both lungs at the same time	bacterial infection
pneumoncystis carinii pneumonia	lungs	usually seen in AIDS patients
viral pneumonia	lungs	caused by viral infection

Several environmental agents cause **pneumoconiosis,** a lung condition caused by dust in the lungs. **Black lung** or **anthracosis** is caused by coal dust and is, therefore, a threat to coal miners; **asbestosis** is caused by asbestos particles released during construction of ships and buildings; **silicosis** is caused by the silica dust from grinding rocks or glass, and other manufacturing materials, such as pipe, building, and roofing products.

Disorders of the pleura, other than pleuritis, include **pneumothorax,** an accumulation of air or gas in the pleural cavity; **empyema,** pus in the pleural cavity; **hemothorax,** blood in the pleural cavity; **pleural effusion,** an escape of fluid into the pleural cavity; and, rarely, **mesothelioma,** a cancer associated with asbestosis.

The respiratory system may be disturbed by spasms that cause coughing or constriction. When severe, these spasms can be life-threatening. **Bronchospasms** occur in the bronchi (as seen in asthma), and **laryngospasms** occur in the larynx.

VOCABULARY REVIEW

In the previous section, you learned terms relating to pathology. Before going on to the exercises, review the terms below and refer to the previous section if you have questions. Pronunciations are provided for certain terms. Sometimes information about where the word came from is included after the term. The etymologies (word histories) are for your information only. You do not need to memorize them.

Term	Definition
adenoiditis [ĂD-ĕ-nŏy-DĪ-tĭs] adenoid-, adenoids + -itis, inflammation	Inflammation of the adenoids.
anthracosis [ăn-thră-KŌ-sĭs] anthrac-, coal + -osis, condition	Lung disease caused by long-term inhalation of coal dust; black lung disease.
apnea [ĂP-nē-ă] Greek *apnoia*, lack of breath	Cessation of breathing.

Term	Definition
asbestosis [ăs-bĕs-TŌ-sĭs] asbest(os) + -osis	Lung disorder caused by long-term inhalation of asbestos (as in construction work).
asthma [ĂZ-mă] Greek, difficult breathing	Chronic condition with obstruction or narrowing of the bronchial airways.
atelectasis [ăt-ĕ-LĚK-tă-sĭs]	Collapse of a lung or part of a lung.
bacilli (*sing.,* **bacillus**) [bă-SĬL-ī (bă-SĬL-ĭs)] Latin, *bacillum*, walking stick	A type of bacteria.
black lung	*See* anthracosis.
bradypnea [brăd-ĭp-NĒ-ă] brady-, slow + -pnea, breathing	Abnormally slow breathing.
bronchitis [brŏng-KĪ-tĭs] bronch-, bronchus + -itis	Inflammation of the bronchi.
bronchospasm [BRŎNG-kō-spăzm] broncho-, bronchus + -spasm, contraction	Sudden contraction in the bronchi that causes coughing.
Cheyne-Stokes respiration [chān stōks rĕs-pĭ-RĀ-shŭn]	Irregular breathing pattern with a period of apnea followed by deep, labored breathing that becomes shallow, then apneic.
chronic bronchitis	Recurring or long-lasting bouts of bronchitis.
chronic obstructive pulmonary disease	Disease of the bronchial tubes or lungs with chronic obstruction.
crackles [KRĂK-ls]	Popping sounds heard in lung collapse or other conditions; rales.
croup [krūp]	Acute respiratory syndrome in children or infants accompanied by seal-like coughing.
cystic fibrosis [SĬS-tĭk fī-BRŌ-sĭs]	Disease that causes chronic airway obstruction and also affects the bronchial tubes.
diphtheria [dĭf-THĒR-ē-ă] Greek *diphthera*, leather	Acute infection of the throat and upper respiratory tract caused by bacteria.
dysphonia [dĭs-FŌ-nē-ă] dys-, abnormal + Greek *phone*, voice	Hoarseness usually caused by laryngitis.
dyspnea [dĭsp-NĒ-ă, DĬSP-nē-ă] Greek *dyspnoia*, bad breathing	Difficult breathing.
emphysema [ĕm-fă-SĒ-mă, ĕm-fă-ZĒ-mă] Greek, inflation of the stomach	Chronic condition of hyperinflation of the air sacs; often caused by prolonged smoking.
empyema [ĕm-pī-Ē-mă] Greek, formation of pus	Pus in the pleural cavity.
epiglottitis [ĕp-ĭ-glŏt-Ī-tĭs] epiglott(is) + -itis	Inflammation of the epiglottis.

Term	Definition
epistaxis [ĔP-ĭ-STĂK-sĭs] Greek, nosebleed	Bleeding from the nose, usually caused by trauma or a sudden rupture of the blood vessels of the nose.
eupnea [yūp-NĒ-ă, YŪP-nē-ă] Greek *eupnoia*, good breath	Normal breathing.
hemoptysis [hē-MŎP-tĭ-sĭs] hemo-, blood + Greek *ptysis*, spitting	Lung or bronchial hemorrhage resulting in the spitting of blood.
hemothorax [hē-mō-THŌR-ăks] hemo- + thorax	Blood in the pleural cavity.
hypercapnia [hī-pĕr-KĂP-nē-ă] hyper-, excessive + Greek *kapnos*, smoke	Excessive buildup of carbon dioxide in lungs, usually associated with hypoventilation.
hyperpnea [hī-pĕrp-NĒ-ă] hyper- + -pnea, breathing	Abnormally deep breathing.
hyperventilation [HĪ-pĕr-vĕn-tĭ-LĀ-shŭn] hyper- + ventilation	Abnormally fast breathing in and out, often associated with anxiety.
hypopnea [hī-PŎP-nē-ă] hypo-, below normal + -pnea	Shallow breathing.
hypoventilation [HĪ-pō-vĕn-ĭ-LĀ-shŭn] hypo- + ventilation	Abnormally low movement of air in and out of the lungs.
hypoxemia [hī-pŏk-SĒ-mē-ă] hyp-, below normal + ox(ygen) + -emia, blood	Deficient amount of oxygen in the blood.
hypoxia [hī-PŎK-sē-ă] hyp- + ox(ygen) + -ia, condition	Deficient amount of oxygen in tissue.
laryngitis [lăr-ĭn-JĪ-tĭs] laryng-, larynx + -itis	Inflammation of the larynx.
laryngospasm [lă-RĬNG-gō-spăsm] laryngo-, larynx + -spasm	Sudden contraction of the larynx, which may cause coughing and may restrict breathing.
laryngotracheobronchitis [lă-RĬNG-gō-TRĀ-kē-ō-brŏng-KĪ-tĭs] laryngo- + tracheo-, trachea + bronch- + -itis	Inflammation of the larynx, trachea, and bronchi.
mesothelioma [MĔZ-ō-thē-lē-Ō-mă] mesotheli(um), layer of cells as in the pleura + -oma, tumor	Rare cancer of the lungs associated with asbestosis.
nasopharyngitis [NĀ-zō-fă-rĭn-JĪ-tĭs] naso- + pharyng-, pharynx + -itis	Inflammation of the nose and pharynx.
nosebleed	*See* epistaxis.
orthopnea [ōr-thŏp-NĒ-ă, ōr-THŎP-nē-ă] ortho-, straight + -pnea	Difficulty in breathing, especially while lying down.

Term	Definition
pansinusitis [păn-sī-nŭ-SĪ-tĭs] pan-, all + sinusitis	Inflammation of all the sinuses.
paroxysmal [păr-ŏk-SĪZ-măl] Greek *paroxysmos*, spasm	Sudden, as a spasm or convulsion.
pertussis [pĕr-TŬS-ĭs] Latin *per*, intensive + *tussis*, cough	Severe infection of the pharynx, larynx, and trachea caused by bacteria; whooping cough.
pharyngitis [făr-ĭn-JĪ-tĭs] pharyng- + -itis	Inflammation of the pharynx; sore throat.
pleural effusion [PLŬR-ăl ĕ-FYŪ-zhŭn]	Escape of fluid into the pleural cavity.
pleuritis, pleurisy [plū-RĪ-tĭs, PLŬR-ĭ-sē] pleur-, pleura + -itis	Inflammation of the pleura.
pneumoconiosis [NŪ-mō-kō-nē-Ō-sĭs] pneumo-, lung + Greek *konis*, dust + -osis	Lung condition caused by inhaling dust.
pneumonia [nū-MŌ-nē-ă] Greek, lung condition	Acute infection of the alveoli.
pneumonitis [nū-mō-NĪ-tĭs] pneumon-, lung + -itis	Inflammation of the lung.
pneumothorax [nū-mō-THŌR-ăks] pneumo- + thorax	Accumulation of air or gas in the pleural cavity.
pulmonary abscess [PŬL-mō-nār-ē ĂB-sĕs]	Large collection of pus in the lungs.
pulmonary edema [PŬL-mō-nār-ē ĕ-DĒ-mă]	Fluid in the air sacs and bronchioles usually caused by failure of the heart to pump enough blood to and from lungs.
rales [răhlz]	*See* crackles.
rhinitis [rī-NĪ-tĭs] rhin-, nose + -itis	Nasal inflammation.
rhinorrhea [rīn-nō-RĒ-ă] rhino-, nose + -rrhea, discharge	Nasal discharge.
rhonchi [RŎNG-kī]	*See* wheezes.
silicosis [sĭl-ĭ-KŌ-sĭs]	Lung condition caused by silica dust from grinding rocks or glass or other materials used in manufacturing.
singultus [sĭng-GŬL-tŭs]	Hiccuping.
sinusitis [sī-nū-SĪ-tĭs] sinus + -itis	Inflammation of the sinuses.
stridor [STRĪ-dōr] Latin, a harsh sound	High-pitched crowing sound heard in certain respiratory conditions.

Term	Definition
tachypnea [tăk-ĭp-NĒ-ă] tachy-, fast + -pnea	Abnormally fast breathing.
tonsillitis [TŎN-sĭ-LĪ-tĭs] tonsill-, tonsils + -iti	Inflammation of the tonsils.
tracheitis [trā-kē-Ī-tĭs] trache-, trachea + -itis	Inflammation of the trachea.
tuberculosis [tū-bĕr-kyū-LŌ-sĭs] Latin *tuberculum*, small nodule + -osis	Acute infectious disease caused by bacteria called bacilli.
upper respiratory infection	Infection of all or part of upper portion of respiratory tract.
wheezes [HWĒZ-ĕz]	Whistling sounds heard on inspiration in certain breathing disorders, especially asthma.
whooping cough [HŎOP-ĭng kăwf]	*See* pertussis.

CASE STUDY

X-rays for Pneumonia

Many of the elderly patients admitted to the hospital through the emergency room are suffering from pneumonia. Their chest x-rays will show evidence of the disease. Usually, after a course of antibiotics, the patients are x-rayed again. If the x-rays are not clear a second time, some other underlying problem, such as an abnormal growth or latent disease, may be suspected. Elderly patients, particularly those who are bedridden, are particularly susceptible to pneumonia.

Critical Thinking

128. Why is a bedridden person more susceptible to pneumonia than a patient who is ambulatory?
129. Patients with any kind of respiratory infection often have breathing problems when lying down, even for weeks after the infection has begun to subside. Why can lying down cause breathing problems?

PATHOLOGICAL TERMS EXERCISES

Match the Condition

Match the words in the column on the left with the definition in the column on the right.

130. _____ pleurisy, pleuritis
131. _____ epistaxis
132. _____ dysphonia
133. _____ hypoxemia
134. _____ hypercapnia
135. _____ anthracosis
136. _____ pleural effusion
137. _____ pertussis
138. _____ tachypnea
139. _____ apnea

a. whooping cough
b. deficient oxygen in blood
c. black lung
d. pleural inflammation
e. hoarseness
f. inability to breathe
g. nosebleed
h. fast breathing
i. too much carbon dioxide
j. fluid in the pleural cavity

Check Your Knowledge

Circle T for true or F for false.

140. Foreign material comes into the body during internal respiration. T F

141. Dysphonia is associated with laryngitis. T F

142. Diphtheria, pertussis, and tuberculosis are all caused by bacteria. T F

143. A pleural effusion is a type of cancer. T F

144. Respiratory spasms may cause uncontrollable coughing. T F

145. Bronchospasms occur during tonsillitis. T F

146. Tuberculosis cannot be passed from one person to another. T F

147. Atelectasis is another name for a nosebleed . T F

148. Inflammation of the voice box is called laryngitis. T F

149. Hypopnea is abnormally deep breathing. T F

Fill in the Blanks

150. Inflammation of the throat is called _____.

151. Any lung condition caused by dust is called _____.

152. Chronic bronchial airway obstruction is a symptom of _____.

153. The sounds heard in atelectasis are _____ or _____.

154. Many respiratory conditions are caused or made worse by _____, an addictive habit.

Surgical Terms

When breathing is disrupted or chronic infections of the respiratory tract occur, surgical procedures can provide relief. Ear, nose, and throat (ENT) doctors or **otorhinolaryngologists** specialize in disorders of the upper respiratory tract. Sometimes it is necessary to remove parts of the respiratory system, either to relieve constant infections or to remove abnormal growths. A **tonsillectomy** is excision of the tonsils (often to stop recurrent tonsillitis). An **adenoidectomy** is removal of the adenoids; a **laryngectomy** removes the larynx (usually to stop cancerous growth); a **pneumonectomy** is the excision of a lung; and a **lobectomy** is the excision of a lobe of a lung (as when cancer is present).

Surgical repair can relieve respiratory problems caused by trauma, abnormalities, growths, or infections. A **bronchoplasty** is the repair of a bronchus; **laryngoplasty** is the repair of the larynx; **rhinoplasty** is the repair of the bones of the nose; **septoplasty** is the repair of the nasal septum; and **tracheoplasty** is the repair of the trachea.

Incisions into parts of the respiratory system are sometimes necessary. **Thoracic surgeons** are the specialists who usually perform such procedures. A **laryngotracheotomy** is an incision of the larynx and trachea; **pneumobronchotomy** is an incision of the lung and bronchus; **septostomy** is the creation of an opening in the nasal septum; **sinusotomy** is an incision of a sinus; **thoracotomy** is an incision into the chest cavity; **thoracostomy** is the establishment of an opening in the chest cavity to drain fluid; and **tracheotomy** is an incision into the trachea, usually to provide an airway (Figure 7-8). Surgical punctures provide a means to aspirate or remove fluid. **Laryngocentesis** is a surgical puncture of the larynx; **pleurocentesis** is a surgical puncture of pleural space; and **thoracocentesis** is a surgical puncture of the chest cavity.

Artificial openings into the respiratory tract may allow for alternative airways as in a **tracheostomy** (artificial tracheal opening) or a **laryngostomy** (artificial laryngeal opening). An **endotracheal intubation** is the insertion of a tube through the nose or mouth, pharynx, and larynx and into the trachea to establish an airway. A **pleuropexy** is performed to attach the pleura in place surgically, usually in case of injury or deterioration.

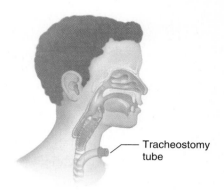
Tracheostomy tube

FIGURE 7-8 A tracheotomy provides an emergency airway.

Vocabulary Review

In the previous section, you learned terms relating to surgery. Before going on to the exercises, review the terms below and refer to the previous section if you have questions. Pronunciations are provided for certain terms. Sometimes information about where the word came from is included after the term. The etymologies (word histories) are for your information only. You do not need to memorize them.

Term	Definition
adenoidectomy [ĂD-ĕ-nŏy-DĔK-tō-mē] adenoid-, adenoids + -ectomy, removal	Removal of the adenoids.
bronchoplasty [BRŎNG-kō-plăs-tē] broncho-, bronchus + -plasty, repair	Surgical repair of a bronchus.
endotracheal intubation (ET) [ĔN-dō-TRĀ-kē-ăl ĭn-tū-BĀ-shŭn] endo- within + trache-, trachea + -al, pertaining to	Insertion of a tube through the nose or mouth, pharynx, and larynx and into the trachea to establish an airway.
laryngectomy [LĂR-ĭn-JĔK-tō-mē] laryng-, larynx + -ectomy	Removal of the larynx.
laryngocentesis [lă-RĬNG-gō-sĕn-TĒ-sĭs] laryngo- , larynx + -centesis, puncture	Surgical puncture of the larynx.
laryngoplasty [lă-RĬNG-gō-plăs-tē] laryngo- + -plasty	Repair of the larynx.
laryngostomy [LĂR-ĭng-GŎS-tō-mē] laryngo- + -stomy, mouth	Creation of an artificial opening in the larynx.
laryngotracheotomy [lă-RĬNG-gō-trā-kē-ŎT-ō-mē] laryngo- + tracheo-, trachea + -tomy, cutting	Incision into the larynx and trachea.
lobectomy [lō-BĔK-tō-mē] lob-, lobe + -ectomy	Removal of one of the lobes of a lung.
otorhinolaryngologist [ō-tō-RĪ-nō-lăr-ĭng-GŎL-ō-jĭst] oto-, ear + rhino-, nose + laryngo- + -logist, specialist	Medical doctor who diagnoses and treats disorders of the ear, nose, and throat.

Term	Definition
pleurocentesis [PLŪR-ō-sĕn-TĒ-sĭs] pleuro-, pleura + -centesis	Surgical puncture of pleural space.
pleuropexy [PLŪR-ō-PĚK-sē] pleuro- + -pexy, a fixing	Fixing in place of the pleura surgically, usually in case of injury or deterioration.
pneumobronchotomy [NŪ-mō-brŏng-KŎT-ō-mē] pneumo-, lung + broncho- + -tomy	Incision of the lung and bronchus.
pneumonectomy [NŪ-mō-NĔK-tō-mē] pneumon-, lung + -ectomy	Removal of a lung.
rhinoplasty [RĪ-nō-plăs-tē] rhino-, nose + -plasty	Surgical repair of the bones of the nose.
septoplasty [SĔP-tō-plăs-tē] sept(um) + -plasty	Surgical repair of the nasal septum.
septostomy [sĕp-TŎS-tō-mē] sept(um) + -stomy	Creation of an opening in the nasal septum.
sinusotomy [sĭn-ū-SŎT-ō-mē] sinus + -tomy	Incision of a sinus.
thoracic [thō-RĂS-ĭk] **surgeon**	Surgeon who specializes in surgery of the thorax.
thoracocentesis [THŌR-ă-kō-sĕn-TĒ-sĭs] thoraco-, thorax + -centesis	Surgical puncture of the chest cavity.
thoracostomy [thōr-ă-KŎS-tō-mē] thoraco- + -stomy	Establishment of an opening in the chest cavity.
thoracotomy [thōr-ă-KŎT-ō-mē] thraco- + -tomy	Incision into the chest cavity.
tonsillectomy [TŎN-sĭ-LĔK-tō-mē] tonsill-, tonsils + ectomy	Removal of the tonsils.
tracheoplasty [TRĀ-kē-ō-PLĂS-tē] tracheo-, trachea + plasty	Repair of the trachea.
tracheostomy [TRĀ-kē-ŎS-tō-mē] tracheo- + -stomy	Creation of an artificial opening in the trachea.
tracheotomy [trā-kē-ŎT-ō-mē] tracheo- + -tomy	Incision into the trachea.

SURGICAL TERMS EXERCISES

Check Your Knowledge

Match the terms in the left column with the definitions in the right column.

155. _____ rhinoplasty   **a.** artificial laryngeal opening

156. _____ pleuropexy   **b.** removal of a lobe of the lung

157. ____ adenoidectomy

158. ____ tracheostomy

159. ____ tracheotomy

160. ____ laryngectomy

161. ____ lobectomy

162. ____ laryngostomy

163. ____ pleurocentesis

164. ____ septostomy

c. puncture of the pleura

d. creation of an opening in the nasal septum

e. incision into the trachea

f. removal of the adenoids

g. repair of the nose

h. attaching of the pleura

i. removal of the larynx

j. artificial tracheal opening

Fill in the Blanks

165. An incision into the chest cavity is a _____.

166. An airway can be provided by an emergency _____.

167. Cancer of the lung may require a _____.

168. Surgical attaching of the pleura in place is called _____.

169. The nasal septum is repaired during _____.

CASE STUDY

Asthma Emergencies

Emergency rooms are also visited frequently by people with asthma. A severe asthmatic attack requires medication and close monitoring or it can be fatal. Once the patient is stabilized, various tests may be necessary to determine the pathology in the lungs. June Lytel is a 10-year-old who has asthma. Recently she has had tonsillitis. Four months ago, another case of tonsillitis caused inflammation of her upper respiratory tract. She had two emergency room visits for asthma attacks during the URI. Her physician, an ENT, is also a surgeon.

Critical Thinking

170. Why is it important that her doctor is a surgeon?

171. How might surgery help avoid future URIs?

Pharmacological Terms

Antibiotics, antihistamines, and anticoagulants are used for respiratory system disorders just as with other system disorders. Specific to respiratory problems are **bronchodilators,** drugs that dilate the walls of the bronchi (as during an asthmatic attack), and **expectorants,** drugs that promote coughing and the expulsion of mucus. **Antitussives** relieve coughing, and **decongestants** help congestion of the upper respiratory tract. Table 7-3 lists some medications commonly prescribed for respiratory disorders.

Two mechanical devices aid in respiration. Mechanical **ventilators** (Figure 7.9) actually serve as a breathing substitute for patients who cannot breathe on their own. **Nebulizers** deliver medication through the nose or mouth to ease breathing problems. Some nebulizers are MDI (metered dose inhalers) that deliver a specific amount of spray with each puff of the inhaler.

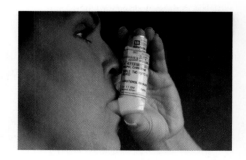

FIGURE 7-9 An inhaler is often used to treat asthma.

TABLE 7-3 Some Common Agents Used to Treat the Respiratory System

Drug Class	Purpose	Generic	Trade Name
antitussives	to relieve coughing	codeine	none except in combination
		dextromethorphan	Benylin, Pertussin, Robitussin, and others
		diphenhydramine	Allermax, Benadryl, and many others
bronchodilators	to dilate the walls of the bronchi and prevent spasms	albuterol	Ventolin, Proventil
		ephedrine	Bronkaid, Primatene
		epinephrine	Bronkaid Mist, Primatene Mist
		terbutaline	Brethaire, Brethine
		omalizumab	Xolair
		theophylline	Theo-Dur, Slo-Bid
decongestants	to lower and prevent mucus buildup	pseudoephedrine	Drixoral, Sudafed, and others
		xylometazoline	Otrivin
expectorants	to promote coughing and expelling of mucus	guaifenesin	Humibid, Robitussin

Recently, new medications have become available to control asthma attacks. Traditionally, asthmatics used ventilators or nebulizers to control the occurrence or intensity of attacks. Now it is possible to take medication in pill form to avoid most attacks.

VOCABULARY REVIEW

In the previous section, you learned terms relating to pharmacology. Before going on to the exercises, review the terms below and refer to the previous section if you have any questions. Pronunciations are provided for certain terms. Sometimes information about where the word came from is included after the term. The etymologies (word histories) are for your information only. You do not need to memorize them.

Term	Definition
antitussives [ăn-tē-TŬS-sĭvs] anti-, against + Latin *tussis*, cough	Agents that control coughing.
bronchodilators [brŏng-kō-dĭ-LĀ-tŏrz] broncho- + dilator, agent that dilates	Agents that dilate the walls of the bronchi.
decongestants [dē-kŏn-JĚST-ănts]	Agents that relieve mucus congestion of the upper respiratory tract.
expectorants [ĕk-SPĚK-tō-rănts] ex-, out of + Latin *pectus*, chest	Agents that promote the coughing and expelling of mucus.

Term	Definition
nebulizers [NĔB-yū-līz-ĕrz]	Devices that deliver medication through the nose or mouth in a fine spray to the respiratory tract.
ventilators [VĔN-tĭ-lā-tŏrz]	Mechanical breathing devices.

CASE STUDY

Mechanical Breathing Apparatus

Missy Ruiz, a 24-year-old mother of two, was admitted to Midvale's trauma center after a serious car accident. Melissa could not breathe on her own because of trauma to her windpipe. A tracheotomy was performed so that she could be connected to a ventilator. Brain scans showed little activity, and doctors gave her only a slight chance for recovery. With intravenous feeding and the ventilator, Melissa could survive in a vegetative state for a long time.

Critical Thinking

172. Melissa cannot breathe unassisted. What organ directs the breathing process? Why is Melissa's breathing process interrupted?
173. Melissa is bedridden. What respiratory disease might she contract?

PHARMACOLOGICAL TERMS EXERCISES

Check Your Knowledge

Complete the sentences below by filling in the blanks.

174. Coughing can be controlled with _____.
175. Insufficiently dilated bronchi can be treated with _____.
176. Productive coughing is helped with _____.
177. Medication is delivered in a fine spray by means of a _____.
178. A person who cannot breathe on his or her own may be kept alive on a _____.

CHALLENGE SECTION

The following chest x-ray report is from a patient who received x-rays during an emergency room visit.

Patient: Marina Sanchez
Age: 55
Physician: Dr. J. Woo

CHEST: 11/6/XXXX:

PA and lateral views of the chest show evidence of patchy alveolar density in the right midlung field, inferior to minor fissure on PA view. It appears to be located in the lateral segment of

(continued)

the right middle lobe, which may represent infiltrate. However, the possibility of a pulmonary neoplasm cannot be excluded. Suggest follow-up chest x-ray after 1 to 2 weeks to confirm its resolution. Remainder of right and left lung are free of any acute pathology. The cardiovascular silhouette shows normal heart size with normal pulmonary vasculature. Both hemidiaphragms are unremarkable. The visualized bony thorax is unremarkable.

In the hospital patient was examined for coronary artery disease. Doctors are now discussing recommendation for a CABG.

Critical Thinking

This patient currently has a high fever and chest tightness. He will be treated for infection. What else did the radiologist suggest as a possible cause of his pulmonary problems? Why do you think a follow-up chest x-ray is necessary?

_____

_____

_____

_____

_____

_____

_____

_____

_____

TERMINOLOGY IN ACTION

Shown below is a referral letter for a 65-year-old patient with severe emphysema. Write a brief description of the disease and discuss the most likely cause of the disease.

Dr. Youssef Muhammed
12 Park Street
Dexter, MI 99999
Dear Dr. Mohammed:

Mr. Alima will be making an appointment to see you in the very near future. He is a 65-year-old male who has had emphysema for many years. Recently it has become quite severe. At this time, he presents with complaints of weakness, even with the most minimal exertion.

I have not instituted any change in his therapy as he plans to see you within the week and will follow your recommendations.

I am enclosing my office notes for your review. Please do not hesitate to contact me if you need further information.

Sincerely,

Allison Jankman, MD

Enclosure

USING THE INTERNET

Go to the American Lung Association's Web site (http://www.lungusa.org). Write a short paragraph about research being done on one disease of the respiratory system.

CHAPTER REVIEW

The material that follows is to help you review all the material in this chapter.

Remembering the Word Parts

Put the letter of the correct definition for each of the following respiratory word parts in the space provided. Answers may be used more than once or not used at all.

179. adenoid(o) _____
180. phren(o) _____
181. alveol(o) _____
182. phon(o) _____
183. bronch(o) _____
184. pharyng(o) _____
185. capn(o) _____
186. ox(o) _____
187. oxi- _____
188. epiglott(o) _____
189. or(o) _____
190. laryng(o) _____
191. nas(o) _____
192. lob(o) _____
193. mediastin(o) _____
194. pleur(o) _____
195. rhin(o) _____
196. pneum(o) _____
197. steth(o) _____
198. -pnea _____
199. pneumon(o) _____
200. thorac(o) _____
201. tonsil(o) _____
202. trache(o) _____

a. air sac
b. throat
c. adenoids
d. carbon dioxide
e. diaphragm
f. nose
g. pleura
h. tonsil
i. lobe
j. area between lungs, middle of thoracic cavity
k. mouth
l. oxygen
m. voice, sound
n. sinus
o. flap that closes over the trachea during swallowing
p. bronchi
q. voicebox
r. bronchus, tube going to lung
s. airway, tube connecting throat to bronchi
t. chest
u. tongue
v. breathing
w. air/lung
x. lining of the lungs

Using Your Allied Health Dictionary

For each of the following word parts, find a respiratory term in your allied health dictionary. Give the meaning of the term.

203. eu-, good, normal _____

204. dys-, bad, difficult, abnormal _____

205. -itis, inflammation _____

206. -ectomy, removal, surgical removal_____

207. -tomy_____ cutting into, incision

208. -(o)stomy_____ new opening, creation of new opening

209. -meter_____ instrument to measure

210. -scope_____ instrument to view

211. brady-_____ slow

212. tachy-_____ fast

213. hyper-_____ above, beyond, too much

214. hyp(o)-_____ below, not enough, deficient

215. a-_____ not, absence of

216. orth(o)-_____ straight, upright

217. -rrhea_____ discharge, runny discharge

218. -plasty_____ surgical repair

219. -pexy_____ fixation

220. -centesis_____ surgical puncture to remove fluid

Understanding Respiratory Terms

Put the letter of the correct definition in the space provided.

221. pneumothorax _____   **a.** runny nose

222. hyperpnea _____   **b.** whooping cough

223. CPR _____   **c.** inflammation of the adenoids

224. Abdominal thrust maneuver _____   **d.** voice box

225. spirometer _____   **e.** saliva and mucus from the lung

226. rhinorrhea _____   **f.** air sacs

227. sputum _____   **g.** instrument for measuring breathing

228. alveoli _____   **h.** inflammation of the parasinuses

229. larynx _____   **i.** cardiopulmonary resuscitation

230. epiglottis _____   **j.** air in the pleura

231. parasinusitis _____   **k.** abnormally fast breathing

232. nasopharynx _____   **l.** Heimlich maneuver

233. pertussis _____   **m.** removal of a lung

234. pneumonectomy _____   **n.** flap of cartilage

235. adenoiditis _____   **o.** just above the soft palate

DEFINITIONS

Define the following terms and combining forms. Review the chapter before starting. Make sure you know how to pronounce each term as you define it. The blue words in curly brackets are references to the Spanish glossary available online at www.mhhe.com/medterm3e.

236. Adam's apple
237. adenoid(o)
238. adenoidectomy [ĂD-ĕ-nŏy-DĔK-tō-mē] {adenoidectomía}
239. adenoiditis [ĂD-ĕ-nŏy-DĪ-tĭs] {adenoiditis}
240. adenoids [ĂD-ĕ-nŏydz] {adenoides}
241. alveol(o)
242. alveolus (pl., alveoli) [ăl-VĒ-ō-lŭs (ăl-VĒ-ō-lī)] {alvéolo}
243. anthracosis [ăn-thră-KŌ-sĭs] {antracosis}
244. antitussives [ăn-tē-TŬS-sĭvs]
245. apex [Ā-pĕks] {apex}
246. apnea [ĂP-nē-ă] {apnea}
247. arterial blood gases
248. asbestosis [ăs-bĕs-TŌ-sĭs] {asbestosis}
249. asthma [ĂZ-mă] {asma}
250. atelectasis [ăt-ĕ-LĔK-tă-sĭs] {atelectasia}
251. auscultation [ăws-kŭl-TĀ-shŭn] {auscultación}
252. bacilli (sing., bacillus) [bă-SĬL-Ī (bă-SĬL-ĭs)] {bacilo}
253. base [bās] {base}
254. black lung
255. bradypnea [brăd-ĭp-NĒ-ă] {bradipnea}
256. bronch(o), bronchi(o)
257. bronchial alveolar lavage [BRŎNG-kē-ăl ăl-VĒ-ō-lăr lă-VĂZH]
258. bronchial brushing
259. bronchiol(o)
260. bronchiole [BRŎNG-kē-ōl] {bronquiolo}
261. bronchitis [brŏng-KĪ-tĭs] {bronquitis}
262. bronchodilators [brŏng-kō-dī-LĀ-tŏrz]
263. bronchography [brŏng-KŎG-ră-fē] {broncografía}
264. bronchoplasty [BRŎNG-kō-plăs-tē]
265. bronchoscope [BRŎNG-kō-skōp] {broncoscopio}
266. bronchospasm [BRŎNG-kō-spăzm] {broncoespasmo}
267. bronchus (pl., bronchi) [BRŎNG-kŭs (BRŎNG-kī)] {bronquio}
268. capn(o)
269. Cheyne-Stokes respiration [chān stōks rĕs-pĭ-RĀ-shŭn]
270. chronic bronchitis
271. chronic obstructive pulmonary disease
272. cilia [SĬL-ē-ă]
273. crackles [KRĂK-ls]
274. croup [krūp] {crup}
275. cystic fibrosis [SĬS-tĭk fī-BRŌ-sĭs]
276. decongestants [dē-kŏn-JĔST-ănts]
277. diaphragm [DĪ-ă-frăm] {diafragma}
278. diphtheria [dĭf-THĒR-ē-ă] {difteria}
279. dysphonia [dĭs-FŌ-nē-ă] {dissfonía}
280. dyspnea [dĭsp-NĒ-ă, DĬSP-nē-ă] {disnea}
281. emphysema [ĕm-fă-SĒ-mă, ĕm-fă-ZĒ-mă] {enfisema}
282. empyema [ĕm-pī-Ē-mă] {empiema}
283. endoscope [ĔN-dō-skōp] {endoscopio}
284. endotracheal intubation [ĕn-dō-TRĀ-kē-ăl ĭn-tū-BĀ-shŭn] (ET)
285. epiglott(o)
286. epiglottis [ĔP-ĭ-GLŎT-ĭs] {epiglotis}
287. epiglottitis [ĕp-ĭ-glŏt-Ī-tĭs] {epiglotitis}
288. epistaxis [ĔP-ĭ-STĂK-sĭs]
289. eupnea [yūp-NĒ-ă, YŪP-nē-ă] {eupnea}
290. exhalation [ĕks-hă-LĀ-shŭn] {exahalación}
291. expectorants [ĕk-SPĔK-tō-rănts]
292. expiration [ĕks-pĭ-RĀ-shŭn] {espiración}
293. external nares [ĕks-TĔR-năl NĀR-ēz]
294. external respiration
295. glottis [GLŎT-ĭs] {glotis}
296. hemoptysis [hē-MŎP-tĭ-sĭs]
297. hemothorax [hē-mō-THŌR-ăks] {hemotórax}
298. hilum (also hilus) [HĪ-lŭm (HĪ-lŭs)] {hilio}
299. hypercapnia [hī-pĕr-KĂP-nē-ă]
300. hyperpnea [hī-pĕrp-NĒ-ă]
301. hyperventilation [HĪ-pĕr-vĕn-tĭ-LĀ-shŭn] {hiperventilación}
302. hypopharynx [HĪ-pō-FĂR-ĭngks] {hipofaringe}
303. hypopnea [hī-PŎP-nē-ă]
304. hypoventilation [HĪ-pō-vĕn-tĭ-LĀ-shŭn] {hipoventilación}
305. hypoxemia [hī-pŏk-SĒ-mē-ă] {hipoxemia}
306. hypoxia [hī-PŎK-sē-ă] {hypoxia}
307. inferior lobe [ĭn-FĒ-rē-ōr lōb]
308. inhalation [ĭn-hă-LĀ-shŭn] {inhalación}
309. inspiration [ĭn-spĭ-RĀ-shŭn] {inspiración}
310. intercostal muscles [ĭn-tĕr-KŎS-tăl MŬS-ĕlz]
311. internal respiration
312. laryng(o)
313. laryngectomy [LĂR-ĭn-JĔK-tō-mē]

314. laryngitis [lăr-ĭn-JĪ-tĭs] {laryngitis}

315. laryngocentesis [lă-RĬNG-gō-sĕn-TĒ-sĭs]

316. laryngopharynx [lă-RĬNG-gō-făr-ĭngks]

317. laryngoplasty [lă-RĬNG-gō-plăs-tē] {laringoplastia}

318. laryngoscopy [LĂR-ĭng-GŎS-kō-pē] {laringoscopia}

319. laryngospasm [lă-RĬNG-gō-spăsm]

320. laryngostomy [LĂR-ĭng-GŎS-tō-mē] {laringostomía}

321. laryngotracheobronchitis [lă-RĬNG-gō-TRĀ-kē-ō-brŏng-KĪ-tĭs]

322. laryngotracheotomy [lă-RĬNG-gō-trā-kē-ŏT-ō-mē]

323. larynx [LĂR-ĭngks] {laringe}

324. lob(o)

325. lobectomy [lō-BĔK-tō-mē] {lobectomía}

326. lung [lŭng] {pulmón}

327. mediastin(o)

328. mediastinoscopy [MĒ-dē-ăs-tĭ-NŎS-kō-pē]

329. mediastinum [MĒ-dē-ăs-TĪ-nŭm] {mediastino}

330. mesothelioma [MĔZ-ō-thē-lē-Ō-mă] {mesotelioma}

331. middle lobe

332. nas(o)

333. nasal cavity [NĀ-zăl KĂV-ĭ-tē]

334. nasal septum [NĀ-zăl SĔP-tŭm]

335. nasopharyngitis [NĀ-zō-fă-rĭn-JĪ-tĭs]

336. nasopharyngoscopy [NĀ-zō-fă-rĭng-GŎS-kō-pē] {nasofaringoscopio}

337. nasopharynx [NĀ-zō-FĂR-ĭngks] {nasofaringe}

338. nebulizers [NĔB-yū-līz-ĕrz]

339. nose [nōz] {nariz}

340. nosebleed {epistaxis}

341. nostrils [NŎS-trĭlz] {naris}

342. or(o)

343. oropharynx [ŌR-ō-FĂR-ĭngks] {orofaringe}

344. orthopnea [ōr-thŏp-NĒ-ă, ōr-THŎP-nē-ă] {ortopnea}

345. otorhinolaryngologist [ō-tō-RĪ-nō-lăr-ĭng-GŎL-ō-jĭst]

346. ox(o), oxi, oxy

347. palatine tonsils [PĂL-ă-tīn TŎN-sĭlz]

348. pansinusitis [păn-sĭ-nŭ-SĪ-tĭs]

249. paranasal sinuses [păr-ă-NĀ-săl SĪ-nŭs-ĕz]

350. parietal pleura [pă-RĪ-ĕ-tăl PLŪR-ă]

351. paroxysmal [păr-ŏk-SĬZ-măl] {paraxístico}

352. peak flow meter

353. percussion [pĕr-KŬSH-ŭn] {percusión}

354. pertussis [pĕr-TŬS-ĭs] {pertussis}

355. pharyng(o)

356. pharyngeal tonsils [fă-RĬN-jē-ăl TŎN-sĭlz]

257. pharyngitis [făr-ĭn-JĪ-tĭs] {faringitis}

358. pharynx [FĂR-ĭngks] {faringe}

359. phon(o)

360. phren(o)

361. pleur(o)

362. pleura (pl., pleurae) [PLŪR-ă (PLŪR-ē)] {pleura}

363. pleural cavity [PLŪR-ăl KĂV-ĭ-tē]

364. pleural effusion [PLŪR-ăl ĕ-FYŪ-zhŭn]

365. pleuritis, pleurisy [plū-RĪ-tĭs, PLŪR-ĭ-sē] {pleuritis}

366. pleurocentesis [PLŪR-ō-sĕn-TĒ-sĭs]

367. pleuropexy [PLŪR-ō-PĔK-sē]

368. pneum(o), pneumon(o)

369. pneumobronchotomy [NŪ-mō-brŏng-KŎT-ō-mē]

370. pneumoconiosis [NŪ-mō-kō-nē-Ō-sĭs] {neumoconiosis}

371. pneumonectomy [NŪ-mō-NĔK-tō-mē] {neumonectomía}

372. pneumonia [nū-MŌ-nē-ă] {neumonía}

373. pneumonitis [nū-mō-NĪ-tĭs] {neumonitis}

374. pneumothorax [nū-mō-THŌR-ăks] {neumotórax}

375. pulmonary abscess [PŬL-mō-nār-ē ĂB-sĕs]

376. pulmonary edema [PŬL-mō-nār-ē ĕ-DĒ-mă]

377. pulmonary function tests

378. rales [răhlz] {rales}

379. respiratory [RĔS-pĭ-ră-tōr-ē, rĕ-SPĪR-ă-tōr-ē] system

380. respiratory tract

381. rhin(o)

382. rhinitis [rī-NĪ-tĭs] {rinitis}

383. rhinoplasty [RĪ-nō-plăs-tē] {rinoplastia}

384. rhinorrhea [rī-nō-RĒ-ă] {rinorrea}

385. rhonchi [RŎNG-kī] {ronquidos}

386. septoplasty [SĔP-tō-plăs-tē] {septoplastia}

387. septostomy [sĕp-TŎS-tō-mē] {septostomía}

388. septum [SĔP-tŭm] {tabique}

389. silicosis [sĭl-ĭ-KŌ-sĭs]

390. singultus [sĭng-GŬL-tŭs] {singulto}

391. sinusitis [sī-nŭ-SĪ-tĭs] {sinusitis}

392. sinusotomy [sĭn-ū-SŎT-ō-mē] {sinosotomía}

393. soft palate [sŏft PĂL-ăt]

394. spir(o)

395. spirometer [sĭ-RŎM-ĕ-tĕr] {espirómetro}

396. sputum [SPŬ-tūm] sample or culture

397. steth(o)

398. stridor [STRĪ-dōr] {estridor}

399. superior lobe

400. sweat test

401. tachypnea [tăk-ĭp-NĒ-ă] {taquipnea}

402. thorac(o)

403. thoracic [thō-RĂS-ĭk] surgeon

404. thoracocentesis [THŌR-ă-kō-sĕn-TĒ-sĭs] {toracocentesis}

405. thoracostomy [thōr-ă-KŎS-tō-mē] {torascostomía}

406. thoracotomy [thōr-ă-KŎT-ō-mē] {toracotomía}

407. thorax [THŌ-răks] {tórax}

408. throat [thrōt] {garganta}

409. throat culture

410. thyroid cartilage [THĪ-rŏyd KĂR-tĭ-lĭj]

411. tonsill(o)

412. tonsillectomy [TŎN-sĭ-LĔK-tō-mē] {tonsilectomía}

413. tonsillitis [TŎN-sĭ-LĪ-tĭs] {tonsilitis}

414. trache(o)

415. trachea [TRĀ-kē-ă] {tráquea}

416. tracheitis [trā-kē-Ī-tĭs]

417. tracheoplasty [TRĀ-kē-ō-PLĂS-tē] {traqueoplastia}

418. tracheostomy [TRĀ-kē-ŎS-tō-mē] {traquestomía}

419. tracheotomy [trā-kē-ŎT-ō-mē] {traqueotomia}

420. tuberculosis [tū-bĕr-kyū-LŌ-sĭs] {tuberculosis}

421. upper respiratory infection

422. ventilators [VĔN-tĭ-lā-tōrz]

423. visceral pleura [VĬS-ĕr-ăl PLŪR-ă]

424. vocal cords

425. voice box

426. wheezes [HWĒZ-ĕz] {sibilancias}

427. whooping cough [HŎOP-ĭng kăwf]

428. windpipe

Abbreviations

Write out the full meaning of each abbreviation.

429. ABG

430. AFB

431. A&P

432. AP

433. ARD

434. ARDS

435. ARF

436. BS

437. COLD

438. COPD

439. CPR

440. CTA

441. CXR

442. DOE

443. DPT

444. ENT

445. ET tube

446. FEF

447. FEV

448. FVC

449. HBOT

450. IMV

451. IPPB

452. IRDS

453. IRV

454. LLL

455. LUL

456. MBC

457. MDI

458. PA

459. PCP

460. PEEP

461. PFT

462. PND

463. RD

464. RDS

465. RLL

466. RUL

467. SARS

468. SIDS

469. SOB

470. T&A

471. TB

472. TLC

473. TPR

474. URI

475. VC

476. V/Q SCAN

Answers to Chapter Exercises

1. Muscles in the diaphragm control the amount of air inhaled and exhaled. Weakened muscles may lead to shallow breathing.
2. oxygen
3. a. Trachea
   b. Lungs
   c. Alveoli
4. external respiration
5. cilia
6. nasal septum
7. epiglottis
8. abdominal thrust maneuver
9. air sacs/alveoli
10. three
11. two
12. diaphragm
13. intercostal
14. F
15. T
16. F
17. T
18. T
19. F
20. T
21. F
22. F
23. F
24. nasopharynx
25. trachea
26. respiration
27. C
28. diaphragm
29. epiglottis
30. pharynx
31. C
32. tonsils
33. bronchus
34. f
35. g
36. k
37. c
38. i
39. b
40. a
41. e
42. h
43. d
44. j
45. chronic obstructive pulmonary disease; smoking, sedentary, weight, heart disease, age.

46. Internal respiration is the exchange of oxygen and carbon dioxide between the blood and the cells. The heart pumps oxygenated blood throughout the body, and internal respiration requires an efficient cardiovascular system.
47. adenoidectomy
48. thoracocentesis
49. tracheotomy
50. tonsillitis
51. mediastinopericarditis
52. pneumonorrhaphy
53. oronasal
54. pharyngitis
55. phonopathy
56. capnogram
57. bronchitis
58. peribronchitis
59. pericardiopleural
60. lobotomy
61. oximetry
62. oxychloride
63. bronchoedema
64. alveoloclasia
65. thoracalgia
66. sinusotomy
67. d
68. f
69. g
70. i
71. a
72. j
73. e
74. h
75. c
76. b
77. LLL
78. LUL
79. ARD
80. A&P
81. MDI
82. SARS
83. SOB
84. SIDS
85. URI
86. acute respiratory failure
87. breath sounds
88. chronic obstructive lung disease
89. cardiopulmonary resuscitation
90. chest x-ray

91. arterial blood gasses
92. diphtheria, pertussis, tetanus
93. ear, nose, and throat
94. hyperbaric oxygen therapy
95. respiratory disease
96. respiratroy distress syndrome
97. tonsillectomy and adenoidectomy
98. tuberculosis
99. temperature, pulse, respiration
100. inflammation of the larynx, trachea, and bronchi: laryngo-, larynx; tracheo, trachea, bronch-, bronchi, -itis, inflammation.
101. surgical incision into the trachea; tracheo-, trachea; -tomy, incision.
102. surgical opening in to the trachea; tracheo-, trachea; -stomy, artificial opening.
103. nose inflammation; rhin(o)-, nose; -itis, inflammation.
104. deficiency of oxygen; hyp(o)-, low; -oxia, oxygen.
105. ear, nose, throat specialist; oto-, ear; rhino-, nose, laryngo-, throat, -logist, specialist.
106. narrowing of the bronchi; broncho-, bronchi; -stenosis, narrowing.
107. puncture of the pleura; pleuro-, pleura; -centesis, puncture.
108. inflammation of the alveoli; alveol(o)-, alveoli; -itis, inflammation.
109. softening of the bronchi; broncho-, bronchi; -malacia, softening.
110. inflammation of the sinuses; sinus, sinus; -itis, inflammation.
111. Mr. DiGiorno has both cardiovascular and respiratory problems. Blood gas tests show how his internal respiration is working.
112. WBC or white blood count
113. pulmonary function
114. sweat test
115. endoscope
116. forced vital
117. auscultation

118. throat culture
119. percussion
120. peak flow meter
121. sputum sample or culture
122. spirometer
123. pharyngo
124. capno
125. laryng
126. lob
127. laryngo
128. The bedridden person's muscles are weaker; breathing is shallower; there is reduced fresh air.
129. Fluids from the infection may still reside in the respiratory system. Lying down causes them to collect rather than to be expelled.
130. d
131. g
132. e
133. b
134. i
135. c
136. j
137. a
138. h
139. f
140. F
141. T
142. T
143. F
144. T
145. F
146. F
147. F
148. T
149. F
150. pharyngitis
151. pneumoconiosis
152. asthma
153. crackles/rales
154. smoking
155. g
156. h
157. f
158. j
159. e

160. i
161. b
162. a
163. c
164. d
165. thoracotomy
166. tracheotomy
167. lobectomy or pneumonectomy
168. pleuropexy
169. septoplasty
170. She may need a tonsillectomy.
171. If the tonsils are removed, they cannot spread infection.
172. brain; Missy's brain trauma affects her breathing process.
173. Pneumonia infections may result from long periods spent in bed and lack of exercise of muscles and lungs.
174. antitussives
175. bronchodilators
176. expectorants
177. nebulizer
178. ventilator
179. c
180. e
181. a
182. m
183. p, r
184. b
185. d
186. l
187. l
188. o
189. k
190. q
191. f
192. i
193. j
194. g
195. f
196. w
197. t
198. v
199. w
200. t
201. h
202. s.

NOTE: 203–220 are sample answers; answers may vary.
203. eupnea, normal breathing
204. dyspnea, abnormal breathing
205. sinusitis, sinus inflammation
206. lobectomy, removal of a lobe of the lung
207. tracheotomy, incision into the trachea
208. tracheostomy, artifical opening into the trachea
209. phonometer, instrument for sound measurement
210. bronchoscope, instrument for viewing the bronchi
211. bradypnea, slow breathing
212. tachypnea, fast breathing
213. hyperventilation, abnormally deep, fast breathing
214. hypopnea, shallow breathing
215. apnea, lack of breath
216. orthopnea, trouble breathing while lying down
217. rhinorrhea, runny nose
218. rhinoplasty, surgical nose repair
219. pleuropexy, surgical attachment of the pleura
220. pleurocentesis, surgical puncture of the pleura
221. j
222. k
223. i
224. l
225. g
226. a
227. e
228. f
229. d
230. n
231. h
232. o
233. b
234. m
235. c
236–476. Answers are available in the vocabulary reviews in this chapter.

The Nervous System

CHAPTER
8

► **NEUROLOGY**
► **ANESTHESIOLOGY**

After studying this chapter, you will be able to:

8.1 Name the parts of the nervous system and discuss the function of each part

8.2 Define the combining forms used in building words that relate to the nervous system

8.3 Identify the meaning of related abbreviations

8.4 Name the common diagnoses, laboratory tests, and clinical procedures used in testing and treating disorders of the nervous system

8.5 List and define the major pathological conditions of the nervous system

8.6 Define surgical terms related to the nervous system

8.7 Recognize common pharmacological agents used in treating disorders of the nervous system

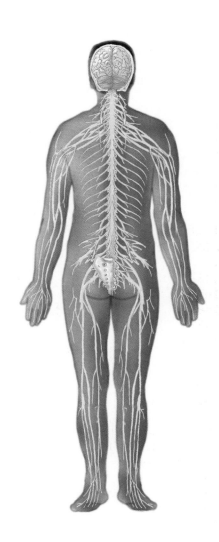

Structure and Function

The nervous system directs the function of all the human body systems (Figure 8-1). Every activity, whether voluntary or involuntary, is controlled by some of the more than 100 billion nerve cells throughout the body. The nervous system is divided into two subsystems: the central nervous system (CNS) and the peripheral nervous system (PNS).

A **nerve cell** or **neuron** (Figure 8-2) is the basic element of the nervous system. Neurons are highly specialized conducting cells and vary greatly in function, shape, and size. All neurons have three parts:

1. The **cell body,** which has branches or fibers that reach out to send or receive impulses. The cell body contains all the biological structures that are common to all human cells.
2. **Dendrites,** which are thin branching extensions of the cell body. They conduct nerve impulses *toward* the cell body.
3. The **axon,** which conducts nerve impulses *away* from the cell body. It is generally a single branch covered by fatty tissue called the **myelin sheath.** This protective sheath prevents the nerve impulse from transmitting in the wrong direction.

Outside the myelin sheath is a membranous covering called the **neurilemma.** At the end of the axon, there are **terminal end fibers** through which pass the impulses leaving the neuron. The nerve impulse then jumps from one neuron to the next over a space called a **synapse.** The nerve impulse is

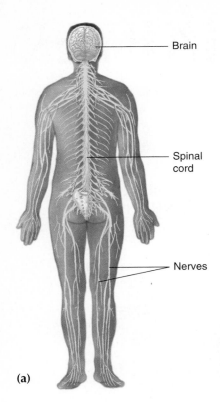

Brain

Spinal
cord

Nerves

(a)

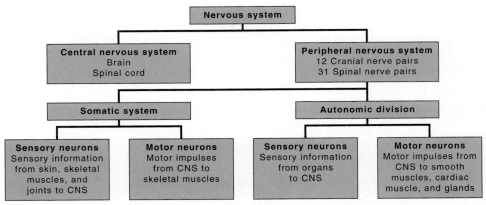

(b)

FIGURE 8-1 **(a)** The nervous system directs the function of all the human body systems. **(b)** The chart illustrates the functions controlled by the various parts of the nervous system.

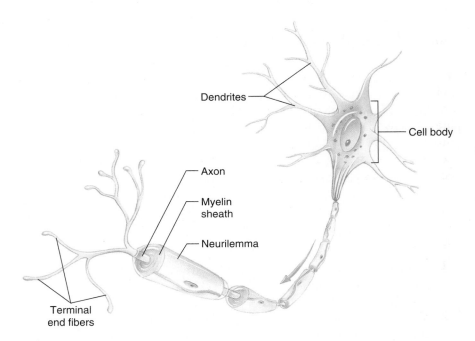

Dendrites

Cell body

Axon

Myelin sheath

Neurilemma

Terminal end fibers

FIGURE 8-2 Parts of a neuron.

stimulated to jump over the synapse by a **neurotransmitter,** any of various substances produced by and located in tiny sacs at the end of the terminal end fibers. Table 8-1 lists some common neurotransmitters.

All neurons also have two basic properties—**excitability,** the ability to respond to a **stimulus** (anything that arouses a response), and **conductivity,**

TABLE 8-1 Some Common Neurotransmitters

Neurotransmitter Group	Compounds in Neurotransmitter	Probable Nervous System Functions
acetylcholine	acetylcholine (ACH)	excites and inhibits muscular and glandular activity; affects memory
amino acids	gamma-aminobutyric acid (GABA) glutamic acid aspartic acid glycine	inhibits certain brain activity excites certain brain activity excites certain brain activity inhibits certain spinal cord activity
monoamines	dopamine histamine norepinephrine (NE) serotonin	involved in brain and motor activity involved in brain activity involved in heat regulation, arousal, motor activity, reproduction; acts as hormone in bloodstream involved in sleep, mood, appetite, and pain
neuropeptides	somatostatin endorphins	involved in secretion of growth hormone have pain-relieving properties

the ability to transmit a signal. The three types of neurons are classified by the direction in which they transmit impulses:

1. **Efferent (motor) neurons,** which convey information to the muscles and glands from the central nervous system
2. **Afferent (sensory) neurons,** which carry information from sensory receptors to the central nervous system
3. **Interneurons,** which carry and process sensory information and make possible more complex types of reflexes.

Some nerves contain combinations of at least two types of neurons.

Neurons are microscopic entities that form bundles called **nerves,** the bearers of electrical messages to the organs and muscles of the body. The body's cells contain stored electrical energy that is released when the cells receive outside stimuli or when internal chemicals (for example, **acetylcholine**) stimulate the cells. The released energy passes through the nerve cell, causing a **nerve impulse.** Nerve impulses are received or transmitted by tissue or organs called **receptors.** These impulses are then transmitted to other receptors throughout the body.

In addition to nerve cells, other cells in the nervous system support, connect, protect, and remove debris from the system. These cells, **neuroglia** or **neuroglial cells,** do not transmit impulses. Each of the three types of neuroglia serves different purposes.

1. Star-shaped **astroglia** (or **astrocytes**) maintain nutrient and chemical levels in neurons and form a supporting network in the brain and spinal cord.
2. **Oligodendroglia** produce myelin and help in supporting neurons by forming rows between neurons in the brain and spinal cord.
3. **Microglia** are phagocytes—small cells that remove debris.

Certain neuroglia, along with the almost solid walls of the brain's capillaries, form what is known as the *blood-brain barrier,* the barrier that permits some chemical substances to reach the brain's neurons, but blocks most others, thereby protecting vital brain tissue. Figure 8-3 shows neuroglia.

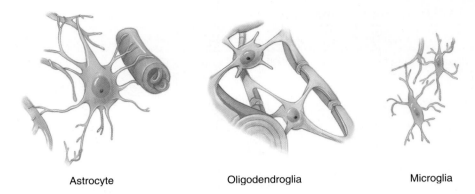

Astrocyte   Oligodendroglia   Microglia

Central Nervous System

The **central nervous system (CNS)** consists of the brain and spinal cord. The word *central* is the key to understanding the purpose of this subsystem. It is located centrally along the midsagittal plane of the body and is the center of control, receiving and interpreting all stimuli and sending nerve impulses to instruct muscles and glands to take or respond to certain actions. Designated actions throughout the body include both voluntary and involuntary movement, sight, hearing, thinking, secretion of hormones, memory, and responses to outside stimuli. The *meninges* (described later) are a covering crucial to the protection of the brain and spinal cord.

Brain

The human adult **brain** weighs about three pounds, is 75 percent water, has the consistency of gelatin, contains over 100 billion neurons, and is responsible for controlling the body's many functions and interactions with the outside world. The brain has four major divisions:

1. the brainstem
2. the cerebrum
3. the cerebellum
4. the diencephalon

The brainstem   The **brainstem** is made up of the **midbrain** (involved with visual reflexes), the **pons** (controls certain respiratory functions), and the **medulla oblongata** (contains centers that regulate heart and lung functions, swallowing, vomiting, coughing, and sneezing). The brainstem connects the brain to the spinal cord and even small areas of damage can be devastating, even fatal. The midbrain connects the pons beneath it with the cerebellum and cerebrum above. The pons lies between the midbrain and the medulla oblongata, which connects the pons to the spinal cord (see Figure 8-4).

The cerebellum   The **cerebellum** is the area that coordinates musculoskeletal movement to maintain posture, balance, and muscle tone.

The cerebrum   Above the cerebellum lies the **cerebrum,** the third major brain structure. The cerebrum is the largest area of the brain, taking up about 85 percent of its mass. The cerebrum has two hemispheres, with an outer portion called the **cerebral cortex.** The inner portion is divided into two hemispheres—one on the left and one on the right.

The cerebral cortex (area of conscious decision making) has many **fissures** (also called **sulci**) and **convolutions** (also called **gyri**) and is composed

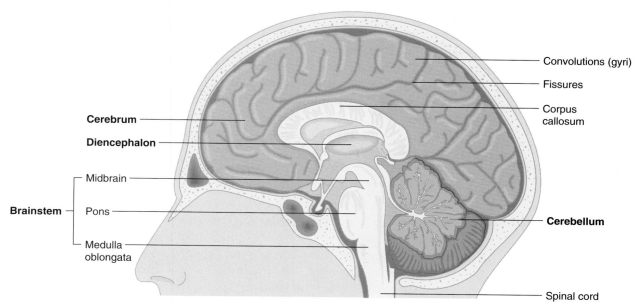

FIGURE 8-4   The parts of the brain.

of gray matter, the substance in the brain composed mainly of nerve cells and dendrites.

Below the cerebral cortex are white matter, substance in the brain composed mainly of nerve fibers, and masses of gray matter called the **basal ganglia** (involved with musculoskeletal movement). The left and right hemispheres of the cerebrum are each divided into four parts or lobes.

1. The **frontal lobe** controls voluntary motor movements, emotional expression, and moral behavior.
2. The **parietal lobe** controls and interprets the senses and taste.
3. The **temporal lobe** controls memory, equilibrium, emotion, and hearing.
4. The **occipital lobe** controls vision and various forms of expression.

The two hemispheres of the cerebrum are connected by the **corpus callosum,** a bridge of nerve fibers that relays information between the two hemispheres.

The diencephalon   The **diencephalon** is the deep portion of the brain containing the **thalamus, hypothalamus, epithalamus,** and the **ventral thalamus.** These parts of the diencephalon serve as relay centers for sensations. They also integrate with the autonomic nervous system in the control of heart rate, blood pressure, temperature regulation, water and electrolyte balance, digestive functions, behavioral responses, and glandular activities.

The brain sits inside the **cranium,** a strong bony structure that protects it. The area between the brain and the cranium is filled with **cerebrospinal fluid (CSF),** a watery fluid that contains various compounds and flows throughout the brain and around the spinal cord delivering essential nutrients. This watery fluid cradles and cushions the brain. The fluid acts as a shock absorber in the event of head trauma. **Ventricles** or cavities in the brain also contain this fluid. The cranial meninges have the same structure as the spinal meninges (described next) and also protect the brain. Figure 8-4 illustrates the brain.

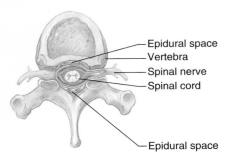

FIGURE 8-5 A section of the spinal column showing a vertebra.

- Epidural space
- Vertebra
- Spinal nerve
- Spinal cord
- Epidural space

Severe spinal cord injuries usually result in some type of paralysis. Research is under way to grow replacement cells for injured nerves. It is expected that some types of paralysis will be cured by 2010.

For an easy way to remember and even test your cranial nerves, go to http://faculty.washington.edu/chudler/cranial.html.

FIGURE 8-6 The brain and spinal cord are protected by the meninges.

Spinal Cord

The **spinal cord** extends from the medulla oblongata of the brain to the area around the second lumbar vertebra in the lower back. The spinal cord is contained within the vertebral column. The space that contains the spinal column is called the vertebral canal. The spinal cord is protected by the bony structure of the vertebral column, by the cerebrospinal fluid that surrounds it, and by the spinal meninges. Figure 8-5 illustrates a section of the spinal cord. Extending out from the spinal cord are the nerves of the peripheral nervous system.

Meninges

The **meninges** (Figure 8-6) are three layers of connective tissue membranes that cover the brain and spinal cord. The outer layer, the **dura mater** (from Latin, "hard mother"), is a tough, fibrous membrane that covers the entire length of the spinal cord and contains channels for blood to enter brain tissue. The middle layer, the **arachnoid,** is a weblike structure that runs across the space (called the **subdural space**) containing cerebrospinal fluid. The **pia mater** (Latin, "tender mother"), the innermost layer of meninges, is a thin membrane containing many blood vessels that nourish the spinal cord. The space between the pia mater and the bones of the spinal cord is called the **epidural space.** It contains blood vessels and some fat. It is the space into which anesthetics may be injected to dull pain (as during childbirth and some pelvic operations) or contrast material for certain diagnostic procedures.

Peripheral Nervous System

The peripheral nervous system includes the 12 pairs of **cranial nerves** that carry impulses to and from the brain and the 31 pairs of **spinal nerves** that carry messages to and from the spinal cord and the torso and extremities of the body. Table 8-2 lists the cranial nerves and their functions.

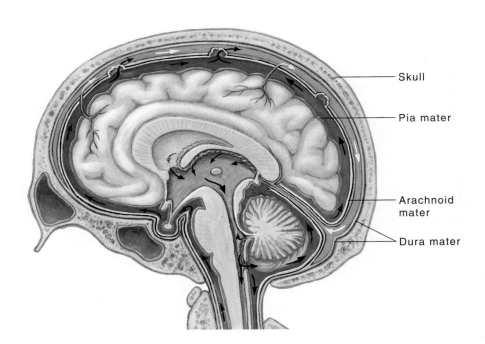

- Skull
- Pia mater
- Arachnoid mater
- Dura mater

TABLE 8-2 The Twelve Pairs of Cranial Nerves and Their Function

Pair of Cranial Nerves	Primary Type of Nerve	Function
I olfactory	sensory	involved in sense of smell
II optic	sensory	involved in sense of vision
III oculomotor	motor	involved in movement of eyes, controlling both the exterior and interior parts
IV trochlear	motor	involved in muscles that move the eyes
V trigeminal	sensory and motor	involved in eyes, tear glands, scalp, forehead, teeth, gums, lips, and muscles of the mouth
VI abducens	motor	involved with muscle conditioning
VII facial	sensory and motor	involved with taste, facial expressions, tear glands, and salivary glands
VIII vestibulocochlear	sensory	involved in equilibrium and hearing
IX glossopharyngeal	sensory and motor	involved in pharynx, tonsils, tongue, and carotid arteries; stimulates salivary glands
X vagus	sensory and motor	involved in speech, swallowing, heart muscles, smooth muscles, and certain glands
XI accessory (cranial and spinal)	motor	involved in muscles of the soft palate, pharynx, larynx, neck, and back
XII hypoglossal	motor	involved in muscles that move the tongue

TABLE 8-3 Major Spinal Nerve Divisions and Their Functions

Region of Spinal Cord	Location	Functions of Nerves
cervical	neck	involved in muscles of the back of the head and neck and in the diaphragm
brachial	lower neck, axilla	involved in the muscles and skin of the neck, shoulder, arm, and hand
lumbar	posterior abdominal wall	involved in abdominal skin and muscles
sacral	posterior pelvic wall	involved in the muscles of the buttocks, thighs, feet, legs, and voluntary sphincters
coccygeal	coccyx and surrounding area	skin in coccyx region

The 31 pairs of spinal nerves are grouped according to the segments of the spinal cord out of which they extend. Table 8-3 lists those groups and the regions served by the nerves of each group. The peripheral nerves are further divided into two subsystems—the somatic and autonomic nervous systems—according to their function.

Somatic Nervous System

Nerves of the **somatic nervous system** receive and process sensory input from the skin, muscles, tendons, joints, eyes, tongue, nose, and ears. They also excite the voluntary contraction of skeletal muscles.

Autonomic Nervous System

Nerves of the **autonomic nervous system** carry impulses from the central nervous system to glands, various smooth (involuntary) muscles, cardiac muscle, and various membranes. The autonomic nervous system stimulates organs, glands, and senses by stimulating secretions of various substances.

The autonomic nerves are further divided into the **sympathetic nervous system** and the **parasympathetic nervous system.** In general, the two systems play opposite roles. The sympathetic system operates when the body is awakening, increasing activity, or under stress. It helps to activate responses necessary to react to sudden changes in activity level or to dangerous or abnormal situations. These nerves control the "fight or flight" reaction to stress—that means it tells the body when to fight back or to flee in dangerous situations. The parasympathetic system, on the other hand, operates to keep the body in homeostasis or balance under normal conditions, as in the "rest and digest" activity of the body.

VOCABULARY REVIEW

In the previous section, you learned terms relating to the nervous system. Before going on to the exercises, review the terms below and refer to the previous section if you have any questions. Pronunciations are provided for certain terms. Sometimes information about where the word came from is included after the term. These etymologies (word histories) are for your information only. You do not need to memorize them.

Term	Definition
acetylcholine [ăs-ē-tĭl-KŌ-lēn]	Chemical that stimulates cells.
afferent [ĂF-ĕr-ĕnt] **(sensory) neuron**	Neuron that carries information from the sensory receptors to the central nervous system.
arachnoid [ă-RĂK-nŏyd] Greek *arachne*, spider + -oid, resembling	Middle layer of meninges.
astrocyte, astroglia [ĂS-trō-sīt], [ăs-TRŎG-lē-ă] Greek *astron*, star + -cyte, cell	A type of neuroglia that maintains nutrient and chemical levels in neurons.
autonomic [ăw-tō-NŎM-ĭk] **nervous system** auto-, self + Greek *nomos*, law	Part of the peripheral nervous system that carries impulses from the central nervous system to glands, smooth muscles, cardiac muscle, and various membranes.
axon [ĂK-sŏn] Greek, axis	Part of a nerve cell that conducts nerve impulses away from the cell body.
basal ganglia [BĀ-săl GĂNG-glē-ă]	Large masses of gray matter within the cerebrum.
brain [brān] Old English *braegen*	Body organ responsible for controlling the body's functions and interactions with outside stimuli.
brainstem	One of the four major divisions of the brain; division that controls certain heart, lung, and visual functions.
cell body	Part of a nerve cell that has branches or fibers that reach out to send or receive impulses.

Term	Definition
central nervous system	The brain and spinal cord.
cerebellum [sĕr-ĕ-BĔL-ūm] Latin, little brain	One of the four major divisions of the brain; division that coordinates musculoskeletal movement.
cerebral cortex [SĔR-ĕ-brăl KŌR-tĕks]	Outer portion of the cerebrum.
cerebrospinal [SĔR-ĕ-brō-spī-năl] **fluid (CSF)** cerebro-, cerebrum + spinal	Watery fluid that flows throughout the brain and around the spinal cord.
cerebrum [SĔR-ĕ-brŭm, sĕ-RĒ-brŭm] Latin, brain	One of the four major divisions of the brain; division involved with emotions, memory, conscious thought, moral behavior, sensory interpretations, and certain bodily movement.
conductivity [kŏn-dŭk-TĬV-ĭ-tē]	Ability to transmit a signal.
convolutions [kŏn-vō-LŪ-shŭnz]	Folds in the cerebral cortex; gyri.
corpus callosum [KŌR-pŭs kă-LŌ-sŭm] Latin, body with a thick skin	Bridge of nerve fibers that connects the two hemispheres of the cerebrum.
cranial [KRĀ-nē-ăL] **nerves**	Any of 12 pairs of nerves that carry impulses to and from the brain.
cranium [KRĀ-nē-ŭm]	Bony structure that the brain sits in.
dendrite [DĔN-drīt]	A thin branching extension of a nerve cell that conducts nerve impulses toward the cell body.
diencephalon [dī-ĕn-SĔF-ă-lŏn] di-, separated + Greek *enkephalos*, brain	One of the four major structures of the brain; it is the deep portion of the brain and contains the thalamus.
dura mater [DŪ-ră MĀ-tĕr] Latin, hard mother	Outermost layer of meninges.
efferent [ĔF-ĕr-ĕnt] **(motor) neuron**	Neuron that carries information to the muscles and glands from the central nervous system.
epidural [ĕp-ĭ-DŪ-răl] **space** epi-, upon + dur(a mater)	Area between the pia mater and the bones of the spinal cord.
epithalamus [ĔP-ĭ-THĂL-ă-mŭs] epi- + thalamus	One of the parts of the diencephalon; serves as a sensory relay station.
excitability [ĕk-SĪ-tă-BĬL-ĭ-tē]	Ability to respond to stimuli.
fissure [FĬSH-ŭr]	One of many indentations of the cerebrum; sulcus.
frontal lobe	One of the four parts of each hemisphere of the cerebrum.
gyrus (*pl.,* gyri) [JĪ-rŭs (JĪ-rī)]	*See* convolution.
hypothalamus [HĪ-pō-THĂL-ă-mŭs] hypo-, below + thalamus	One of the parts of the diencephalon; serves as a sensory relay station.
interneuron [ĬN-tĕr-NŪ-rŏn] inter-, between + neuron	Neuron that carries and processes sensory information.

Term	Definition
medulla oblongata [mĕ-DŪL-ă ŏb-lŏng-GĂ-tă] Latin, long marrow	Part of the brain stem that regulates heart and lung functions, swallowing, vomiting, coughing, and sneezing.
meninges (*sing.*, meninx) [mĕ-NĬN-jēz (MĔ-nĭngks)] Greek, plural of *meninx*, membrane	Three layers of membranes that cover and protect the brain and spinal cord.
microglia [mī-KRŎG-lē-ă] micro-, small + Greek *glia*, glue	A type of neuroglia that removes debris.
midbrain mid-, middle + brain	Part of the brainstem involved with visual reflexes.
myelin sheath [MĪ-ĕ-lĭn shēth]	Fatty tissue that covers axons.
nerve [nĕrv]	Bundle of neurons that bear electrical messages to the organs and muscles of the body.
nerve cell	Basic cell of the nervous system having three parts: cell body, dendrite, and axon; also called a neuron.
nerve impulse	Released energy that is received or transmitted by tissue or organs and that usually provokes a response.
neurilemma [nūr-ĭ-LĔM-ă] neuri-, nerve + Greek *lemma*, husk	Membranous covering that protects the myelin sheath.
neuroglia [nū-RŎG-lē-ă], **neuroglial** [nū-RŎG-lē-ăl] **cell** neuro-, nerve + Greek *glia*, glue	Cell of the nervous system that does not transmit impulses.
neuron [NŪR-ŏn] Greek, nerve	Basic cell of the nervous system having three parts; also called a nerve cell.
neurotransmitters [NŪR-ō-trăns-MĬT-ĕrz] neuro- + transmitter	Various substances located in tiny sacs at the end of the axon.
occipital lobe [ŏk-SĬP-ĭ-tăl lōb]	One of the four parts of each hemisphere of the cerebrum.
oligodendroglia [ŌL-ĭ-gō-dĕn-DRŎG-lē-ă] oligo-, few + Greek *dendron*, tree + *glia*, glue	A type of neuroglia that produces myelin and helps to support neurons.
parasympathetic nervous system para-, beside + sympathetic	Part of the autonomic nervous system that operates when the body is in a normal state.
parietal lobe [pă-RĪ-ĕ-tăl lōb]	One of the four parts of each hemisphere of the cerebrum.
pia mater [PĪ-ă, PĒ-ă MĀ-tĕr, MĂ-tĕr] Latin, tender mother	Innermost layer of meninges.
pons [pŏnz] Latin, bridge	Part of the brainstem that controls certain respiratory functions.
receptor [rē-SĔP-tĕr]	Tissue or organ that receives nerve impulses.

Term	Definition
somatic [sō-MĂT-ĭk] **nervous system**	Part of the peripheral nervous system that receives and processes sensory input from various parts of the body.
spinal cord	Ropelike tissue that sits inside the vertebral column and from which spinal nerves extend.
spinal nerves	Any of 31 pairs of nerves that carry messages to and from the spinal cord and the torso and extremities.
stimulus (*pl.*, **stimuli**) [STĬM-yū-lŭs (STĬM-yū-lī)]	Anything that arouses a response.
subdural [sŭb-DŪR-ăl] **space** sub-, under + dur(a mater)	Area between the dura mater and the pia mater across which the arachnoid runs.
sulcus (*pl.*, **sulci**) [SŬL-kŭs (SŬL-sī)]	*See* fissure.
sympathetic [sĭm-pă-THĔT-ĭk] **nervous system**	Part of the autonomic nervous system that operates when the body is under stress.
synapse [SĬN-ăps]	Space over which nerve impulses jump from one neuron to another.
temporal lobe [TĔM-pŏ-răl lōb]	One of the four parts of each hemisphere of the cerebrum.
terminal end fibers	Group of fibers at the end of an axon that passes the impulses leaving the neuron to the next neuron.
thalamus [THĂL-ă-mŭs]	One of the four parts of the diencephalon; serves as a sensory relay station.
ventral thalamus	One of the four parts of the diencephalon; serves as a sensory relay station.
ventricle [VĔN-trĭ-kl]	Cavity in the brain for cerebrospinal fluid.

CASE STUDY

Neurological Problem

Jose Gutierrez is a patient of Dr. Marla Chin, an internist. He is scheduled for his six-month checkup and medication review. Mr. Gutierrez has a history of heart disease and skin carcinoma. In the past few months he has been having trouble buttoning his shirts and remembering things. He has also developed a limp. Dr. Chin orders some tests.

Critical Thinking

1. Mr. Gutierrez has some new problems. According to his symptoms, what areas of the brain might have been affected by some disorder?

2. Dr. Chin does a thorough checkup and asks both Mr. Gutierrez and his wife many questions about such things as respiratory function, sleep habits, and so on. How will the answers to the questions help Dr. Chin determine the next steps to take?

STRUCTURE AND FUNCTION EXERCISES

Know the Position

3. The brain and spinal cord are protected by three layers of meninges. Name the three layers in order from inside the skull to the brain and describe the structure of each.

    a. _____

    b. _____

    c. _____

Find a Match

Match the definition in the right-hand column to the word in the left-hand column.

4. _____ neuroglia

5. _____ meninges

6. _____ neuron

7. _____ acetylcholine

8. _____ excitability

9. _____ ventricle

10. _____ basal ganglia

11. _____ sulci

12. _____ arachnoid

13. _____ epidural space

a. gray matter

b. weblike meningeal layer

c. internal chemical

d. cell that does not transmit impulses

e. fissures

f. area between pia mater and spinal bones

g. responsiveness to stimuli

h. protective membranes

i. cell that transmits impulses

j. cavity for fluid

Complete the Thought

Fill in the blanks.

14. Organs that receive [or transmit] nerve impulses are called _____.

15. Each axon is covered by a _____ _____.

16. Neuron structures that conduct nerve impulses toward the cell body are called _____.

17. Neuron structures that conduct nerve impulses away from the cell body are called _____.

18. The spinal cord connects to the brain at the _____ _____.

19. The part of the brain with two hemispheres is called the _____.

20. The part of the brainstem that controls certain respiratory functions is called the _____.

21. The bony structure protecting the brain is the _____.

22. Ventricles hold _____ _____.

23. The deep portion of the brain is called the _____.

Spell It Correctly

Write the correct spelling in the blank to the right of each word. If the word is already correctly spelled, write C.

24. meninxes _____

25. thalomus _____

26. ganoglia _____

27. gyri _____

28. synapse _____

29. axen _____

30. neurilemma _____

31. acetycholine _____

32. neurglia _____

33. cerebrellum _____

Combining Forms and Abbreviations

The lists below include combining forms and abbreviations that relate specifically to the nervous system. Pronunciations are provided for the examples.

COMBINING FORM	MEANING	EXAMPLE
cerebell(o)	cerebellum	*cerebellitis* [sĕr-ĕ-bĕl-Ī-tĭs], inflammation of the cerebellum
cerebr(o), cerebri	cerebrum	*cerebralgia* [sĕr-ĕ-BRĂL-jē-ă], pain in the head
crani(o)	cranium	*craniofacial* [KRĀ-nē-ō-FĀ-shăl], relating to the face and the cranium
encephal(o)	brain	*encephalitis* [ĕn-sĕf-ă-LĪ-tĭs], inflammation of the brain
gangli(o)	ganglion	*gangliform* [GĂNG-glē-fŏrm], having the shape of a ganglion
gli(o)	neuroglia	*gliomatosis* [glī-ō-mă-TŌ-sĭs], abnormal growth of neuroglia in the brain or spinal cord
mening(o), meningi(o)	meninges	*meningocele* [mĕ-NĬNG-gō-sēl], protrusion of the spinal meninges above the surface of the skin; *meningitis* [mĕn-ĭn-JĪ-tĭs], inflammation of the meninges
myel(o)	bone marrow, spinal cord	*myelomalacia* [MĪ-ĕ-lō-mă-LĀ-shē-ă], softening of the spinal cord
neur(o), neuri	nerve	*neuritis* [nū-RĪ-tĭs], inflammation of a nerve
spin(o)	spine	*spinoneural* [spī-nō-NŪ-răl], relating to the spine and the nerves that extend from it
thalam(o)	thalamus	*thalamotomy* [thăl-ă-MŎT-ō-mē], incision into the thalamus to destroy a portion causing or transmitting sensations of pain
vag(o)	vagus nerve	*vagectomy* [vā-JĔK-tō-mē], surgical removal of a portion of the vagus nerve; *vagotomy* [vā-GŎT-ō-mē], surgical severing of the vagus nerve
ventricul(o)	ventricle	*ventriculitis* [vĕn-trĭk-yū-LĪ-tĭs], inflammation of the ventricles of the brain

ABBREVIATION	MEANING	ABBREVIATION	MEANING
Ach	acetylcholine	CSF	cerebrospinal fluid
ALS	amyotrophic lateral sclerosis	CT or CAT scan	computerized (axial) tomography
BBB	blood-brain barrier	CVA	cerebrovascular accident
CNS	central nervous system	CVD	cerebrovascular disease
CP	cerebral palsy	PNS	peripheral nervous system

CASE STUDY

Referral to a Neurologist

Dr. Chin takes some blood tests and decides to send Mr. Gutierrez to a neurologist, Dr. Martin Stanley, for an evaluation. Dr. Stanley reviews Dr. Chin's notes and finds that Mr. Gutierrez has no history of CVA, but is experiencing numbness in his fingers and has some difficulty walking. Dr. Stanley will test for CVA, but since Mr. Gutierrez has a history of normal blood pressure, he suspects another disorder.

Critical Thinking

34. Why is Mr. Gutierrez referred to a neurologist?
35. What nerves might affect Mr. Gutierrez's walking?

COMBINING FORMS AND ABBREVIATIONS EXERCISES

Root Out the Meaning

Find at least two nervous system combining forms in each word. Write the combining forms and their definitions in the space provided.

36. encephalomyelitis: _____
37. craniomeningocele: _____
38. glioneuroma: _____
39. cerebromeningitis: _____
40. spinoneural: _____
41. neuroencephalomyelopathy: _____

Trace the Root

Add the combining form that completes the word.

42. Acting upon the vagus nerve: _____tropic.
43. Tumor consisting of ganglionic neurons: ganglio _____oma.
44. Myxoma containing glial cells: _____myxoma.
45. Relating to nerves and meninges: neuro _____eal.

In each word, find the combining form that relates to the nervous system and give its definition.

46. parencephalia _____
47. angioneurectomy _____
48. cephalomegaly _____
49. myelitis _____
50. meningocyte _____
51. neurocyte _____
52. craniomalacia _____
53. vagotropic _____
54. glioblast _____
55. cerebrosclerosis _____

Reviewing Combining Forms

Match the following word parts with the correct meanings. Some answers may be used more than once or not at all.

56. _____ encephal(o)
57. _____ gli(o)
58. _____ myel(o)
59. _____ spin(o)
60. _____ cerebell(o)
61. _____ mening(o), meningi(o)
62. _____ neur(o), neuri
63. _____ gangli(o)
64. _____ crani(o)
65. _____ cerebr(o), cerebri
66. _____ myel(o)
67. _____ ventricul(o)
68. _____ radic(o), radicul(o), rhiz(o)
69. _____ thalam(o)
70. _____ dur(o)
71. _____ esthesi(o)
72. _____ mon(o)
73. _____ hemi-
74. _____ ment(o), psych(o)
75. _____ quadra, quadri
76. _____ -plegia

a. sensation, sensitivity, feeling
b. cerebrum
c. one, single
d. paralysis
e. ganglion
f. neuroglia
g. meninges
h. bone marrow, spinal cord
i. nerve
j. spine
k. four
l. vagus nerve
m. half, on one side
n. hard, dura mater
o. mind
p. cerebellum
q. cranium
r. ventricle
s. nerve root
t. thalamus
u. brain

Knowing Nervous System Abbreviations

Match the following abbreviations with their correct meaning.

77. _____ CVA
78. _____ ALS
79. _____ CSF
80. _____ BBB
81. _____ CVD
82. _____ CNS
83. _____ PNS
84. _____ CP
85. _____ CT scan, CAT scan
86. _____ Ach
87. _____ AD
88. _____ MS
89. _____ EP

a. electroencephalography
b. central nervous system
c. attention deficit hyperactivity disorder
d. Alzheimer disease
e. amyotrophic lateral sclerosis, Lou Gehrig's disease
f. polysomnography
g. acetylocholine
h. evoked potential (studies)
i. computerized (axial) tomography
j. obsessive-compulsive disorder
k. positron emission tomography
l. multiple sclerosis
m. Parkinson's disease

90. _____ MRI

91. _____ PET

92. _____ EEG

93. _____ LP

94. _____ EMG

95. _____ PSG

96. _____ ADHD

97. _____ OCD

98. _____ PD

99. _____ PTSD

100. _____ TIA

n. blood-brain barrier

o. peripheral nervous system

p. transient ischemic attack

q. cerebrovascular disease

r. lumbar puncture

s. posttraumatic stress disorder

t. cerebrovascular accident, stroke

u. cerebrospinal fluid

v. magnetic resonance imaging

w. cerebral palsy

x. electromyogram

Remembering Suffixes

Match the following suffixes commonly used with nervous system terms with their correct meaning.

101. _____ -iatry

102. _____ -iatrist

103. _____ -paresis

104. _____ -logy

105. _____ -algia

106. _____ -cele

107. _____ -itis

108. _____ -osis

109. _____ -phasia

110. _____ -plegia

a. physician, specialist

b. inflammation

c. pain

d. paralysis

e. slight paralysis

f. abnormal condition

g. speech

h. treatment

i. study of

j. hernia

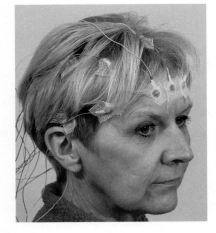

FIGURE 8-7 An electroencephalogram (EEG) records the brain's impulses. The impulses are collected from electrodes placed around the patient's head.

Diagnostic, Procedural, and Laboratory Terms

Neurologic assessment is a step-by-step process of evaluating function, reviewing specific problems, and eliminating some causes while building a case for others. Many of the diagnostic tests used to examine the nervous system include electrodiagnostic procedures. An **electroencephalogram (EEG)** is a record of the electrical impulses of the brain (Figure 8-7). This record can detect abnormalities that signal certain neurological conditions. **Evoked potentials** are electrical waves observed in an electroencephalogram. Abnormal wave patterns can help in the diagnosis of auditory, visual, and sensory disorders. Peripheral nervous system diseases can sometimes be detected by shocking the peripheral nerves and timing the conductivity of the shock. This procedure is called **nerve conduction velocity** or *electromyogram*. **Polysomnography (PSG)** is a recording of electrical and movement patterns during sleep to diagnose sleep disorders, such as *sleep apnea*, a dangerous breathing disorder.

Various types of imaging are used to visualize the structures of the brain and spinal cord. *Magnetic resonance imaging (MRI)* is the use of magnetic fields and radio waves to visualize structures. *Magnetic resonance angiography (MRA)* is the imaging of blood vessels to detect various abnormalities. *Intracranial MRA* is the visualizing of the head to check for aneurysms and other abnormalities. *Extracranial MRA* is the imaging of the neck to check the carotid artery for abnormalities. **SPECT (single photon emission computed tomography) brain scan** is a procedure that produces brain images in various colors using radioactive isotopes. **PET (positron emission tomography)** is a procedure that produces brain images using radioactive isotopes and tomography. It gives highly accurate images in various colors of the brain structures and physiology and can provide diagnoses of various brain disorders. **Computerized (axial) tomography (CT or CAT) scans** use tomography to show cross-sectional radiographic images.

X-rays are used to diagnose specific malformations or structural disorders. A **myelogram** is an x-ray of the spinal cord after a contrast medium is injected. A **cerebral angiogram** is an x-ray of the brain's blood vessels after a contrast medium is injected. *Encephalography* is the radiographic study of the ventricles of the brain. The record made by this study is called an **encephalogram.** Sound waves are used to create brain images in a **transcranial sonogram** for diagnosing and managing head and stroke trauma. Ultrasound is also used in *echoencephalography,* encephalography using ultrasound waves.

Reflexes are involuntary muscular contractions in response to a stimulus. Reflex testing can aid in the diagnosis of certain nervous system disorders. **Babinski's reflex** is a reflex on the plantar surface of the foot used to evaluate weakness on one side of the body. In most physical examinations, the reflex of each knee is tested for responsiveness (Figure 8-8).

Cerebrospinal fluid that has been withdrawn from between two lumbar vertebrae during a **lumbar (spinal) puncture** can be studied for the presence of various substances, which may indicate certain diseases. Blood tests are also used to diagnose nervous system disorders.

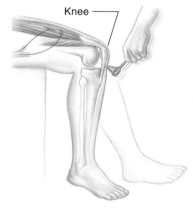

Knee

FIGURE 8-8 Tapping just below the knee usually causes a reflex reaction similar to the one shown here.

VOCABULARY REVIEW

In the previous section, you learned terms relating to diagnosis, clinical procedures, and laboratory tests. Before going on to the exercises, review the terms below and refer to the previous section if you have any questions. Pronunciations are provided for certain terms. Sometimes information about where the word came from is included after the term. These etymologies (word histories) are for your information only. You do not need to memorize them.

Term	Definition
Babinski's [bă-BĬN-skēz] **reflex** After Joseph F. Babinski, French neurologist (1857–1932)	Reflex on the plantar surface of the foot.
cerebral angiogram	X-ray of the brain's blood vessels after a dye is injected.
computerized (axial) tomography [(ĂKS-ē-ăl) tō-MŎG-ră-fē] **(CT or CAT) scan**	Radiographic imaging that produces cross-sectional images.

Term	Definition
electroencephalogram [ē-LĔK-trō-ĕn-SĔF-ă-lō-grăm] **(EEG)** electro-, electrical + encephalo-, brain + -gram, a recording	Record of the electrical impulses of the brain.
encephalogram [ĕn-SĔF-ă-lō-grăm] encephalo- + -gram	Record of the radiographic study of the ventricles of the brain.
evoked potentials [ē-VŌKT pō-TĔN- shălz]	Record of the electrical wave patterns observed in an EEG.
lumbar [LŬM-băr] **(spinal) puncture**	Withdrawal of cerebrospinal fluid from between two lumbar vertebrae.
myelogram [MĪ-ĕ-lō-grăm] myelo-, spinal cord + -gram	X-ray of the spinal cord after a contrast medium has been injected.
nerve conduction velocity	Timing of the conductivity of an electrical shock administered to peripheral nerves.
PET (positron emission tomography) [pet (PŎZ-Ĭ-trŏn ē-MĬ-shŭn tō-MŎG-ră-fē)]	Imaging of the brain using radioactive isotopes and tomography.
polysomnography [PŎL-ē-sŏm-NŎG-ră-fē] **(PSG)** poly-, many + somno-, sleep + -graphy, recording	Recording of electrical and movement patterns during sleep.
reflex [RĒ-flĕks]	Involuntary muscular contraction in response to a stimulus.
SPECT (single photon emission computed tomography) brain scan	Brain image produced by the use of radioactive isotopes.
transcranial sonogram [trănz-KRĀ-nē-ăl SŎN-ō-grăm] trans-, across + cranial	Brain images produced by the use of sound waves.

CASE STUDY

Ordering Treatment

Dr. Stanley orders an electroencephalogram of Mr. Gutierrez's brain. He also orders some additional blood tests. Dr. Stanley performs a number of reflex tests. The abnormalities present confirm Dr. Stanley's initial suspicion of Parkinson's disease. He prescribes several medications and schedules a visit for Mr. Gutierrez in three weeks to discuss his progress. He asks Mr. Gutierrez to keep a daily log of his walking ability, any vision changes, his speech, and tremors for the three weeks until his appointment.

Critical Thinking

111. Why does Dr. Stanley want Mr. Gutierrez to keep a log?
112. What might Mr. Gutierrez's abnormal reflex tests indicate?

DIAGNOSTIC, PROCEDURAL, AND LABORATORY TERMS EXERCISES

Check Your Knowledge

Circle T for true and F for false.

113. Extracranial MRA is imaging of the spinal cord. T F
114. Reflexes are voluntary muscular contractions. T F
115. An encephalogram is a record of a study of the ventricles of the brain. T F
116. A lumbar puncture removes blood. T F
117. PET is an extremely accurate imaging system. T F
118. Evoked potentials are electrical waves. T F
119. A myelogram and an angiogram are both taken after injection of a contrast medium. T F
120. PSG is taken during waking hours. T F
121. Encephalography uses sound waves to produce brain images. T F

Understanding Terms

Match the following diagnostic, procedural, and laboratory terms with their correct definitions.

122. _____ reflex
123. _____ lumbar puncture
124. _____ Babinski's reflex
125. _____ SPECT
126. _____ cerebral angiogram
127. _____ myelogram
128. _____ encephalogram
129. _____ evoked potentials
130. _____ PET
131. _____ nerve conduction velocity
132. _____ CT scan, CAT scan
133. _____ polysomnography
134. _____ transcranial sonogram
135. _____ electroencephalogram
136. _____ extracranial MRA

a. brain images produced by using sound waves
b. record of the electrical wave patterns observed in an EEG
c. timing of the conductivity of an electrical shock to the peripheral nerves
d. record of the electrical impulses of the brain
e. imaging of the brain using radioactive isotopes and tomography
f. involuntary muscular contraction in response to a stimulus
g. x-ray of the brain's blood vessels using contrast dye
h. recording of electrical and movement patterns during sleep
i. record of the radiographic study of the brain's ventricles
j. reflex to stimulus on the plantar surface of the foot
k. collection of cerebrospinal fluid from between two lumbar vertebrae
l. imaging of the neck to check the carotid artery for abnormalities
m. radiographic imaging that produces cross-sectional images
n. brain image produced by the use of radioactive isotopes
o. x-ray of the spinal cord using contrast dye

Pathological Terms

Neurologial disorders can be caused by trauma, congenital abnormalities, infectious disorders, degenerative diseases, or vascular conditions. Bones, cerebrospinal fluid, and the meninges protect the nervous system from most types of external trauma, but not all, and the blood-brain barrier protects the brain from most infectious diseases.

Trauma Disorders

A **concussion** is an injury to the brain from an impact with an object. Cerebral concussions usually clear within 24 hours. Concussions may be followed by nausea, disorientation, dizziness, double vision (diplopia), sensitivity to light (photophobia), and/or vomiting. A severe concussion can lead to **coma,** abnormally deep sleep with little or no response to stimuli. Coma can also result from other causes, such as stroke. A more serious trauma than concussion is a **brain contusion,** a bruising of the surface of the brain without penetration into the brain. Brain contusions can result in extreme disorientation, listlessness, and even death. Traumatic injury, as during a car accident, may also cause the brain to hit the skull and then to rebound to the other side of the skull. This is called a *closed head trauma,* because there is no penetration of the skull. *Shaken baby syndrome* is a severe form of closed head trauma in which a young child experiences head trauma (as a result of falling, being shaken, or other trauma), causing the brain to hit the sides of the skull and causing potentially fatal damage.

A *subdural hematoma* (between the dura mater and the arachnoid or at the base of the dura mater) is a tumorlike collection of blood often caused by trauma. Other types of cranial hematomas are *epidural hematomas* (located on the dura mater) and *intracerebral hematomas* (within the cerebrum).

Injuries that result in penetration of the brain through the skull are usually extremely serious and often fatal. Depending on the degree of penetration and the place penetrated, brain damage may result. Bleeding in the brain from an injury can also cause brain damage resulting in inability to function normally.

Congenital Disorders

Congenital diseases of the brain or spinal cord can be devastating and have an impact on the activities of daily living. **Spina bifida** is a defect in the spinal column. *Spina bifida occulta* is a covered lesion of the vertebra that is generally visible only by x-ray. This is the least severe form of spina bifida. *Spina bifida cystica* is a more severe form of the condition, usually with a **meningocele** (protrusion of the spinal meninges above the surface of the skin) or a **meningomyelocele** (protrusion of the meninges and spinal cord).

Tay-Sachs disease is a hereditary disease found primarily in the descendants of Eastern European Jews. It is a genetic disease characterized by an enzyme deficiency that causes deterioration in the central nervous system's cells. **Hydrocephalus** is an overproduction of fluid in the brain. It usually occurs at birth (although it can occur in adults with infections or tumors) and is treated with a shunt placed from the ventricle of the brain to the peritoneal space to relieve pressure by draining fluid. Figure 8-9 illustrates an infant with a shunt for relief of the pressure of hydrocephalus. See the

Trauma to the brain can occur by breaking down of the blood-brain barrier. Go to http://faculty.washington.edu/chudler/bbb.html for some of the ways this can happen.

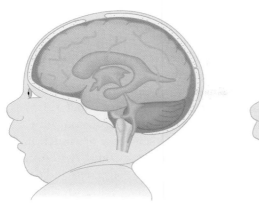
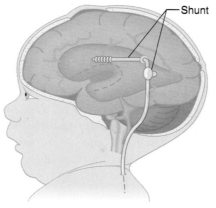

Shunt

section on nondegenerative disorders, which discusses *cerebral palsy*, a disease caused by damage during gestation.

Degenerative Diseases

Degenerative diseases of the central nervous system can affect almost any part of the body. Deterioration in mental capacity is found in **dementia** and **Alzheimer's disease,** a progressive degeneration of neurons in the brain, eventually leading to death. Some symptoms that worsen as Alzheimer's disease progresses are **amnesia** (loss of memory), **apraxia** (inability to properly use familiar objects), and **agnosia** (inability to receive and understand outside stimuli).

    Amyotrophic lateral sclerosis (ALS) is a degenerative disease of the motor neurons leading to loss of muscular control and death. It is also known as **Lou Gehrig's disease.** Several other degenerative diseases are not necessarily fatal. **Huntington's chorea** is a hereditary disease with uncontrollable, jerking movements and progressive loss of neural control. **Multiple sclerosis (MS)** is the destruction of the myelin sheath, called **demyelination,** leading to muscle weakness, unsteady **gait** (walking), **paresthesias** (odd sensations, of tingling, stinging, etc.), extreme fatigue, and some paralysis. In certain cases, it can lead to death. **Myasthenia gravis,** a disease with muscle weakness, can be treated to avoid the overproduction of antibodies that block neurotransmitters from sending proper nerve impulses to skeletal muscles. **Parkinson's disease,** a degeneration of nerves in the brain, causes tremors, weakness of muscles, and difficulty in walking. It is treated with drugs that increase the levels of **dopamine** in the brain. Treatment helps relieve symptoms but does not cure the disease. Parkinson's can become severe and lead to death.

Nondegenerative Disorders

Severe neurological disorders cause paralysis, convulsions, and other symptoms, but are not necessarily degenerative or congenital. **Palsy** is partial or complete paralysis. **Cerebral palsy** includes lack of motor coordination from cerebral damage during gestation or birth (Figure 8-10). **Bell's palsy** is paralysis of one side of the face. It usually disappears after treatment. **Ataxia** is lack of voluntary muscle coordination resulting from disorders of the cerebellum, pons, or spinal cord.

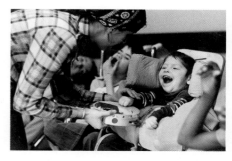

FIGURE 8-10 Cerebral palsy often leads to significant disabilities.

Most neurological disorders and diseases are helped by national organizations that maintain Web sites. See www.alz.org for information on Alzheimer's disease and www.nmss.org for information on multiple sclerosis. For other diseases, use a search engine and type in the name of the disease to find the Web site for the organization.

Epilepsy is chronic, recurrent seizure activity. Epilepsy has been known since ancient times, when victims were thought to be under the influence of outside forces. Now it is understood that this disease occurs because of abnormal conditions in the brain that cause sudden excessive electrical activity. The seizures caused by this activity can be preceded by an **aura,** a collection of symptoms felt just before the actual seizure. Seizures may be mild or intense. **Absence seizures (petit mal seizures)** are mild and usually include only a momentary disorientation with the environment. **Tonic-clonic seizures (grand mal seizures)** are much more severe and include loss of consciousness, convulsions, and twitching of limbs. The most serious form of seizure is called *status epilepticus* and occurs when one seizure follows another with no recovery period or ability to regain consciousness between attacks. This is considered a medical emergency that requires immediate advanced medical care. In any form of seizure, it is not uncommon for the individual to experience *amnesia* (loss of memory) of the attack.

Tourette syndrome is a neurological disorder that causes uncontrollable sounds and twitching (**tics**). Some drugs are helpful in controlling symptoms and allowing sufferers to lead normal lives.

Infectious Diseases

Infectious diseases of the nervous system include **shingles** and **meningitis.** Shingles is a viral disease caused by the herpes zoster virus. Its symptoms include pain in the peripheral nerves and blisters on the skin.

Several types of meningitis, inflammation of the meninges, can be infectious. **Pyrogenic meningitis** (also called **bacterial meningitis**) is caused by bacteria and includes such symptoms as fever, headache, and stiff neck. It is usually treated with antibiotics. In some severe cases, it can be fatal. **Viral meningitis** is caused by viruses and, although it has the same symptoms as pyrogenic meningitis, it is usually allowed to run its course. Medication can be given for some of the more uncomfortable symptoms (fever, headache). Inflammation can also occur in the nerves (**neuritis**), the spinal cord (**myelitis**), the brain (**encephalitis**), the cerebellum (**cerebellitis**), the dura mater (**duritis**), the ganglion (**gangliitis**), or the spinal nerve roots (**radiculitis**). Some specific nerve inflammations, such as **sciatica,** cause pain in the area served by the nerve. This is a common cause of lower back and leg pain.

Abnormal Growths

Abnormal growths in the nervous system usually occur in the brain or the meninges. About one-third of all brain tumors are growths that spread from cancers in other parts of the body (lungs, breasts, skin, and so on). The remaining growths can be benign or malignant. In either case, the pressure and distortion of the brain caused by a tumor may result in many other neurological symptoms. **Gliomas** (tumors that arise from neuroglia) and **meningiomas** (tumors that arise from the meninges) can be either benign or malignant. Both may be removed surgically. **Astrocytoma, oligodendroglioma,** and **glioblastoma multiforme** are all types of gliomas, with the latter being the most malignant. Tumors can be treated surgically if they have not infiltrated or affected certain essential areas of the brain. Radiation and medication may be used to try to reduce tumor growth. Some nontumorous growths can cause pain from pressure on nerves. A **ganglion** is any group of nerve cells bunched together to form a growth or a cyst, usually arising from a wrist tendon.

Vascular Disorders

Vascular problems, such as *arteriosclerosis*, may cause a **cerebrovascular accident or CVA**, a disruption in the normal blood supply to the brain. Various types of **strokes (cerebral infarctions)** result from this disruption. A **thrombus** (stationary blood clot) may cause **occlusion** (blocking of a blood vessel), which in turn may cause a **thrombotic stroke.** As the blockage grows, the person may experience milder symptoms before a major stroke. These short incidents are known as **transient ischemic attacks (TIAs).** TIAs may be symptomless or may cause brief disorientation and speech and motor difficulty. An **embolic stroke** is caused by an **embolus,** a clot that travels from somewhere in the body to the cerebral arteries and blocks a small vessel, causing a sudden stroke. A **hemorrhagic stroke** is caused by blood escaping from a damaged cerebral artery. It may be caused by sudden trauma or an **aneurysm,** an abnormal bulge in the wall of a blood vessel resulting from weaking of the blood vessel wall.

Strokes can be mild and result in complete recovery, or they can range from mild to severe, with symptoms that remain permanently. Common symptoms are thought disorders, **dysphasia** (speech difficulty), **aphasia,** (loss of speech), loss of muscular control, some paralysis, and disorientation. Note that dysphasia is different from *dysphagia*, difficulty in swallowing, discussed in Chapter 14.

Some states of consciousness are changed by lack of oxygen or brain abnormalities that affect the flow of blood and oxygen to the brain. **Fainting** or **syncope** is caused by lack of oxygen to the brain. **Somnolence** (extreme sleepiness), **somnambulism** (sleepwalking), and **narcolepsy** (uncontrollable, sudden lapses into deep sleep) are all altered states of consciousness.

MORE ABOUT . . .

Tourette Syndrome

Medications for Tourette syndrome do not always work. People who have Tourette syndrome may not be able to function in social and work environments because of their inability to control sounds, often inappropriate in nature, and twitching, often extreme and repetitive. The National Tourette Syndrome Association publicizes information about the syndrome, holds conventions for people with the syndrome, and provides information and support to its members. This large support group holds social events where members feel comfortable with their fellow sufferers. More information is available from the Association's Web site (www.tsa-usa.org) or from conducting a search for the word *tourette*.

VOCABULARY REVIEW

In the previous section, you learned terms relating to pathology. Before going on to the exercises, review the terms below and refer to the previous section if you have questions. Pronunciations are provided for certain terms. Sometimes information about where the word came from is included after the term. These etymologies (word histories) are for your information only. You do not need to memorize them.

Term	Definition
absence seizure [SĒ-zhŭr]	Mild epileptic seizure consisting of brief disorientation with the environment.
agnosia [ăg-NŌ-zhē-ă] Greek, ignorance	Inability to receive and understand outside stimuli.
Alzheimer's [ĂLTS-hī-mĕrz] **disease** After Alois Alzheimer (1864–1915), German neurologist	A type of degenerative brain disease causing thought disorders, gradual loss of muscle control, and, eventually, death.
amnesia [ăm-NĒ-zhē-ă] Greek, forgetfulness	Loss of memory.
amyotrophic lateral sclerosis [ă-mī-ō-TRŌ-fĭk LĂT-ĕr-ăl sklĕ-RŌ-sĭs] **(ALS)**	Degenerative disease of the motor neurons leading to loss of muscular control and death.
aneurysm [ĂN-yū-rĭzm] Greek *aneurysma*, dilation	Abnormal widening of an artery wall that bursts and releases blood.
aphasia [ă-FĀ-zhē-ă] a-, without + -phasia, speech	Loss of speech.
apraxia [ă-PRĂK-sē-ă] a- + Greek *pratto*, to do	Inability to properly use familiar objects.
astrocytoma [ĂS-trō-sī-TŌ-mă] Greek *astron*, star + cyt-, cell + -oma, tumor	Type of glioma formed from astrocytes.
ataxia [ă-TĂK-sē-ă] a- + Greek *taxis*, order	Condition with uncoordinated voluntary muscular movement, usually resulting from disorders of the cerebellum or spinal cord.
aura [ĂW-ră] Latin, breeze	Group of symptoms that precede a seizure.
bacterial meningitis [mĕn-ĭn-JĪ-tĭs]	Meningitis caused by a bacteria; pyrogenic meningitis.
Bell's palsy [PĂWL-zē] After Sir Charles Bell, Scottish surgeon (1774–1842)	Paralysis of one side of the face; usually temporary.
brain contusion [kŏn-TŪ-zhŭn]	Bruising of the surface of the brain without penetration.
cerebellitis [sĕr-ĕ-bĕl-Ī-tĭs] cerebell-, cerebellum + -itis, inflammation	Inflammation of the cerebellum.
cerebral infarction [SĔR-ē-brăl ĭn-FĂRK-shŭn]	*See* cerebrovascular accident.

Term	Definition
cerebral palsy [PĂWL-zē]	Congenital disease caused by damage to the cerebrum during gestation or birth and resulting in lack of motor coordination.
cerebrovascular [SĔR-ē-brō-VĂS-kyū-lăr] **accident (CVA)** cerebro-, brain + vascular	Neurological incident caused by disruption in the normal blood supply to the brain; stroke.
coma [KŌ-mă] Greek *koma*, trance	Abnormally deep sleep with little or no response to stimuli.
concussion [kŏn-KŬSH-ŭn]	Brain injury due to trauma.
dementia [dē-MĔN-shē-ă]	Deterioration in mental capacity, usually in the elderly.
demyelination [dē-MĪ-ĕ-lĭ-NĀ-shŭn]	Destruction of myelin sheath, particularly in MS.
dopamine [DŌ-pă-mēn]	Substance in the brain or manufactured substance that helps relieve symptoms of Parkinson's disease.
duritis [dū-RĪ-tĭs] dur(a mater) + -itis	Inflammation of the dura mater.
dysphasia [dĭs-FĀ-zhē-ă] dys-, difficult + -phasia	Speech difficulty.
embolic [ĕm-BŎL-ĭk] **stroke**	Sudden stroke caused by an embolus.
embolus [ĔM-bō-lŭs]	Clot from somewhere in the body that blocks a small blood vessel in the brain.
encephalitis [ĕn-sĕf-ă-LĪ-tĭs] encephal-, brain + -itis	Inflammation of the brain.
epilepsy [ĔP-ĭ-LĔP-sē]	Chronic recurrent seizure activity.
fainting	*See* syncope.
gait [gāt]	Manner of walking.
gangliitis [găng-glē-Ī-tĭs] gangli(on) + -itis	Inflammation of a ganglion.
ganglion (*pl.*, ganglia, ganglions) [GĂNG-glē-ŏn (-a, -ons)]	Any group of nerve cell bodies forming a mass or a cyst in the peripheral nervous system; usually forms in the wrist.
glioblastoma multiforme [GLĪ-ō-blăs-TŌ-mă MŬL-tĭ-fŏrm]	Most malignant type of glioma.
glioma [glī-Ō-mă] Greek *glia*, glue + -oma	Tumor that arises from neuroglia.
grand mal [măhl] **seizure**	*See* tonic-clonic seizure.
hemorrhagic [hĕm-ō-RĂJ-ĭk] **stroke**	Stroke caused by blood escaping from a damaged cerebral artery.

Term	Definition
Huntington's chorea [kōr-Ē-ă] After George Huntington (1850–1916), U.S. physician	Hereditary disorder with uncontrollable, jerking movements.
hydrocephalus [hī-drō-SĔF-ă-lŭs] hydro-, water + Greek *kephale*, head	Overproduction of fluid in the brain.
Lou Gehrig's [GĔR-ĭgz] **disease**	*See* amyotrophic lateral sclerosis.
meningioma [mĕ-NĬN-jē-Ō-mă] meningi-, meninges + -oma, tumor	Tumor that arises from the meninges.
meningitis [mĕ-nĭn-JĪ-tĭs] mening-, meninges + -itis	Inflammation of the meninges.
meningocele [mĕ-NĬNG-gō-sēl] meningo-, meninges + -cele, hernia	In spina bifida cystica, protrusion of the spinal meninges above the surface of the skin.
meningomyelocele [mĕ-nĭng-gō-MĪ-ĕ-lō-sēl] meningo- + myelo-, spinal cord + -cele	In spina bifida cystica, protrusion of the meninges and spinal cord above the surface of the skin.
multiple sclerosis [MŬL-tĭ-pŭl sklĕ-RŌ-sĭs] **(MS)**	Degenerative disease with loss of myelin, resulting in muscle weakness, extreme fatigue, and some paralysis.
myasthenia gravis [mī-ăs-THĒ-nē-ă GRĂV-ĭs]	Disease involving overproduction of antibodies that block certain neurotransmitters; causes muscle weakness.
myelitis [mī-ĕ-LĪ-tĭs] myel-, spinal cord + -itis	Inflammation of the spinal cord.
narcolepsy [NĂR-kō-lĕp-sē] narco, sleep + -lepsy, condition with seizures	Nervous system disorder that causes uncontrollable, sudden lapses into deep sleep.
neuritis [nū-RĪ-tĭs] neur-, nerve + -itis	Inflammation of the nerves.
occlusion [ō-KLŪ-zhŭn]	Blocking of a blood vessel.
oligodendroglioma [ŎL-ĭ-gō-DĔN-drŏ-glī-Ō-mă] oligodendrogli(a) + -oma	Type of glioma formed from oligodendroglia.
palsy [PĂWL-zē]	Partial or complete paralysis.
paresthesia [păr-ĕs-THĒ-zhē-ă] para-, beside + Greek *aisthesia*, sensation	Abnormal sensation, such as tingling.
Parkinson's disease After James Parkinson (1755–1824), British physician	Degeneration of nerves in the brain caused by lack of sufficient dopamine.
petit mal [PĔ-tē măhl] **seizure**	*See* absence seizure.
pyrogenic [pī-rō-JĔN-ĭk] **meningitis** pyro-, fever + -genic, producing	Meningitis caused by bacteria; can be fatal; bacterial meningitis.
radiculitis [ră-dĭk-yū-LĪ-tĭs] radicul-, root + -itis	Inflammation of the spinal nerve roots.

Term	Definition
sciatica [sī-ĂT-ĭ-kă]	Inflammation of the sciatic nerve.
shingles [SHĬNG-glz]	Viral disease affecting the peripheral nerves.
somnambulism [sŏm-NĂM-byū-lĭzm] somno-, sleep + Latin *ambulo*, to walk	Sleepwalking.
somnolence [SŎM-nō-lĕns] Latin, sleepiness	Extreme sleepiness caused by a neurological disorder.
spina bifida [SPĪ-nă BĬF-ĭ-dă] Latin, cleft spine	Congenital defect of the spinal column.
stroke [strōk]	*See* cerebrovascular accident (CVA).
syncope [SĬN-kŏ-pē]	Loss of consciousness due to a sudden lack of oxygen in the brain.
Tay-Sachs [TĀ-săks] **disease**	Hereditary disease that causes deterioration in the central nervous system and, eventually, death.
thrombotic [thrŏm-BŎT-ĭk] **stroke**	Stroke caused by a thrombus.
thrombus [THRŎM-bŭs]	Blood clot.
tics [tĭks]	Twitching movements that accompany some neurological disorders.
tonic-clonic [TŎN-ĭk KLŎN-nĭk] **seizure**	Severe epileptic seizure accompanied by convulsions, twitching, and loss of consciousness.
Tourette [tū-RĔT] **syndrome** After Gilles de la Tourette (1857–1904), French physician	Neurological disorder that causes uncontrollable speech sounds and tics.
transient ischemic [ĭs-KĒ-mĭk] **attack (TIA)**	Short neurological incident usually not resulting in permanent injury, but usually signaling that a larger stroke may occur.
viral meningitis	Meningitis caused by a virus and not as severe as pyrogenic meningitis.

PATHOLOGICAL TERMS EXERCISES

Check Your Knowledge

Fill in the blanks.

137. Palsy is partial or complete _____.

138. Dopamine sometimes helps the symptoms of _____ disease.

139. Inflammation of the spinal nerve roots is called _____.

140. A stationary blood clot is called a(n) _____.

141. A blood clot that moves is called a(n) _____.

142. Abnormally deep sleep with lack of responsiveness is a(n) _____.

143. A mild stroke that may be a signal that a larger stroke will occur is called a(n) _____

_____ _____.

144. _____ seizures are milder than _____ seizures.

145. Multiple sclerosis is usually associated with loss of _____, a covering for nerves.

146. ALS is a disease of the _____ neurons.

Make a Match

Match the definition in the right-hand column with the correct word in the left-hand column.

147. _____ coma
148. _____ shaken baby syndrome
149. _____ glioma
150. _____ duritis
151. _____ aphasia
152. _____ CVA
153. _____ spina bifida
154. _____ TIA
155. _____ syncope
156. _____ dysphasia

a. speech difficulty
b. fainting
c. disruption in brain's blood supply
d. loss of speech
e. short, mild stroke
f. congenital spinal cord disorder
g. abnormally deep sleep
h. brain damage caused by rough handling
i. neurological tumor
j. meningeal inflammation

CASE STUDY

Adjusting the Dosage

When Mr. Gutierrez returns to Dr. Stanley's office after three weeks, he reports that he can button his shirt again and that his walking has improved. He complains, however, that some of his cognitive symptoms have not improved. Dr. Stanley is encouraged that some of the physical symptoms have begun to improve. He will increase the dosage of the anti-Parkinson's medication he has prescribed. He is confident that Mr. Gutierrez will stabilize and possibly even gain strength.

Critical Thinking

157. Many medications cure the symptoms, but not the disease. How might exercise help Mr. Gutierrez regain mobility?

158. What compound does Mr. Gutierrez's medication contain?

Surgical Terms

Neurosurgeons are the specialists who perform surgery on the nervous system, especially on the brain and spinal cord. Neurosurgery is considered high risk because the potential for permanent injury is great. When some brain diseases, such as epilepsy, do not respond well to drugs, they may, in extreme cases, require surgery. A **lobectomy** is removal of a portion of the brain to treat epilepsy and other disorders, such as brain cancer. A **lobotomy,** severing of nerves in the frontal lobe of the brain, was once considered a primary method for treating mental illness. Now it is rarely used. Laser surgery to destroy damaged parts of the brain is also used to treat some neurological disorders. Often, treatment is a combined approach, using surgery, radiation therapy, chemotherapy, and other medications.

When it is necessary to operate directly on the brain (as in the case of a tumor), a **craniectomy,** removal of part of the skull, or a **craniotomy,** incision into the skull, may be performed. **Trephination** (or **trepanation**) is a circular opening into the skull to operate on the brain or to relieve pressure when there is fluid buildup. **Stereotaxy** or **stereotactic surgery** is the destruction of deep-seated brain structures using three-dimensional coordinates to locate the structures.

Neuroplasty is the surgical repair of a nerve. **Neurectomy** is the surgical removal of a nerve. A **neurotomy** is the dissection of a nerve. A **neurorrhaphy** is the suturing of a severed nerve. A **vagotomy** is the severing of the vagus nerve to relieve pain. **Cordotomy** is an operation to resect (remove part of) the spinal cord.

> Brain surgery is often performed using computers and minimal incisions. For up-to-date information, go to www.brain-surgery.com.

VOCABULARY REVIEW

In the previous section, you learned terms relating to surgery. Before going on to the exercises, review the terms below and refer to the previous section if you have questions. Pronunciations are provided for certain terms. Sometimes information about where the word came from is included after the term. These etymologies (word histories) are for your information only. You do not need to memorize them.

Term	Definition
cordotomy [kŏr-DŎT-ō-mē] Greek *chorde,* cord + -tomy, a cutting	Removing part of the spinal cord.
craniectomy [krā-nē-ĔK-tō-mē] crani-, cranium + -ectomy, removal	Removal of a part of the skull.
craniotomy [krā-nē-ŎT-ō-mē] cranio-, cranium + -tomy	Incision into the skull.
lobectomy [lō-BĔK-tō-mē] lob-, lobe + -ectomy	Removal of a portion of the brain to treat certain disorders.
lobotomy [lō-BŎT-ō-mē] lobo-, lobe + -tomy	Incision into the frontal lobe of the brain.
neurectomy [nū-RĔK-tō-mē] neur-, nerve + -ectomy	Surgical removal of a nerve.
neuroplasty [NŪR-ō-PLĂS-tē] neuro-, nerve + -plasty, repair	Surgical repair of a nerve.
neurorrhaphy [nur-ŎR-ă-fē] neuro- + -rrhaphy, a suturing	Suturing of a severed nerve.
neurosurgeon [nūr-ō-SĔR-jŭn] neuro- + surgeon	Medical specialist who performs surgery on the brain and spinal cord.
neurotomy [nū-RŎT-ō-mē] neuro- + -tomy	Dissection of a nerve.
stereotaxy, stereotactic [stĕr-ē-ō-TĂK-sē, stĕr-ē-ō-TĂK-tĭk] **surgery** Greek *stereos,* solid + *taxis,* orderly arrangement	Destruction of deep-seated brain structures using three-dimensional coordinates to locate the structures.

Term	Definition
trephination, trepanation [trĕf-ĭ-NĀ-shŭn, trĕp-ă-NĀ-shŭn]	Circular incision into the skull.
vagotomy [vā-GŎT-ō-mē] vag-, vagus nerve + -tomy	Surgical severing of the vagus nerve.

CASE STUDY

Repairing a Neurological Injury

Later in the year, Mr. Gutierrez was seriously injured in a car accident. He experienced some nerve damage in his leg. A neurosurgeon was called in to see if she could repair enough of the leg nerves to allow Mr. Gutierrez to walk. She operated, and the results were mixed. The trauma of the accident seemed to worsen some of the symptoms of Parkinson's disease, but Mr. Gutierrez experienced improvement with his walking after undergoing physical therapy. The neurologist decided not to increase Mr. Gutierrez's medication and to give him time to overcome the trauma.

Critical Thinking

159. The damaged leg nerves could actually be a result of an injury elsewhere in the body. What particular nerves or areas might the neurosurgeon examine before determining exactly where to operate?

160. Traumas can temporarily change body chemistry. The body produces dopamine naturally. Why did the doctor not increase the dosage?

SURGICAL TERMS EXERCISES

Check Your Knowledge

Fill in the blanks.

161. An incision into the skull is a(n) _____.

162. Removal of a portion of the skull is a(n) _____.

163. A circular skull incision is _____.

164. The incision into the frontal lobe is called a(n) _____.

165. The removal of a portion of the brain is called a(n) _____.

166. Suturing of a severed nerve is _____.

167. Removal of a nerve is _____.

168. Repair of a nerve is _____.

169. Vagotomy is severing the _____ nerve.

170. Removing a part of the spinal cord is a _____.

Pharmacological Terms

The nervous system can be the site of severe pain. **Analgesics** relieve pain. Other problems of the nervous system may be associated with diseases such as epilepsy. **Anticonvulsants** are often used to treat epilepsy and other disorders to lessen or prevent convulsions. **Narcotics** relieve pain by inducing a stuporous or euphoric state. **Sedatives** and **hypnotics** relax the nerves and sometimes induce sleep. **Anesthetics** block feelings or sensation and are used in surgery. Anesthetics can be given *locally* (to numb sensation to one section of the body) or *generally* (to numb sensation to the entire body).

TABLE 8-4 Medications for the Nervous System

Drug Class	Purpose	Generic	Trade Name
analgesic	relieves or eliminates pain	salicylates (aspirin) acetaminophen acetaminophen and codeine ibuprofen	various Tylenol, various Tylenol #3 Advil, Motrin, Nuprin
local anesthetic	causes loss of sensation in a localized area of the body	lidocaine procaine	Lidoderm Novocain
general anesthetic	causes loss of senstion over the whole body	enflurane propofol ketamine midazolam	Ethrane Diprivan Ketalar Versed
anticonvulsant	lessens or prevents convulsions	phenobarbital carbamazeprine clonazepam phenytoin	Luminal, Solfoton Tegretol Klonopin Dilantin
sedative/hypnotic	relieves feeling of agitation; induces sleepiness	diazepam zolpidem methaqualone meprobamate	Valium Ambien Quaalude Miltown

Table 8-4 lists some of the common pharmacological agents prescribed for the nervous system.

VOCABULARY REVIEW

In the previous section, you learned terms relating to pharmacology. Before going on to the exercises, review the terms below and refer to the previous section if you have questions. Pronunciations are provided for certain terms. Sometimes information about where the word came from is included after the term. These etymologies (word histories) are for your information only. You do not need to memorize them.

Term	Definition
analgesic [ăn-ăl-JĒ-zĭk] Greek *analgesia*, insensibility	Agent that relieves or eliminates pain.
anesthetic [ăn-ĕs-THĔT-ĭk] Greek *anaisthesia*, without sensation	Agent that causes loss of feeling or sensation.
anticonvulsant [ĂN-tē-kŏn-VŬL-sănt] anti-, against + convulsant	Agent that lessens or prevents convulsions.
hypnotic [hĭp-NŎT-ĭk] Greek *hypnotikos*, inducing sleep	Agent that induces sleep.
narcotic [năr-KŎT-ĭk] Greek *narkotikos*, numbing	Agent that relieves pain by inducing a stuporous or euphoric state.
sedative [SĔD-ă-tĭv] Latin *sedativus*	Agent that relieves feelings of agitation.

CASE STUDY

Easing Pain with Medication

Mr. Gutierrez's internist, Dr. Chin, visited him in the hospital daily. She reconsidered all his medications in light of his trauma. She checked all the medications for any side effects that might be harmful and for any possible interactions among the medications. She ordered a sedative and a mild painkiller, to be taken as needed. Dr. Chin also made notes for the nutritionist, now that Mr. Gutierrez will have to stay in the hospital for at least three more weeks.

Critical Thinking

171. Pain management is a delicate art. Physicians have to consider the addictive nature and strong side effects of many painkillers while at the same time making the patient comfortable enough to recover. Many physicians and medical ethicists have endorsed the unlimited use of pain medication for those with terminal diseases. What might explain the reluctance of some practitioners to allow unlimited painkillers?

172. What might Dr. Chin ask the nutritionist to consider for Mr. Gutierrez in the next three weeks?

PHARMACOLOGICAL TERMS EXERCISES

Check Your Knowledge

Fill in the blanks.

173. An agent that induces sleep is called a(n) _____.

174. An agent that causes loss of feeling is called a(n) _____.

175. An agent that relieves nervousness is called a(n) _____.

176. A drug prescribed for epilepsy is probably a(n) _____.

177. Pain is relieved with a(n) _____.

178. A pain reliever that induces a euphoric state is a(n) _____.

CHALLENGE SECTION

Dr. Stanley has a 72-year-old patient whose diagnosis of a sleep disorder does not fit with some of the symptoms she is now experiencing. Dr. Stanley gives the patient, Mary Carpenter, a full physical exam and records notes on her chart.

The patient has had sleep difficulties since her CABG (coronary artery bypass graft) in 2004. She falls asleep easily but awakens 1 to 2 hours later and then sleeps little through the night. In the last two years she has noted increased difficulty in remembering names, numbers, and how to do things. She lost her way while driving, and her family wishes her to surrender her license. She has had intermittent numbness in her fingers and legs and seems more unsteady on her feet.

Objective:

General: very slow and wobbly gait.

Vitals: Wt. 160 P 56 BP 112/72 R 16 Temp. 97.3

Chest: Clear to percussion and auscultation

Neurologic: Cereb: F-F H-K doing well.; Motor: Symmetric strength and tone; Reflex: Symmetric; Sense: Normal vibratory sense; Gave date; Cannot spell easy words backwards.

Critical Thinking

Dr. Stanley tested physical and cognitive functions. He noted that Mary's family wanted her license surrendered and seemed to be legitimately worried about her ability to concentrate. What disease might Dr. Stanley be considering as a diagnosis? Does a sleep disorder affect cognitive functioning?

TERMINOLOGY IN ACTION

The following chart is for a 30-year-old. Write a brief paragraph discussing his current health and what steps he should be taking in light of his genetic profile.

Patient: Elijah Cannon   December 24, 2XXX

SUBJECTIVE: Patient has had daily headaches for 5 days. He has intermittent nausea and vomiting with the headaches. He also complains of flashing lights in the right eye for a few minutes before the onset of a headache. The headaches are not associated with any time of the day or activity. He is in general good health. Anti-inflammatory medications do not offer improvement. Cafergot has been prescribed in the past. Mother died after complications following a CVA at age 55.

OBJECTIVE:

EARS: TMs are clear.

EYES: Normal discs and venous pulsations.

MOUTH AND THROAT: Clear.

FACE: Sinus percussion reveals no tenderness.

NECK: Supple without tenderness or rigidity.

NEUROLOGIC: Cranial nerves II-XII are intact. Muscle strength and coordination normal.

ASSESSMENT: Vascular, cluster, or migraine variant.

PLAN: Midrin capsules two q.4h. p.r.n. at first sign of headache. Recheck p.r.n. or immediately if symptoms worsen. Discuss long-term issues relating to mother's early death following a CVA.

USING THE INTERNET

Go to the Alzheimer's Association Web site (http://www.alz.org) and write a paragraph on recent developments in Alzheimer's research. Also, list the stages of Alzheimer's disease.

CHAPTER REVIEW

The material that follows is to help you review all the material in this chapter.

Understanding Nervous Systems Terms

For the following definitions, write the correct term in the space provided.

179. star-shaped neuroglia; maintain nutrient and chemical levels in the neurons _____

180. conveys information to the muscles and glands from CNS _____

181. thin branching extensions of the cell body _____

182. portion of the brain that controls voluntary movements, emotional expression, and moral behavior _____

183. consists of the brain and spinal cord _____

184. made up of the midbrain, pons, and medulla oblongata _____

185. the largest portion of the brain, with two hemispheres _____

186. strong bony structure that protects the brain _____

187. the three layers of connective tissue membranes that cover the brain and spinal cord _____

188. carries impulses to and from the brain and includes 12 pairs of cranial nerves and 31 pairs of spinal nerves _____

189. receives and process sensory input from the skin, muscles, tendons, joints, eyes, tongue, nose, and ears _____

190. chemical that stimulates cells _____

191. considered the "basic element" of the nervous system _____

192. conducts nerve impulses away from the cell body _____

193. neurons that carry information from sensory receptors to the central nervous system

    _____

194. produce myelin and help support neurons _____

195. permits some chemical substances to reach the brain's neurons but blocks others _____

196. portion of the brain that controls and interprets the senses and taste _____

197. area of the brain that coordinates musculoskeletal movement to maintain posture, balance, and muscle tone _____

198. congenital disease causing a defect in the spinal column _____

199. overproduction of fluid in the brain _____

200. hereditary disease with uncontrollable, jerking movements and progressive loss of neural control _____

201. a degeneration of nerves in the brain, causing tremors, weakness of muscles, and difficulty in walking _____

202. viral disease caused by the herpes zoster virus _____

203. mild epileptic seizure consisting of brief disorientation _____

204. abnormally deep sleep with little or no response to stimuli _____

205. deterioration in mental capacity, usually in the elderly _____

206. brain injury due to trauma _____

207. sleepwalking _____

208. twitching movements that accompany some neurological conditions _____

True or False

Circle T for true or F for false.

209. Spina bifida may cause paralysis. T F

210. A transient ischemic attack (TIA) causes death of affected brain cells. T F

211. CT stands for carinothoracic. T F

212. Epilepsy is a brain disorder characterized by recurrent seizures. T F

213. Sciatica causes nerve pain in the legs. T F

214. A CVA causes death of the affected brain cells. T F

215. A form of facial paralysis affecting one or both sides of the face and usually temporary is called Bell's palsy. T F

216. Medications prescribed to relieve pain are called analgesics. T F

217. A surgical procedure to sever nerves in the frontal lobe of the brain is called a lobectomy. T F

Remembering Prefixes

Match the following prefixes commonly used with nervous system terms with their correct meaning.

218. _____ hemi-   a. positioned beneath

219. _____ poly-   b. half

220. _____ dys-   c. four

221. _____ eu-   d. equal

222. _____ iso-   e. without

223. _____ bi-   f. difficult, abnormal

224. _____ infra-   g. beside, involving two parts

225. _____ para-   h. normal

226. _____ a-, an-   i. many

227. _____ quadri-, quadra-   j. two

Word Building

Using word parts you have learned in this chapter, build the correct medical terms for the following definitions.

228. any disease of the mind _____

229. condition of difficulty speaking _____

230. pertaining to below the dura mater _____

231. paralysis of four limbs _____

232. record of the electrical impulses of the brain _____

233. excision of a nerve _____

234. tumor of the meninges _____

235. nerve weakness _____

236. softening of the brain _____

237. protrusion of the meninges _____

238. disease of nerves and joints _____

239. recording of impulses of the brain _____

240. inflammation of a nerve _____

241. pertaining to within the cerebrum _____

242. physician who treats and studies diseases of the nervous system _____

243. paralysis of one limb _____

244. inflammation of many nerves _____

245. disease of the nerves _____

246. incision into a nerve root _____

247. slight paralysis of one limb _____

248. originating in the mind _____

249. specialist of the mind _____

250. pain in a nerve _____

251. process of recording the electrical impulses of the brain _____

252. pertaining to the mind and the body _____

253. protrusion of the meninges and spinal cord _____

254. the study of nerves _____

255. paralysis of half of the body _____

256. loss of feeling or sensation _____

257. pertaining to the cerebrum _____

DEFINITIONS

Define the following terms and combining forms. Review the chapter before starting. Make sure you know how to pronounce each term as you define it. The blue words in curly brackets are references to the Spanish glossary is available online at www.mhhe.com/medterm3e.

WORD

258. absence seizure [SĔ-zhŭr]

259. acetylcholine [ăs-ē-tĭl-KŌ-lēn] {acetilcolina}

260. afferent [ĂF-ĕr-ĕnt] (sensory) neuron

261. agnosia [ăg-NŌ-zhē-ă] {agnosia}

262. Alzheimer's [ĂLTS-hī-mĕrz] disease

263. amnesia [ăm-NĒ-zhē-ă] {amnesia}

264. amyotrophic lateral sclerosis [ă-mī-ō-TRŌ-fĭk LĂT-ĕr-ăl sklĕ-RŌ-sĭs] (ALS)

265. analgesic [ăn-ăl-JĒ-zĭk]

266. anesthetic [ăn-ĕs-THĔT-ĭk]

267. aneurysm [ĂN-yū-rĭzm] {aneurisma}

268. anticonvulsant [ĂN-tē-kŏn-VŬL-sănt]

269. aphasia [ă-FĀ-zhē-ă] {afasia}

270. apraxia [ă-PRĂK-sē-ă] {apraxia}

271. arachnoid [ă-RĂK-nŏyd] {aracnoideo}

272. astrocyte [ĂS-trō-sīt], astroglia [ăs-TRŎG-lē-ă] {astrocito, astroglia}

273. astrocytoma [ĂS-trō-sī-TŌ-mă] {astrocitoma}

274. ataxia [ă-TĂK-sē-ă] {ataxia}

275. aura [ĂW-ră] {aura}

276. autonomic [ăw-tō-NŎM-ĭk] nervous system

277. axon [ĂK-sŏn] {axón}

278. bacterial meningitis [mĕn-ĭn-JĪ-tĭs]

279. Babinski's [bă-BĬN-skēz] reflex

280. basal ganglia [BĀ-săl GĂNG-glē-ă]

281. Bell's palsy [PĂWL-zē]

282. brain [brān] {cerebro}

283. brain contusion [kŏn-TŪ-zhŭn]

284. brainstem {tronco encefálico}

285. cell body

286. central nervous system

287. cerebell(o)

288. cerebellitis [sĕr-ĕ-bĕl-Ī-tĭs] {cerebelitis}

289. cerebellum [sĕr-ĕ-BĔL-ŭm]

290. cerebr(o), cerebri

291. cerebral [SĔR-ē-brăl] angiogram

292. cerebral cortex [KŌR-tĕks]

293. cerebral infarction [ĭn-FĂRK-shŭn]

294. cerebral palsy [PĂWL-zē]

295. cerebrospinal [SĔR-ĕ-brō-spī-năl] fluid (CSF)

296. cerebrovascular [SĔR-ĕ-brō-VĂS-kyū-lăr] accident (CVA)

297. cerebrum [SĔR-ĕ-brŭm, sĕ-RĒ-brŭm] {cerebrum}

298. coma [KŌ-mă] {coma}

299. computerized (axial) tomography [(ĂKS-ē-ăl) tō-MŎG-ră-fē] (CT or CAT) scan

300. concussion [kŏn-KŬSH-ŭn] {concusión}

301. conductivity [kŏn-dŭk-TĬV-ĭ-tē] {conductividad}

302. convolution [kŏn-vō-LŪ-shŭn] {circunvolución}

303. cordotomy [kōr-DŎT-ō-mē] {cordotomía}

304. corpus callosum [KŌR-pŭs kă-LŌ-sŭm]

305. crani(o)

306. cranial [KRĀ-nē-ăl] nerves

307. craniectomy [krā-nē-ĔK-tō-mē] {craniectomía}

308. craniotomy [krā-nē-ŎT-ō-mē] {craneotomía}

309. cranium [KRĀ-nē-ŭm] {cráneo}

310. dementia [dē-MĔN-shē-ă] {demencia}

311. demyelination [dē-MĪ-ĕ-lĭ-NĀ-shŭn] {desmielinación}

312. dendrite [DĔN-drīt] {dendrita}

313. diencephalon [dī-ĕn-SĔF-ă-lŏn] {diencéfalo}

314. dopamine [DŌ-pă-mēn] {dopamina}

315. dura mater [DŪ-ră MĀ-tĕr]

316. duritis [dū-RĪ-tĭs]

317. dysphasia [dĭs-FĀ-zhē-ă] {disfasia}

318. efferent [ĔF-ĕr-ĕnt] (motor) neuron

319. electroencephalogram [ē-LĔK-trō-ĕn-SĔF-ă-lō-grăm] (EEG) {electroencefalógrafo}

320. embolic [ĕm-BŌL-ĭk] {émbolo} stroke

321. embolus [ĔM-bō-lŭs]

322. encephal(o)

323. encephalitis [ĕn-sĕf-ă-LĪ-tĭs] {encefalitis}

324. encephalogram [ĕn-SĔF-ă-lō-grăm] {encefalograma}

325. epidural [ĕp-ĭ-DŪ-răl] space

326. epilepsy [ĔP-ĭ-LĔP-sē] {epilepsia}

327. epithalamus [ĔP-ĭ-THĂL-ă-mŭs] {epitálamo}

328. evoked potentials [ē-VŌKT pō-TĔN-shălz]

329. excitability [ĕk-SĪ-tă-BĬL-ĭ-tē] {excitabilidad}

330. fainting

331. fissure [FĬSH-ŭr] {fisura}

332. frontal lobe

333. gait [gāt] {marcha}

334. gangli(o)

335. gangliitis [găng-glē-Ī-tĭs] {ganglitis}

336. ganglion (*pl.* ganglia, ganglions) [GĂNG-glē-ŏn (-a, -ons)] {ganglio}

337. gli(o)

338. glioblastoma multiforme [GLĪ-ō-blăs-TŌ-mă MŬL-tĭ-fŏrm]

339. glioma [glī-Ō-mă] {glioma}

340. grand mal [măhl] seizure

341. gyrus (*pl.*, gyri) [JĪ-rŭs (JĪ-rī)] {circunvolución}

342. hemorrhagic [hĕm-ō-RĂJ-ĭk] stroke

343. Huntington's chorea [kōr-Ē-ă]

344. hydrocephalus [hī-drō-SĔF-ă-lŭs] {hidrocefalia}

345. hypnotic [hĭp-NŎT-ĭk]

346. hypothalamus [HĪ-pō-THĂL-ă-mŭs] {hipotálamo}

347. interneuron [ĬN-tĕr-NŪ-rŏn] {interneurona}

348. lobectomy [lō-BĔK-tō-mē] {lobotomía}

349. lobotomy [lō-BŎT-ō-mē]

350. Lou Gehrig's [GĔR-ĭgz] disease

351. lumbar [LŬM-bǎr] (spinal) puncture

352. medulla oblongata [mě-DŪL-ă ŏb-lŏng-GĂ-tă]

353. mening(o), meningi(o)

354. meninges (*sing.*, meninx) [mě-NĬN-jēz (MĒ-nĭngks)] {meninges}

355. meningioma [mě-NĬN-jē-Ō-mă] {meningioma}

356. meningitis [měn-ĭn-JĪ-tĭs] {meningitis}

357. meningocele [mě-NĬNG-gō-sēl] {meningocele}

358. meningomyelocele [mě-nĭng-gō-MĪ-ě-lō-sēl] {meningomielocele}

359. microglia [mī-KRŎG-lē-ă] {microglia}

360. midbrain {cerebro medio}

361. multiple sclerosis [MŬL-tĭ-pŭl sklě-RŌ-sĭs] (MS)

362. myasthenia gravis [mī-ăs-THĒ-nē-ă GRĂV-ĭs]

363. myel(o)

364. myelin sheath [MĪ-ě-lĭn shēth]

365. myelitis [mī-ě-LĪ-tĭs]

366. myelogram [MĪ-ě-lō-grăm] {mielograma}

367. narcolepsy [NĂR-kō-lěp-sē] {narcolepsia}

368. narcotic [năr-KŎT-ĭk]

369. nerve [něrv] {nervio}

370. nerve cell

371. nerve conduction velocity

372. nerve impulse

373. neur(o), neuri

374. neurectomy [nū-RĔK-tō-mē] {neurectomía}

375. neurilemma [nūr-ĭ-LĔM-ă] {neurilema}

376. neuritis [nū-RĪ-tĭs] {neuritis}

377. neuroglia [nū-RŎG-lē-ă], neuroglial [nū-RŎG-lē-ăl] cell

378. neuron [NŪR-ŏn] {neurona}

379. neuroplasty [NŪR-ō-PLĂS-tē]

380. neurorrhaphy [nūr-ŌR-ă-fē]

381. neurosurgeon [nūr-ō-SĔR-jŭn] {neurocirujano}

382. neurotomy [nū-RŎT-ō-mē]

383. neurotransmitter [NŪR-ō-trăns-MĬT-ěr] {neurotramisor}

384. occipital lobe [ŏk-SĬP-ĭ-tăl lōb]

385. occlusion [ō-KLŪ-zhŭn] {oclusión}

386. oligodendroglia [ŌL-ĭ-gō-děn-DRŎG-lē-ă] {oligodendroglia}

387. oligodendroglioma [ŌL-ĭ-gō-DĔN-drŏ-glī-Ō-mă] {oligodendroglioma}

388. palsy [PĂWL-zē] {parálisis}

389. parasympathetic [păr-ă-sĭm-pă-THĒT-ĭk] nervous system

390. paresthesia [pār-ěs-THĒ-zhē-ă]

391. parietal lobe [pă-RĪ-ě-tăl lōb]

392. Parkinson's disease

393. PET (positron emission tomography) {TEP}

394. petit mal [PĔ-tē măhl] seizure

395. pia mater [PĪ-ă, PĒ-ă MĀ-těr, MĂ-těr)] {piamadre}

396. polysomnography [PŎL-ē-sŏm-NŎG-ră-fē] (PSG)

397. pons [pŏnz] {pons}

398. pyrogenic [pī-rō-JĔN-ĭk] meningitis

399. radiculitis [ră-dĭk-yū-LĪ-tĭs] {radiculitis}

400. receptor [rē-SĔP-těr] {receptor}

401. reflex [RĒ-flěks] {reflejo}

402. sciatica [sī-ĂT-ĭ-kă] {ciática}

403. sedative [SĔD-ă-tĭv]

404. shingles [SHĬNG-glz] {culebrilla}

405. somatic [sō-MĂT-ĭk] nervous system

406. somnambulism [sŏm-NĂM-byū-lĭzm] {sonambulismo}

407. somnolence [SŎM-nō-lěns] {somnolencia}

408. SPECT (single photon emission computed tomography) brain scan

409. spin(o)

410. spina bifida [SPĪ-nă BĬF-ĭ-dă]

411. spinal cord

412. spinal nerves

413. stereotaxy [stĕr-ē-ō-TĂK-sē], stereotactic [stĕr-ē-ō-TĂK-tĭk] surgery

414. stimulus (*pl.*, stimuli) [STĬM-yū-lŭs (STĬM-yū-lī)] {estimulo}

415. stroke [strōk] {accidente cerebrovascular}

416. subdural [sŭb-DŪR-ăl] space

417. sulcus (*pl.*, sulci) [SŬL-kŭs (SŬL-sī)] {surco}

418. sympathetic [sĭm-pă-THĔT-ĭk] nervous system

419. synapse [SĬN-ăps] {sinapsis}

420. syncope [SĬN-kŏ-pē] {síncope}

421. Tay-Sachs [TĀ-săks] disease

422. temporal lobe [TĔM-pō-răl lōb]

423. terminal end fibers

424. thalam(o)

425. thalamus [THĂL-ă-mŭs] {tálamo}

426. thrombotic [thrŏm-BŎT-ĭk] stroke

427. thrombus [THRŎM-bŭs] {trombo}

428. tic [tĭk] {tic}

429. tonic-clonic [TŎN-ĭk KLŎN-nĭk] seizure

430. transcranial sonogram [trănz-KRĀ-nē-ăl SŎN-ō-grăm]

431. trephination [trĕf-ĭ-NĀ-shŭn], trepanation [trĕp-ă-NĀ-shŭn]

432. Tourette [tū-RĔT] syndrome

433. transient ischemic [ĭs-KĒ-mĭk] attack (TIA)

434. vag(o)

435. vagotomy [vā-GŎT-ō-mē]

436. ventral thalamus

437. ventricle [VĔN-trĭ-kl] {ventrículo}

438. ventricul(o)

439. viral meningitis

Abbreviation

Write out the full meaning of each abbreviation.

440. ACH

441. ALS

442. BBB

443. CNS

444. CP

445. CSF

446. CT OR CAT SCAN

447. CVA

448. CVD

449. PNS

Answers to Chapter Exercises

1. brainstem, frontal lobe, temporal lobe
2. symptoms may point to one or two specific disorders
3. a. dura mater, tough fibrous membrane
   b. arachnoid, weblike structure across a space
   c. pia mater, thin membrane containing blood vessels
4. d
5. h
6. i
7. c
8. g
9. j
10. a
11. e
12. b
13. f
14. receptors
15. myelin sheath
16. dendrites
17. axons
18. medulla oblongata
19. cerebrum
20. pons
21. cranium
22. cerebrospinal fluid
23. diencephalon
24. meninges
25. thalamus
26. ganglia
27. C
28. C
29. axon
30. C
31. acetylcholine
32. neuroglia
33. cerebellum
34. Mr. Gutierrez has normal blood pressure and no history of CVA. He does, however, have neurological impairments and may well have a neurological disorder.
35. sacral, sciatic, spinal, leg
36. encephalo-, brain; myelo-, spinal cord
37. cranio-, skull; meningo-, meninges
38. glio-, neuroglia; neuro-, nerve

39. cerebro-, cerebrum; meningo-, meninges
40. spino-, spine; neur-, nerve
41. neuro-, nerve, encephalo-, brain, myelo-, spinal cord
42. vago-
43. neur-
44. glio-
45. mening-
46. encephal-, brain
47. neur-, nerve
48. cephalo-, head
49. myel-, spinal cord
50. meningo-, meninges
51. neuro-, nerve
52. cranio-, cranium
53. vago-, vagus nerve
54. glio-, neuroglia
55. cerebro-, cerebrum
56. u
57. f
58. h
59. j
60. p
61. g
62. i
63. e
64. q
65. b
66. h
67. r
68. s
69. t
70. n
71. a
72. c
73. m
74. o
75. k
76. d
77. t
78. e
79. u
80. n
81. q
82. b
83. o
84. w
85. i
86. g
87. d
88. l

89. h
90. v
91. k
92. a
93. r
94. x
95. f
96. c
97. j
98. m
99. s
100. p
101. h
102. a
103. e
104. i
105. c
106. j
107. b
108. f
109. g
110. d
111. to see how the medicine is helping to reduce symptoms and to adjust the dosage as necessary
112. weakened reflexes, particularly in the legs and hands
113. F
114. F
115. T
116. F
117. T
118. T
119. T
120. F
121. F
122. f
123. k
124. j
125. n
126. g
127. o
128. i
129. b
130. e
131. c
132. m
133. h
134. a
135. d
136. l
137. paralysis

138. Parkinson's
139. radiculitis
140. thrombus
141. embolus
142. coma
143. transient ischemic attack
144. absence, tonic-clonic (or petit mal, grand mal)
145. myelin
146. motor
147. g
148. h
149. i
150. j
151. d
152. c
153. f
154. e
155. b
156. a
157. Once the weakness symptoms are relieved, exercise can strengthen muscles in the legs and arms
158. dopamine
159. spinal, brainstem
160. because Mr. Gutierrez may normalize within a short time and an overdose might cause other problems
161. craniotomy
162. craniectomy
163. trephination (or trepanation)
164. lobotomy
165. lobectomy
166. neurorrhaphy
167. neurectomy
168. neuroplasty
169. vagus
170. cordotomy
171. Some physicians feel that the addictive nature of painkillers and the strong side effects change the patient's ability to relate normally to family
172. a lower-calorie diet because of his lack of exercise

173. hypnotic (or sedative)
174. anesthetic
175. sedative (or hypnotic)
176. anticonvulsant
177. analgesic
178. narcotic
179. astroglia, astrocytes
180. efferent (motor) neurons
181. dendrites
182. frontal lobe
183. central nervous system (CNS)
184. brainstem
185. cerebrum
186. cranium
187. meninges
188. peripheral nervous system (PNS)
189. somatic nervous system
190. acetylcholine (Ach)
191. nerve cell or neuron
192. axon
193. afferent (sensory) neurons
194. oligodendroglia
195. blood-brain barrier
196. parietal lobe
197. cerebellum
198. spina bifida
199. hydrocephalus
200. Huntington's chorea
201. Parkinson's disease
202. shingles
203. absence seizure
204. coma
205. dementia
206. concussion
207. somnambulism
208. tics
209. T
210. F
211. F
212. T
213. T
214. T
215. T
216. T
217. F
218. b

219. i
220. f
221. h
222. d
223. j
224. a
225. g
226. e
227. c
228. psychopathy
229. dysphasia
230. subdural
231. quadriplegia
232. electroencephalogram
233. neurectomy
234. meningioma
235. neurasthenia
236. encephalomalacia
237. meningocele
238. neuroarthropathy
239. electroencephalograph
240. neuritis
241. intracerebral
242. neurologist
243. monoplegia
244. polyneuritis
245. neuropathy
246. radicotomy
247. monoparesis
248. psychogenic
249. psychologist
250. neuralgia
251. electroencephalography
252. psychosomatic
253. meningomyelocele
254. neurology
255. hemiparesis
256. anesthesia
257. cerebral
258–449. Answers are available in the vocabulary reviews in this chapter.

CHAPTER
9

The Urinary System

▶ UROLOGY

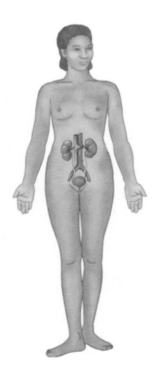

After studying this chapter, you will be able to:

9.1 Name the parts of the urinary system and discuss the function of each part

9.2 Define combining forms used in building words that relate to the urinary system

9.3 Identify the meaning of related abbreviations

9.4 Name the common diagnoses, clinical procedures, and laboratory tests used in treating disorders of the urinary system

9.5 List and define the major pathological conditions of the urinary system

9.6 Explain the meaning of surgical terms related to the urinary system

9.7 Recognize common pharmacological agents used in treating disorders of the urinary system

Structure and Function

The **urinary system** (also called the *renal system* or *excretory system*) maintains the proper amount of water in the body and removes waste products from the blood by excreting them in the urine. The urinary system consists of:

- Two **kidneys,** organs that remove dissolved waste and other substances from the blood and urine
- Two **ureters,** tubes that transport urine from the kidneys to the bladder
- The **bladder,** the organ that stores urine
- The **urethra,** a tubular structure that transports urine through the **meatus,** the external opening of a canal, to the outside of the body

Figure 9-1a shows the urinary system, and Figure 9-1b diagrams the path of urine through the system.

Kidneys

Each kidney is a bean-shaped organ about the size of a human fist, weighs about 4 to 6 ounces, and is about 12 centimeters long, 6 centimeters wide, and 3 centimeters thick. The kidneys are located in the **retroperitoneal** (posterior to the peritoneum) space behind the abdominal cavity on either side of the vertebral column. The kidneys sit against the deep muscles of the back surrounded by fatty and connective tissue. The left kidney is usually slightly higher than the right one.

The kidneys serve two functions—to form urine for excretion and to retain essential substances the body needs in the process called *reabsorption.*

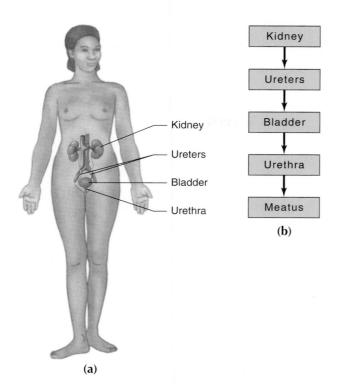

(a)

Kidney

↓

Ureters

↓

Bladder

↓

Urethra

↓

Meatus

(b)

— Kidney

— Ureters

— Bladder

— Urethra

FIGURE 9-1 (a) An illustration of the urinary system; (b) a diagram of the path of urine through the system.

Urine is produced by **filtration** of water, salts, sugar, **urea,** and other nitrogenous waste materials such as **creatine** (and its component **creatinine**) and **uric acid.** The excretion rate of creatinine is measured in urinary tests because it is an indicator of how the kidney is functioning. Kidneys, in the average adult, will filter about 1700 liters of blood per day. Urine output is the only means for the body to remove toxic nitrogenous wastes from the body.

The kidneys have an outer protective portion, the **cortex,** and an inner soft portion, the **medulla,** which is a term used for the inner, soft portion of any organ. In the middle of the concave side of the kidney is a depression, the **hilum,** through which the blood vessels, the nerves, and the ureters enter and exit the kidney.

The functional unit of the kidney is the **nephron** (Figure 9-2). The nephron removes waste products from the blood and produces **urine.** Each kidney contains about one million nephrons, more nephrons than one person needs. That is why people can live a normal life with only one kidney.

Blood enters each kidney through the *renal artery* and leaves through the *renal vein*. Once inside the kidney, the renal artery branches into smaller arteries called *arterioles*. Each arteriole leads into a nephron. Each nephron contains a *renal corpuscle* made up of a group of capillaries called a **glomerulus** (*pl.*, **glomeruli**) (Figure 9-3). The glomerulus filters fluid from the blood and is the first place where urine is formed in the kidney. Each nephron also contains a *renal tubule*, which carries urine to ducts in the kidney's cortex. Blood flows through the kidneys at a constant rate. If the blood flow is decreased, the kidney automatically produces **renin,** a substance that causes an increase in the blood pressure in order to maintain the filtration rate of blood. The wall of each glomerulus is thin enough to allow water, salts, sugars, urea, and certain wastes to pass through. Each glomerulus is surrounded by a capsule, **Bowman's capsule,** where this fluid collects. The filtered substances that are removed from the blood then pass into the renal tubules.

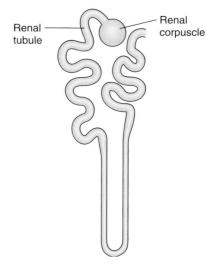

Renal tubule

Renal corpuscle

FIGURE 9-2 A nephron contains both a renal corpuscle and a renal tubule.

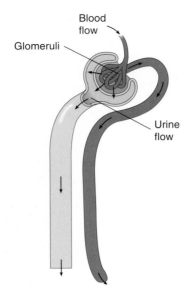

Blood flow

Glomeruli

Urine flow

FIGURE 9-3 Blood flows into the glomeruli where urine is excreted and moved to the kidney's cortex.

FIGURE 9-4 The kidneys form urine for excretion and retain essential substances for reabsorption.

MORE ABOUT . . .

Blood Pressure and the Kidneys

The kidneys have mechanisms to maintain *homeostasis* (equilibrium) in the filtration rate of the glomeruli. The constant flow of water and its substances back into the bloodstream and the flow of water and waste substances into the renal tubule maintain the body's balance of water, salts (the most common salt in the body is sodium chloride), sugars (the most common sugar in the body is glucose), and other substances. To do this, the kidneys have two lines of defense. The first is the automatic dilating and constricting of the arterioles as needed to increase or decrease the flow of blood into the glomeruli. The second is to release renin to increase the blood pressure and thus the filtration rate of blood to maintain a constant supply. Maintaining homeostasis affects blood pressure either by lowering it when blood is flowing too quickly or by increasing it when blood is flowing too slowly. Some forms of high blood pressure are caused by the effort of poorly functioning kidneys to maintain homeostasis.

Substances held in the renal tubule that can be used by the body are reabsorbed back to the bloodstream. During this **reabsorption,** most of the water, nutrients including glucose, and selected electrolytes move back to the blood. Any substance *not* reabsorbed will become urine. Urine travels to the **renal pelvis,** a collecting area in the center of the kidney. Pelvis is a general term for the collecting area of an organ or system. The renal pelvis

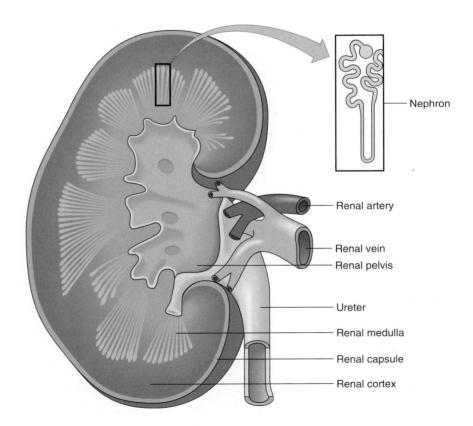

Nephron

Renal artery

Renal vein

Renal pelvis

Ureter

Renal medulla

Renal capsule

Renal cortex

contains small cuplike structures called **calices** (also spelled **calyces;** singular **calyx**) that collect urine. Figure 9-4 shows the parts of a kidney involved in urine flow.

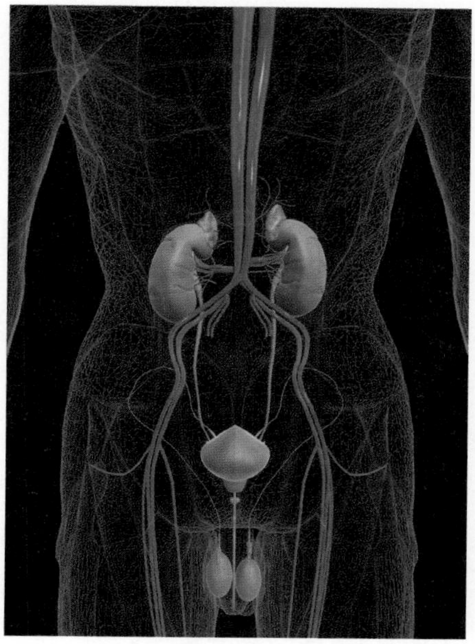

Ureters

Attached to each kidney is a *ureter,* a tube (usually 16 to 18 centimeters long) that transports urine from the renal pelvis to the urinary bladder. The two ureters are made up of three layers of tissue—smooth muscle, fibrous tissue, and a mucous layer. *Peristalsis,* a rhythmic contraction of the smooth muscle, helps to move urine into the urinary bladder.

Bladder

The **urinary bladder** is a hollow, muscular organ that stores urine until it is ready to be excreted from the body. *Bladder* is a general term meaning a receptacle. Urine is pumped into the bladder every few seconds. The *sphincter muscles,* muscles that encircle a duct to contract or expand the duct, hold the urine in place. Control of urination has to be taught to young children (usually between the ages of one and three), while in adults it is usually easily controlled. The bladder can hold from 300 to 400 milliliters of urine before emptying. The bladder's walls contain epithelial tissue that can stretch and allow the bladder to hold twice as much as it does when normally full. The walls also contain three layers of muscle that help in the emptying process. The base of the bladder (Figure 9-5) contains a triangular area, the **trigone,** where the ureters enter the bladder and the urethra exits it.

Urethra

Urine is excreted outside the body through the urethra, a tube of smooth muscle with a mucous lining. The female urethra is only about 4 centimeters [1.5 inches] long. It opens through the meatus, which is located at the distal end of the urethra between the clitoris and the vagina. The male urethra is about 20 centimeters [8 inches] long and passes through three different regions. The first region is the **prostate,** a gland where the urethra and the ejaculatory duct meet. Thus, the urethra in the male is part of the urinary system as well as part of the reproductive system. The second region is a membranous portion, after which urine passes into the third part, the penis, and is excreted through the meatus at the distal end of the penis. Excreting urine is called *voiding* or *micturition*.

FIGURE 9-5   A photograph showing the male urinary system with the ureters leading from the kidneys to the bladder in which urine is stored and then released into the urethra to exit the body.

VOCABULARY REVIEW

In the previous section, you learned terms relating to the urinary system. Before going on to the exercises, review the terms below and refer to the previous section if you have any questions. Pronunciations are provided for certain terms. Sometimes information about where the word came from is included after the term. These etymologies (word histories) are for your information only. You do not need to memorize them.

Term	Definition
bladder [BLĂD-ĕr] Old English *blaedre*	Organ where urine collects before being excreted from the body.
Bowman's [BŌ-măns] **capsule** After Sir William Bowman (1816–1892), English anatomist	Capsule surrounding a glomerulus and serving as a collection site for urine.
calices, calyces (*sing.*, calix, calyx) [KĂL-ĭ-sēz (KĀ-lĭks)] From Greek *kalyx*, cup of a flower	Cup-shaped structures in the renal pelvis for the collection of urine.
cortex [KŌR-tĕks] Latin, bark	Outer portion of the kidney.
creatine [KRĒ-ă-tēn] From Greek *kreas*, flesh	Substance found in urine; elevated levels may indicate muscular dystrophy.
creatinine [krē-ĂT-ĭ-nēn]	A component of creatine.
filtration [fĭl-TRĀ-shŭn]	Process of separating solids from a liquid by passing it through a porous substance.
glomerulus (*pl.*, glomeruli) [glō-MĂR-yū-lŏs (glō-MĂR-yū-lī)] From Latin *glomus*, ball of yarn	Group of capillaries in a nephron.
hilum [HĪ-lŭm] Latin, a small bit	Portion of the kidney where blood vessels and nerves enter and exit.
kidney [KĬD-nē] Middle English, *kidenei*	Organ that forms urine and reabsorbs essential substances back into the bloodstream.
meatus [mē-Ă-tŭs] Latin, passage	External opening of a canal, such as the urethra.
medulla [mĕ-DŪL-ă] Latin, marrow	Soft, central portion of the kidney.
nephron [NĚF-rŏn] From Greek *nephros*, kidney	Functional unit of a kidney.
prostate [PRŎS-tāt] Greek *prostates*, one that protects	Gland surrounding the urethra in the male; active in ejaculation of semen.
reabsorption [rē-ăb-SŎRP-shŭn] re + absorption	Process of returning essential elements to the bloodstream after filtration.
renal pelvis	Collecting area for urine in the center of the kidney.
renin [RĚ-nĭn] Latin *ren*, kidney	Enzyme produced in the kidneys to regulate the filtration rate of blood by increasing blood pressure as necessary.
retroperitoneal [RĚ-trō-PĚR-ĭ-tō-nē-ăl] retro-, behind + peritoneal	Posterior to the peritoneum.
trigone [TRĪ-gōn] Latin *trigonum*, triangle	Triangular area at the base of the bladder through which the ureters enter and the urethra exits the bladder.

Term	Definition
urea [yū-RĒ-ă] Greek *ouron*, urine	Waste product of nitrogen metabolism excreted in normal adult urine.
ureter [yū-RĒ-tēr] Greek *oureter*, urinary canal	One of two tubes that conduct urine from the kidney to the bladder.
urethra [yū-RĒ-thră] Greek *ourethra*	Tube through which urine is transported from the bladder to the exterior of the body.
uric [YŪR-ĭk] **acid** ur-, urine + -ic, pertaining to	Nitrogenous waste excreted in the urine.
urinary [YŪR-ĭ-nār-ē] **bladder**	*See* bladder.
urinary system	Body system that forms and excretes urine and helps in the reabsorption of essential substances.
urine [YŪR-ĭn] Greek *ouron*, urine	Fluid excreted by the urinary system.

CASE STUDY

Visiting a Clinic

Central Valley HMO is located in a large medical office building next to a hospital complex. The first floor is a large clinic where patients are evaluated first. Later, they may be referred to specialists located in the same building.

Three of the morning patients complained of problems relating to the urinary system. The first, Mr. Delgado, was having difficulty urinating. The second, Ms. Margolis, showed blood in her urine, and the third, Ms. Jones, complained of frequent, painful, and scanty urination.

All three were seen by Dr. Chorzik, a family practitioner employed by the HMO.

Critical Thinking

1. Is blood normally seen in the urine? Why or why not?
2. Does the fact that Mr. Delgado and Ms. Jones are of different sexes make the diagnosis of their urinary problems different?

STRUCTURE AND FUNCTION EXERCISES

Check Your Knowledge

Fill in the blanks.

3. Urine is transported within the urinary system via the _____.

4. Urine is transported to the outside of the body via the _____.

5. Each kidney has about one million _____.

6. The renal corpuscle contains a mass of capillaries termed a _____.

7. The collecting area in the center of the kidney is called the _____.

8. The return of essential substances to the bloodstream is called _____.

9. The urethra draws urine from the _____.

10. Two words meaning excreting urine are _____ and _____.

11. A fluid collection site in a nephron is called a _____.

12. A triangular area at the base of the bladder is called a _____.

Check Your Accuracy

Circle T for true or F for false.

13. The loss of one kidney is fatal. T F

14. The urethra transports urine from the kidney to the bladder. T F

15. Most of the water and sugar filtered in the kidney are reabsorbed. T F

16. Renin increases blood flow through the kidneys. T F

17. Two fluid collection sites within the kidney are the calices and the Bowman's capsule. T F

18. The female urethra is longer than the male urethra. T F

19. The female urethra opens into the vagina. T F

20. The prostate gland ejects semen into the male urethra. T F

21. The left kidney is usually slightly higher than the right one. T F

22. Blood flows through the kidney at varying intervals. T F

Go with the Flow

Put the following steps, which describe the flow of urine, in order by placing the letters a through g in the space provided.

23. Urine flows from the ureters into the bladder. _____

24. Fluid collects in the Bowman's capsule. _____

25. Urine flows through the renal tubules to ducts in the kidney. _____

26. Urine exits the body. _____

27. Urine flows from the bladder to the urethra. _____

28. Urine flows from the kidneys into the ureter. _____

29. Fluid flows from the Bowman's capsule to the renal tubule. _____

Combining Forms and Abbreviations

The lists below include combining forms and abbreviations that relate specifically to the urinary system. Pronunciations are provided for the examples.

COMBINING FORM	MEANING	EXAMPLE
cali(o), calic(o)	calix	*calioplasty* [KĂ-lē-ō-plăs-tē], surgical reconstruction of a calix
cyst(o)	bladder, especially the urinary bladder	*cystitis* [sĭs-TĪ-tĭs], bladder inflammation
glomerul(o)	glomerulus	*glomerulitis* [glō-MĀR-yū-LĪ-tĭs], inflammation of the glomeruli
meat(o)	meatus	*meatotomy* [mē-ă-TŎT-ō-mē], surgical enlargement of the meatus

COMBINING FORM	MEANING	EXAMPLE
nephr(o)	kidney	*nephritis* [nĕ-FRĪ-tĭs], kidney inflammation
pyel(o)	renal pelvis	*pyeloplasty* [PĪ-ĕ-lō-plăs-tē], surgical repair of the renal pelvis
ren(o)	kidney	*renomegaly* [RĒ-nō-MĔG-ă-lē], enlargement of the kidney
trigon(o)	trigone	*trigonitis* [TRĪ-gō-NĪ-tĭs], inflammation of the trigone of the bladder
ur(o), urin(o)	urine	*uremia* [yū-RĒ-mē-ă], excess of urea and other nitrogenous wastes in the blood
ureter(o)	ureter	*ureterostenosis* [yū-RĒ-tĕr-ō-stĕ-NŌ-sĭs], narrowing of a ureter
urethr(o)	urethra	*urethrorrhea* [yū-rē-thrō-RĒ-ă], abnormal discharge from the urethra
-uria	of urine	*anuria* [ăn-yū-RĒ-ă], lack of urine formation
vesic(o)	bladder, generally used when describing something in relation to a bladder	*vesicoabdominal* [VĔS-ĭ-kō-ăb-DŎM-ĭ-năl], relating to the urinary bladder and the abdominal wall

ABBREVIATION	MEANING	ABBREVIATION	MEANING
ADH	antidiuretic hormone	IVP	intravenous pyelogram
A/G	albumin/globulin	K+	potassium
AGN	acute glomerulonephritis	KUB	kidney, ureter, bladder
ARF	acute renal failure	Na+	sodium
BNO	bladder neck obstruction	pH	power of hydrogen concentration
BUN	blood urea nitrogen	PKU	phenylketonuria
CAPD	continuous ambulatory perito-neal dialysis	RP	retrograde pyelogram
Cath	catheter	SG	specific gravity
CRF	chronic renal failure	UA	urinalysis
ESRD	end-stage renal disease	UTI	urinary tract infection
ESWL	extracorporeal shock wave lithotripsy	VCU, VCUG	voiding cystourethrogram
HD	hemodialysis		

CASE STUDY

Using Tests for Diagnosis

Dr. Chorzik ordered a urinalysis for two of his patients. The results give some clues to a possible diagnosis (see chart below and on p. 299). Note that the column marked Flag indicates when something is out of the range of normal. The reference column gives the normal ranges, and the results column gives the actual readings for the patients' tests. A clean catch urine test is one in which the urine is collected once the area has been cleaned and some urine has been excreted first.

Critical Thinking

30. Whose tests had the most abnormal readings?

31. Spell out at least three of the items being tested for.

Dr. Joel Chorzik
1420 Glen Road
Meadowvale, OK 44444
111-222-3333

Run Date: 09/22/XX			Page 1
Run Time: 1507			Specimen Report

Patient: James Delgado	Acct #: A994584732	Loc: ED	U #:
Reg Dr: S. Anders, M.D.	Age/Sx: 55/M	Room:	Reg: 09/22/XX
	Status: Reg ER	Bed:	Des:

Spec #: 0922 : U0009A	Coll: 09/22/XX	Status: Comp	Req #: 77744444
	Recd.: 09/22/XX	Subm Dr:	

Entered: 09/22/XX–0841   Other Dr:
Ordered: UA with micro
Comments: Urine Description: Clean catch urine

Test	Result	Flag	Reference
Urinalysis			
UA with micro			
COLOR	YELLOW		
APPEARANCE	HAZY	**	
SP GRAVITY	1.018		1.001-1.030
GLUCOSE	NORMAL		NORMAL mg/dl
BILIRUBIN	NEGATIVE		NEG
KETONE	NEGATIVE		NEG mg/dl
BLOOD	2+	**	NEG
PH	5.0		4.5-8.0
PROTEIN	TRACE	**	NEG mg/dl
UROBILINOGEN	NORMAL		NORMAL-1.0 mg/dl
NITRITES	NEGATIVE		NEG
LEUKOCYTES	2+	**	NEG
WBC	20-50	**	0-5 /HPF
RBC	2-5		0-5 /HPF
EPI CELLS	20-50		/HPF
BACTERIA	2+	**	
MUCUS			

Patient 1

COMBINING FORMS AND ABBREVIATIONS EXERCISES

Build Your Medical Vocabulary

Complete the words by adding combining forms, suffixes, or prefixes you have learned in this chapter and in Chapters 1, 2, and 3.

32. Lack of urination: _____urea.

33. Inflammation of the renal pelvis: _____itis

CASE STUDY

Run Date: 09/22/XX	Dr. Joel Chorzik	Page 1
Run Time: 1507	1420 Glen Road	Specimen Report
	Meadowvale, OK 44444	
	111-222-3333	

Patient: Sarah Margolis	Acct #: E005792849	Loc:	U #:
Reg Dr: S. Anders, M.D.	Age/Sx: 45/F	Room:	Reg: 09/22/XX
	Status: Reg ER	Bed:	Des:

| Spec #: 0922 : U00010R | Coll 09/22/XX | Status: Comp | Req #: 00704181 |
| | Recd.: 09/22/XX | Subm Dr: | |

Entered: 09/22/XX–0936
Ordered: UA with micro
Comments: Urine Description: Clean catch urine

Other Dr:

Test	Result	Flag	Reference
Urinalysis			
UA with micro			
COLOR	BROWNISH	***	
APPEARANCE	HAZY	***	
SP GRAVITY	1.017		1.001-1.030
GLUCOSE	NORMAL		NORMAL mg/dl
BILIRUBIN	NEGATIVE		NEG
KETONE	NEGATIVE		NEG mg/dl
BLOOD	TRACE	**	NEG
PH	5.0		4.5-8.0
PROTEIN	NEGATIVE		NEG mg/dl
UROBILINOGEN	NORMAL		NORMAL-1.0 mg/dl
NITRITES	NEGATIVE		NEG
LEUKOCYTES	NEGATIVE		NEG
WBC	NO CELLS		0-5 /HPF
RBC	2-5		0-5 /HPF
EPI CELLS	0-2		/HPF
MUCUS	1+		

Patient 2

34. Excessive urination: _____uria

35. Kidney disease: _____pathy

36. Scanty urination: _____

37. Bladder paralysis: olig_____plegia

38. Lipids in the urine: lip_____

39. Abnormally large bladder: mega_____

40. Relating to the bladder and the urethra: vesico_____al

41. Kidney enlargement: reno_____

42. Inflammation of the tissues surrounding the bladder: _____cystitis

43. Medical specialty concerned with kidney disease: _____logy

44. Inflammation of the renal pelvis and other kidney parts: pyelo_____itis

45. Suturing of a calix: calio_____

46. Between the two kidneys: inter_____

47. Abnormal urethral discharge: urethro_____

48. Hemorrhage from a ureter: _____rrhagia

49. Softening of the kidneys: nephro_____

50. Within the urinary bladder: _____cystic

51. Removal of a kidney stone: _____litho_____

52. Imaging of the kidney: _____graphy

53. Kidney-shaped: reni_____

Root Out the Meaning

Divide the following words into parts. Write the urinary combining forms in the space at the right and define the word shown.

54. glomuleronephritis

55. nephrocystosis

56. urethrostenosis

57. ureterovesicostomy

58. urocyanosis

59. urolithology

60. pyeloureterectasis

61. calicotomy

62. cystolithotomy

63. nephroma

64. meatorrhaphy

65. nephrosclerosis

66. renopulmonary

67. trigonitis

Find the Right Words

Define the following abbreviations.

68. ADH

69. pH

70. CAPD

71. VCU

72. HD

73. PKU

74. BUN

75. KUB

76. ESWL

77. UTI

78. RP

Reviewing Word Parts

Write the letter of the correct definition in the space provided. Letters may be used more than once or not at all.

79. _____ ur(o)

80. _____ ureter

81. _____ –uria

82. _____ ren(o)

83. _____ meat(o)

84. _____ nephr(o)

85. _____ pyel(o)_

86. _____ cyst(o)

87. _____ urin(o)

88. _____ vesic(o)

a. many

b. flowing

c. urine

d. bladder

e. enlargement

f. bladder

g. renal pelvis

h. kidney

i. opening

j. tube from kidney to bladder

89. _____ –megaly
90. _____ -rrhea
91. _____ oligo-
92. _____ poly-
93. _____ –itis

k. inflammation
l. scanty
m. blood
n. urethra
o. nephron

Building Words

Complete each of the following urinary terms by putting a word part in the blank.

94. bladder inflammation: cyst_____.

95. removal of a kidney: _____ectomy.

96. hernia in the bladder: _____cele.

97. blood in the urine: hemat_____.

98. common urinary test: _____alysis.

99. bladder tumor: cyst_____.

100. enlargement of the kidneys: nephro_____.

Diagnostic, Procedural, and Laboratory Terms

Specialists in the urinary system are *urologists*, who treat disorders of the male and female urinary tracts and the male reproductive system, and *nephrologists*, who treat disorders of the kidneys. **Urinalysis** is the most common diagnostic and laboratory test of the urinary system. It involves the examination of urine for the presence of normal or abnormal amounts of various elements. Substances in the urine are a prime factor in the diagnosis of diseases of the urinary system as well as of other body systems. In addition, various imaging and blood tests help diagnose conditions or diseases.

Urinalysis

Urinalysis is the examination of urine for its physical and chemical and microscopic properties (Figure 9-6). Urine is gathered from clients who fill a specimen bottle by themselves or whose urine is obtained by *urinary catheterization*, the insertion of a flexible tube through the meatus and into the urinary bladder. Some patients do not have bladder control or may have certain conditions that require catheters to aid in urination. A **Foley catheter** (Figure 9-7) is **indwelling** (left in the bladder) and is held in place by a balloon inflated in the bladder. Foley catheters are also known as *retention catheters*. Other types of catheters may be disposable units. **Condom catheters** (also called *Texas catheters*, *external urinary drainage* [EUD] *catheters*, or *latex catheters*) are changed at least once a day (Figure 9-8). A condom catheter consists of a rubber sheath placed over the penis with tubing connected to a drainage or leg bag where the urine collects.

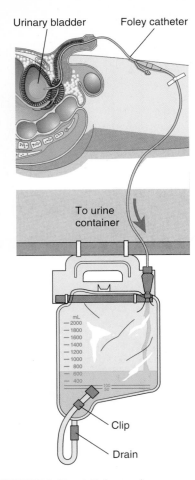

FIGURE 9-7 A Foley catheter remains in place; the collection bag is drained and cleaned.

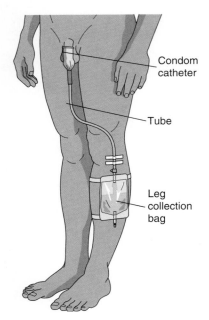

FIGURE 9-8 A condom catheter is changed daily.

	Meadow Health Systems, Inc.		
Run Date: 02/22/XX	1420 Glen Road		Page 1
Run Time: 1632	Meadowvale, OK 44444		Specimen Report
	111-222-3333		

Patient: Maria Bozutti	Acct #: C038642	Loc:	U #:
Reg Dr: S. Anders, M.D.	Age/Sx: 28/F	Room:	Reg: 02/22/XX
	Status: Reg ER	Bed:	Des:

Spec #: 0222 : U00022	Coll: 02/22/XX	Status: Comp	Req #: 77744590
	Recd.: 02/22/XX	Subm Dr:	

Entered: 02/22/XX–0841   Other Dr:
Ordered: UA with micro
Comments: Urine Description: Clean catch urine

Test	Result	Flag	Reference
Urinalysis			
UA with micro			
COLOR	YELLOW		
APPEARANCE	HAZY		
SP GRAVITY	1.018		1.001-1.030
GLUCOSE	2.604	***	NORMAL mg/dl
BILIRUBIN	NEGATIVE		NEG
KETONE	NEGATIVE		NEG mg/dl
BLOOD	NEGATIVE		NEG
PH	5.0		4.5-8.0
PROTEIN	NEGATIVE		NEG mg/dl
UROBILINOGEN	NORMAL		NORMAL-1.0 mg/dl
NITRITES	NEGATIVE		NEG
LEUKOCYTES	NEGATIVE		NEG
WBC	3		0-5 /HPF
RBC	3.5		0-5 /HPF
EPI CELLS	20-50		/HPF
BACTERIA	NEGATIVE		
MUCUS			

FIGURE 9-6 Urinalysis is a crucial diagnostic test. Dissolved wastes in the urine may reveal any of a number of diseases. For example, in the test results shown here, the patient's glucose is higher than normal, indicating possible diabetes.

There are three phases of a complete urinalysis:

1. The first phase is the *macroscopic* or *physical phase*. During this phase, the color, turbidity (cloudiness caused by suspended sediment), and **specific gravity** (ratio of density of a substance) of urine give certain diagnostic clues. Normal urine is straw-colored and clear. Blood in the urine may darken it, or show up clearly as blood. Pus or infection may make the urine cloudy. Low specific gravity may indicate kidney disease, and high specific gravity may indicate diabetes.

2. The second phase is the *chemical phase*, which determines what chemicals are present in the urine. It also determines the **pH** range of urine. The normal pH range is from 5 to 7. A reading above 7 indicates alkaline urine; a reading below 7 indicates acid urine. Alkaline urine may indicate the presence of an infection. Acidic urine controls the bacteria

entering the urethra. High uric acid may indicate gout, a metabolic disorder.

3. The third phase is the *microscopic phase* during which urine sediment is examined for solids (including cellular material) or **casts,** which are formed when protein accumulates in the urine. This may indicate the presence of kidney disease. The casts are often composed of pus or fats. The amount of wastes, minerals, and solids in urine is measured as the specific gravity.

Appendix E gives the chemical analyses and ranges commonly used in urinalysis.

In addition, tests of urine are designed to detect various substances indicative of specific conditions. The presence of high quantities of **acetones** usually occurs in diabetes. **Ketones** in the urine may indicate starvation or diabetes. Ketones in the urine can lead to dangerously high levels of acid in the blood, a potential cause of coma and/or death. The presence of the serum protein **albumin** in urine may indicate a leakage of blood proteins through the renal tubules, an indicator of *nephron disease*. **Glucose** in the urine usually indicates diabetes. Pus in the urine makes the urine cloudy and indicates an infection or inflammation in the urinary system. Bacteria in the urine elevates the nitrite result on the urinalysis. This indicates a urinary tract infection. Blood in the urine usually indicates bleeding in the urinary tract. Calcium in the urine is abnormal and indicates one of several conditions, such as rickets. **Bilirubin** in the urine indicates liver disease, such as obstructive disease of the biliary tract and liver cancer.

Blood Tests

Two important blood tests of kidney function are the *blood urea nitrogen* (*BUN*) and the *creatinine clearance test*. The presence of high amounts of urea or creatinine in the kidney shows that the kidney is not filtering and removing these toxic substances from the blood. If this is not treated and kidney failure persists, death may result.

Phenylketones in the blood show a lack of an important enzyme that can lead to mental retardation in infants unless a strict diet is followed into adulthood. Infants are routinely tested for this deficiency at birth by taking a blood sample (using a heel stick), which is analyzed for presence of the enzyme.

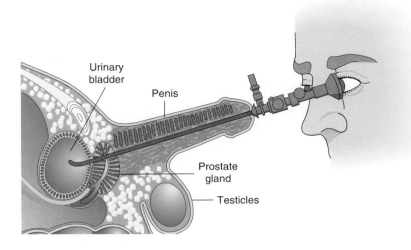

Imaging Tests

Various tests are used to visually diagnose stones, growths, obstructions, or abnormalities in the urinary system. A **cystoscopy** is the insertion of a tubular instrument (a **cystoscope**) to examine the bladder with a light (Figure 9-9). An *intravenous pyelogram* (*IVP*) and an *intravenous urogram* are x-rays of the urinary tract after a contrast medium is injected into the bloodstream. A **kidney, ureter, bladder (KUB)** is an x-ray of three parts of the urinary tract. A *renal angiogram* is an x-ray of the renal artery after a contrast medium is injected into the artery. A **retrograde pyelogram (RP)** is an x-ray of the kidney, bladder, and ureters taken after a cystoscope is used to introduce a contrast medium. A **voiding (urinating) cystourethrogram (VCU, VCUG)** is an x-ray taken during urination to examine the flow of urine through the system. An *abdominal sonogram* is the production of an image of the urinary tract using sound waves.

Radioactive imaging is also used to diagnose kidney disorders via a renal scan. A **renogram** is used to study kidney function.

Urinary Tract Procedures

Certain procedures, particularly **dialysis,** can mechanically maintain kidney or renal function when kidney failure occurs. **Hemodialysis** is the process of filtering blood outside the body in an artificial kidney machine and returning it to the body after filtering (Figure 9-10). **Peritoneal dialysis** is the insertion and removal of a dialysis solution into the peritoneal cavity (Figure 9-11). The action of this type of dialysis causes the wastes in the capillaries of the peritoneum to be released and drained out of the body. Peritoneal dialysis is used for patients who are able to have dialysis while ambulatory. The patient attaches a bag containing the dialysis solution to an opening in the peritoneum and fills the peritoneal cavity. The fluid is retained for several hours. During that time, waste products will move from the blood into the fluid through osmosis. Once empty, the bag is removed and replaced by a drainage bag into which the solution flows gradually.

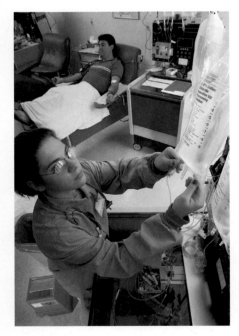

FIGURE 9-10   Hemodialysis is the removal of waste from the bloodstream by passing blood through a filtering machine.

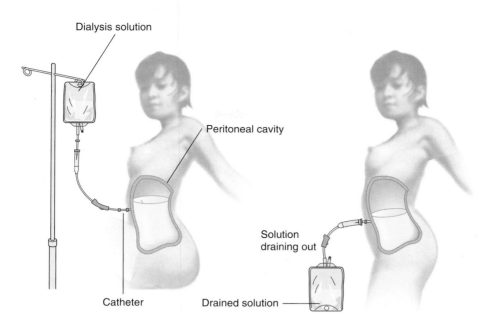

Dialysis solution

Peritoneal cavity

Solution draining out

Catheter

Drained solution

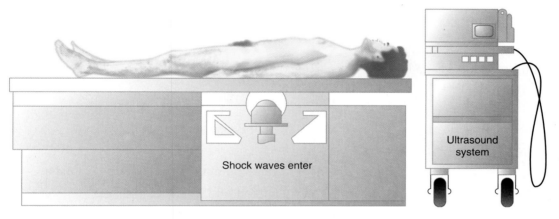

Shock waves enter

Ultrasound system

FIGURE 9-12 ESWL is the use of shock waves to break up urinary stones.

Extracorporeal shock wave lithotripsy (ESWL) is the breaking up of urinary stones by using shock waves from outside the body. Figure 9-12 shows a patient undergoing this procedure. The stones are broken into fragments that can then pass through the urine. This procedure is often used for kidney stones. There are other methods for treating stones or *calculi*. Some involve surgery; others involve medication and/or waiting for smaller stones to pass through the urinary tract.

VOCABULARY REVIEW

In the previous section, you learned terms relating to diagnosis, clinical procedures, and laboratory tests. Before going on to the exercises, review the terms below and refer to the previous section if you have any questions. Pronunciations are provided for certain terms. Sometimes information about where the word came from is included after the term. These etymologies (word histories) are for your information only. You do not need to memorize them.

Term	Definition
acetone [ĂS-ĕ-tōn]	Type of ketone normally found in urine in small quantities; found in larger quantities in diabetic urine.
albumin [ăl-BYŪ-mĭn] Latin *albumen*, egg white	Simple protein; when leaked into urine, may indicate a kidney problem.
bilirubin [bĭl-ĭ-RŪ-bĭn] bil(e) + Latin *ruber*, red	Substance produced in the liver; elevated levels may indicate liver disease or hepatitis when found in urine.
casts	Materials formed in urine when protein accumulates; may indicate renal disease.
condom catheter [KŎN-dŏm KĂTH-ĕ-tĕr]	Disposable catheter for urinary sample collection or incontinence.
cystoscope [SĬS-tō-skōp] cysto-, bladder + -scope, instrument for viewing	Tubular instrument for examining the interior of the bladder.
cystoscopy [sĭs-TŎS-kō-pē] cysto- + -scopy, use of an instrument for viewing	The insertion of a cystoscope to examine the bladder with light.
dialysis [dī-ĂL-ĭ-sĭs] Greek, a separation	Method of filtration used when kidneys fail.
extracorporeal shock wave lithotripsy [ĔKS-tră-kōr-PŌR-ē-ăl shŏk wāv LĬTH-ō-trĭp-sē] **(ESWL)**	Breaking of kidney stones by using shock waves from outside the body.
Foley [FŌ-lē] **catheter** After F. E. B. Foley (1891–1966), American urologist	Indwelling catheter held in place by a balloon that inflates inside the bladder.
glucose [GLŪ-kōs] Greek *gleukos*, sweetness	Form of sugar found in the blood; may indicate diabetes when found in the urine.
hemodialysis [HĒ-mō-dī-ĂL-ĭ-sĭs] hemo-, blood + dialysis	Dialysis performed by passing blood through a filter outside the body and returning filtered blood to the body.
indwelling [ĬN-dwĕ-lĭng] in + dwelling	Of a type of catheter inserted into the body.
ketone [KĒ-tōn]	Substance that results from the breakdown of fat; indicates diabetes or starvation when present in the urine.
kidney, ureter, bladder (KUB)	X-ray of three parts of the urinary system.
peritoneal [PĔR-ĭ-tō-NĒ-ăl] **dialysis**	Type of dialysis in which liquid that extracts substances from blood is inserted into the peritoneal cavity and later emptied outside the body.
pH	Measurement of the acidity or alkalinity of a solution such as urine.
phenylketones [FĔN-ĭl-KĒ-tōns]	Substances that, if accumulated in the urine of infants, indicate phenylketonuria (PKU), a disease treated by diet.

Term	Definition
renogram [RĒ-nō-grăm] reno-, kidney + -gram, a recording	Radioactive imaging of kidney function after introduction of a substance that is filtered through the kidney while it is observed.
retrograde pyelogram [RĔT-rō-grād PĪ-ĕl-ō-grăm] **(RP)**	X-ray of the bladder and ureters after a contrast medium is injected into the bladder.
specific gravity	Measurement of the concentration of wastes, minerals, and solids in urine.
urinalysis [yū-rĭ-NĂL-ĭ-sĭs] urin-, urine + (an)alysis	Examination of the properties of urine.
voiding (urinating) cystourethrogram [sĭs-tō-yū-RĒ-thrō-grăm] **(VCU, VCUG)**	X-ray image made after introduction of a contrast medium and while urination is taking place.

CASE STUDY

Examining the Symptoms

Ms. Jones is a 77-year-old female who complained to Dr. Chorzik of painful, scanty, and frequent urination for the past two days. She says that she normally drinks 7 to 8 glasses of water a day, but lately has cut down because of the frequent urination. Her urine was cloudy with a strong odor.

Critical Thinking

101. What did the cloudy urine most likely indicate?

102. What might be present in cloudy urine to indicate infection?

DIAGNOSTIC, PROCEDURAL, AND LABORATORY TERMS EXERCISES

Find the Test

In the space provided, put Y for those properties or substances tested for in urinalysis and N for those substances that are not tested for in urinalysis.

103. glucose _____

104. sodium _____

105. albumin _____

106. cholesterol _____

107. protein _____

108. lipids _____

109. specific gravity _____

110. pH _____

111. bilirubin _____

112. acetone _____

113. phenylketones _____

114. ketones _____

115. homocysteine _____

Finish the Thought

Fill in the blanks.

116. Removing wastes from the blood outside the body is called _____.

117. Removing wastes from the peritoneal cavity using a portable apparatus is called _____
_____.

118. A type of indwelling catheter is a(n) _____ catheter.

119. A catheter changed at least once a day is called a(n)_____ _____ catheter.

120. Two substances found in the urine that may indicate diabetes are _____ and _____.

121. Lithotripsy is used to break up _____ that have formed.

122. Solids found in urine are called _____.

123. Dialysis is a method of _____ used in _____ failure.

124. Kidney disorders may be diagnosed by blood tests such as the _____ _____
_____ or _____ _____ _____.

125. An x-ray image taken during urination is a(n) _____ _____.

Pathological Terms

The National Kidney and Urologic Diseases Information Clearinghouse gives facts about UTI prevention and treatment on their Web site (http://kidney.niddk.nih.gov/kudiseases/pubs/utiadult/index.htm).

Some additional photos of interesting kidney stones can be seen at http://www.herringlab.com/photos/.

Infections can occur anywhere in the urinary tract. A **urinary tract infection (UTI)** commonly refers to a bladder or urethra infection. Symptoms include painful and frequent urination and a general feeling of malaise (general discomfort). Treatment generally includes antibiotics. Fully emptying the bladder during urination, emptying the bladder after intercourse, adequate water intake, and careful maintenance of cleanliness around the urethra can help in preventing UTIs.

Hardened lumps of matter (*calculi* or *stones*) tend to form in the kidneys and other parts of the urinary system. The stone may cause bleeding that shows up as blood in the urine. Stones can be extremely painful. If possible, the stones are allowed to pass into the urine; otherwise, lithotripsy (the use of sound waves aimed at the stone to break it up) or surgery may be required. The patient's urine is then filtered through something (such as gauze) that retains the solid material. The solid material is analyzed for content, and a diet or medication is prescribed to prevent the occurrence of further stones. Kidney stones are also known as *nephrolithiasis*.

A number of infections and inflammations affect the urinary system. **Nephritis** is the general term for inflammation of the kidney. **Glomerulonephritis** refers to a kidney inflammation located in the glomeruli. This inflammation, known as **Bright's disease,** can be acute, as after a systemic infection, or may become chronic. When chronic, high blood pressure, kidney failure, and other conditions can result. *Interstitial nephritis* is an inflammation of the connective tissue between the renal tubules. **Pyelitis** is an inflammation of the renal pelvis. *Pyelonephritis* is a bacterial infection in the renal pelvis with abscesses.

Nephrosis or *nephrotic syndrome* is a group of symptoms usually following or related to another illness that causes protein loss in the urine (**proteinuria**). **Edema** (swelling) may result from this syndrome. Such swelling may adversely affect blood pressure. **Hydronephrosis** is the collection of urine in the kidneys without release due to a blockage. **Polycystic kidney disease** is a progressive, hereditary condition in which numerous kidney cysts form that can cause other conditions in adults, such as high blood pressure and excess blood and waste in the urine.

Renal hypertension may result from other kidney or systemic diseases. **Kidney** (*renal*) **failure,** the loss of kidney function, may result from other conditions—some chronic, such as diabetes, and some acute, such as a kidney infection. Kidney failure can be treated with dialysis and medications. **Uremia** and **azotemia,** excesses of urea and other nitrogenous wastes in the blood, may result from kidney failure. **End-stage renal disease** (**ESRD**) is severe, and fatal if not treated. *Renal cell carcinoma* or kidney cancer is usually treated by surgery. **Wilms' tumor** or a **nephroblastoma** is a malignant tumor of the kidneys found primarily in children. It is usually treated with surgery, radiation, and chemotherapy. A **nephroma** is any renal tumor.

Cystitis is an inflammation of the bladder. Aside from urinary tract infections, the bladder may be the site of **bladder cancer.** Various tumors can be removed or treated. In cases of extensive malignancy, the bladder may need to be surgically removed. Other bladder problems include a **cystocele,** a hernia of the bladder, and a **cystolith,** a stone in the bladder.

Inflammations can also occur in the urethra (*urethritis*), the urethra and bladder together (*urethrocystitis*), or the ureters (*ureteritis*). *Urethral stenosis* is a narrowing of the urethra that causes voiding difficulties.

Difficulties in urination are often a symptom of another systemic disease, such as diabetes, or a localized infection (UTI). Such difficulties can include no urine output (**anuria**), painful urination (**dysuria),** lack of bladder control (**enuresis,** including *nocturnal enuresis*, nighttime bed-wetting), frequent nighttime urination (**nocturia**), scanty urination (**oliguria**), excessive urination (**polyuria**), or urination during sneezing or coughing (*stress incontinence*). The general term **incontinence** refers to the involuntary discharge of urine or feces.

Abnormal substances or specific levels of substances in the urine indicate either urinary tract disorders or systemic disorders. Some can be minor infections or major problems. **Albuminuria** or *proteinuria* indicates the presence of albumin in the urine; **hematuria** indicates the presence of blood in the urine. **Ketonuria** indicates the presence of ketone bodies in the urine. **Pyuria** indicates the presence of pus and white blood cells in the urine.

Diabetes is a name for several metabolic diseases that both affect, and are diagnosed, in part, through observation of, the urinary system. Diabetes is covered in detail in Chapter 15.

Many congenital problems can occur in the urinary system. Surgery can correct many of these. *Hypospadias* is a congenital problem and is discussed in Chapters 10 and 11. It is a defect in which the urinary meatus opens at a place other than the distal end of the penis in males or between the clitoris and vagina in females. **Atresia** (narrowing) of the ureters or urethra may also be present at birth.

MORE ABOUT . . .

Bed-wetting

Some children, particularly boys, may wet their beds at night (a condition called *nocturnal enuresis*) up to their teenage years. For years, parents have tried everything from humiliation and restricting fluids, to some sort of shock therapy, such as awakening with a loud sound. Most of these methods have not worked. Usually the problem resolves by itself by the teenage years or earlier. In most cases, the children are found to have immature development of the urinary tract, allergies, or such sound sleep habits that they are unable to awaken. Medications are now available to control or treat enuresis.

VOCABULARY REVIEW

In the previous section, you learned terms relating to pathology. Before going on to the exercises, review the terms below and refer to the previous section if you have any questions. Pronunciations are provided for certain terms. Sometimes information about where the word came from is included after the term. These etymologies (word histories) are for your information only. You do not need to memorize them.

Term	Definition
albuminuria [ăl-byū-mĭ-NŪ-rē-ă] albumin + -uria, urine	Presence of albumin in urine, usually indicative of disease.
anuria [ăn-YŪ-rē-ă] an- + -uria	Lack of urine formation.
atresia [ă-TRĒ-zhē-ă] a-, without + Greek *tresis*, hole	Abnormal narrowing, as of the ureters or urethra.
azotemia [ăz-ō-TĒ-mē-ă] French *azote*, nitrogen + -emia, blood	*See* uremia.
bladder cancer	Malignancy of the bladder.
Bright's disease After Richard Bright (1789–1858), English internist	Inflammation of the glomeruli that can result in kidney failure.
cystitis [sĭs-TĪ-tĭs] cyst-, bladder + -itis, inflammation	Inflammation of the bladder.
cystocele [SĬS-tō-sēl] cysto-, bladder + -cele, hernia	Hernia of the bladder.
cystolith [SĬS-tō-lĭth] cysto- + -lith, stone	Bladder stone.
dysuria [dĭs-YŪ-rē-ă] dys-, difficult + -uria	Painful urination.
edema [ĕ-DĒ-mă] Greek *oidema*, a swelling	Retention of water in cells, tissues, and cavities, sometimes due to kidney disease.
end-stage renal disease (ESRD)	The last stages of kidney failure.
enuresis [ĕn-yū-RĒ-sĭs] Greek *enoureo*, to urinate in + -sis, condition	Urinary incontinence.

Term	Definition
glomerulonephritis [glō-MĀR-yū-lō-nĕf-RĪ-tĭs] glomerulo-, glomerulus + nephr-, kidney + -itis	Inflammation of the glomeruli of the kidneys.
hematuria [hē-mă-TŪ-rē-ă] hemat-, blood + -uria	Blood in the urine.
hydronephrosis [HĬ-drō-nĕ-FRŌ-sĭs] hydro-, water + nephr- + -osis, condition	Abnormal collection of urine in the kidneys due to a blockage.
incontinence [ĭn-KŎN-tĭ-nĕns] From in-, not + Latin *contineo*, to hold together	Inability to prevent excretion of urine or feces.
ketonuria [kē-tō-NŪ-rē-ă] keton(e) + -uria	Increased urinary excretion of ketones, usually indicative of diabetes or starvation.
kidney failure	Loss of kidney function.
nephritis [nĕ-FRĪ-tĭs] nephr- + -itis	Inflammation of the kidneys.
nephroblastoma [NĚF-rō-blăs-TŌ-mă] nephro-, kidney + blastoma	*See* Wilms' tumor.
nephroma [nĕ-FRŌ-mă] nephr- + -oma, tumor	Any renal tumor.
nephrosis [nĕ-FRŌ-sĭs] nephr- + -osis	Disorder caused by loss of protein in the urine.
nocturia [nŏk-TŪ-rē-ă] noct-, night + -uria	Frequent nighttime urination.
oliguria [ŏl-ĭ-GŪ-rē-ă] olig-, scant + -uria	Scanty urine production.
polycystic [pŏl-ē-SĬS-tĭk] **kidney disease**	Condition with many cysts on and within the kidneys.
polyuria [pŏl-ē-ŪR-ē-ă] poly-, much + -uria	Excessive urination.
proteinuria [prō-tē-NŪ-rē-ă] protein + -uria	Abnormal presence of protein in the urine.
pyelitis [pī-ĕ-LĪ-tĭs] pyel-, pelvis + -itis	Inflammation of the renal pelvis.
pyuria [pī-YŪ-rē-ă] py-, pus + -uria	Pus in the urine.
uremia [yū-RĒ-mē-ă] ur-, urine + -emia, blood	Excess of urea and other nitrogenous wastes in the blood.
urinary tract infection (UTI)	Infection of the urinary tract.
Wilms' [vĭlmz] **tumor** After Max Wilms (1867–1918), German surgeon	Malignant kidney tumor found primarily in young children; nephroblastoma.

PATHOLOGICAL TERMS EXERCISES

Build Your Medical Vocabulary

Using the combining forms in this chapter, complete the names of the disorders.

126. Inflammation of the urethra: _____ itis

127. Inflammation of the ureter: _____ itis

128. Inflammation of the bladder and urethra: _____ itis

129. Inflammation of the kidneys: _____ itis

130. Tumor in the kidneys: _____ oma

Spell It Correctly

Check the spelling of the following words. Write C if the spelling is correct. If it is incorrect, write the correct spelling in the space provided.

131. ureteritis _____

132. cystitis_____

133. dysuria_____

134. uretheritis_____

135. cytorrhaphy_____

Check Your Knowledge

Circle T for true or F for false.

136. Wilms' tumor is found only in middle-aged adults. T F

137. Urine collects in the renal pelvis. T F

138. Edema is swelling that may be due to kidney disease. T F

139. Oliguria is abnormally high production of urine. T F

140. Anuresis means the same as enuresis. T F

CASE STUDY

Seeing a Specialist

Mr. Delgado had a fairly normal urinalysis, but restricted urination indicated some other urinary tract problem. Dr. Chorzik referred Mr. Delgado to a urologist. Ms. Margolis had blood in her urine and some signs of infection. Ms. Jones had pus in her urine, and it was cloudy. She had complained about painful, scanty, and excessive urination at various times. Dr. Chorzik concluded that she had a urinary tract infection.

Critical Thinking

141. What are the medical terms for the symptoms Ms. Jones experienced?

142. What course of treatment will likely be prescribed for Ms. Jones?

Surgical Terms

Urology is the practice of medicine specializing in the urinary tract. The practitioner is called a urologist. Urologists diagnose, treat, and perform surgery on the urinary system in the female and on the urinary and reproductive system in the male.

Parts of the urinary system may be surgically removed. A person can live with only one kidney, so a diseased kidney may be removed in a **nephrectomy.** Diseased kidneys are removed before a *kidney* or *renal transplant*. Other surgical procedures on the kidney include **nephrolysis,** the removal of adhesions in the kidney; **nephrostomy,** the creation of an opening in the kidney leading to the outside of the body; **nephrolithotomy,** surgical removal of a kidney stone; **nephropexy,** surgical affixing in place of a floating kidney; and **nephrorrhaphy,** suturing of a damaged kidney.

An incision into the renal pelvis is called a **pyelotomy.** A **pyeloplasty** is the surgical repair of the renal pelvis. Surgical repair of a ureter is **ureteroplasty. Ureterorrhaphy** is the suture of a damaged ureter. **Ureterectomy** is the surgical removal of a diseased ureter.

The urinary bladder can be the site of stones, which are removed during a **lithotomy.** A **cystectomy** is the removal of the bladder (usually when cancer is present). Surgical fixing of the bladder to the abdominal wall is **cystopexy,** an operation to help correct urinary incontinence. **Cystoplasty** is the surgical repair of a bladder, and **cystorrhaphy** is the suturing of a damaged bladder.

The urethra may also need surgical repair (**urethroplasty**), surgical fixation (**urethropexy**), or suturing (**urethrorrhaphy**). A **urethrostomy** is the surgical creation of an opening between the urethra and the skin, while a **meatotomy** is the surgical enlargement of the opening of the meatus. Either of these operations may be necessary when certain birth defects are present. A narrowing in the urethra may require a **urethrotomy,** a surgical incision to enlarge the narrowed area.

Sometimes an opening is made to bypass diseased parts of the urinary tract. A **urostomy** is the creation of an artificial opening in the abdomen through which urine exits the body. **Intracorporeal electrohydraulic lithotripsy** is the use of an endoscope, an instrument for examining an interior canal or cavity, to break up stones in the urinary tract. A **resectoscope** is an endoscope used to cut and remove lesions in parts of the urinary system. An instrument called a *stone basket* may be attached to an endoscope and used for retrieving stones through a body cavity.

VOCABULARY REVIEW

In the previous section, you learned terms relating to surgery. Before going on to the exercises, review the terms below and refer to the previous section if you have any questions. Pronunciations are provided for certain terms. Sometimes information about where the word came from is included after the term. These etymologies (word histories) are for your information only. You do not need to memorize them.

Term	Definition
cystectomy [sĭs-TĔK-tō-mē] cyst-, bladder + -ectomy, removal	Surgical removal of the bladder.
cystopexy [SĬS-tō-pĕk-sĕ] cysto-, bladder +-pexy, fixing	Surgical fixing of the bladder to the abdominal wall.
cystoplasty [SĬS-tō-plăs-tē] cysto- + -plasty, repair	Surgical repair of the bladder.
cystorrhaphy [sĭs-TŌR-ă-fē] cysto- + -rrhaphy, suturing	Suturing of a damaged bladder.

Term	Definition
intracorporeal electrohyrdraulic lithotripsy [ĬN-tră-kōr-PŌ-rē-ăl ē-LĔK-trō-hĭ-DRŌ-lĭk LĬTH-ō-trĭp-sē]	Use of an endoscope to break up stones.
lithotomy [lĭ-THŎT-ō-mē] litho-, stone + -tomy, a cutting	Surgical removal of bladder stones.
meatotomy [mē-ă-TŎT-ō-mē] meat(us) + -tomy	Surgical enlargement of the meatus.
nephrectomy [nĕ-FRĔK-tō-mē] nephr-, kidney + -ectomy	Removal of a kidney.
nephrolithotomy [NĔF-rō-lĭ-THŎT-ō-mē] nephro-, kidney + litho-, stone + -tomy	Surgical removal of a kidney stone.
nephrolysis [nĕ-FRŎL-ĭ-sĭs] nephro- + -lysis, dissolving	Removal of kidney adhesions.
nephropexy [NĔF-rō-pĕk-sē] nephro- + -pexy	Surgical fixing of a kidney to the abdominal wall.
nephrorrhaphy [nĕf-RŌR-ă-fē] nephro- + -rrhaphy	Suturing of a damaged kidney.
nephrostomy [nĕ-FRŎS-tō-mē] nephro- + -stomy, opening	Establishment of an opening from the renal pelvis to the outside of the body.
pyeloplasty [PĪ-ĕ-lō-PLĂS-tē] pyelo-, pelvis + -plasty	Surgical repair of the renal pelvis.
pyelotomy [pī-ĕ-LŎT-ō-mē] pyelo- + -tomy	Incision into the renal pelvis.
resectoscope [rē-SĔK-tō-skōp] Latin *reseco*, to cut off + scope, instrument for viewing	Type of endoscope for removal of lesions.
ureterectomy [yū-rē-tĕr-ĔK-tō-mē] ureter + -ectomy	Surgical removal of all or some of a ureter.
ureteroplasty [yū-RĒ-tĕr-ō-PLĂS-tē] uretero-, ureter + -plasty	Surgical repair of a ureter.
ureterorrhaphy [yū-rē-tĕr-ŌR-ă-fē] uretero- + -rrhaphy	Suturing of a ureter.
urethropexy [yū-RĒ-thrō-pĕk-sē] urethro-, urethra + -pexy	Surgical fixing of the urethra.
urethroplasty [yū-RĒ-thrō-PLĂS-tē] urethro- + -plasty	Surgical repair of the urethra.
urethrorrhaphy [yū-rē-THRŌR-ă-fē] urethro- + -rrhaphy	Suturing of the urethra.
urethrostomy [yū-rē-THRŎS-tō-mē] urethro- + -stomy	Establishment of an opening between the urethra and the exterior of the body.
urethrotomy [yū-rē-THRŎT-ō-mē] urethro- + -tomy	Surgical incision of a narrowing in the urethra.
urology [yū-RŎL-ō-jē] uro-, urine + -logy, study of	Medical specialty that diagnoses and treats the urinary system and the male reproductive system.
urostomy [yū-RŎS-tō-mē] uro- + -stomy	Establishment of an opening in the abdomen to the exterior of the body for the release of urine.

CASE STUDY

Getting the Diagnosis

Patient #1: Mr. Delgado's appointment with the urologist was scheduled for the next day. During a physical examination, the urologist noticed some swelling in the prostate gland, but did not think this was enough to cause Mr. Delgado's difficulties. The urologist ordered a blood test (PSA) to determine if there were another possible cause. The PSA results were normal. The urologist then ordered imaging tests. One test showed a narrowing of the urethra.

Patient #2: Ms. Margolis, a 69-year-old female, had additional tests and was found to have serious kidney disease in one kidney. A nephrectomy was performed, and eventually her symptoms subsided.

Critical Thinking

143. What procedure might relieve Mr. Delgado's symptoms?
144. Ms. Margolis had one kidney removed. The other one is healthy. Does she need dialysis?

SURGICAL TERMS EXERCISES

Build Your Medical Vocabulary

Complete the name of the operation by adding one or more combining forms.

145. Removal of kidney stones: _____ tomy

146. Removal of kidney adhesions: _____ lysis

147. Removal of a kidney: _____ ectomy

148. Removal of a ureter: _____ ectomy

149. Creation of an artificial opening in the urinary tract: _____ stomy

Check Your Knowledge

Circle T for true or F for false.

150. Surgical repair of the urethra is ureteroplasty. T F

151. Several organs and structures in the urinary system may need surgical attaching to be held in position. T F

152. A resectoscope is an instrument used to remove lesions. T F

153. A urethrostomy and a urostomy serve the same function. T F

154. A cystopexy can help urinary incontinence. T F

Pharmacological Terms

Medications for the urinary tract can relieve pain (analgesics), relieve spasms (**antispasmodics**), or inhibit the growth of microorganisms (*antibiotics*). They may also increase (**diuretics**) or decrease (*antidiuretics*) the secretion of urine. Table 9-1 shows some common medications prescribed for urinary tract disorders.

TABLE 9-1 Some Common Medications Used to Treat the Urinary System

Drug Class	Purpose	Generic	Trade Name
analgesic	to relieve pain	phenazopyridine	Pyridium, Urogesic
antibiotic	to treat infections (especially UTIs) including ones with a fungal cause	trimethoprim amoxicillin tetracycline ciprofloxacin levofloxacin	Trimpex Amoxil, Wymox Sumycin Cipro Levaquin
antidiuretic	to control secretion of urine	vasopressin	Pitressin
antispasmodic	to relax muscles so as to relieve pain and decrease urgency to urinate	oxybutynin tolteridine	Ditropan Detrol
diuretic	to increase urination	bethanecol	Duvoid, Urecholine

VOCABULARY REVIEW

In the previous section, you learned terms relating to pharmacology. Before going on to the exercises, review the terms below and refer to the previous section if you have any questions. Pronunciations are provided for certain terms. Sometimes information about where the word came from is included after the term. These etymologies (word histories) are for your information only. You do not need to memorize them.

Agent	Purpose
antispasmodic [ĂN-tē-spăz-MŎD-ĭk] anti-, against + spasmodic	Pharmacological agent that relieves spasms; also decreases frequency of urination.
diuretic [dī-yū-RĔT-ĭk] From Greek *dia-*, through + *ouresis*, urine	Pharmacological agent that increases urination.

CASE STUDY

Receiving Treatment

Ms. Jones recovered from her urinary tract infection but came in a few months later with swollen feet and high blood pressure. She was given a prescription, a list of dietary changes she should observe, and a course of mild, daily exercise to follow.

Critical Thinking

155. What type of medication do you think was prescribed for Ms. Jones?

156. How might diet help reduce swelling?

PHARMACOLOGICAL TERMS EXERCISES

Know the Right Medication

Fill in the blanks.

157. To help relieve edema, a(n) _____ may be prescribed.

158. For dysuria, a(n) _____ may be prescribed.

159. For cystitis a(n) _____ may be prescribed.

160. Sudden contractions may lead to urinary incontinence and, therefore, a(n) _____ may be prescribed.

CHALLENGE SECTION

Review the following doctor's notes and test results for a patient hospitalized with an unusually high fever, dysuria, and general malaise.

Critical Thinking

What do the abnormal results of the urinalysis indicate?
What other tests might be necessary to reach a diagnosis?

	Meadow Health Systems, Inc.		
	1420 Glen Road		
Run Date: 09/22/XX	Meadowvale, OK 44444		Page 1
Run Time: 1507	111-222-3333		Specimen Report

Patient: Dexter Judge	Acct #: E115592848	Loc:	U #:
Reg Dr: S. Anders, M.D.	Age/Sx: 40/M	Room:	Reg: 06/10/XX
	Status: Reg ER	Bed:	Des:

Spec #: 0922 : U00010R	Coll: 09/22/XX	Status: Comp	Req #: 00704169
	Recd.: 09/22/XX	Subm Dr:	

Entered: 06/10/XX–0936   Other Dr:
Ordered: UA with micro
Comments: Urine Description: Clean catch urine

Test	Result	Flag	Reference
Urinalysis			
UA with micro			
COLOR	YELLOW		
APPEARANCE	CLEAR		
SP GRAVITY	1.017		1.001-1.030
GLUCOSE	4.7	**	NEG
BILIRUBIN	NEGATIVE		NEG
KETONE	NEGATIVE		NEG mg/dl
BLOOD	NEGATIVE		NEG
PH	5.0		4.5-8.0
PROTEIN	NEGATIVE		NEG mg/dl
UROBILINOGEN	NORMAL		NORMAL-1.0 mg/dl
NITRITES	NEGATIVE		NEG
LEUKOCYTES	NEGATIVE		NEG
WBC	8-10	**	0-5 /HPF
RBC	2-5		0-5 /HPF
EPI CELLS	0-2		/HPF
MUCUS	1+		

Patient 4

MEDICAL RECORD	PROGRESS NOTES

DATE	
9/22/XX	*Patient is a forty-year-old male admitted yesterday with symptoms including high fever and dysuria. Blood*
	pressure normal; lungs clear. Urinalysis positive for glucose and white blood count. Test for infection. Talk
	to patient about high glucose reading. —Steve Anders, M.D.

PATIENT'S IDENTIFICATION (For typed or written entries give: Name—last, first, middle; grade; rank; hospital or medical facility)

Judge, Dexter
000-000-000

REGISTER NO.	WARD NO.

PROGRESS NOTES
STANDARD FORM 509

TERMINOLOGY IN ACTION

Below is a urinalysis for a 55-year old woman. Write a short paragraph explaining what pathology the abnormal readings might indicate.

Meadow Health Systems, Inc.
1420 Glen Road
Meadowvale, OK 44444
111-222-3333

Run Date: 09/22/XX			Page 1
Run Time: 1507			Specimen Report

Patient: Mary Langado	Acct #: E115592848	Loc:	U #:
Reg Dr: S. Anders, M.D.	Age/Sx: 55/F	Room:	Reg: 06/10/XX
	Status: Reg ER	Bed:	Des:

Spec #: 0922 : U00010R	Coll: 09/22/XX	Status: Comp	Req #: 00704181
	Recd.: 09/22/XX	Subm Dr:	

Entered: 06/10/XX–0936   Other Dr:
Ordered: UA with micro
Comments: Urine Description: Clean catch urine

Test	Result	Flag	Reference
Urinalysis			
UA with micro			
COLOR	BROWNISH	***	
APPEARANCE	HAZY	***	
SP GRAVITY	1.017		1.001-1.030
GLUCOSE	5.2	**	NEG
BILIRUBIN	NEGATIVE		NEG
KETONE	NEGATIVE		NEG mg/dl
BLOOD	TRACE	***	NEG
PH	5.0		4.5-8.0
PROTEIN	NEGATIVE		NEG mg/dl
UROBILINOGEN	NORMAL		NORMAL-1.0 mg/dl
NITRITES	NEGATIVE		NEG
LEUKOCYTES	NEGATIVE		NEG
WBC	8-10	**	0-5 /HPF
RBC	2-5		0-5 /HPF
EPI CELLS	0-2		/HPF
MUCUS	1+		

Patient 5

USING THE INTERNET

Go to the National Kidney Foundation's Web site (http://www.kidney.org) and enter the cyberNephrology site by typing *cybernephrology* in the search window. Write a short paragraph on what's new in transplantation or dialysis.

CHAPTER REVIEW

The material that follows is to help you review all the material in this chapter.

Using Your Allied Health Dictionary

Build a urinary term using each of the following word parts; define the word part and the term.

161. –ectomy: _____

162. –emia: _____

163. dips/o: _____

164. glycos/o: _____

165. –lithiasis: _____

166. –lith: _____

167. cyst/o: _____

168. nephr/o: _____

169. olig/o: _____

170. py/o: _____

171. ren/o: _____

172. –rrhaphy: _____

173. ur/o: _____

174. –plasty: _____

175. –scope: _____

176. –stenosis: _____

177. urethr/o: _____

178. ureter/o: _____

179. noct(o): _____

180. –megaly: _____

181. dys-: _____

182. anti-: _____

183. poly-: _____

184. retro-: _____

185. a-, an-: _____

186. –lysis: _____

187. urin/o: _____

Spelling Correctly

Circle the correct spelling.

188. polydipsia   pollydipsia

189. urethra   uretha

190. urination   urinetion

191. absces   abscess

192. cathater   catheter

193. bacteriuria   bacteruria

194. nephrolithisis   nephrolithiasis

DEFINITIONS

Define the following terms and combining forms. Review the chapter before starting. Make sure you know how to pronounce each term as you define it. The blue words in brackets are references to the Spanish glossary available online at www.mhhe.com/medterm3e.

195. acetone [ĂS-ĕ-tŌn] {acetona}
196. albumin [ăl-BYŪ-mĭn] {albúmina}
197. albuminuria [ăl-byū-mĭ-NŪ-rē-ă] {albuminuria}
198. antispasmodic [ĂN-tē-spăz-MŎD-ĭk]
199. anuria [ăn-YŪ-rē-ă] {anuria}
200. atresia [ă-TRĒ-zhē-ă] {atresia}
201. azotemia [ăz-ō-TĒ-mē-ă] {azoemia}
202. bilirubin [bĭl-ĭ-RŪ-bĭn] {bilirrubina}
203. bladder [BLĂD-ĕr] {vejiga}
204. bladder cancer
205. Bowman's capsule
206. Bright's disease
207. cali(o), calic(o)
208. calices, calyces (sing. calix, calyx) [KĂL-ĭ-sēz (KĀ-lĭks)] {calices}
209. casts
210. condom catheter [KŎN-dŏm KĂTH-ĕ-tĕr]
211. cortex [KŌR-tĕks] {corteza}
212. creatine [KRĒ-ă-tēn] {creatina}
213. creatinine [krē-ĂT-ĭ-nēn] {creatinina}
214. cyst(o)
215. cystectomy [sĭs-TĔK-tō-mē] {cistectomía}
216. cystitis [sĭs-TĪ-tĭs] {cistitis}
217. cystocele [SĬS-tō-sēl] {cistocele}
218. cystolith [SĬS-to-lĭth] {cistolito}
219. cystopexy [SĬS-tō-pĕk-sē]
220. cystoplasty [SĬS-tō-plăs-tē]

221. cystorrhaphy [sĭs-TŌR-ă-fē] {cistorrafia}
222. cystoscope [SĬS-tō-skōp] {cistoscopio}
223. cystoscopy [sĭs-TŎS-kō-pē]
224. dialysis [dī-ĂL-ĭ-sĭs] {dialysis}
225. diuretic [dī-yū-RĔT-ĭk]
226. dysuria [dĭs-YŪ-rē-ă] {disuria}
227. edema [ĕ-DĒ-mă] {edema}
228. end-stage renal disease (ESRD)
229. enuresis [ĕn-yū-RĒ-sĭs] {enuresis}
230. extracorporeal shock wave lithotripsy [ĔKS-tră-kōr-PŌR-ē-ăl shŏk wāv LĬTH-ō-trip-sē] (ESWL)
231. filtration [fĭl-TRĀ-shŭn] {filtración}
232. Foley [FŌ-lē] catheter
233. glomerul(o)
234. glomerulonephritis [glō-MĂR-yū-lō-nĕf-RĪ-tĭs]
235. glomerulus (pl., glomeruli) [glō-MĂR-yū-lŏs (glō-MĂR-yū-lī)] {glomérulo}
236. glucose [GLŪ-kōs] {glucose}
237. hematuria [hē-mă-TŪ-rē-ă] {hematuria}
238. hemodialysis [HĒ-mō-dī-ĂL-ĭ-sĭs] {hemodiálisis}
239. hilum [HĪ-lŭm] {hilio}
240. hydronephrosis [HĪ-drō-nĕ-FRŌ-sĭs]
241. incontinence [ĭn-KŎN-tĭ-nĕns] {incontinecia}
242. indwelling [ĬN-dwĕ-lĭng]
243. intracorporeal electro-hydraulic lithotripsy [ĬN-tră-kōr-PŌ-rē-ăl ē-LĔK-trō-hī-DRŌ-lĭk LĬTH-ō-trip-sē]

244. ketone [KĒ-tōn] {cetona}
245. ketonuria [kē-tō-NŪ-rē-ă] {cetonuria}
246. kidney [KĬD-ne] {riñón}
247. kidney failure
248. kidney, ureter, bladder (KUB)
249. lithotomy [lĭ-THŎT-ō-mē]
250. meat(o)
251. meatotomy [mē-ă-TŎT-ō-mē]
252. meatus [mē-Ă-tŭs] {meato}
253. medulla [mĕ-DŪL-ă] {médula}
254. nephrectomy [nĕ-FRĔK-tō-mē]
245. nephritis [nĕ-FRĪ-tĭs] {nefritis}
246. nephr(o)
247. nephroblastoma [NĔF-rō-blăs-TŌ-mă]
248. nephrolithotomy [NĔF-rō-lĭ-THŎT-ō-mē]
249. nephrolysis [nĕ-FRŎL-ĭ-sĭs] {nefrólisis}
250. nephroma [nĕ-FRŌ-mă] {nefroma}
251. nephron [NĔF-rŏn] {nefrona}
252. nephropexy [NĔF-rō-pĕk-sē]
253. nephrorrhaphy [nĕf-RŌR-ă-fē]
254. nephrosis [nĕ-FRŌ-sĭs] {nefrosis}
255. nephrostomy [nĕ-FRŎS-tō-mē]
256. nocturia [nŏk-TŪ-rē-ă] {nocturia}
257. oliguria [ŏl-ĭ-GŪ-rē-ă] {oliguria}
258. peritoneal [PĔR-ĭ-tō-NĒ-ăl] dialysis
259. pH {pH}
260. phenylketones [FĔN-ĭl-KĒ-tōns] (PKU)

261. polycystic [pŏl-ē-SĬS-tĭk] kidney disease
262. polyuria [pŏl-ē-ŬR-ē-ă] {poliuria}
263. prostate [PRŎS-tāt] {próstata}
264. proteinuria [prō-tē-NŪ-rē-ă]
265. pyel(o)
266. pyelitis [pī-ĕ-LĪ-tĭs] {pielitis}
267. pyeloplasty [PĪ-ĕ-lō-PLĂS-tē]
268. pyelotomy [pi-ĕ-LŎT-ō-mē]
269. pyuria [pī-YŪ-rē-ă] {piuria}
270. reabsorption [rē-ăb-SŌRP-shŭn]
271. ren(o)
278. renal pelvis
279. renin [RĔ-nĭn] {renina}
280. renogram [RĒ-nō-grăm] {renograma}
281. resectoscope [rē-SĔK-tō-skōp] {resectoscopio}
282. retrograde pyelogram [RĔT-rō-grād PĪ-ĕl-ō-grăm] (RP)

283. retroperitoneal [RĔ-trō-PĔR-ĭ-tō-nē-ăl] {retroperitoneal}
284. specific gravity
285. trigon(o)
286. trigone [TRĪ-gōn] {trígono}
287. ur(o), urin (o)
288. urea [yū-RĒ-ă] {urea}
289. uremia [yū-RĒ-mē-ă] {uremia}
290. ureter(o)
291. ureter [yū-RĒ-tĕr] {uréter}
292. ureterectomy [yū-rē-tĕr-ĔK-tō-mē]
293. ureteroplasty [yū-RĒ-tĕr-ō-PLĂS-tē]
294. ureterorrhaphy [yū-rē-tĕr-ŌR-ă-fē]
295. urethr(o)
296. urethra [yū-RĒ-thră] {uretra}
297. urethropexy [yū-RĒ-thrō-pĕk-sē]
298. urethroplasty [yū-RĒ-thrō-PLĂS-tē]

299. urethrorrhaphy [yū-rē-THRŌR-ă-fē]
300. urethrostomy [yū-rē-THRŎS-tō-mē]
301. urethrotomy [yū-rē-THRŎT-ō-mē]
302. -uria
303. uric [YŪR-ĭk] acid
304. urinalysis [yū-rĭ-NĂL-ĭ-sĭs] {análisis de orina}
305. urinary [YŪR-ĭ-nār-ē] bladder
306. urinary system
307. urinary tract infection (UTI)
308. urine [YŪR-ĭn] {orina}
309. urology [yū-RŎL-ō-jē] {urología}
310. urostomy [yū-RŎS-tō-mē]
311. vesic(o)
312. voiding (urinating) cystourethrogram [sĭs-tō-yū-RĒ-thrō-grăm] (VCU, VCUG)
313. Wilms' [vĭlmz] tumor

Abbreviations

Write the full meaning of each abbreviation.

314. ADH
315. A/G
316. AGN
317. ARF
318. BNO
319. BUN
320. CAPD
321. Cath

322. CRF
323. ESRD
324. ESWL
325. HD
326. IVP
327. K +
328. KUB
329. Na +

330. PH
331. PKU
332. RP
333. SG
334. UA
335. UTI
336. VCU, VCUG

CHAPTER
10

► OBSTETRICS
► GYNECOLOGY

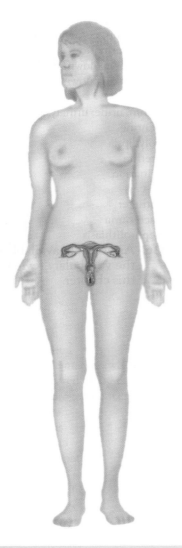

Fertility Friend is a commercial Web site (www.fertilityfriend.com) that has good information about tracking ovulation for people who are trying to get pregnant.

The Female Reproductive System

After studying this chapter, you will be able to:

10.1 Name the parts of the female reproductive system and discuss the function of each part

10.2 Define combining forms used in building words that relate to the female reproductive system

10.3 Identify the meaning of related abbreviations

10.4 Name the common diagnoses, clinical procedures, and laboratory tests used in treating disorders of the female reproductive system

10.5 List and define the major pathological conditions of the female reproductive system

10.6 Explain the meaning of surgical terms related to the female reproductive system

10.7 Recognize common pharmacological agents used in treating disorders of the female reproductive system

Structure and Function

The female reproductive system is a group of organs and glands that produce **ova** (singular, **ovum**) or *egg cells* (female sex cells), move them to the site of fertilization, and, if they are fertilized by a sperm (male sex cell), nurture them until birth. The major parts of the female reproductive system (Figure 10-1) are the ovaries, fallopian tubes, uterus, and vagina.

Reproductive Organs

The **ovaries** (also known as the female **gonads**) are two small, solid, oval structures in the pelvic cavity that produce ova and secrete female hormones. The ovaries lie on either side of the uterus. In the monthly cycle of egg production described below, one ovary usually releases only one mature ovum. In most women, the ovaries alternate this release, called **ovulation,** each month. In rare cases more eggs are released. In some women, the ovaries do not alternate regularly or do not alternate at all. The monthly production of ova or sex cells is fairly regular in most women. In males, the production of sex cells is not cyclical.

Within the ovaries are sex cells, also known as **gametes.** Before being released from an ovary, the cells develop in a part of the ovary called the **graafian follicle.** These sex cells have the potential to become fertilized and

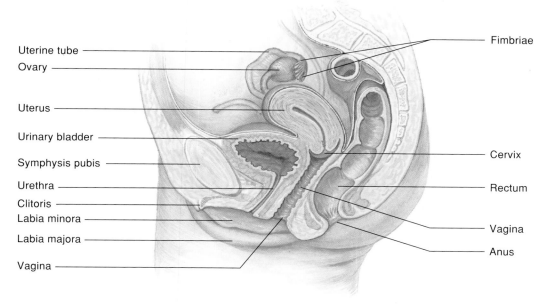

FIGURE 10-1   The female reproductive system has cycles that determine fertility.

develop. In their immature stage, they are called **oocytes;** once mature (normally 5-7 days), they are known as ova. The ovum is then released from the graafian follicle to the **uterine** or **fallopian tubes,** the two tubes that lead from the ovaries to the uterus (Figure 10-2).

The **uterus** is the female reproductive organ in which a fertilized ovum implants and develops. When the ovum is not fertilized, the lining of the uterus is released during the monthly cycle, known as *menstruation*. This cycle is described later in this chapter.

The fertilized ovum attaches to the lining of the uterus where it develops during pregnancy (discussed later in this chapter). At the end of its development, the infant is born through the **vagina** or birth canal (the canal leading from the uterus to the *vulva*) in a routine delivery or surgically through the abdomen in a *Caesarean delivery*. The organs and structures described above form the basic reproductive structure. The female breast, the **mammary gland** (Figure 10-3), is also part of the female reproductive system as an *accessory organ,* providing milk to nurse the infant (*lactation*) after birth. The breast was also discussed in Chapter 4 as an apocrine gland. In addition to fertilization, female reproduction is controlled by hormones, such as estrogen and progesterone.

At birth, most females have from 200,000 to 400,000 immature ova (oocytes) in each ovary. Many of these disintegrate before the female reaches **puberty,** the stage at which ovulation and **menarche** (first menstruation) and the **menstruation** cycle occur (usually between 10 and 14 years of age). Menstruation is the cyclical release of the uterine lining usually occurring every 28 days. Most women menstruate monthly (except during pregnancy) for about 30 to 40 years. **Menopause** signals the end of the ovulation/menstruation cycle and, therefore, the end of the childbearing years.

After release, the ovum next enters the uterine or fallopian tubes, which have fingerlike ends called **fimbriae** that sweep the ovum further

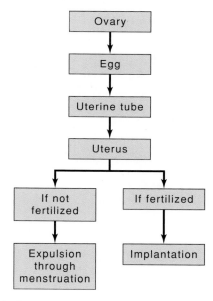

FIGURE 10-2   The path of an egg in the ovarian cycle.

The Museum of Menstruation and Women's Health online (www.mum .org) has many facts about menstruation and how it has been regarded throughout history.

FIGURE 10-3 The female breast has mammary glands and ducts through which nourishment is provided to the infant.

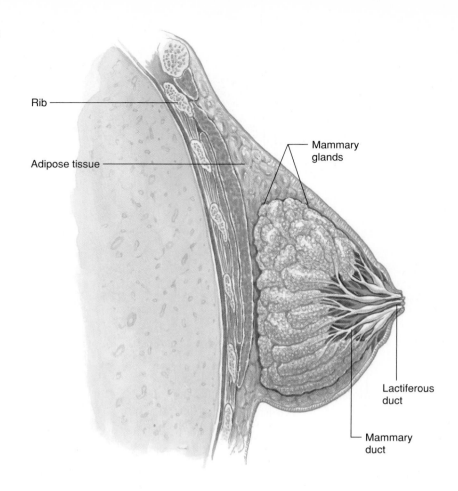

Rib

Adipose tissue

Mammary glands

Lactiferous duct

Mammary duct

down into one of the fallopian tubes, where it may be fertilized by a sperm. Fertilized or not, the ovum moves by contractions of the tube to the uterus (Figure 10-4). The uterus is pear-shaped and about the size of the fist. It is wider at the top than at the bottom, where it attaches to the vagina. Once inside the uterus, a fertilized ovum attaches to the uterine wall, where it will be nourished for about 40 weeks of development (**gestation**). The upper portion of the uterus, the **fundus,** is where a nutrient-rich organ (the **placenta**) grows in the uterine wall. An ovum that has not been fertilized is released along with the lining of the uterus (*endometrium*) during menstruation.

The middle portion of the uterus is called the **body.** It leads to a narrow region, the **isthmus.** The neck or lower region of the uterus is the **cervix.** The cervix is a protective body with glands that secrete mucous substances into the vagina. The cervical canal is the opening leading to the uterine cavity. Cells from the distal part of the cervical canal are collected during a routine Pap smear. The opening of the cervical canal into the vagina is called the *cervical os.* Cervical cancers are more likely to occur in the distal third of the cervical canal and os, accessible during routine PAP smears.

The vagina has small transverse folds called *rugae* that can expand to accommodate an erect penis during intercourse or the passage of a baby during childbirth. A fold of mucous membranes, the **hymen,** partially covers the external opening (**introitus**) of the vagina. It is usually ruptured during the female's first sexual intercourse, but may be broken earlier during physical activity or because of use of a tampon. It may also be congenitally absent.

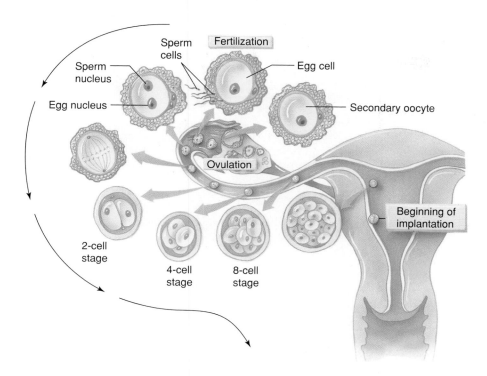

FIGURE 10-4 Movement of an oocyte during the female cycle.

The uterus (Figure 10-5) is made up of three layers of tissue—the **perimetrium,** the outer layer; the **myometrium,** the middle layer; and the **endometrium,** the inner mucous layer. The outer layer is a protective layer of membranous tissue. The middle layer is really three layers of smooth muscle that move in strong downward motions. The uterus stretches during pregnancy. The endometrium is deep and velvety, has an abundant supply of blood vessels and glands, and is built up and broken down during the ovulation/menstruation cycle.

The external genitalia (Figure 10-6), collectively known as the **vulva,** consist of a mound of soft tissue, the **mons pubis,** which is covered by pubic hair after puberty. Two folds of skin below the mons pubis, the **labia majora,** form the borders of the vulva. Between the labia majora lie two smaller skin folds, the **labia minora,** which merge at the top to form the **foreskin** of the **clitoris,** the primary female organ of sexual stimulation. The **Bartholin's glands** are embedded in the vaginal tissue near the introitus. The duct from these glands is located between the labia minora. The glands produce a lubricating fluid that bathes the vagina and surrounding vulva.

The space between the bottom of the labia majora and the anus is called the **perineum.** During childbirth, it is possible for the perineum to become torn. A surgical procedure (*episiotomy*) is commonly done before childbirth to avoid tearing the perineum, because an even surgical incision is easier to repair.

The mammary glands or breasts are full of glandular tissue that is stimulated by hormones after puberty to grow and respond to the cycles of menstruation and birth. During pregnancy, hormones stimulate the **lactiferous** (milk-producing) ducts and **sinuses** that transport milk to the **nipple** (or *mammary papilla*). The dark-pigmented area surrounding the nipple is called the **areola.** After birth (**parturition**), the mammary glands experience a *letdown reflex,* which allows milk to flow through the nipples (lactation) when the infant suckles.

FIGURE 10-5 The uterine wall has several layers.

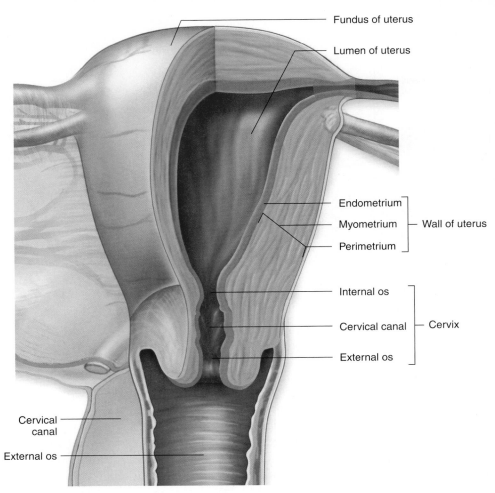

Fundus of uterus

Lumen of uterus

Endometrium
Myometrium — Wall of uterus
Perimetrium

Internal os
Cervical canal — Cervix
External os

Cervical canal

External os

FIGURE 10-6 External female genitalia.

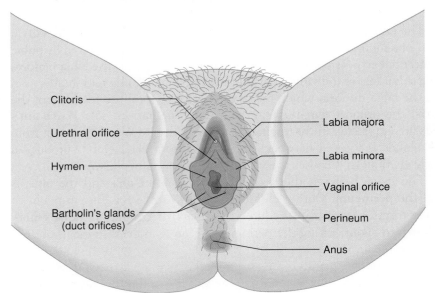

Clitoris
Urethral orifice
Hymen
Bartholin's glands (duct orifices)

Labia majora
Labia minora
Vaginal orifice
Perineum
Anus

Hormones and Cycles

The ovaries secrete **estrogen** and **progesterone,** the primary female **hormones.** In the stages before and during puberty, estrogen and progesterone play an important role in the development of mature genitalia and of secondary sex characteristics, such as pubic hair and breasts. Other hormones help in childbirth

TABLE 10-1 Major Reproductive Hormones

Hormone	Purpose	Source
estrogen	stimulates development of female sex characteristics and uterine wall thickening; inhibits FSH and increases LH	ovarian follicle; corpus luteum
progesterone	stimulates uterine wall thickening and formation of mammary ducts	corpus luteum
prolactin	promotes lactation	pituitary gland
oxytocin	stimulates labor and lactation	pituitary gland
FSH (follicle-stimulating hormone)	stimulates oocyte maturation; increasing estrogen	pituitary
HCG (human chorionic gonadotropin)	stimulates estrogen and progesterone from corpus luteum	placenta, embryo
LH (luteinizing hormone)	stimulates oocyte maturation; increases progesterone	pituitary

and milk production. Table 10-1 lists the major reproductive hormones and their functions. In the chapter on the endocrine system (Chapter 15), hormones that stimulate glands in the female reproductive system are discussed.

Ovulation and Menstruation

Ovulation and menstruation are contained within the average 28-day female cycle (Figure 10-7). Although the timing of cycles may vary, the average female cycle is divided into four phases as follows:

1. Days 1-5. Menstruation takes place during the first five days. The endometrial lining sloughs off and is released, causing generally slow bleeding through the vagina.
2. Days 6-12. The **follicle-stimulating hormone (FSH)** is released from the anterior pituitary. The body reactions take place in the ovary where an immature ovum is matured in the graafian follicle and in the uterus where the endometrial lining that has been passed out of the body during menstruation is built up again. The rebuilding of the lining is prompted by the production of estrogen. During this time, menstruation has stopped.
3. Days 13-14. The next two days, approximately two weeks after the beginning of menstruation, is the time of ovulation or the egg's release from the graafian follicle and the beginning of its trip down the fallopian tube. This release is stimulated by the pituitary's release of **luteinizing hormone (LH)**, which prompts the fimbriae to swell and wave to entice the newly released ovum toward the fallopian tube. Meanwhile, the graafian follicle fills with a yellow substance that secretes estrogen and progesterone. This secreting structure is known as the **corpus luteum.** The secreted hormones encourage the uterus to prepare for a pregnancy by growing the endometrium into a thick, nutritive layer.
4. Days 15-28. In the second 14 days of the cycle, either fertilization occurs or the built-up endometrium starts to break down as estrogen and progesterone levels drop. The symptoms (bloating, cramps, nervousness, and depression) of the hormonal changes during the phase leading to menstruation (*premenstrual syndrome [PMS]*) appear.

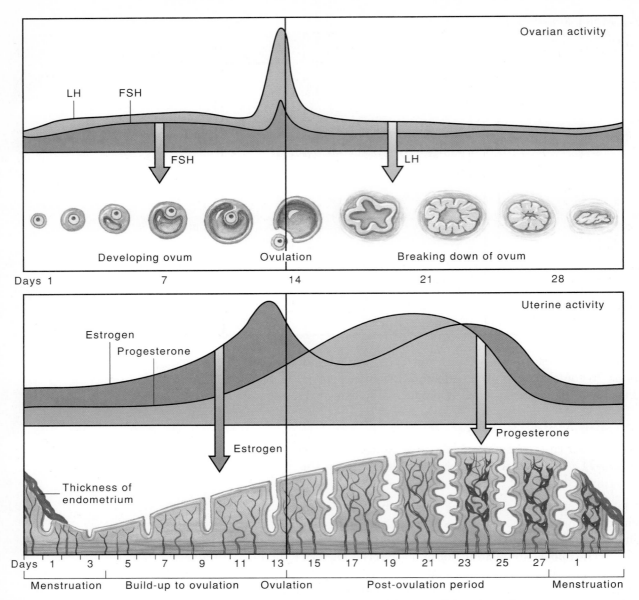

FIGURE 10-7 The cycles of ovulation and menstruation are parts of the overall female cycle.

It is at the point of ovulation that fertilization can occur or be prevented. Prevention of fertilization is accomplished with **contraception.** Contraceptive methods include the **intrauterine device (IUD), intravaginal ring, condom** (both male and female), **spermicide, diaphragm,** *cervical cap,* or **sponge.**

Some forms of hormone interaction will also prevent fertilization. A combination of estrogen and progesterone in varying levels of strengths shut off production of follicle-stimulating hormone (FSH) and luteinizing hormone (LH), without which ovulation cannot occur. These doses are taken in pill form, by injection, via a patch, or through a ring that is inserted in the vagina. The *rhythm method* is another method that may be used. It involves knowing one's cycle carefully and abstaining from intercourse for a few days before, during, and after the time of ovulation—about 2 days.

Other female hormones, such as *oxytocin,* aid in the birth process by intensifying contractions of the uterus. Release of hormones is a function of the endocrine system, discussed in Chapter 15.

Pregnancy

As a result of contact between the sperm and an ova usually through sexual intercourse (**coitus** or **copulation**), fertilization may occur. Fertilization should take place soon after ovulation and high in the fallopian tube to ensure the cells are at the proper stage of development when entering the uterus. If fertilized, implantation in the uterus takes place, the placenta forms, and pregnancy begins. Fertilization may also take place through *artificial insemination*. This can take place either by mechanical insertion of sperm from a sperm donor or by *in vitro* fertilization, which occurs in a laboratory that harvests ova and fertilizes them in the laboratory before implanting them into the uterus. A pregnant woman is known as a **gravida,** with gravida I being the first pregnancy, gravida II being the second, and so on.

An **umbilical cord** connects the placenta to the navel of the fetus so that the mother's blood and the fetal blood do not mix, but nutrients and waste products are exchanged. The fetus develops in a sac containing the **chorion,** the outermost membrane covering the fetus, and the **amnion,** the innermost membrane next to the fluid surrounding the fetus (**amniotic fluid**). The birth process usually begins when the sac breaks naturally or is broken by medical intervention.

The placenta separates from the uterus after delivery and is expelled from the body as the **afterbirth.** The umbilical cord is then severed and tied so that the infant is physically separated from its mother. At the end of this process, the woman is known as a **para** (one who has maintained a pregnancy to the point of viability). Para I refers to the first such pregnancy, para II the second, and so on. The period of time immediately after the birth (parturition) of the infant is known as *postpartum*.

> Baby Center (www.babycenter.com) is a commercial site that shows fetal development during pregnancy.

Menopause

Menopause, the cessation of menstruation, takes place after levels of estrogen decline. Most women experience menopause between the ages of 45 and 55. However, some women may experience it earlier than that or later. The period of hormonal changes leading up to menopause is called the **climacteric.** The three to five years of decreasing estrogen levels prior to menopause is called **perimenopause.** The hormonal changes cause symptoms in some women that can be uncomfortable, such as night sweats, fatigue, irritability, or vaginal dryness. Hormone replacement therapy is sometimes used. Some women find relief from increasing their intake of natural plant estrogens found in such products as soy.

Postmenopausal women are at greater risk for osteopenia and osteoporosis (discussed in Chapter 5) because estrogen has been shown to help in maintaining and increasing bone mass. It is suggested that all women monitor their intake of calcium starting in their early years of menstruation and continuing throughout their lives to help avoid bone loss after menopause.

> The North American Menopause Society (www.menopause.org) provides information to consumers and health professionals regarding menopause.

VOCABULARY REVIEW

In the previous section, you learned terms relating to the female reproductive system. Before going on to the exercises, review the terms below and refer to the previous section if you have any questions. Pronunciations are provided for certain terms. Sometimes information about where the word came from is included after the term. These etymologies (word histories) are for your information only. You do not need to memorize them.

Term	Definition
afterbirth [ĂF-tĕr-bĕrth] after + birth	Placenta and membranes that are expelled from the uterus after birth.
amnion [ĂM-nē-ŏn] From Greek *amnios*, lamb	Innermost membrane of the sac surrounding the fetus during gestation.
amniotic [ăm-nē-ŎT-ĭk] **fluid**	Fluid surrounding the fetus and held by the amnion.
areola [ă-RĒ-ō-lă] Latin, small area	Darkish area surrounding the nipple on a breast.
Bartholin's [BĂR-thō-lĕnz] **gland** After Casper Bartholin (1655–1738), Danish anatomist	One of two glands on either side of the vagina that secrete fluid into the vagina.
body	Middle portion of the uterus.
cervix [SĔR-vĭks] Latin, neck	Protective part of uterus, located at the bottom and protruding through the vaginal wall; contains glands that secrete fluid into the vagina.
chorion [KŌ-rē-ŏn]	Outermost membrane of the sac surrounding the fetus during gestation.
climacteric [klī-MĂK-tĕr-ĭk, klī-măk-TĔR-ĭk] Greek *klimakter*, the rung of a ladder	Period of hormonal changes just prior to menopause.
clitoris [KLĬT-ō-rĭs] Greek *kleitoris*	Primary organ of female sexual stimulation, located at the top of the labia minora.
coitus [KŌ-ĭ-tŭs] Latin	Sexual intercourse.
condom [KŎN-dŏm]	Contraceptive device consisting of a rubber or vinyl sheath placed over the penis or as a lining that covers the vaginal canal, blocking contact between the sperm and the female sex organs.
contraception [kŏn-tră-SĔP-shŭn] contra-, against + conceptive, able to conceive	Method of controlling conception by blocking access or interrupting reproductive cycles; birth control.
copulation [kŏp-yū-LĀ-shŭn] Latin *copulatio*, a joining	Sexual intercourse.
corpus luteum [KŌR-pŭs LŪ-tē-ŭm] Latin, yellow body	Structure formed after the graafian follicle fills with a yellow substance that secretes estrogen and progesterone.
diaphragm [DĪ-ă-frăm] Greek *diaphragma*, partition	Contraceptive device that covers the cervix and blocks sperm from entering; used in conjunction with spermicide.
endometrium [ĔN-dō-MĒ-trē-ŭm] endo-, within + Greek *metra*, uterus	Inner mucous layer of the uterus.
estrogen [ĔS-trō-jĕn] estr(us), sexual cycle phase in female animals + -gen, producing	One of the primary female hormones produced by the ovaries.

Term	Definition
fallopian [fă-LŌ-pē-ăn] **tube** After Gabriele Fallopio (1523–1562), Italian anatomist	One of the two tubes that lead from the ovaries to the uterus; uterine tube.
fimbriae [FĬM-brē-ē] Latin, fringes	Hairlike ends of the uterine tubes that sweep the ovum into the uterus.
follicle [FŎL-Ĭ-kl] **-stimulating hormone (FSH)**	Hormone necessary for maturation of oocytes and ovulation.
foreskin [FŌR-skĭn] fore-, in front + skin	Fold of skin at the top of the labia minora.
fundus [FŬN-dŭs] Latin, bottom	Top portion of the uterus.
gamete [GĂM-ēt] Greek, wife or *gametes*, husband	Sex cell; *see* ovum.
gestation [jĕs-TĀ-shŭn] Latin *gestation*	Period of fetal development in the uterus; usually about 40 weeks.
gonad [GŌ-năd] From Greek *gone*, seed	Male or female sex organ; *see* ovary.
graafian follicle [gră-FĒ-ăn FŎL-ĭ-kl] After Reijnier de Graaf (1641–1673), Dutch physiologist	Follicle in the ovary that holds an oocyte during development and then releases it.
gravida [GRĂV-ĭ-dă] Latin, from *gravis*, heavy	Pregnant woman.
hormone [HŌR-mōn] Greek *hormon*, one that rouses	Chemical secretion from glands such as the ovaries.
hymen [HĪ-mĕn] Greek, membrane	Fold of mucous membranes covering the vagina of a young female; usually ruptures during first intercourse.
intrauterine [ĬN-tră-YŪ-tĕr-ĭn] **device (IUD)** intra-, within + uterine	Contraceptive device consisting of a coil placed in the uterus to block implantation of a fertilized ovum.
introitus [ĭn-TRŌ-ĭ-tŭs] Latin, entrance	External opening or entrance to a hollow organ, such as a vagina.
isthmus [ĬS-mŭs] Greek, narrow area	Narrow region at the bottom of the uterus opening into the cervix.
labia majora [LĀ-bē-ă mă-JŌR-ă] Latin, larger lips	Two folds of skin that form the borders of the vulva.
labia minora [mĭ-NŌR-ă] Latin, smaller lips	Two folds of skin between the labia majora.
lactiferous [lăk-TĬF-ĕr-ŭs] lacti-, milk + -ferous, bearing	Producing milk.
luteinizing [LŪ-tē-ĭn-Ī-zĭng] **hormone (LH)** From Latin *luteus*, dark yellow	Hormone essential to ovulation.
mammary [MĂM-ă-rē] **glands** From Latin *mamma*, breast	Glandular tissue that forms the breasts, which respond to cycles of menstruation and birth.

Term	Definition
menarche [mĕ-NĂR-kē] meno-, menstruation + Greek *arche*, beginning	First menstruation.
menopause [MĔN-ō-păwz] meno- + pause	Time when menstruation ceases; usually between ages 45 and 55.
menstruation [mĕn-strū-Ā-shŭn] Latin *menstruo*, to menstruate	Cyclical release of uterine lining through the vagina; usually every 28 days.
mons pubis [mŏnz pyū-BĬS]	Mound of soft tissue in the external genitalia covered by pubic hair after puberty.
myometrium [MĪ-ō-MĒ-trē-ŭm] myo-, muscle + Greek *metrium*, uterus	Middle layer of muscle tissue of the uterus.
nipple [NĬP-l]	Projection at the apex of the breast through which milk flows during lactation.
oocyte [Ō-ō-sīt] oo-, egg + -cyte, cell	Immature ovum produced in the gonads.
ovary [Ō-vă-rē] From Latin *ovum*, egg	One of two glands that produce ova.
ovulation [ŎV-yū-LĀ-shŭn]	Release of an ovum (or rarely, more than one ovum) as part of a monthly cycle that leads to fertilization or menstruation.
ovum (*pl.*, **ova**) [Ō-vŭm (Ō-vă)] Latin, egg	Mature female sex cell produced by the ovaries, which then travels to the uterus. If fertilized, it implants in the uterus; if not, it is released during menstruation to the outside of the body.
para [PĂ-ră] Latin *pario*, to bring forth	Woman who has given birth to one or more viable infants.
parturition [păr-tūr-ĬSH-ŭn] Latin *parturition*	Birth.
perimenopause [pĕr-ĭ-MĔN-ō-păws] peri-, around + menopause	Three- to five-year period of decreasing estrogen levels prior to menopause.
perimetrium [pĕr-ĭ-MĒ-trē-ŭm] peri- + Greek *metra*, uterus	Outer layer of the uterus.
perineum [PĔR-ĭ-NĒ-ŭm]	Space between the labia majora and the anus.
placenta [plă-SĔN-tă] Latin, flat cake	Nutrient-rich organ that develops in the uterus during pregnancy; supplies nutrients to the fetus.
progesterone [prō-JĔS-tĕr-ōn] pro-, before + gest(ation)	One of the primary female hormones.
puberty [PYŪ-bĕr-tē] Latin *pubertas*	Preteen or early teen period when secondary sex characteristics develop and menstruation begins.
sinus [SĪ-nŭs] Latin, cavity	Space between the lactiferous ducts and the nipple.
spermicide [SPĔR-mĭ-sīd] sperm + -cide, killing	Contraceptive chemical that destroys sperm; usually in cream or jelly form.

Term	Definition
sponge [spŭnj] Greek *spongia*, sea sponge	Polyurethane contraceptive device filled with spermicide and placed in the vagina near the cervix.
umbilical [ŭm-BĬL-ĭ-kăl] **cord** From Latin *umbilicus*, navel	Cord that connects the placenta in the mother's uterus to the navel of the fetus during gestation for nourishment of the fetus.
uterine [YŪ-tĕr-ĭn] **tube**	One of two tubes through which ova travel from an ovary to the uterus.
uterus [YŪ-tĕr-ŭs] Latin	Female reproductive organ; site of implantation after fertilization or release of the lining during menstruation.
vagina [vă-JĪ-nă] Latin	Genital canal leading from the uterus to the vulva.
vulva [VŬL-vă] Latin	External female genitalia.

CASE STUDY

Examining the Patient

Dr. Liana Malvern is an internist on the staff of Crestwood HMO. She examined Jane Smits and entered the following notes on Jane's record.

Critical Thinking

1. The patient was afebrile. What does afebrile mean?

   _____

2. The patient has normal menstruation, but she has only one ovary. How is that possible?

   _____

S: Patient is a 29-year-old female who reports generalized lower abdominal pain for the past three days, which seems to have worsened today. She had trouble sleeping last night because of it. States she threw up one time last night but it was after she coughed. She ate today, had no problems digesting her food. She has been afebrile, not taking any medicines. Patient admits to having unprotected sexual intercourse with a new partner. Patient denies burning upon urination; no appreciable vaginal discharge. Her last menstrual period was eleven days ago.

Past history—she has had ovarian cysts on the right ovary. The right ovary and right fallopian tube were removed surgically. She states that her appendix was removed ten years ago. She states she has fairly normal periods.

O: Exam shows her to be afebrile. She has bilateral lower quadrant discomfort but no rebound and no remarkable guarding. Pelvic exam done. Normal appearing introitus; cervix is viewed. No remarkable discharge. She is minimally uncomfortable to manipulation of the cervix but does have more discomfort with palpation toward the uterus. Rectal exam is negative.

Lab: White count: 15,500 with 70 segs. UA: 3-5 red cells, no white cells.

A: Probable pelvic inflammatory disease

P: Prescription for Doxycycline (antibiotic) for infection and recommended ibuprofen for pain. To return to office if any increased symptoms appear such as fever, nausea, vomiting, or increased pain.

STRUCTURE AND FUNCTION EXERCISES

Follow the Path

Using letters a through d, put the following in order according to the path of an ovum from its production to implantation.

3. uterine tube _____

4. ovary _____

5. fimbriae _____

6. uterus _____

Check Your Knowledge

Fill in the blanks.

7. The oocyte is first released from the _____.

8. Implantation usually takes place in the _____.

9. The release of an ovum from the ovary is called _____.

10. The release of the uterine lining on a cyclical basis is called _____.

11. The upper portion of the uterus where the placenta usually develops is the _____.

12. The opening at the bottom of the uterus into the vagina is called the _____.

13. The outermost layer of the uterus is the _____.

14. The mammary glands make up the tissue of the _____.

15. The first menstruation is known as _____.

16. The time when menstruation is beginning to cease is called _____.

17. The primary female hormones are _____ and _____.

18. Birth control pills or implants are chemical forms of _____.

19. The fetus gestates in a sac containing the _____, the outermost membrane, and the _____, the innermost membrane.

20. When the placenta is expelled from the body, it is called the _____.

21. The period after the birth of a baby is known as _____.

Combining Forms and Abbreviations

The lists below include combining forms and abbreviations that relate specifically to the female reproductive system. Pronunciations are provided for the examples.

COMBINING FORM	MEANING	EXAMPLE
amni(o)	amnion	*amniocentesis* [ĂM-nē-ō-sĕn-TĒ-sĭs], test of amniotic fluid by insertion of a needle into the amnion
cervic(o)	cervix	*cervicitis* [sĕr-vĭ-SĪ-tĭs], inflammation of the cervix

Combining Form	Meaning	Example
colp(o)	vagina	*colporrhagia* [kōl-pō-RĀ-jē-ǎ], vaginal hemorrhage
episi(o)	vulva	*episiotomy* [ě-pĭz-ē-ŌT-tō-mē] surgical incision into the perineum to prevent tearing during childbirth
galact(o)	milk	*galactopoiesis* [gǎ-LĂK-tō-pǒy-Ē-sǐs], milk production
gynec(o)	female	*gynecology* [gī-ně-KŎL-ō-jē], medical specialty that diagnoses and treats disorders of the female reproductive system
hyster(o)	uterus	*hysterectomy* [hǐs-těr-ĚK-tō-mē], surgical removal of the uterus
lact(o), lacti	milk	*lactogenesis* [lǎk-tō-JĚN-ē-sǐs], milk production
mamm(o)	breast	*mammography* [mǎ-MŎG-rǎ-fē], imaging of the breast
mast(o)	breast	*mastitis* [mǎs-TĪ-tǐs], inflammation of the breast
men(o)	menstruation	*menopause* [MĚN-ō-pǎwz], cessation of menstruation
metr(o)	uterus	*metropathy* [mě-TRŎP-ǎ-thē], disease of the uterus
oo	egg	*oogenesis* [ō-ō-JĚN-ē-sǐs], production of eggs
oophor(o)	ovary	*oophoritis* [ō-ǒf-ōr-Ī-tǐs], inflammation of an ovary
ov(i), ov(o)	egg	*ovoid* [Ō-vǒyd], egg-shaped
ovari(o)	ovary	*ovariocele* [ō-VĂR-ē-ō-sēl], hernia of an ovary
perine(o)	perineum	*perineocele* [pěr-ǐ-NĒ-ō-sēl], hernia in the perineum
salping(o)	fallopian tube	*salpingoplasty* [sǎl-PĬNG-ō-plǎs-tē], surgical repair of a fallopian tube
uter(o)	uterus	*uteroplasty* [YŪ-těr-ō-plǎs-tē], surgical repair of the uterus
vagin(o)	vagina	*vaginitis* [vǎj-ǐ-NĪ-tǐs], inflammation of the vagina
vulv(o)	vulva	*vulvitis* [vŭl-VĪ-tǐs], inflammation of the vulva

ABBREVIATION	MEANING	ABBREVIATION	MEANING
AB	abortion	HRT	hormone replacement therapy
AFP	alpha-fetoprotein	HSG	hysterosalpingography
AH	abdominal hysterectomy	HSO	hysterosalpingo-oophorectomy
CIS	carcinoma in situ	IUD	intrauterine device
CS	caesarean section	LH	luteinizing hormone
C-section	caesarean section	LMP	last menstrual period
Cx	cervix	multip	multiparous
D & C	dilation and curettage	OB	obstetrics
DES	diethylstilbestrol	OCP	oral contraceptive pill
DUB	dysfunctional uterine bleeding	P	para (live births)
ECC	endocervical curettage	Pap smear	Papanicolaou smear
EDC	expected date of confinement (delivery)	PID	pelvic inflammatory disease
EMB	endometrial biopsy	PMP	previous menstrual period
ERT	estrogen replacement therapy	PMS	premenstrual syndrome
FHT	fetal heart tones	primip	primiparous (having one child)
FSH	follicle-stimulating hormone	TAH-BSO	total abdominal hyster-ectomy with bilateral salpingo-oophorectomy
G	gravida (pregnancy)		
gyn	gynecology	TSS	toxic shock syndrome
HCG	human chorionic gonadotropin	UC	uterine contractions

CASE STUDY

Treating an Unusual Occurrence

Dr. Alvino's next patient, Sarah Messer, was having a heavier than usual menstrual flow. After the visit, her record read as follows.

Critical Thinking

22. Did the laboratory tests confirm that the patient was pregnant?
23. What do BP and P mean, and were Sarah Messer's BP and P normal?

S: Patient is a 22-year-old female who presents with a heavier than usual menstrual flow. Patient states she is using 12–15 pads per day. She states her period started two days ago but is much heavier than usual. Period was about two days late. She is sexually active, no form of birth control, does not think she could be pregnant. She is worried about going to work where she is on her feet all day, and that she seems to flow heavier when she is on her feet. Patient reports cramping

O: Examination shows a young, white female who does not appear in any remarkable distress. She is afebrile. BP 122/70, P 80. Abdomen is soft, no remarkable discomfort, no guarding or rebound present. Pelvic exam was performed. Cervix was closed, significant amount of blood in the cervical vault. There was no remarkable discharge otherwise noted. No discomfort at cervix. No remarkable discomfort or mass in the LLQ on bimanual exam. Lab shows negative serum pregnancy. Noticeable discomfort on RLQ exam. White count 5500 with 62 segs, HCG 11.5. She has had a persistent problem with her right ovary. A previous ultrasound showed problems with the ovary, most likely benign ovarian cysts.

A: Menorrhagia. Persistent right ovarian pain.

P: Prescribed Naprosyn 250 mg., one b.i.d. for pain. Provided patient with note to take off work for next two days. Patient to rest and report blood flow tomorrow. Patient to return if problems continue; will monitor HCG.

COMBINING FORMS AND ABBREVIATIONS EXERCISES

Build Your Medical Vocabulary

For the following definitions, provide a medical term. Use the combining forms listed in this chapter and in Chapters 1, 2, and 3.

24. narrowing of the vulva _____

25. x-ray of the breast _____

26. production of milk _____

27. hernia of an ovary _____

28. agent that stimulates milk production _____

29. suture of the perineum _____

30. vaginal infection due to a fungus _____

31. uterine pain _____

32. inflammation of the vulva _____

33. vaginal hemorrhage _____

34. formation and development of the egg _____

35. any disease of the breast _____

36. plastic surgery of the uterus _____

37. inflammation of a fallopian tube _____

38. removal of the cervix _____

39. ovarian tumor _____

40. incision into an ovary _____

41. narrowing of the uterine cavity _____

42. resembling a woman _____

43. rupture of the amniotic membrane _____

Make a Match

Match the definition in the right-hand column with the correct term in the left-hand column.

44. ____ episioperineorrhapy

45. ____ galactophoritis

46. ____ ovariorrhexis

47. ____ oviduct

48. ____ colpodynia

49. ____ metritis

50. ____ perineoplasty

51. ____ ookinesis

52. ____ amniorrhea

53. ____ metrosalpingitis

a. rupture of an ovary

b. vaginal pain

c. surgical repair of the perineum

d. egg movement

e. inflammation of the milk ducts

f. escape of amniotic fluid

g. uterine tube

h. inflammation of the uterus and fallopian tubes

i. inflammation of the uterus

j. surgical repair of a tear in the vulva and perineum

Diagnostic, Procedural, and Laboratory Terms

An e-mail can be sent to you regularly to remind you when you need a Pap smear or mammogram. Go to www .myhealthtestreminder.com and register to get the regular e-mails.

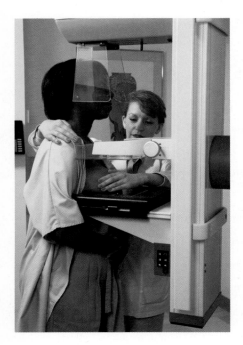

FIGURE 10-8 Early breast cancer detection has been increased by mammography, which can locate a cancerous growth up to two years earlier than it can be felt by palpation.

The major function of the female reproductive system is to bear children. There are several basic tests for pregnancy. Diagnosis of fertility problems involves more sophisticated technology. Aside from pregnancy, the health of the female reproductive system is monitored on a regular basis by a **gynecologist,** a physician who diagnoses and treats disorders of the female reproductive system. An **obstetrician** diagnoses and treats both normal and abnormal pregnancies and childbirths.

A routine gynecological exam usually includes a **Papanicolaou (Pap) smear,** a gathering of cells from the cervix to detect cervical or vaginal cancer or other anomalies. The vagina is held open by a vaginal *speculum*, a device that holds open any cavity or canal for examination. The cervix and vagina may also be examined by **colposcopy,** use of a lighted instrument (a *colposcope*) for viewing into the vagina. The colposcope is used for almost all vaginal examinations and is a very common instrument in a gynecologyical or obstetrical office.

Hysteroscopy is the use of a *hysteroscope*, a lighted instrument for examination of the interior of the uterus. **Culdoscopy** is the use of an endoscope to examine the contents of the pelvic cavity. These tests can determine whether masses, tumors, or other abnormalities are present. Some abnormalities are caused by sexually transmitted diseases.

Depending on a woman's age, a routine gynecological exam usually includes a prescription for a *mammogram*, a cancer screening test that can detect tumors before they can be felt. **Mammography** is a procedure that provides images of breast tissue (Figure 10-8). The age recommended for routine mammography differs according to family history, physical condition, and the recommending body. (Recommendations from the American Medical Association, American Cancer Society, and the National Institutes for Health vary.)

A pregnancy test is a blood or urine test to detect *human chorionic gonadotropin* (*HCG*), a hormone that stimulates growth during the first trimester of pregnancy. A pregnancy test may also involve palpation of the uterus during an internal examination by the gynecologist or an obstetrician.

Several tests for fertility problems include **hysterosalpingography,** a procedure to x-ray the uterus and uterine tubes after a contrast medium is injected; *pelvic ultrasonography*, imaging of the pelvic region using sound waves (used both for detection of tumors and for examination of the fetus); and *transvaginal ultrasound*, also a sound wave image of the pelvic area but done with a probe inserted into the vagina. Male fertility tests are discussed in Chapter 11.

During pregnancy, the dimensions of the pelvis are measured during **pelvimetry,** an examination to see if the pelvis is large enough to allow delivery. *Fetal monitoring* records an infant's heart rate and other functions during labor. There is also a simple blood test recently developed to detect pregnant women at risk for preeclampsia (see the pathological terms section below), a potentially fatal condition. The birth process is discussed in Chapter 17.

VOCABULARY REVIEW

In the previous section, you learned terms related to diagnosis, clinical procedures, and laboratory tests. Before going on to the exercises, review the terms below and refer to the previous section if you have any questions. Pronunciations are provided for certain terms. Sometimes information about where the word came from is included after the term. The etymologies (word histories) are for your information only. You do not need to memorize them.

Term	Definition
colposcopy [kŏl-PŎS-kō-pē] colpo-, vagina + -scopy, a viewing	Examination of the vagina with a colposcope.
culdoscopy [kŭl-DŎS-kō-pē] French cul-d(e-sac), bottom of a sack + -scopy	Examination of the pelvic cavity using an endoscope.
gynecologist [gī-nĕ-KŎL-ō-jĭst] gyneco-, female + -logy, study of	Specialist who diagnoses and treats the processes and disorders of the female reproductive system.
hysterosalpingography [HĬS-tĕr-ō-săl-pĭng- GŎG-ră-fē] hystero-, uterus + salpingo-, fallopian tube + -graphy, a recording	X-ray of the uterus and uterine tubes after a contrast medium has been injected.
hysteroscopy [hĭs-tĕr-ŎS-kō-pē] hystero- + -scopy	Examination of the uterus using a hysteroscope.
mammography [mă-MŎG-ră-fē] mammo-, breast + -graphy	X-ray imaging of the breast as a cancer screening method.
obstetrician [ŏb-stĕ-TRĬSH-ŭn] Latin obstetrix, midwife	Physician who specializes in pregnancy and childbirth care.
Papanicolaou [pă-pă-NĒ-kō-lū] **(Pap) smear** After George N. Papanicolaou (1883–1962), Greek-American physician	Gathering of cells from the cervix and vagina to observe for abnormalities.
pelvimetry [pĕl-VĬM-ĕ-trē] pelvi(s) + -metry, measurement	Measurement of the pelvis during pregnancy.

CASE STUDY

Seeing a Specialist

The first patient, Jane Smits, called two days after her visit to say that the pain in her lower abdomen seemed to have increased. Also, she said that she had had some unusual bleeding from her vagina yesterday. She was told to come in and see Dr. Maurice Alvino, a gynecologist. He discussed her health history, examined her with a colposcope, and scheduled her for x-rays.

Critical Thinking

54. Why did Dr. Alvino use a colposcope?
55. What are some of the specific areas he might want to view on an x-ray?

Check Your Knowledge

Fill in the blanks.

56. Viewing of the cervix and vagina may be done with a _____.

57. Viewing of the uterus may be done with a _____.

58. Pap smears and mammograms are both _____ screening tests.

59. A pregnancy test can be performed on _____ or _____.

60. Presence of HCG indicates _____.

Pathological Terms

Pregnancy is a normal process, with gestation taking about 40 weeks and ending in the birth of an infant. Some pregnancies are not in themselves normal and spontaneously end in **abortion.** Abortion is a controversial term in public discourse, but in medicine, it simply means the premature end of a pregnancy, whether spontaneously during a **miscarriage,** or surgically. There are several types of abortion, such as *habitual abortion*—three or more consecutive abortions; *spontaneous abortions*—those that appear to occur for no specific medical reason; and *missed abortion,* an abortion in which the fetus is dead in the womb and must be removed surgically.

Complications of Pregnancy and Birth

Pregnancies can involve many complications. The initial pregnancy can implant abnormally outside the uterus as in an *ectopic pregnancy,* which requires surgery to remove the fetus because it will die due to lack of nourishment. A *tubal pregnancy* is implantation of the fertilized egg within the fallopian tube or partially within the tube and partially within the abdominal cavity or uterus, and also requires immediate surgical intervention to avoid rupture as the fertilized egg grows.

The Preeclampsia Foundation (www .preeclampsia.org) gives helpful information about this disease of pregnancy.

The placenta may break away from the uterine wall (**abruptio placentae**) and require immediate delivery of the infant. **Placenta previa** is a condition in which the placenta blocks the birth canal, and usually requires a caesarean delivery. Even though a pregnancy appears normal, a *stillbirth,* birth of a dead fetus, may occur. The typical pregnancy lasts from 37 to 40 weeks. An infant may be born *prematurely,* before 37 week's gestation. A toxic condition during pregnancy is called **preeclampsia.** Symptoms are sudden hypertension with proteinuria and/or edema. Left untreated, preeclampsia can lead to *eclampsia* or *toxemia,* which can be fatal. Routine prenatal care includes screening for the early warning signs of toxemia. Treatment is symptomatic and can halt progress of the condition. If symptoms persist, the fetus can be delivered early to prevent malignant hypertension and possible life-threatening complications. Routine care also screens for gestational diabetes. A urine test for glucose and GTT can reveal this condition.

One of the most dangerous conditions if untreated in pregnancy occurs when a mother has a different Rh factor from the father (blood types are discussed in Chapter 12). The fetus may then carry an Rh factor different from the mother's, in which case *Rh incompatibility* or *erythroblastosis fetalis,* a potentially dangerous fetal condition, may occur.

Normal delivery of an infant is with a *cephalic presentation*, in which the head appears first, but a fetus may have to be delivered in *breech presentation*, in which the buttocks or feet appear first.

Fetal birth defects can occur in any of the body's systems. The heart can have serious congenital defects. The lungs may not develop properly. In the reproductive system, abnormalities such as *hypospadias*, a defect in which the urethra opens below its normal position, can occur. Other malformations, such as of the uterus or uterine tubes, may cause fertility problems later in life.

Abnormalities in the Female Cycle

Menstrual abnormalities sometimes occur. **Amenorrhea,** the absence of menstruation, may result from a normal condition (pregnancy or menopause) or an abnormal condition (excessive dieting or extremely strenuous exercise). It may also occur for no apparent reason. **Dysmenorrhea** is painful cramping associated with menstruation. **Menorrhagia** is excessive menstrual bleeding. **Oligomenorrhea** is a scanty menstrual period. **Menometrorrhagia** is irregular and often excessive bleeding during or between menstrual periods. **Metro-rrhagia** is uterine bleeding between menstrual periods.

Other abnormal conditions in the female cycle also occur. **Anovulation** is the absence of ovulation. **Oligo-ovulation** is irregular ovulation. **Leukorrhea** is an abnormal vaginal discharge.

Abnormalities and Infections in the Reproductive System

Dyspareunia is painful sexual intercourse, usually due to some condition, such as dryness, inflammation, or other disorder, in the female reproductive system.

The uterus normally sits forward over the bladder. Abnormal positioning of the uterus includes **anteflexion,** a bending forward. **Retroflexion** is a bending backward of the uterus so that it is angled, and **retroversion** is a backward turn of the uterus (sometimes called a *tipped uterus*) so that it faces toward the back.

Various inflammations and infections occur in the female reproductive system. **Cervicitis** is an inflammation of the cervix. **Mastitis** is a general term for inflammation of the breast, particularly during lactation. **Salpingitis** is an inflammation of the fallopian tubes. **Vaginitis** is an inflammation of the vagina. *Toxic shock syndrome* is a rare, severe infection that occurs in menstruating women and is usually associated with tampon use. *Pelvic inflammatory disease* (PID) is a bacterial infection anywhere in the female reproductive system.

Organs of the reproductive system may suffer from muscle weakness. A *prolapsed uterus* is a condition where the uterine muscles cause the cervix to protrude into the vaginal opening. Perineal muscles can be strengthened using **Kegel exercises,** alternately contracting and releasing the perineal muscles.

Growths in the female reproductive system are benign or malignant and either one can cause pain, abnormal bleeding, infertility, and pregnancy complications. *Cervical polyps* usually start out benign, but can become malignant. If the accompanying bleeding is troublesome or if there is danger of their becoming malignant, polyps can be removed surgically. Cysts can form in any part of the female reproductive system. *Polycystic ovaries* are ovaries with many small cysts inside them. A *teratoma* is a type of germ cell tumor that is most often found in the ovaries. A benign teratoma of the ovary is known as a *dermoid cyst*.

A **condyloma** is a growth on the outside of the genitalia that may be a result of an infection by the human papilloma virus (HPV). An *ovarian cyst*

The Website www.endometriosis.org has information about the prevalence of endometriosis.

The National Breast Cancer Foundation (www.nationalbreastcancer.org) discusses the myths and truths about breast cancer.

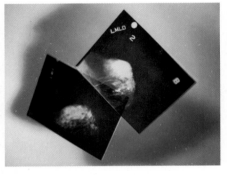

FIGURE 10-9 Healthy breast (left) and cancerous breast (right).

develops on or in the ovaries. **Fibroid**s are common benign tumors found in the uterus. They may cause pain and bleeding. Some growths occur when normal tissue is found in abnormal areas; for example, **endometriosis** is an abnormal condition in which uterine lining tissue (endometrium) is found in the pelvis or on the abdominal wall. This results in the endometrial cells growing and shedding with each menstrual cycle, making the problem worse with each passing month. Any symptom that is new or unusual should be watched and checked with a health care provider.

Malignant growths found in the reproductive system can be fatal unless detected early. Cervical cancer is often detected early with Pap smears before having spread (**carcinoma in situ**). *Endometrial cancer* occurs in the endometrium of the uterus. *Ovarian cancer* is a potentially fatal cancer of the ovary; it is difficult to diagnose in its earliest stages and often spreads to other organs before it is detected. Figure 10-9 shows two mammograms—the one on the left is of a healthy breast and the one on the right is a cancerous breast.

Breast cancer can be found locally in one site without spreading (*carcinoma in situ*) or may require more extensive treatment if it has spread to the lymph nodes. Breast cancer may sometimes be related to overproduction of estrogen. An important chemical test for estrogen receptors (cells that bind to estrogen) indicates whether hormone therapy is an option for women in perimenopause or menopause.

Sexually Transmitted Diseases

Sexually transmitted diseases (STDs) are diseases that are transmitted primarily through sexual contact. **Syphilis,** an infectious disease treatable with antibiotics; **gonorrhea,** a contagious infection of the genital mucous membrane; *Genital Herpes (HSV)*, a contagious and recurring infection with lesions on the genitalia; *human papilloma virus (HPV)*, a contagious infection that causes genital warts; **chlamydia,** a microorganism that causes several sexually transmitted diseases; and *HIV* (which leads to *AIDS*) are some common sexually transmitted diseases. HPV is sometimes associated with cervical cancer and is typically diagnosed by abnormal Pap test results. A new vaccine, Giardisil, is now available to protect women who have not been infected by HPV. *Trichomoniasis*, an infection, often in the vaginal tract, may also be transmitted through sexual contact.

The American Social Health Association (www.ashastd.org) gives information about the ways to avoid STDs.

VOCABULARY REVIEW

In the previous section, you learned terms related to pathology. Before going on to the exercises, review the terms below and refer to the previous section if you have any questions. Pronunciations are provided for certain terms. Sometimes information about where the word came from is included after the term. The etymologies (word histories) are for your information only. You do not need to memorize them.

Term	Definition
abortion [ă-BŎR-shŭn] From Latin *abortus*, abortion	Premature ending of a pregnancy.
abruptio placentae [ăb-RŬP-shē-ō plă-SĔN-tē] Latin, a breaking off of the placenta	Breaking away of the placenta from the uterine wall.
amenorrhea [ă-mĕn-ō-RĒ-ă] a-, without + meno-, menstruation + -rrhea, flow	Lack of menstruation.
anovulation [ăn-ŏv-yū-LĀ-shŭn] an-, without + ovulation	Lack of ovulation.
anteflexion [ăn-tē-FLĔK-shŭn] ante-, before + flexion, a bending	Bending forward, as of the uterus.
carcinoma in situ [kăr-sĭ-NŌ-mă ĭn SĪ-tū]	Localized malignancy that has not spread.
cervicitis [sĕr-vĭ-SĪ-tĭs] cervico-, cervix + -itis, inflammation	Inflammation of the cervix.
chlamydia [klă-MĬD-ē-ă] Greek *chlamys*, cloak	Sexually transmitted bacterial infection affecting various parts of the male or female reproductive systems; the bacterial agent itself.
condyloma [kŏn-dĭ-LŌ-mă] Greek *kondyloma*, knob	Growth on the external genitalia.
dysmenorrhea [dĭs-mĕn-ōr-Ē-ă] dys-, abnormal + meno- + -rrhea	Painful menstruation.
dyspareunia [dĭs-pă-RŪ-nē-ă] dys- + Greek *pareumos*, lying beside	Painful sexual intercourse due to any of various conditions, such as cysts, infection, or dryness, in the vagina.
endometriosis [ĔN-dō-mē-trē-Ō-sĭs] endometri(um) + -osis, condition	Abnormal condition in which uterine wall tissue is found in the pelvis or on the abdominal wall.
fibroid [FĪ-brŏyd]	Benign tumor commonly found in the uterus.
gonorrhea [gŏn-ō-RĒ-ă] Greek *gonorrhoia*, from *gone*, seed + -rrhea	Sexually transmitted inflammation of the genital membranes.
Kegel [KĒ-gĕl] **exercises** After A. H. Kegel, U. S. gynecologist	Exercises to strengthen perineal muscles.
leukorrhea [lū-kō-RĒ-ă] leuko-, white + -rrhea	Abnormal vaginal discharge; usually whitish.
mastitis [măs-TĪ-tĭs] mast-, breast + -itis	Inflammation of the breast.
menometrorrhagia [MĔN-ō-mĕ-trō-RĀ-jē-ă] meno- + metro-, uterus + -rrhagia	Irregular or excessive bleeding between or during menstruation.

Term	Definition
menorrhagia [měn-ō-RĀ-jē-ă] meno- + -rrhagia	Excessive menstrual bleeding.
metrorrhagia [mě-trŏ-RĀ-jē-ă] metro- + -rrhagia	Uterine bleeding between menstrual periods.
miscarriage [mǐs-KĂR-ăj]	Spontaneous, premature ending of a pregnancy.
oligomenorrhea [ŎL-ǐ-gō-měn-ō-RĒ-ă] oligo-, scanty + meno- + -rrhea	Scanty menstrual period.
oligo-ovulation [ŎL-ǐ-gō-ŎV-ū-LĀ-shŭn] oligo- + ovulation	Irregular ovulation.
placenta previa [plă-SĔN-tă PRĒ-vē-ă] placenta + Latin *prae*, before + *via*, the way	Placement of the placenta so it blocks the birth canal.
preeclampsia [prē-ě-KLĂMP-sē-ă] pre-, before + eclampsia, convulsion	Toxic infection during pregnancy.
retroflexion [rě-trō-FLĔK-shŭn] retro-, toward the back + flexion, a bending	Bending backward of the uterus.
retroversion [rě-trō-VĔR-zhŭn] retro- + version, a change of position	Backward turn of the uterus.
salpingitis [săl-pǐn-JĪ-tǐs] salping-, fallopian tube + -itis	Inflammation of the fallopian tubes.
syphilis [SĬF-ǐ-lǐs]	Sexually transmitted infection.
vaginitis [văj-ǐ-NĪ-tǐs] vagin-, vagina + -itis	Inflammation of the vagina.

PATHOLOGICAL TERMS EXERCISES

Check Your Knowledge

Fill in the blanks.

61. If an ovum is not fertilized, _____ usually occurs within two weeks.

62. Amenorrhea can result from two normal conditions: _____ and _____.

63. Painful menstruation is called _____.

64. Toxic shock syndrome is a rare infection that usually occurs during _____.

65. Pap smears test for _____ cancer.

66. Benign tumors found in the uterus are _____.

67. Perineal muscles can be strengthened using _____ exercises.

68. Chlamydia is an agent that can cause a _____ _____ disease.

69. An abortion is the premature ending of a _____, whether spontaneously or by choice.

70. Scanty menstruation is _____.

71. A toxic infection during pregnancy is _____.

72. AIDS is caused by _____, a virus.

73. A localized cancer is called a _____ _____ _____.

74. Uterine bleeding other than that associated with menstruation is called _____.

75. Delivery of the buttocks or feet first is known as a _____ _____.

76. Premature birth occurs before _____ weeks of gestation.

CASE STUDY

Finding the Cause

Sarah Messer recovered from menorrhagia and persistent ovarian pain, and was able to return to work after two days off. Six months later, however, Sarah experienced heavy bleeding and painful cramps after missing one menstrual period. She did not think she was pregnant, but Dr. Alvino had her HCG level checked and it showed that she was indeed pregnant. Sarah's bleeding turned out to be an early miscarriage. Dr. Alvino prescribed medication for the pain, and again told Sarah to take two days off from work, during which the bleeding should stop. If not, she was to call him.

Dr. Alvino talked to Sarah about the benefits of birth control. He particularly thought that condoms would be appropriate for now, while Sarah remains sexually active with more than one partner.

Critical Thinking

77. What diseases might Sarah contract if she does not use condoms?

78. Does the birth control pill protect you from sexually transmitted diseases?

Surgical Terms

Surgery of the female reproductive system is performed for a variety of reasons. During pregnancy, it may be necessary to terminate a pregnancy prematurely (*abortion*), to remove a fetus through an abdominal incision (*caesarean birth*), to open and scrape the lining of the uterus (*dilation and curettage* [*D & C*]), or to puncture the amniotic sac to obtain a sample of the fluid for examination (**amniocentesis**). In **culdocentesis,** a sample of fluid from the base of the pelvic cavity may show if an ectopic pregnancy has ruptured. An ectopic pregnancy can be removed through a *salpingotomy*, an incision into one of the fallopian tubes.

Surgery may also be performed as a form of birth control. *Tubal ligation,* a method of female sterilization, blocks the fallopian tubes by cutting or tying and, therefore, blocking the passage of ova. It is usually performed using a *laparoscope*, a thin tube inserted through a woman's navel during **laparoscopy.**

Cryosurgery and **cauterization** are two methods of destroying tissue (such as polyps), using cold temperatures in the former and burning in the latter. A Loop Electrosurgical Excision Procedure (LEEP) is the removal of precancerous tissue from around the cervix with a wirelike instrument.

Parts of the female reproductive system may have to be removed, usually because of the presence of cancer or benign growths that cause pain or excessive bleeding. A biopsy is usually performed first to determine the spread of cancer. A **conization** is the removal of a cone-shaped section of the cervix for examination. Breast cancer may be diagnosed by **aspiration,** a type of biopsy in which fluid is withdrawn through a needle by suction. A **hysterectomy** is removal of the uterus that may be done through the

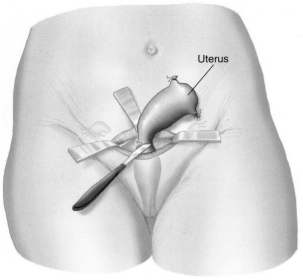

Abdominal hysterectomy

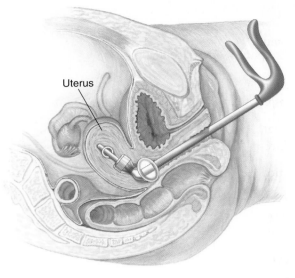

Vaginal hysterectomy

FIGURE 10-10 Hysterectomies can be performed abdominally or vaginally. A surgical instrument is inserted through the cervix in a vaginal hysterectomy.

abdomen (*abdominal hysterectomy*) or through the vagina (*vaginal hysterectomy*). Figure 10-10 shows the two types of hysterectomies. New procedures such as *laparascopic hysterectomies* are reducing recovery time.

A **myomectomy** is the removal of fibroid tumors. An **oophorectomy** is the removal of an ovary. An *ovarian cystectomy* is the removal of an ovarian cyst. A **salpingectomy** is the removal of a fallopian tube. A *salpingo-oophorectomy* is the removal of one ovary and one fallopian tube. A *bilateral salpingo-oophorectomy* is the removal of both ovaries and both fallopian tubes. A **salpingotomy** is an incision into the fallopian tubes (usually to remove blockages).

Breast cancer may be treated surgically. A **lumpectomy** is the removal of the tumor itself along with surrounding tissue. During a **mastectomy,** a breast is removed, which may mean the breast and underlying muscle as in a simple mastectomy; the breast, underlying muscles, and the lymph nodes, as in a *radical mastectomy;* or removal of the breast and lymph nodes, as in a *modified radical mastectomy.*

Breast surgery may include plastic surgery after mastectomy (**mammoplasty**) or reduction of the size of the breast (*reduction mammoplasty*). Some women have pendulous breast tissue raised (**mastopexy**) or have small breasts augmented by surgical insertion of implants (*augmentation mammoplasty*).

VOCABULARY REVIEW

In the previous section, you learned terms relating to surgery. Before going on to the exercises, review the terms below and refer to the previous section if you have any questions. Pronunciations are provided for certain terms. Sometimes information about where the word came from is included after the term. These etymologies (word histories) are for your information only. You do not need to memorize them.

Term	Meaning
amniocentesis [ĂM-nē-ō-sĕn-TĒ-sĭs] amnio-, amnion + -centesis, puncture	Removal of a sample of amniotic fluid through a needle injected in the amniotic sac.
aspiration [ăs-pĭ-RĀ-shŭn] Latin *aspiratio*, breath	Biopsy in which fluid is withdrawn through a needle by suction.
cauterization [kăw-tĕr-ĭ-ZĀ-shŭn] From Greek *kauterion*, a branding iron	Removal or destruction of tissue using chemicals or devices such as laser-guided equipment.
conization [kō-nĭ-ZĀ-shŭn]	Removal of a cone-shaped section of the cervix for examination.
cryosurgery [krī-ō-SĔR-jĕr-ē] cryo-, cold + surgery	Removal or destruction of tissue using cold temperatures.
culdocentesis [KŬL-dō-sĕn-TĒ-sĭs] French *cul-de-sac*, bottom of the sack + -centesis	Taking of a fluid sample from the base of the pelvic cavity to see if an ectopic pregnancy has ruptured.
hysterectomy [hĭs-tĕr-ĔK-tō-mē] hyster-, uterus + -ectomy, removal	Removal of the uterus.
laparoscopy [lăp-ă-RŎS-kō-pē] laparo-, loins + -scopy, a viewing	Use of a lighted tubular instrument inserted through a woman's navel to perform a tubal ligation or to examine the fallopian tubes.
lumpectomy [lŭm-PĔK-tō-mē] lump + -ectomy	Removal of a breast tumor.
mammoplasty [MĂM-ō-plăs-tē] mammo-, breast + -plasty, repair	Plastic surgery to reconstruct the breast, particularly after a mastectomy.
mastectomy [măs-TĔK-tō-mē] mast-, breast + -ectomy	Removal of a breast.
mastopexy [MĂS-tō-pĕk-sē] masto-, breast + -pexy, an attaching	Surgical procedure to attach sagging breasts in a more normal position.
myomectomy [mī-ō-MĔK-tō-mē] myoma, benign tumor + -ectomy	Removal of fibroids from the uterus.
oophorectomy [ō-ŏf-ōr-ĔK-tō-mē] oophor-, ovary + -ectomy	Removal of an ovary.
salpingectomy [săl-pĭn-JĔK-tō-mē] salping-, fallopian tube + -ectomy	Removal of a fallopian tube.
salpingotomy [săl-pĭng-GŎT-ō-mē] salpingo- + -tomy, a cutting	Incision into the fallopian tubes.

CASE STUDY

Treating the Problem

Jane Smits learned in her next exam that she now has some cysts on her left ovary. Her right ovary had been removed earlier because of cysts. Jane wants to have a child and expresses her concern to Dr. Alvino.

Critical Thinking

79. Jane had a surgery in which one ovary and one fallopian tube were removed. What is the medical term for this surgery?

80. Jane wants to have children. How might her current condition present a problem?

SURGICAL TERMS EXERCISES

Know the Parts

Refer to Figure 10-1 is on p. 325. In the following list, write the name of the part(s) to be removed or altered in the surgery indicated.

81. salpingectomy _____

82. hysterectomy _____

83. bilateral salpingo-oophorectomy _____

84. tubal ligation _____

Pharmacological Terms

Various forms of birth control are pharmacological agents. Spermicides destroy sperm in the vagina; **birth control pills** (or oral contraceptives, OCPs), hormonal, patches, vaginal rings, and **implants** control the flow of hormones to block ovulation; and **abortifacients** or **morning-after pills** (or emergency contraception) prevent implantation of an ovum. **Hormone replacement therapy (HRT)** is used during and after menopause to alleviate symptoms, such as hot flashes. **Oxytocin,** another hormone, is used to induce labor. A **tocolytic agent** stops labor contractions. Table 10-2 lists common pharmacological agents used for the female reproductive system.

TABLE 10-2 Some Common Medications Used in Providing Birth Control and in Treating Disorders of the Female Reproductive System

Drug Class	Purpose	Generic	Trade Name
abortifacient emergency contraception or morning-after pill	to prevent implantation of an ovum	mifepristone	Mifeprex
hormone replacement therapy (HRT)	to normalize hormone levels in the body	raloxifene alendronate estrogen estrogen/progestin	Evista Fosamax Premarin Prempro
hormones related to birth	to induce labor to stop labor	oxytocin tocolytic	Pitocin various

VOCABULARY REVIEW

In the previous section, you learned terms related to pharmacology. Before going on to the exercises, review the terms below and refer to the previous section if you have any questions. Pronunciations are provided for certain terms. Sometimes information about where the word came from is included after the term. The etymologies (word histories) are for your information only. You do not need to memorize them.

Agent	Purpose
abortifacient [ă-bŏr-tĭ-FĀ-shĕnt] Latin *abortus*, abortion + *faceo*, to make	Medication to prevent implantation of an ovum.
birth control pills or implants	Medication that controls the flow of hormones to block ovulation.
hormone replacement therapy (HRT)	Treatment with hormones when the body stops or decreases the production of hormones by itself.
morning-after pill	*See* abortifacient.
oxytocin [ŏk-sē-TŌ-sĭn] Greek *okytokos*, quick birth	Hormone given to induce labor.
tocolytic [tō-kō-LĬT-ĭk] **agent** Greek *tokos*, birth + -lytic, loosening	Hormone given to stop labor.

CASE STUDY

Removing a Malignancy

Jane Smits, who had several check-ups over the next few months, eventually required a hysterectomy. Some abnormal cells on her latest Pap smear turned out to be malignant. The cancer was contained, so her prognosis for recovery is excellent.

Critical Thinking

85. Jane, 30 years old at the time of her hysterectomy, was given estrogen and progesterone following her surgery. What is this treatment called?
86. Is it necessary for Jane and her husband to use birth control?

PHARMACOLOGICAL TERMS EXERCISES

Check Your Knowledge

Circle T for true or F for false.

87. An abortifacient is a birth control medication. T F
88. Hormone replacement therapy is generally used around menopause. T F
89. It is never appropriate to induce labor. T F
90. Birth control pills are used to control hormones. T F
91. Tocolytic agents stop labor. T F

CHALLENGE SECTION

Dr. Maya Lundgren, an obstetrician at the HMO, examined Elisa Mayaguez, who is 26 years old. Dr. Lundgren entered the following notes on Elisa's record.

Patient is 26 years old, gravida II, para I, who was seen in the office today with symptoms of preterm labor at 30-weeks' gestation.

Patient reports an uncomplicated prenatal course until two weeks ago. Patient stated that she had some break-through bleeding, which seemed to improve following bed rest. Patient reports mild, regular contractions starting yesterday but diminishing today. Patient reports only mild "twinges" today. No cramping or back pain. She had preterm labor with her first pregnancy. Her first child was born at 32-weeks' gestation.

Physical exam was essentially normal. BP 130/80, P 100. HEENT: PERRLA. Lungs were clear to auscultation. Pelvic exam consistent with gestational dates. Cervix is dilated 2 cm. No edema noted. Her membranes are intact. Fetal heart tones 150s with increases noted to 170s. Baby active.

Patient was placed on strict bed rest. She was prescribed oral terbutaline to suppress labor. Patient to return to office in one week.

Critical Thinking

92. The patient's first child was born at 32-weeks' gestation. What is the period of normal gestation? Was her first child born preterm or postterm?

93. The patient is gravida II, para I. What does this mean?

TERMINOLOGY IN ACTION

The following are chart notes for a routine gynecological exam:

Patient: Marina Telly   March 30, 2XXX

S: Marina is a 47-year-old, gravida 4, para 4-0-0-4, being seen for an annual gynecological exam. She has had amenorrhea for 3 years and has a lot of trouble with hot flashes. She was placed on estrogen 4 months ago but that made her very sick. She has otherwise been well.

Gyn. History: Menses began at age 14 with PMS as a teenager. She has had 2 C-sections: 1 for eclampsia and 1 for cephalopelvic disproportion.

O: Breasts are pendulous with no discernible masses. Abdomen is soft; no organs or masses noted. Pelvic exam shows external genitalia are normal. Vagina and cervix show mild atrophic changes. Uterus is in midposition and feels normal in size. Stool is guaiac negative. Pap smear is done. Mammogram results sent in about two weeks ago are normal.

A: Annual gynecological examination.

P: Patient is undecided about trying another HRT treatment. I gave her all appropriate literature and she will let me know if she wants to try a different hormone. I am scheduling a bone density study.

From the chart, how many children does Marina have? How regular are her periods? What is likely causing her discomfort?

USING THE INTERNET

Go to the Centers for Disease Control site for Women's Health Risks (http://www.cdc.gov/health/womensmenu.htm) and write a paragraph on the latest news in breast and cervical cancer prevention.

CHAPTER REVIEW

The material that follows is to help you review all the material in this chapter.

Understanding Word Parts

For each of the following terms, write the definition and the meaning of each word part.

94. mammogram _____

95. dysmenorrhea _____

96. neonatologist _____

97. amniocentesis _____

98. oligomenorrhea _____

99. metritis _____

100. prenatal _____

101. salpingitis _____

102. uteroplasty _____

103. hysterectomy _____

Understanding Female Reproductive Terms

Complete each of the following terms.

104. breast reconstruction: mamma_____

105. vaginal infection: _____itis

106. first pregnancy: primi_____

107. cervical inflammation: _____itis

108. inflammation of the peritoneum: _____itis

109. ovarian hernia: ovari_____

110. female reproductive system specialist: _____logist

111. uterine hemorrhage: metro_____

112. instrument for uterine examination: hystero_____

113. time just preceding menopause: _____menopause

DEFINITIONS

Define the following terms and combining forms. Review the chapter before starting. Make sure you know how to pronounce each term as you define it. The blue words in brackets are references to the Spanish glossary available online at www.mhhe/medterm3e.

WORD

114. abortion [ă-BŎR-shŭn] {aborto}

115. abortifacient [ă-bŏr-tǐ-FĀ-shĕnt] {abortifaciente}

116. abruptio placentae [ăb-RŬP-shē-ō plă-SĔN-tē]

117. afterbirth [ĂF-tĕr-bĕrth]{secundina}

118. amenorrhea [ā-mĕn-ō-RĒ-ă]{amenorrea}

119. amni(o)

120. amniocentesis [ĂM-nē-ō-sĕn-TĒ-sǐs]{amniocentesis}

121. amnion [ĂM-nē-ŏn]{amnios}

122. amniotic [ăm-nē-ŎT-ĭk] fluid {amniótico}

123. anovulation [ăn-ŏv-yū-LĀ-shŭn]

124. anteflexion [ăn-tē-FLĔK-shŭn] {anteflaxión}

125. areola [ă-RĒ-ō-lă] {areola}

126. aspiration [ăs-pǐ-RĀ-shŭn] {aspiración}

127. Bartholin's [BĂR-thō-lĕnz] gland
128. birth control pills or implants
129. body {cuerpo}
130. carcinoma in situ [kăr-sĭ-NŌ-mă ĭn SĪ-tū]
131. cauterization [kăw-tĕr-ĭ-ZĀ-shŭn] {cauterización}
132. cervic(o)
133. cervicitis [sĕr-vĭ-SĪ-tĭs]
134. cervix [SĔR-vĭks] {cervix}
135. chlamydia [klă-MĬD-ē-ă] {clamidia}
136. chorion [KŌ-rē-ŏn] {corion}
137. climacteric [klī-MĂK-tĕr-ĭk, klī-măk-TĔR-ĭk] {climaterio}
138. clitoris [KLĬT-ō-rĭs] {clítoris}
139. coitus [KŌ-ĭ-tŭs] {coito}
140. colp(o)
141. colposcopy [kōl-PŎS-kō-pē]
142. condom [KŎN-dŏm] {condón}
143. condyloma [kŏn-dĭ-LŌ-mă] {condiloma}
144. conization [kō-nĭ-ZĀ-shŭn] {conización}
145. contraception [kŏn-tră-SĔP-shŭn] {anticoncepción}
146. copulation [kŏp-yū-LĀ-shŭn] {copulación}
147. corpus luteum [KŌR-pŭs LŪ-tē-ŭm]

148. cryosurgery [krī-ō-SĔR-jĕr-ē] {criocirugía}
149. culdocentesis [KŬL-dō-sĕn-tē-sĭs]
150. culdoscopy [kŭl-DŎS-kō-pē]
151. diaphragm [DĪ-ă-frăm] {diafragma}
152. dysmenorrhea [dĭs-mĕn-ōr-Ē-ă] {dismenorrea}
153. dyspareunia [dĭs-pă-RŪ-nē-ă] {dispareunia}
154. endometriosis [ĔN-dō-mē-trē-Ō-sĭs] {endometriosis}
155. endometrium [ĔN-dō-MĒ-trē-ŭm] {endometrio}
156. episi(o)
157. estrogen [ĔS-trō-jĕn] {estrógeno}
158. fallopian [fă-LŌ-pē-ăn] tube
159. fibroid [FĪ-brŏyd] {fibroide}
160. fimbriae [FĬM-brē-ē] {fimbrias}
161. follicle-stimulating hormone (FSH)
162. foreskin [FŌR-skĭn] {prepucio}
163. fundus [FŬN-dŭs] {fondo}
164. galact(o)
165. gamete [GĂM-ēt] {gameto}
166. gestation [jĕs-TĀ-shŭn] {gestación}
167. gonad [GŌ-năd] {gónada}
168. gonorrhea [gŏn-ō-RĒ-ă] {gonorrea}
169. graafian follicle [gră-FĒ-ăn FŎL-ĭ-kl]
170. gravida [GRĂV-ĭ-dă] {grávida}
171. gynec(o)

172. gynecologist [gī-nĕ-KŎL-ō-jĭst] {ginecólogo}
173. hormone [HŌR-mōn] {hormona}
174. hormone replacement therapy (HRT)
175. hymen [HĪ-mĕn] {himen}
176. hyster(o)
177. hysterectomy [hĭs-tĕr-ĔK-tō-mē] {histerectomía}
178. hysterosalpingography [HĬS-tĕr-ō-săl-pĭng-GŎG-ră-fē] {histerosalpingografía}
179. hysteroscopy [hĭs-tĕr-ŎS-kō-pē] {histeroscopia}
180. intrauterine [ĬN-tră-YŪ-tĕr-ĭn] device (IUD)
181. introitus [ĭn-TRŌ-ĭ-tŭs] {introito}
182. isthmus [ĬS-mŭs] {istmo}
183. Kegel [KĒ-gĕl] exercises
184. labia majora [LĀ-bē-ă mă-JŌR-ă]
185. labia minora [mī-NŌR-ă]
186. lact(o), lacti
187. lactiferous [lăk-TĬF-ĕr-ŭs] {lactífero}
188. laparoscopy [lăp-ă-RŎS-kō-pē] {laparoscopia}
189. leukorrhea [lū-kō-RĒ-ă] {leucorrea}
190. lumpectomy [lŭm-PĔK-tō-mē] {nodulectomía}
191. luteinizing [LŪ-tē-ĭn-Ī-zĭng] hormone (LH)
192. mamm(o)
193. mammary [MĂM-ă-rē] glands

194. mammography [mă-MŎG-ră-fē] {mamografía}

195. mammoplasty [MĂM-ō-plăs-tē] {mamoplastia}

196. mast(o)

197. mastectomy [măs-TĔK-tō-mē] {mastectomía}

198. mastitis [măs-TĪ-tĭs] {mastitis}

199. mastopexy [MĂS-tō-pĕk-sē]

200. men(o)

201. menarche [mĕ-NĂR-kē] {menarca}

202. menometrorrhagia [MĔN-ō-mĕ-trō-RĀ-jē-ă]

203. menopause [MĔN-ō-păwz] {menopausia}

204. menorrhagia [mĕn-ō-RĀ-jē-ă] {menorragia}

205. menstruation [mĕn-strū-Ā-shŭn] {menstruación}

206. metr(o)

207. metrorrhagia [mĕ-trō-RĀ-jē-ă] {metrorragia}

208. miscarriage [mĭs-KĂR-ăj] {aborto espontáneo}

209. mons pubis [mŏnz pyū-BĬS]

200. morning-after pill

211. myomectomy [mī-ō-MĔK-tō-mē] {miomectomía}

212. myometrium [MĪ-ō-MĒ-trē-ŭm] {miometrio}

213. nipple [NĬP-l] {pezón}

214. obstetrician [ŏb-stĕ-TRĬSH-ŭn] {obstetra}

215. oligomenorrhea [ŎL-ĭ-gō-mĕn-ō-RĒ-ă] {oligomenorrea}

216. oligo-ovulation [ŎL-ĭ-gō-ŎV-ū-LĀ-shŭn]

217. oo

218. oocyte [Ō-ō-sīt] {oocito}

219. oophor(o)

220. oophorectomy [ō-ŏf-ōr-ĔK-tō-mē] {ooforectomía}

221. ov(i), ov(o)

222. ovari(o)

223. ovary [Ō-vă-rē] {ovario}

224. ovulation [ŎV-yū-LĀ-shŭn] {ovulación}

225. ovum (pl. ova) [Ō-vŭm (Ō-vă)] {óvulo}

226. oxytocin [ŏk-sē-TŌ-sĭn]

227. Papanicolaou [pă-pă-NĒ-kō-lū] (Pap) smear

228. para [PĂ-ră]

229. parturition [păr-tūr-ĬSH-ŭn] {parturición}

230. pelvimetry [pĕl-VĬM-ĕ-trē]

231. perimenopause [pĕr-ĭ-MĔN-ō-păws]

232. perimetrium [pĕr-ĭ-MĒ-trē-ŭm] {perimetrio}

233. perine(o)

234. perineum [PĔR-ĭ-NĒ-ŭm]

235. placenta [plă-SĔN-tă] {placenta}

236. placenta previa [plă-SĔN-tă PRĒ-vē-ă]

237. preeclampsia [prē-ĕ-KLĂMP-sē-ă]

238. progesterone [prō-JĔS-tĕr-ōn] {progesterona}

239. puberty [PYŪ-bĕr-tē] {pubertad}

240. retroflexion [rĕ-trō-FLĔK-shŭn] {retroflexión}

241. retroversion [rĕ-trō-VĔR-zhŭn] {retroversión}

242. salping(o)

243. salpingectomy [săl-pĭn-JĔK-tō-mē]

244. salpingitis [săl-pĭn-JĪ-tĭs] {salpingitis}

245. salpingotomy [săl-pĭng-GŎT-ō-mē]

246. sinus [SĪ-nŭs] {seno}

247. spermicide [SPĔR-mĭ-sīd] {espermicida}

248. sponge {esponja}

249. syphilis [SĬF-ĭ-lĭs] {sífilis}

250. tocolytic [tō-kō-LĬT-ĭk] agent

251. umbilical [ŭm-BĬL-ĭ-kăl] cord

252. uter(o)

253. uterine [YŪ-tĕr-ĭn] tube

254. uterus [YŪ-tĕr-ŭs] {útero}

255. vagin(o)

256. vagina [vă-JĪ-nă] {vagina}

257. vaginitis [văj-ĭ-NĪ-tĭs] {vaginitis}

258. vulv(o)

259. vulva [VŬL-vă] {vulva}

Abbreviations

Write the full meaning of each abbreviation.

260. AB

261. AFP

262. AH

263. CIS

264. CS

265. C-section

266. C_X

267. D & C

268. DES

269. DUB

270. ECC

271. EDC

272. EMB

273. ERT

274. FHT

275. FSH

276. G

277. gyn

278. HCG

279. HRT

280. HSG

281. HSO

282. IUD

283. LH

284. LMP

285. multip

286. OB

287. OCP

288. P

289. Pap smear

290. PID

291. PMP

292. PMS

293. primip

294. TAH-BSO

295. TSS

296. UC

Answers to Chapter Exercises

1. Without fever.
2. Ovaries do not always alternate ovulation by month. Her single ovary has taken over the function of both.
3. c
4. a
5. b
6. d
7. ovary
8. uterus
9. ovulation
10. menstruation
11. fundus
12. cervix
13. perimetrium
14. breasts
15. menarche
16. menopause
17. estrogen, progesterone
18. contraception
19. chorion, amnion
20. afterbirth
21. postpartum
22. no
23. blood pressure, pulse, yes
24. episiostenosis
25. mammogram
26. galactopoiesis
27. ovariocele
28. lactogen
29. perineorrhaphy
30. vaginomycosis
31. metralgia, metrodynia
32. vulvitis
33. colporrhagia
34. oogenesis
35. mastopathy
36. uteroplasty
37. salpingitis
38. cervicectomy
39. oophoroma
40. ovariotomy
41. metrostenosis
42. gynecoid
43. amniorrhexis
44. j
45. e
46. a

47. g
48. b
49. i
50. c
51. d
52. f
53. h
54. Jane's suggested diagnosis was pelvic inflammatory disease (PID). Examination of the vagina is a first step to confirming the diagnosis and seeing if there is an additional problem.
55. uterus, ovaries, fallopian tubes
56. colposcope
57. hysteroscope
58. cancer
59. blood, urine
60. pregnancy
61. menstruation
62. pregnancy, menopause
63. dysmenorrhea
64. menstruation
65. cervical
66. fibroids
67. Kegel
68. sexually transmitted
69. pregnancy
70. oligomenorrhea
71. preeclampsia
72. HIV
73. carcinoma in situ
74. metrorrhagia
75. breech birth
76. 37
77. a sexually transmitted disease, such as HIV, gonorrhea, herpes II, HPV, or chlamydia
78. No; it does not block fluid-tofluid contact.
79. salpingo-oophorectomy
80. If her left ovary needs to be removed, Jane will not be able to get pregnant.
81. uterine/fallopian tube
82. uterus
83. uterine tubes and ovaries
84. uterine tubes
85. hormone replacement therapy

86. No, a hysterectomy means that pregnancy is not possible.
87. T
88. T
89. F
90. T
91. T
92. 37-40 weeks; preterm
93. She is in her second pregnancy and has one other child.
94. breast imaging: mamo-, breast; -gram, recording
95. painful menstruation: dys-, difficult; meno-, menstruation; -rrhea, flow
96. specialist in treating newborns: neo-, new; nat(al), of birth; -ologist, specialist
97. puncture into the amnion to withdraw fluid: amnio-, amnion; -centesis, puncture
98. scanty menstruation: oligo, scanty; meno-, menstruation; -rrhea, flow
99. uterine inflammation: metr-, uterus; itis, inflammation
100. before birth: pre-, before; natal, of birth
101. fallopian tube inflammation: salping-, fallopian tube; -itis, inflammation
102. surgical repair of the uterus: utero-, uterus; -plasty, surgical repair
103. removal of the uterus: hyster-, uterus; -ectomy, removal
104. mammaplasty
105. vaginitis
106. primpara
107. cervicitis
108. peritonitis
109. ovaricele
110. gynecologist
111. metrorrhagia
112. hysteroscope
113. perimenopause
114–296. Answers are available in the vocabulary reviews in this chapter.

CHAPTER 11

▶ UROLOGY

The Male Reproductive System

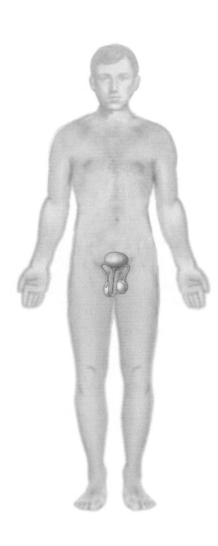

After studying this chapter, you will be able to:

11.1   Name the parts of the male reproductive system and discuss the function of each part

11.2   Define combining forms used in building words that relate to the male reproductive system

11.3   Identify the meaning of related abbreviations

11.4   Name the common diagnoses, clinical procedures, and laboratory tests used in treating disorders of the male reproductive system

11.5   List and define the major pathological conditions of the male reproductive system

11.6   Explain the meaning of surgical terms related to the male reproductive system

11.7   Recognize common pharmacological agents used in treating disorders of the male reproductive system

Structure and Function

The sex cell or **spermatozoon** (plural, **spermatozoa**) or **sperm** is produced in the male gonads or **testes** (singular *testis*). The testes are also called **testicles** and are contained within the **scrotum,** a sac outside the body. The scrotal sack holds and protects the testes as well as regulating the temperature of the testicles. If the testicles are too cold, the scrotum contracts to draw them closer to the body for warmth. If the testicles are too warm, then the scrotum relaxes to draw the testicles away from the body's heat.

The development of sperm (**spermatogenesis**) takes place in the scrotum, where the temperature is lower than inside the body. The lower temperature is necessary for the safe development of sperm. Inside the testes are cells that manufacture the sperm cells. These cells are contained in *seminiferous tubules*. Between the seminiferous tubules lie endocrine cells that produce **testosterone,** the most important male hormone; it is thought to decrease during a stage of life sometimes referred to as "male menopause." Table 11-1 lists the male reproductive hormones and their purpose.

At the top part of each testis is the **epididymis,** a group of ducts for storing sperm. The sperm develop to maturity and become *motile* (able to move) in the epididymis. They leave the epididymis and enter a narrow tube called the **vas deferens.** The sperm then travel to the *seminal vesicles* (which secrete material to help the sperm move) and to the *ejaculatory duct* leading to the **prostate gland** and the urethra. The prostate gland also secretes

TABLE 11-1 Male Reproductive Hormones

Hormone	Purpose	Source
testosterone	stimulates development of male sex characteristics; increases sperm; inhibits LH	testes
FSH (follicle-stimulating hormone)	increases testosterone; aids in sperm production	pituitary gland
LH	stimulates testosterone secretion	pituitary gland
inhibin	inhibits FSH	testes

prostatic fluid, which provides a milky color to **semen** (a mixture of sperm and secretions from the seminal vesicles, Cowper's glands, and prostate) and helps the sperm move. The gland then contracts its muscular tissue during ejaculation to help the sperm exit the body.

Just below the prostate are the two **bulbourethral glands (Cowper's glands)** that also secrete a fluid that neutralizes the acidity of the male urethra prior to ejaculation. The urethra passes through the **penis** to the outside of the body. The tip of the penis is called the **glans penis,** a sensitive area covered by the **foreskin** (*prepuce*). Between the penis and the anus is the area called the **perineum.** Figure 11-1a shows the male reproductive system. Figure 11-1b is a diagram of the path of sperm through the system.

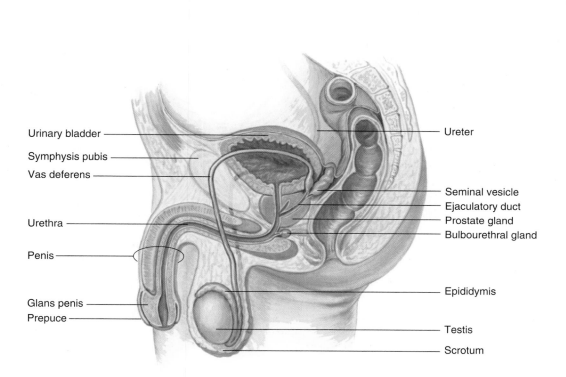

FIGURE 11-1A   The male reproductive system usually maintains fertility well into old age.

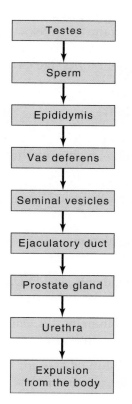

FIGURE 11-1B   A diagram of the path that sperm travel.

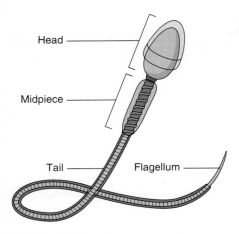

Head

Midpiece

Tail   Flagellum

FIGURE 11-2 Spermatozoa have a flagellum to help propel them forward.

MORE ABOUT . . .

Male Hormones

Traditionally, the term menopause has referred to women only. In recent years, some researchers have studied the hormonal cycle of males. While males do not experience menstruation and its ultimate cessation, they do seem to experience reduced hormone production, particularly testosterone. This can cause symptoms similar to those of female menopause, including mood swings, decreased libido, and increased fatigue. Some men require treatment with hormonal therapy.

The spermatozoon is a microscopic cell, much smaller than an ovum. It has a head region that carries genetic material (*chromosomes*) and a tail (**flagellum**) that propels the sperm forward (Figure 11-2). During **ejaculation,** hundreds of millions of sperm are released. Usually only one sperm can fertilize a single ovum. In rare instances, two or more ova are fertilized at a single time, resulting in twins, triplets, quadruplets, and so on. *Identical twins* are the result of one ovum's splitting after it has been fertilized by a single sperm. *Fraternal twins* are the result of two sperm fertilizing two ova.

VOCABULARY REVIEW

In the previous section, you learned terms relating to the male reproductive system. Before going on to the exercises, review the terms below and refer to the previous section if you have any questions. Pronunciations are provided for certain terms. Sometimes information about where the word came from is included after the term. These etymologies (word histories) are for your information only. You do not need to memorize them.

Term	Definition
bulbourethral [BŬL-bō-yū-RĒ-thrăl] **gland** bulbo-, bulb + urethra	*See* Cowper's gland.
Cowper's [KŎW-pĕrs] **gland** After William Cowper (1666–1709), English anatomist	One of two glands below the prostate that secrete a fluid to lubricate the inside of the urethra.
ejaculation [ē-jăk-yū-LĀ-shŭn] Latin *e-iaculo*, to shoot out	Expulsion of semen outside the body.
epididymis [ĕp-ĭ-DĬD-ĭ-mĭs] Greek, on twins (testes)	Group of ducts at the top of the testis where sperm are stored.
flagellum [flă-JĔL-ŭm] Latin, little whip	Tail at the end of a sperm that helps it move.
foreskin [FŌR-skĭn] fore-, in front + skin	Flap of skin covering the glans penis; removed by circumcision in many cultures.
glans penis [glănz PĒ-nĭs] Latin *glans*, acorn	Sensitive area at the tip of the penis.

Term	Definition
penis [PĒ-nĭs]	Male reproductive part that covers the urethra on the outside of the body.
perineum [PĔR-ĭ-NĒ-ŭm] Greek *perineon*	Area between the penis and the anus.
prostate [PRŎS-tāt] **gland** Greek *prostates*, one that protects	Gland surrounding the urethra that emits a fluid to help the sperm move and contracts its muscular tissue during ejaculation to help the sperm exit the body.
scrotum [SKRŌ-tŭm] Latin, sac	Sac outside the body containing the testicles.
semen [SĒ-mĕn] Latin, seed	Thick, whitish fluid containing spermatozoa and secretions from the seminal vesicles, Cowper's glands, and prostate; ejaculated from the penis.
sperm [spĕrm] Greek *sperma*, seed	Male sex cell that contains chromosomes.
spermatogenesis [SPĔR-mă-tō-JĔN-ĕ-sĭs] spermato-, sperm + -genesis	Production of sperm.
spermatozoon (*pl.*, **spermatozoa**) [SPĔR-mă-tō-ZŌ-ŏn (SPĔR-mă-tō-ZŌ-ă)] spermato- + Greek *zoon*, animal	*See* sperm.
testicle [TĔS-tĭ-kl] Latin *testiculus*, small testis	*See* testis.
testis (*pl.*, **testes**) [TĔS-tĭs (TĔS-tēz)] Latin	One of a pair of male organs that produce sperm and are contained in the scrotum.
testosterone [tĕs-TŎS-tĕ-rōn]	Primary male hormone.
vas deferens [văs DĔF-ĕr-ĕns] Latin, vessel that carries away	Narrow tube through which sperm leave the epididymis and travel to the seminal vesicles and into the urethra.

CASE STUDY

Getting Help

Marta and Luis Consalvo have been trying to have a baby for two years. They are both young and healthy. Recently, Marta's obstetrician-gynecologist referred the couple to an infertility clinic. The doctors at the clinic found nothing in Marta that would cause infertility. They found, however, that Luis had a low sperm count. Marta's ob-gyn referred Luis to a urologist, Dr. Medina, for an examination.

Critical Thinking

1. Why did Marta's physician refer Luis to a urologist?
2. What parts of the male reproductive system might Dr. Medina examine for the cause of Luis's low sperm count?

Check Your Knowledge

Choose answer a, b, or c to identify each of the following parts of the reproductive system.

a. only in males   b. only in females   c. in both males and females

3. sex cell _____

4. prostate gland _____

5. perineum _____

6. foreskin _____

7. scrotum _____

8. epididymis _____

9. fallopian tube _____

10. gamete _____

11. ova _____

12. spermatozoa _____

Put in order the following sites through which sperm travel, starting with the letter a.

13. epididymis _____

14. seminal vesicles _____

15. testes _____

16. ejaculatory ducts _____

17. vas deferens _____

18. urethra _____

Check Your Understanding

Circle T for true or F for false.

19. Urine is stored in the prostate gland. T F

20. Fluid from the seminal vesicles helps the sperm move. T F

21. During ejaculation, about three thousand sperm are released. T F

22. Cowper's gland is another name for the prostate gland. T F

23. Identical twins result from two sperm and one ovum. T F

24. Male genetic material is called testosterone. T F

25. In many cultures, the glans penis is removed during circumcision. T F

Combining Forms and Abbreviations

The lists below include combining forms and abbreviations that relate specifically to the male reproductive system. Pronunciations are provided for the examples.

COMBINING FORM	MEANING	EXAMPLE
andr(o)	men	*andropathy* [ăn-DRŎP-ă-thē], any disease peculiar to men
balan(o)	glans penis	*balanitis* [băl-ă-NĪ-tĭs], inflammation of the glans penis
epididym(o)	epididymis	*epididymoplasty* [ĕp-ĭ-DĬD-ĭ-mō-plăs-tē], surgical repair of the epididymis
orch(o), orchi(o), orchid(o)	testes	*orchitis* [ŏr-KĪ-tĭs], inflammation of the testis

Combining Form	Meaning	Example
prostat(o)	prostate gland	*prostatitis* [prŏs-tă-TĪ-tĭs], inflammation of the prostate
sperm(o), spermat(o)	sperm	*spermatogenesis* [SPĔR-mă-tō-JĔN-ē-sĭs], sperm production

Abbreviation	Meaning	Abbreviation	Meaning
AIH	artificial insemination homologous	SPP	suprapubic prostatectomy
BPH	benign prostatic hypertrophy	TUIP	transurethral incision of the prostate
PED	penile erectile dysfunction	TUNA	transurethral needle ablation
PSA	prostate-specific antigen	TURP	transurethral resection of the prostate

CASE STUDY

Achieving Results

Dr. Medina was able to help Luis by giving him prescription hormones for his low sperm count and telling him about certain techniques that can increase sperm count. Within six months, Marta was pregnant.

As a urologist, Dr. Medina treats both the reproductive and urinary systems of males. Men who have fertility problems account for a small percentage of Dr. Medina's practice. A slightly larger group sees Dr. Medina about difficulties in sexual functioning (PED, ED). Most of Dr. Medina's patients are much older than Luis. Middle-aged and elderly men tend to have urinary tract problems more frequently than younger men.

Bernard McCoy, who is 35 years old, called for an appointment after his urethrogram. The receptionist scheduled a visit for 10:00 a.m. on November 15. McCoy was escorted to the examining room where the nurse made notes about his complaints (difficulty in urination). A digital rectal exam showed extensive swelling but his previous PSA test was normal. The doctor examined Mr. McCoy. The doctor spoke to Mr. McCoy about the results of his urethrogram.

Critical Thinking

26. What part of the urinary tract is tested for by a PSA test?
27. What condition does Dr. Medina think Mr. McCoy has?

11/15/XX TW: Bernard McCoy, age 35, complains of frequent urination, small stream, and stop and start urine flow; inability to achieve erection. RM: Lab: CBC, chem screen panel, PSA normal. Urethrogram showed swelling. Diagnosis: BPH. A. Medina, M.D.

COMBINING FORMS AND ABBREVIATIONS EXERCISES

Build Your Medical Vocabulary

Build words for the following definitions using at least one combining form from this chapter. You can refer to Chapters 1, 2, and 3 for general combining forms.

28. Morbid fear of men: _____

29. Surgical reconstruction of the glans penis: _____

30. Killer of sperm: _____

31. Incision into a testis: _____

32. Abnormal discharge of prostate fluid: _____

Put the reproductive system combining form and its meaning in the space following the sentence.

33. A prostatectomy is usually performed only in cases of cancer. _____

34. Androgens cause the development of male secondary sex characteristics. _____

35. An orchiectomy is done in cases of cancer. _____

36. Balanoplasty may be necessary in cases of injury. _____

Diagnostic, Procedural, and Laboratory Terms

The Prostate Cancer Research Institute www.prostate-cancer.org offers free booklets and a wealth of information about this disease.

A normal male medical checkup may include a *digital rectal exam (DRE)*, the insertion of a finger into the rectum to check the prostate for abnormalities, tenderness, or irregularities. During the DRE, the physician can reach approximately two-thirds of the prostate. A medical check-up for males usually includes a **prostate-specific antigen (PSA) test,** a blood test to screen for abnormal prostatic growth, which can be associated with prostate cancer. The PSA level that is considered normal ranges from 0 to 4 nanograms/milliliter (ng/ml). A PSA level of 4 to 10 ng/ml is considered slightly elevated; levels between 10 and 20 ng/ml are considered moderately elevated; and anything above that is considered highly elevated.

If a couple is having fertility problems, a **semen analysis** is done to determine the quantity and quality of the male partner's sperm. Such an analysis determines the percentage of living and normally developed sperm, the ability of the sperm to move, and the percentage of well-formed sperm. Poor-quality sperm may result from temperature variation of the testicles, illness, the effect of drugs (even over-the-counter medications), and stress.

Visit the American Fertility Association Web site (www.theafa.org) to find out what is normal in a semen analysis.

X-ray or imaging procedures are used to further test for abnormalities or blockages. A **urethrogram** is an x-ray of the urethra and prostate. A sonogram may be used when needle biopsies are taken, as of the testicles or prostate. If cancer is present, surgery, chemotherapy, or radiation may be used. Hormone replacement therapy is given to males who have a deficiency of male hormones. Men who have erectile dysfunction may be treated chemically with medications or with a *penile prosthesis*, a device implanted in the penis to treat impotence.

VOCABULARY REVIEW

In the previous section, you learned terms relating to diagnosis, clinical procedures, and laboratory tests. Before going on to the exercises, review the following terms and refer to the previous section if you have any questions. Pronunciations are provided for certain terms. Sometimes information about where the word came from is included after the term. These etymologies (word histories) are for your information only. You do not need to memorize them.

Term	Definition
prostate-specific [ĂN-tĭ-jĕn] antigen (PSA) test	Blood test for prostate cancer.
semen analysis	Observation of semen for viability of sperm.
urethrogram [yū-RĒ-thrō-grăm] urethro-, urethra + -gram, a recording	X-ray of the urethra and prostate.

CASE STUDY

Testing Further

Alan Salvo is a 58-year-old male with a complaint of difficulty urinating. His blood work is normal including his PSA test. Dr. Medina schedules Mr. Salvo for a urethrogram.

Critical Thinking

37. The normal PSA test virtually eliminated one possible diagnosis. What did it likely eliminate?
38. What might the urethrogram show?

DIAGNOSTIC, PROCEDURAL, AND LABORATORY TERMS EXERCISES

Check Your Knowledge

Fill in the blanks.

39. A semen analysis examines the _____ and _____ of sperm.
40. A DRE is for finding any abnormalities in the _____ and _____.
41. A PSA tests for _____ cancer.
42. Both males and females may need _____ _____ therapy.
43. Erectile problems may be treated chemically or with a _____ _____.

Pathological Terms

Birth or developmental defects affect the functioning of the reproductive system. An *undescended testicle* (**cryptorchism**) means that the normal descending of the testicle to the scrotal sac does not take place during gestation and requires surgery to place it properly (Figure 11-3). **Anorchism** or **anorchia** is the lack of one or both testes.

Hypospadias is an abnormal opening of the urethra on the underside of the penis. **Epispadias** is an abnormal opening on the top side of the penis. Figure 11-4 shows these two abnormal conditions of the urinary meatus. **Phimosis** is an abnormal narrowing of the foreskin over the glans penis (only in uncircumsized males). These conditions are also repaired by surgery (sometimes during circumcision), in which the foreskin is removed and used in the repair.

As the male matures, infections and various other medical conditions may cause **infertility,** an inability to produce enough viable sperm to fertilize an ovum or an inability to deliver sperm to the proper location in the vagina. Several levels of sperm production may be involved in infertility.

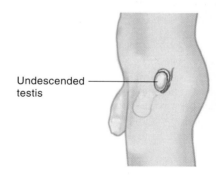

Undescended testis

FIGURE 11-3 Cryptorchism is also known as an undescended testicle.

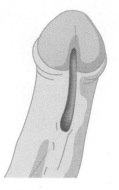
Hypospadias

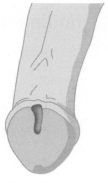
Epispadias

FIGURE 11-4 Hypospadias and epispadias are two congenital urethral abnormalities.

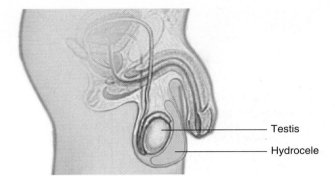
Testis

Hydrocele

FIGURE 11-5 Hydroceles commonly occur in the scrotal sac.

Aspermia is the inability to produce sperm; **azoospermia** is semen without living sperm; and **oligospermia** is the scanty production of sperm. Medical or psychological conditions may cause **impotence** (*penile erectile dysfunction*), inability to maintain an erection for ejaculation. **Priapism** is a persistent, painful erection, usually related to other medical conditions. **Hernias,** abnormal protrusions of part of a tissue or an organ out of its normal space through a barrier, may occur in the male reproductive system. (Hernias are also covered in Chapter 14.) A **hydrocele** is a fluid-containing hernia in a testicle (Figure 11-5); a **varicocele** is a group of herniated veins near the testes. This is a common cause of infertility due to the increased heat that the dilated blood vessel brings to the scrotum. It can be corrected by surgery.

Various inflammations occur in the male reproductive system. **Prostatitis** is any inflammation of the prostate; **balanitis** is an inflammation of the glans penis; and **epididymitis** is an inflammation of the epididymis. Likewise, some diseases and conditions affect the function of the reproductive system. *Benign prostatic hypertrophy* or *hyperplasia (BPH)* is enlargement of the prostate gland not involving cancer but causing some obstruction of the urinary tract. *Testicular torsion* is a surgical emergency caused by the constriction of testicular arteries. Ischemia and infarction result in testicular death if not corrected.

Peyronie's disease is a disorder with curvature of the penis caused by some hardening in the interior structure of the penis. *Prostate cancer* and *testicular cancer* are fairly common malignancies. A common tumor of the testicle is a **seminoma.**

Sexually transmitted diseases are the same for the male as for the female (see Chapters 10, 12, and 13), with males being more susceptible to **chancroids,** venereal sores caused by a bacterial infection on the penis, urethra, or anus.

The National Kidney and Urologic Diseases Clearinghouse (http:// kidney.niddk.nih.gov/kudiseases/ pubs/peyronie/index.htm) provides information about Peyronie's disease.

VOCABULARY REVIEW

In the previous section, you learned terms relating to pathology. Before going on to the exercises, review the terms below and refer to the previous section if you have any questions. Pronunciations are provided for certain terms. Sometimes information about where the word came from is included after the term. These etymologies (word histories) are for your information only. You do not need to memorize them.

Term	Definition
anorchism [ăn-ŌR-kĭzm], **anorchia** [-kē-ă] an-, without + orch-, testicle + -ism, state of being	Congenital absence of one or both testicles.
aspermia [ā-SPĔR-mē-ă] a-, without + sperm + -ia, condition	Inability to produce sperm.
azoospermia [ā-zō-ō-SPĔR-mē-ă] a- + zoo-, life + sperm + -ia	Semen without living sperm.
balanitis [băl-ă-NĪ-tĭs] Greek *balanos*, acorn + -itis, inflammation	Inflammation of the glans penis.
chancroids [SHĂNG-krŏyds] chancr(e) + -oid, like	Bacterial infection that can be sexually transmitted; results in sores on the penis, urethra, or anus.
cryptorchism [krĭp-TŌR-kĭzm] crypto-, hidden + orch- + -ism	Birth defect with the failure of one or both of the testicles to descend into the scrotal sac.
epididymitis [ĕp-ĭ-dĭd-ĭ-MĪ-tĭs] epididym(is) + -itis	Inflammation of the epididymis.
epispadias [ĕp-ĭ-SPĀ-dē-ăs] epi-, upon + Greek *spadon*, a ripping or tearing	Birth defect with abnormal opening of the urethra on the top side of the penis.
hernia [HĔR-nē-ă] Latin, rupture	Abnormal protrusion of tissue through muscle that contains it.
hydrocele [HĪ-drō-sēl] hydro-, water + -cele, hernia	Fluid-containing hernia of the testis.
hypospadias [HĪ-pō-SPĀ-dē-ăs] hypo-, under + Greek *spadon*, a ripping or tearing	Birth defect with abnormal opening of the urethra on the bottom side of the penis.
impotence [ĬM-pō-těns] Latin *impotentia*, inability	Inability to maintain an erection for ejaculation.
infertility [ĭn-fĕr-TĬL-ĭ-tē] in-, not + fertility	Inability to fertilize ova.
oligospermia [ŏl-ĭ-gō-SPĔR-mě-ă] oligo-, few + sperm + -ia	Scanty production of sperm.
Peyronie's [pā-RŌN-ēz] **disease** After Francois de la Peyronie (1678–1747), French surgeon	Abnormal curvature of the penis caused by hardening in the interior of the penis.
phimosis [fĭ-MŌ-sĭs] Greek, a muzzling	Abnormal narrowing of the opening of the foreskin.
priapism [PRĪ-ă-pĭzm] After Priapus, god of procreation	Persistent, painful erection of the penis.
prostatitis [prŏs-tă-TĪ-tĭs] prostat-, prostate + -itis	Inflammation of the prostate.
seminoma [sěm-ĭ-NŌ-mă] Latin *semen*, seed + -oma, tumor	Malignant tumor of the testicle.
varicocele [VĂR-ĭ-kō-sēl] varico(se) + -cele	Enlargement of veins of the spermatic cord.

CASE STUDY

Resolving Problems

Marta and Luis Consalvo's baby, an 8-pound boy, was healthy except for hypospadias. Dr. Medina told the Consalvos that an operation to properly place the urethral opening would be needed, but as long as the baby remained in diapers, they could wait until he was a bit older for the surgery. The parents were also told to delay circumcision, so that any excess skin might be used to repair the penis.

Critical Thinking

44. Why might hypospadias cause urination problems once the baby is out of diapers and trained to use a toilet?
45. Hypospadias, if left untreated, may cause fertility problems later in life. How?

PATHOLOGICAL TERMS EXERCISES

Find a Match

Match the definitions in the right-hand column with the terms in the left-hand column.

46. _____ anorchism
47. _____ aspermia
48. _____ seminoma
49. _____ balinitis
50. _____ hydrocele
51. _____ impotence
52. _____ infertility
53. _____ hypospadias
54. _____ cryptorchism
55. _____ azoospermia

a. inflammation of the glans penis
b. hernia in the testes
c. inability to maintain an erection
d. inability to fertilize an ovum
e. undescended testicle
f. lacking sperm
g. abnormal urethral opening
h. lacking testicles
i. having no living sperm
j. testicular tumor

Surgical Terms

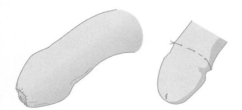

FIGURE 11-6 Circumcision is usually determined by cultural preference.

The most common surgery of the male reproductive system is **circumcision,** the removal of the foreskin or prepuce (Figure 11-6). Various cultures and religions have rituals associated with this removal. Some parents prefer to have it done in the hospital immediately after birth.

Other surgeries are to prevent or enhance the possibility of conception, diagnose or remove cancerous tumors, remove or reduce blockages, and remove or repair parts of the system. Biopsies are commonly taken of the testicles and prostate when cancer is suspected.

Various operations to remove cancerous or infected parts of the reproductive system are an **epididymectomy,** removal of an epididymis; an **orchiectomy** or **orchidectomy,** removal of a testicle; a **prostatectomy,** removal of the prostate gland, which may be done through the perineum or above the pubic bone; and a *transurethral resection of the prostate (TURP)*, removal of

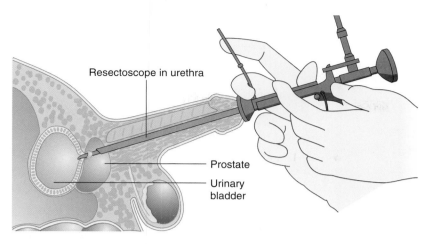

Resectoscope in urethra

Prostate

Urinary bladder

FIGURE 11-7   A TURP (transurethral resection of the prostate) is the removal of some prostate tissue through the urethra.

a portion of the prostate through the urethra (Figure 11-7). A **vasectomy** is the removal of part of the vas deferens as a method of birth control. A **vasovasostomy** is the reversing of a vasectomy so the male regains fertility. **Castration** is the removal of the testicles in the male.

In addition to the TURP, other treatments exist for benign prostatic hypertrophy. In the procedure called *transurethral microwave thermotherapy (TUMT)*, the Prostatron, an FDA-approved device, sends computer-regulated microwaves through a catheter to heat and destroy selected portions of the prostate. A cooling system protects the urinary tract during the procedure. A similar microwave device, the Targis System, also received FDA approval. Like the Prostatron, the Targis System delivers microwaves to destroy selected portions of the prostate and uses a cooling system to protect the urethra. A heat-sensing device inserted in the rectum helps monitor the therapy. Both procedures take about 1 hour and can be performed on an outpatient basis without general anesthesia. Neither procedure has been reported to lead to impotence or incontinence. The *transurethral incision of the prostate (TUIP)* is similar to TURP. It is used on slightly enlarged prostate glands. The surgeon places one or two small cuts in the prostate. This relieves pressure without trimming away tissue. It has a low risk of side effects. Like TURP, this form of BPH treatment helps with urine flow by widening the urethra. The *transurethral needle ablation (TUNA)* burns away excess prostate tissue using radio waves. It helps with urine flow, relieves symptoms, and may have fewer side effects than TURP.

> The practice of circumcising infant males is the subject of controversy. There is a Web site (www.circumcision.org) that gives reasons against the practice, while other Web sites give information about the surgery.

VOCABULARY REVIEW

In the previous section, you learned terms relating to surgery. Before going on to the exercises, review the terms below and refer to the previous section if you have any questions. Pronunciations are provided for certain terms. Sometimes information about where the word came from is included after the term. These etymologies (word histories) are for your information only. You do not need to memorize them.

Term	Definition
castration [kăs-TRĀ-shŭn] Latin *castro*, to deprive of power	Removal of the testicles.
circumcision [sĭr-kŭm-SĬZH-ŭn] Latin *circumcido*, to cut around	Removal of the foreskin.
epididymectomy [ĔP-ĭ-dĭd-ĭ-MĔK-tō-mē] epididym(is) + -ectomy, removal	Removal of an epididymis.
orchidectomy [ōr-kĭ-DĔK-tō-mē] orchid-, testicle + -ectomy	Removal of a testicle.
orchiectomy [ōr-kē-ĔK-tō-mē] orchi-, testicle + -ectomy	Removal of a testicle.
prostatectomy [prŏs-tă-TĔK-tō-mē] prostat- + -ectomy	Removal of the prostate.
vasectomy [vă-SĔK-tō-mē] Latin *vas*, vessel + -ectomy	Removal of part of the vas deferens to prevent conception.
vasovasostomy [VĀ-sō-vă-SŎS-tō-mē] vaso-, vessel + vaso- + -stomy, creation of a hole	Reversal of a vasectomy.

MORE ABOUT . . .

Birth Control

An operation is not necessary for male birth control. Other options available to males are a *condom,* a sheath worn over the penis to collect the semen after ejaculation, *coitus interruptus,* removal of the penis from the vagina before ejaculation (although this is not very safe), and a forthcoming *male birth control pill,* which will block the production of sperm.

CASE STUDY

Surgical Relief

Dr. Medina checked the results of Mr. McCoy's urethrogram. There did not seem to be any abnormalities other than in the prostate. He scheduled Mr. McCoy for a TURP, which is done as cryogenic surgery (surgery using cold to numb an area prior to operating). The procedure is done on an outpatient basis, and one week later, Mr. McCoy is improving rapidly. Dr. Medina wants to wait a while to see if the TURP also helps improve erectile function, before exploring other options. One such option is new medication that can improve erectile function.

Critical Thinking

56. Why did Dr. Medina schedule Mr. McCoy for a TURP?
57. If medication does not work to improve sexual function, what is another option for men with impaired erectile function?

Check Your Knowledge

Fill in the blanks.

58. Circumcision is removal of the _____ and is commonly practiced in various cultures.

59. An _____ or _____ is removal of a testicle.

60. A prostatectomy is a general term for removal of the _____.

61. A contraceptive operation is a(n) _____.

62. An operation to reverse a previously done contraceptive one is a(n) _____.

Pharmacological Terms

Males are sometimes treated with hormone replacement therapy (usually, testosterone). Such treatment can help with sexual problems and with some of the signs of aging. Medications for impotence may help some men restore sexual function. It may also be treated surgically or with mechanical devices. Some erectile disfunction is a vascular problem and may be treated with *transient vasoconstrictors*, medications that cause temporary constriction of the blood vessels in the penis. Table 11-2 lists some of the medications used to treat disorders of the male reproductive system.

Anabolic steroids can help overcome the symptoms of some wasting diseases and build muscle mass. The ability of such drugs to increase muscle mass means that they are important to some athletes. However, the widespread overuse of anabolic steroids by some people has proven to be dangerous, even fatal. Many sports organizations now disqualify athletes who are found using steroids.

> The American Academy of Pediatrics (www.aap.org/family/steroids.htm) discusses the abuse of steroids in children's sports.

TABLE 11-2 Drugs Used to Treat Disorders of the Male Reproductive System

Drug Class	Purpose	Generic	Trade Name
treatments for benign prostatic hypertrophy	to cure or relieve enlargement of the prostate	finasteride dutasteride terazosin doxazosin alfuzosin tamsulosin	Proscar Avodart Hytrin Cardura Uroxatral Flomax
treatments for erectile dysfunction	to achieve or lengthen the duration of erections	sildenafil tadalafil vardenafil	Viagra Cialis Levitra

CASE STUDY

Trying Medication

About a month later, Mr. McCoy is back for an appointment to discuss his sexual dysfunction. He still is having difficulty sustaining erections. Dr. Medina reviews other medications that Mr. McCoy takes to check for possible interactions, prescribes a drug to treat impotence, and asks Mr. McCoy to call him in about a month. The drug works well for Mr. McCoy.

In recent years, Dr. Medina has seen an increase in the number of patients who cite sexual dysfunction as a problem. Often, people would rather accept the condition rather than talk to a doctor openly about it. Media publicity about impotence has made known some of the available treatments.

Critical Thinking

63. Mr. McCoy's impotence existed for about ten years before he told a doctor about it. Do you think all the media coverage of the issue of impotence or PED helps people to discuss this issue with their health care practitioners? Why or why not?

64. Dr. Medina tells Mr. McCoy to call him if his internist prescribes any other drugs for him while he is taking his medication for impotence. Why is Dr. Medina concerned?

PHARMACOLOGICAL TERMS EXERCISES

Check Your Knowledge

Fill in the blanks.

65. Male hormone replacement therapy usually involves the hormone _____.

66. Inability to maintain an erection can be treated with _____.

67. Weight trainers and sports figures sometimes illegally use _____.

CHALLENGE SECTION

William Hartman, 30 years old, has a history of orchialgia, which was usually treatable with a mild painkiller. Lately, he tells his internist, the pain is increasing. He is referred to Dr. Medina. His records are sent to Dr. Medina's office for review. Dr. Medina notes that the patient has an encysted hydrocele that has been aspirated and drained once before. Now it is quite large. He suggests removal of the hernia on an outpatient basis. He explains to the patient that its removal may affect the functioning of his left testicle.

Critical Thinking

68. Should William be worried about fertility issues?

69. What is inside a hydrocele that makes it swell?

TERMINOLOGY IN ACTION

From the following letter, can you determine why the doctor did *not* suspect prostate cancer?

Dr. Robert Thorkild, MD
Department of General Surgery
555 Tenth Avenue
New York, NY 99999

Dear Dr. Thorkild:

Thank you for agreeing to see John Roberts, a patient of mine, on an urgent basis. He is the 30-year-old male I mentioned in my telephone conversation.

Mr. Roberts complains of right inguinal cramping and sharp, constant pain radiating into the scrotum and right testicle. The pain occurred after lifting several heavy objects at work. He works for a moving company and does constant heavy lifting.

On examination, abdomen is soft and non tender. There is fullness in the right groin area. Palpation of the inguinal canal reveals a bulge that is made worse with coughing. It is reducible and there is no question of strangulation. Rectal examination is normal. Prostate is normal in size and texture.

My assessment is right inguinal hernia.

Because of his difficult financial situation, he needs to have this repaired as soon as possible. He agrees to seeing you and having you perform a herniorrhaphy.

Thank you for seeing Mr. Roberts.

Sincerely,

Robert Thorkild, MD

USING THE INTERNET

Google the words "prostate cancer" and write a short paragraph on recent news about prostate cancer.

CHAPTER REVIEW

The material that follows is to help you review all the material in this chapter.

Build Your Medical Vocabulary

Using the combining forms learned in this chapter and in Chapters two and three, build a medical term for each of the following.

70. painful prostate: _____

71. surgical fixation of the testes: _____

72. surgical repair of the glans penis: _____

73. suturing of the testes: _____

74. herniation of the prostate: _____

75. pain in the testes: _____

Root Out the Meaning

Divide each of the following terms into parts and then define the term.

76. orchitis: _____

77. spermatogenesis: _____

78. prostatomegaly: _____

79. prostatorrhea : _____

80. vasectomy: _____

81. perineoplasty : _____

82. spermatocele: _____

Spell It Correctly

Write the correct spelling in the blank to the right of each word. If the word is already correctly spelled, write C.

83. hyospadias _____

84. testosterone _____

85. semin _____

86. epididimis _____

87. semenoma _____

DEFINITIONS

Define the following terms and combining forms. Review the chapter before starting. Make sure you know how to pronounce each term as you define it. The blue words in curly brackets are references to the Spanish glossary available online at www.mhhe.com/medterm3e.

WORD

88. anabolic steroids

89. andr(o)

90. anorchism, anorchia [ăn-ŌR-kĭzm, -kē-ă] {anorquia}

91. aspermia [ā-SPĔR-mē-ă] {aspermia}

92. azoospermia [ā-zō-ŏ-SPĔR-mē-ă] {azoospermia}

93. balan(o)

94. balanitis [băl-ă-NĪ-tĭs] {balanitis}

95. bulbourethral [BŬL-bō-yū-RĒ-thrăl] gland

96. castration [kăs-TRĀ-shŭn] {castración}

97. chancroids [SHĂNG-krŏyds]

98. circumcision [sĕr-kŭm-SĬZH-ŭn] {circuncisión}

99. Cowper's [KŎW-pĕrs] gland

100. cryptorchism [krĭp-TŎR-kĭzm]

101. ejaculation [ē-jăk-yū-LĀ-shŭn] {eyaculación}

102. epididym(o)

103. epididymectomy [ĔP-ĭ-dĭd-ĭ-MĔK-tō-mē]

104. epididymis [ĕp-ĭ-DĬD-ĭ-mĭs] {epidídimo}

105. epididymitis [ĕp-ĭ-dĭd-ĭ-MĪ-tĭs] {epididimitis}

106. epispadias [ĕp-ĭ-SPĀ-dē-ăs] {epispadias}

107. flagellum [flă-JĔL-ŭm] {flagelo}

108. foreskin [FŌR-skĭn] {prepucio}

109. glans penis [glănz PĒ-nĭs]

110. hernia [HĔR-nē-ă] {hernia}

111. hydrocele [HĪ-drō-sēl] {hidrocele}

112. hypospadias [HĪ-pō-SPĀ-dē-ăs] {hipospadias}

113. impotence [ĬM-pō-tĕns] {impotencia}

114. infertility [ĭn-fĕr-TĬL-ĭ-tē] {infertilidad}

115. oligospermia [ŏl-ĭ-gō-SPĔR-mē-ă] {oligospermia}

116. orch(o), orchi(o), orchid(o)

117. orchidectomy [ōr-kĭ-DĔK-tō-mē] {orquidectomía}

118. orchiectomy [ōr-kē-ĔK-tō-mē] {orquietomía}

119. penis [PĒ-nĭs] {pene}

120. perineum [PĔR-ĭ-NĒ-ŭm] {perineo}

121. Peyronie's [pā-RŌN-ēz] disease

122. phimosis [fĭ-MŌ-sĭs] {fimosis}

123. priapism [PRĪ-ă-pĭzm] {priapismo}

124. prostat(o)

125. prostate [PRŎS-tāt] {próstata} gland

126. prostatectomy [prŏs-tă-TĔK-tō-mē] {prostatectomía}

127. prostate-specific antigen [ĂN-tĭ-jĕn] (PSA) test

128. prostatitis [prŏs-tă-TĪ-tĭs] {prostatitis}

129. scrotum [SKRŌ-tŭm] {escroto}

130. semen [SĒ-mĕn] {semen}

131. semen analysis

132. seminoma [sĕm-ĭ-NŌ-mă]

133. sperm [spĕrm] {esperma}

134. sperm(o), spermat(o)

135. spermatogenesis [SPĔR-mă-tō-JĔN-ĕ-sĭs]

136. spermatozoon (pl., spermatozoa) [SPĔR-mă-tō-ZŌ-ŏn (SPĔR-mă-tō-ZŌ-ă)] {espermatozoo}

137. testicle [TĔS-tĭ-kl] {testículo}

138. testis (pl., testes) [TĔS-tĭs (TĔS-tēz)] {testículo}

139. testosterone [tĕs-TŎS-tĕ-rōn] {testosterona}

140. urethrogram [yū-RĒ-thrō-grăm]

141. varicocele [VĂR-ĭ-kō-sēl] {varicocele}

142. vas deferens [văs DĔF-ĕr-ĕns]

143. vasectomy [vă-SĔK-tō-mē] {vasectomía}

144. vasovasostomy [VĀ-sō-vă-SŎS-tō-mē] {vasovasostomía}

Abbreviations

Write the full meaning of each abbreviation.

145. AIH

146. BPH

147. PED

148. PSA

149. SPP

150. TURP

Answers to Chapter Exercises

1. Ob-gyns do not treat male infertility.
2. testicles, seminal vesicles, epididymis, prostate, and vas deferens
3. c
4. a
5. c
6. c
7. a
8. a
9. b
10. c
11. b
12. a
13. b
14. d
15. a
16. e
17. c
18. f
19. F
20. T
21. F
22. F
23. F
24. F
25. F
26. prostate
27. benign prostatic hypertrophy
28. androphobia
29. balanoplasty
30. spermicide, spermatocide
31. orchiotomy
32. prostatorrhea
33. prostat-, prostate
34. andro-, male
35. orchi-, testes
36. balano-, glans penis
37. Prostate cancer is probably not present.

38. swelling or other abnormalities in the urethra or prostate
39. quantity, quality
40. rectum, prostate
41. prostate
42. hormone replacement
43. penile prosthesis
44. If the urethra opens on the bottom, the child will urinate straight down and probably find it difficult to keep his urine from splattering.
45. Delivery of sperm to the cervix during male ejaculation usually requires a centered meatus.
46. h
47. f
48. j
49. a
50. b
51. c
52. d
53. g
54. e
55. i
56. The prostate was enlarged and interfering with urination. A TURP removes some prostate tissue.
57. penile prosthesis
58. foreskin
59. orchidectomy, orchiectomy
60. prostate
61. vasectomy
62. vasovasostomy
63. Most people have the opinion that open discussions of sexual dysfunction make it easier to seek and receive medical help.

64. Dr. Medina does not want his patient to experience drug interactions.
65. testosterone
66. medications for impotence
67. anabolic steroids
68. No, his other testis should be fine.
69. fluid
70. prostatodynia, prostatalgia
71. orchidopexy, orchiopexy
72. balanoplasty
73. orchidorrhaphy, orchiorrhaphy
74. prostatocele
75. testalgia
76. orch-, testis, -itis, inflammation; inflammation of a testis
77. spermato-, sperm, -genesis, producing; producing or forming sperm
78. prostato-, prostate, -megaly, enlargement; enlargement of the prostate
79. prostato-, prostate, -rrhea, flowing; discharge of the prostate
80. vas-, blood vessel, duct, -ectomy, removal; excision (removal) of the vas deferens
81. perineo-, perineum, -plasty, repair; surgical repair of the perineum
82. spermato-, sperm, -cele, hernia; hernia or cyst in the epididymis or testes
83. hypospadias
84. C
85. semen
86. epididymis
87. seminoma
88–150. Answers are available in the vocabulary reviews of this chapter.

CHAPTER
12

▶ HEMATOLOGY

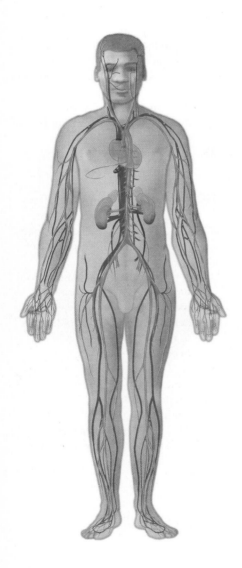

To learn more about blood donation, go to the National Heart, Lung, and Blood Institute's Web site (www.nhlbi.nih.gov).

The Blood System

After studying this chapter, you will be able to:

12.1 Name the parts of the blood system and discuss the function of each part

12.2 Define combining forms used in building words that relate to the blood system

12.3 Identify the meaning of related abbreviations

12.4 Name the common diagnoses, clinical procedures, and laboratory tests used in treating disorders of the blood system

12.5 List and define the major pathological conditions of the blood system

12.6 Explain the meaning of surgical terms related to the blood system

12.7 Recognize common pharmacological agents used in treating disorders of the blood system

Structure and Function

Blood is a complex mixture of cells, water, and various biochemical agents, such as proteins and sugars. It transports life-sustaining nutrients, oxygen, and hormones to all parts of the body. As a transport medium for waste products from cells of the body, it prevents toxic buildup. It helps maintain the stability of the fluid volume that exists within body tissues (a form of *homeostasis*, the maintaining of a balance), and it helps regulate body temperature. Without blood, human life is not possible. Figure 12-1a illustrates the blood system, with arteries shown in red and veins shown in blue. Figure 12-1b is a schematic showing the path of blood through the body.

An average adult has about 5 liters of blood circulating within the body. The volume of blood changes with body size, usually equaling about 8 percent of body weight. If a person loses blood, either through bleeding or by donating blood, most of the blood volume is replaced within 24 hours. If bleeding is extensive, blood transfusions may be necessary.

Blood is a thick liquid made up of a fluid part, **plasma,** and a solid part containing **red blood cells, white blood cells,** and **platelets.** Plasma (the liquid portion of unclotted blood) consists of water, proteins, salts, nutrients, vitamins, and hormones. If some proteins and blood cells are removed from plasma, as happens during coagulation (clotting), the resulting fluid is called **serum.** Serum is the liquid portion of clotted blood. *Serology* is the science that deals with the properties of serum, such as the presence of immunity-provoking agents.

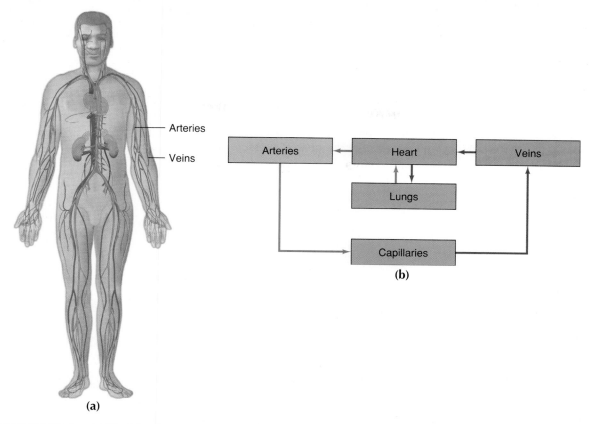

(a)

FIGURE 12-1 **(a)** The blood system transports life-sustaining nutrients to all parts of the body; **(b)** a schematic showing the path of blood through the body.

Plasma

When blood is separated, the plasma (about 55 percent of the blood) is the clear liquid made up of 92 percent water and 8 percent organic and inorganic chemicals. The 8 percent consists of proteins, nutrients, gases, electrolytes, and other substances.

The main groups of plasma proteins are **albumin, globulin, fibrinogen,** and **prothrombin.** Albumin helps regulate water movement between blood and tissue. Plasma proteins cannot pass through capillaries, and, in order to maintain a balance of fluids on both sides of the capillary walls, they create pressure that forces water into the bloodstream. Leakage of water out of the bloodstream can cause edema. An injury can upset the balance of water in the blood and, if too much water is lost, can eventually lead to shock.

Globulins have different functions, depending on their type. The *alpha* and *beta globulins,* which are joined in the liver, transport lipids and fat-soluble vitamins. **Gamma globulins** arise in the lymphatic tissues and function as part of the immune system. Globulins can be separated from each other when plasma is placed in a special solution and electrical currents attract the different proteins to move in the direction of the electricity through a process called **electrophoresis.** Blood may also be *centrifuged,* put in a device that separates blood elements by spinning. **Plasmapheresis** is a process that uses centrifuging to take a patient's blood and return only red cells to that patient.

Fibrinogen and prothrombin are essential for blood **coagulation,** the process of *clotting.* The clot is formed by platelets that rush to the site of an

MORE ABOUT . . .

Blood

In an emergency situation, in which a person is hemorrhaging, a quick response can save a life. First, make sure the person can breathe. The most effective way to control hemorrhaging is to apply direct pressure on the wound, elevate the area (whenever possible, to a level above the heart), and apply pressure to the nearest pressure point. The points shown here are just some of the most common pressure points.

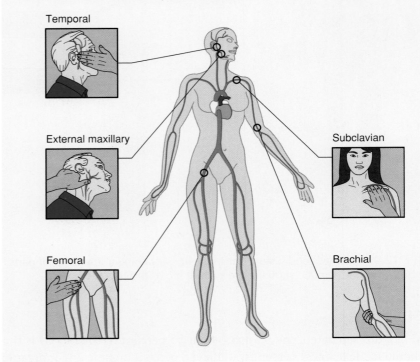

Temporal

External maxillary

Femoral

Subclavian

Brachial

injury. They clump at the site and release a protein, **thromboplastin,** which combines with calcium and various clotting factors (I-V and VII-XIII) to form the **fibrin clot** (Figure 12-2). **Thrombin,** an enzyme, helps in formation of the clot. The clot tightens while releasing serum, a clear liquid. Blood clotting at the site of a wound is essential. Without it, one would bleed to death. Blood clotting inside blood vessels, however, can cause major cardiovascular problems. Some elements of the blood, such as **heparin,** prevent clots from forming during normal circulation.

Blood Cells

The solid part of the blood that is suspended in the plasma consists of the red blood cells (RBCs), also called **erythrocytes,** white blood cells (WBCs), also called **leukocytes,** and platelets, also referred to as **thrombocytes.** These cells or the solids in the blood make up about 45 percent of the blood. The measurement of the percentage of packed red blood cells is known as the **hematocrit.** Most blood cells are formed as **stem cells** (**hematocytoblasts**) or immature blood cells in the bone marrow. Stem cells mature in the bone marrow before entering the bloodstream and becoming *differentiated*, specialized in their purpose. Figure 12-3 shows the stages of

Stem cells can be gotten from umbilical cord blood. To find out about how to donate cord blood once a baby is born, go to the NIH website on stem cells (http://stemcells.nih.gov).

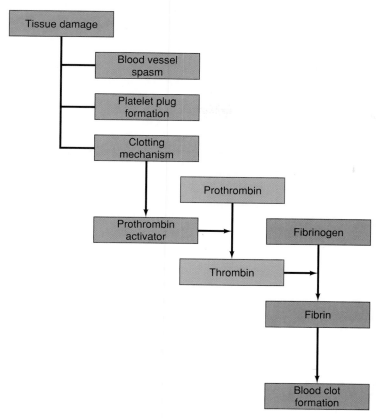

FIGURE 12-2 A fibrin clot is formed at the site of an injury.

blood cell development. The term *differential*, which you will see on written orders for blood tests, refers to the percentage of each type of white blood cell in the bloodstream.

MORE ABOUT . . .

Stem Cells

Stem cells are the foundation cells for all other cells in the body. As a new individual develops, the process of differentiation begins by designating certain cells to become specific cell types within the body. It is the stem cell's ability to be manipulated that is believed to hold the key to engineering new tissues to repair diseases or injuries. There are two types of stem cells that are at the center of this bioethical debate; embryonic and adult stem cells. Embryonic stem cells tend to be the preferred cell due to their genetic ability to easily divide and develop into all types of cells within the body. An adult stem cell found in a person or umbilical cord has a limited ability to form only certain types of cells.

Controversy about the use of embryonic stem cells arises because an embryo is used in the process. Some individuals who believe that human life begins at conception are strongly opposed to using embryos in research and development. Others counter that these cells are harvested for the purpose of reproduction by artificial means and unused embryos will be destroyed if not used. Why not use them for the benefit of those individuals whose disease processes could be treated or possibly cured?

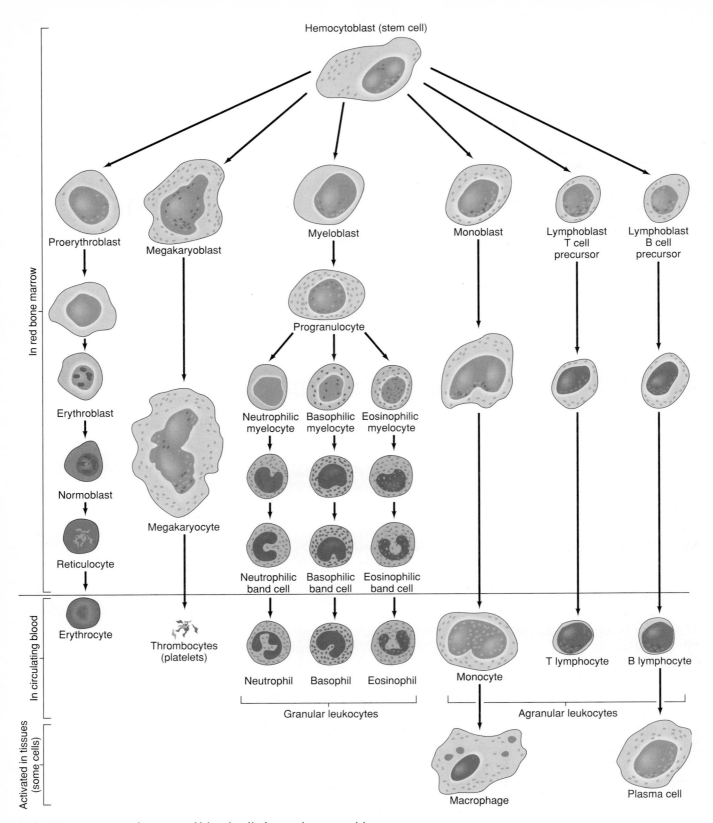

FIGURE 12-3 Development of blood cells from a hemocytoblast.

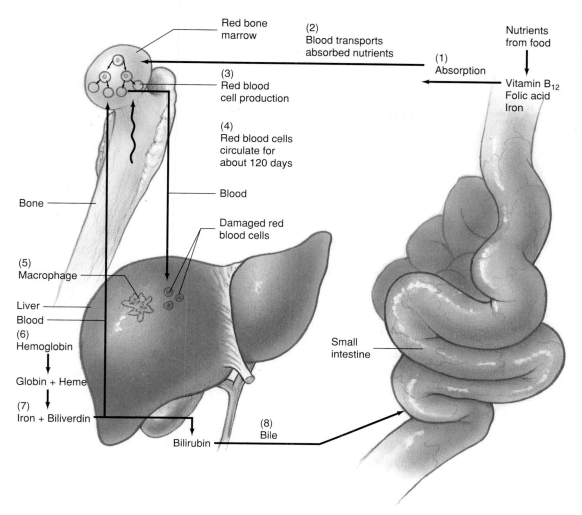

FIGURE 12-4 Life cycle of a red blood cell. Nutrients taken into the small intestine are then supplied to the bone marrow where red blood cells are produced. These cells then circulate in the body for approximately 120 days.

Erythrocytes or Red Blood Cells

A hormone produced in the kidneys, **erythropoietin,** stimulates the production of red blood cells in the bone marrow. When stem cells mature into erythrocytes, they lose their nucleus and become bi-concave.

A protein within red blood cells, **hemoglobin,** aids in the transport of oxygen to the cells of the body. Oxygen molecules have the ability to bond with hemoglobin molecules. When a red blood cell has oxygen on board, it becomes bright red in color. Oxygen-poor red blood cells are a deep burgundy color.

About one-third of each red blood cell is made up of hemoglobin. Hemoglobin is composed of **heme,** a pigment containing iron, and **globin,** a protein. Erythrocytes live for about 120 days. Some are removed from circulation each day to maintain a steady concentration of red blood cells. *Macrophages* are cells formed from stem cells that consume damaged or aged cells. The average number of red blood cells in a cubic millimeter of blood is 4.6 to 6.4 million for adult males and 4.2 to 5.4 million for adult females. This measurement is known as the **red blood cell count.** Figure 12-4 tracks the life cycle of a **red blood cell.**

Erythropoietin is used in the treatment of AIDS patients to encourage red blood cell production.

TABLE 12-1 Types of Leukocytes

Leukocytes	Percentage of Leukocytes in Blood	Function
granulocytes		
basophils	minimal—under 1 percent	release heparin and histamine
eosinophils	minimal—under 3 percent	kill parasites and help control inflammation
neutrophils	most plentiful—over 50 percent	remove unwanted particles
agranulocytes		
lymphocytes	plentiful—25 to 33 percent	important to immune system
monocytes	minimal—3 to 9 percent	destroy large unwanted particles

Leukocytes

Leukocytes or white blood cells protect against disease in various ways—for example, by destroying foreign substances. Leukocytes are transported in the bloodstream to the site of an infection. There are two main groups of leukocytes—granulocytes and agranulocytes.

The first group, **granulocytes,** have a granular cytoplasm and have nuclei with several lobes when viewed under a microscope and when stain is used. There are three types of granulocytes:

1. **Neutrophils** are the most plentiful leukocytes (over half of the white blood cells in the bloodstream). They do not stain distinctly with either an acidic or an alkaline dye. Their purpose is to remove small particles of unwanted material from the bloodstream.
2. **Eosinophils** are only about 1 to 3 percent of the leukocytes in the bloodstream. Their granules stain bright red in the presence of an acidic red dye called eosin. Their purpose is to kill parasites and to help control inflammations and allergic reactions.
3. **Basophils** are less than 1 percent of the leukocytes in the bloodstream. Their granules stain dark purple in the presence of alkaline dyes. They release heparin, an anticlotting factor, and **histamine,** a substance involved in allergic reactions.

The second group of leukocytes, **agranulocytes,** have cytoplasm with no granules. Their single nucleus does not have the dark-staining elements of granulocytes. There are two types of agranulocytes:

1. **Monocytes,** the largest blood cells, make up about 3 to 9 percent of the leukocytes in the bloodstream. They destroy large particles of unwanted material (such as old red blood cells) in the bloodstream.
2. **Lymphocytes** make up about 25 to 33 percent of the leukocytes in the bloodstream. They are essential to the immune system, discussed in Chapter 13.

Table 12-1 lists the types of white blood cells.

Platelets

Platelets or thrombocytes are fragments that break off from large cells in red bone marrow called **megakaryocytes.** Platelets live for about 10 days and

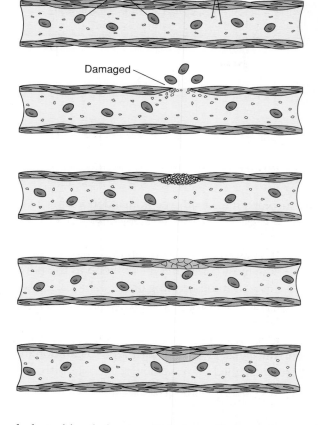

Red blood cells   Platelets

Damaged

Platelets begin to adhere to tissue edges and to each other as blood escapes.

They form a soft platelet plug.

Other clotting factors make this a stable plug or clot.

Tissue mends and anti-thrombin and other agents break down clot.

FIGURE 12-5 Platelets clumping together to form a clot.

help in blood clotting. Platelets adhere to damaged tissue and to each other and group together to control blood loss from a blood vessel. Figure 12-5 shows platelets clumping together.

Blood Types

When blood is needed for **transfusion,** the blood being donated is tested for type and put into one of four human **blood types** or **groups.** The donated

---

MORE ABOUT . . .

Transfusions

Two early scientists attempted various experimental transfusions. Sir Christopher Wren (1632–1723), a famous English architect and scientist, did biological experiments in which he injected fluids into the veins of animals. This process is regarded as an early attempt at blood transfusions. During the same century, a French physician, Jean Baptiste Denis (1643–1704), tried unsuccessfully to transfuse sheep's blood into a human. Later, experiments with transfusing human blood succeeded somewhat, but the majority of people receiving transfusions died, until the advent of blood typing in the twentieth century. Once blood factors and typing became routine, transfusions were widely used in surgery. Later, it was found that some infections (hepatitis, AIDS) were transmitted by blood. Now, donated blood is carefully screened for infections.

TABLE 12-2 Blood Types

Blood Type	Antigen	Antibody	Percent of Population with This Type
A	A	Anti-B	41
B	B	Anti-A	10
AB	A and B	Neither anti-A nor anti-B	4
O	Neither A nor B	Both anti-A and anti-B	45

The lives of some animals are saved by blood transfusions. Go to www.cvm.uiuc.edu/petcolumns/showarticle.cfm?id=114 and search the term "transfusions" to read about the similarities between human and some pet transfusions.

blood must be tested since an incompatible blood type from a donor can cause adverse reactions. Blood typing is based on the antigens (substances that promote an immune response) and antibodies (special proteins in the blood) present in the blood. (Chapter 13 describes the work of antigens and antibodies in the immune system.) The most common type of blood in the population is O, followed by A, B, and AB in descending order. Table 12-2 lists the four blood types and their characteristics.

The danger in transfusing blood of a different type is that **agglutination** or clumping of the antigens stops the flow of blood, which can be fatal. People with type O blood have no antigens, so people with type O can donate to all other types and are, therefore, called *universal donors*. People with AB blood are called *universal recipients* because they can receive blood from people with all the other types and not experience clotting.

In addition to the four human blood types, there is a positive or negative element in the blood. **Rh factor** is a type of antigen first identified in rhesus monkeys. **Rh-positive** blood contains this factor and **Rh-negative** blood does not. The factor contains any of more than 30 types of **agglutinogens,** substances that cause agglutination, and can be fatal to anyone who receives blood with a factor different from the donor.

Rh factor is particularly important during pregnancy. The fetus of parents with different Rh factors could be harmed by a fatal disease or a type of anemia if preventive measures are not taken prior to birth. The problem arises

FIGURE 12-6 How the Rh factor affects pregnancy.

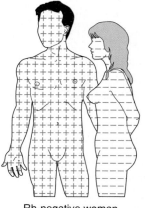
Rh-negative woman and Rh-positive man conceive a child.

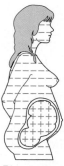
Rh-negative woman with Rh-positive fetus

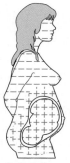
Cells from Rh-positive fetus enter mother's bloodstream.

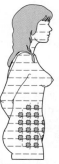
Woman becomes sensitized—antibodies (✱) form to fight Rh-positive blood cells.

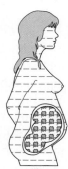
In the next Rh-positive pregnancy, maternal antibodies attack fetal blood cells.

when the mother is Rh-negative and produces antibodies to the father's Rh-positive factor present in the fetus. When the Rh-negative mother becomes exposed to the Rh-positive blood, usually during childbirth, antibodies are formed by the mother. The problem does not arise during a first pregnancy but will arise in each subsequent pregnancy because the antibodies that arise after the first birth would carry a risk for an Rh-positive fetus. Treatment with Rhogam, a gamma globulin, during each pregnancy usually prevents the problem. Figure 12-6 shows how a combination of Rh factors affects pregnancy.

VOCABULARY REVIEW

In the previous section, you learned terms relating to the blood system. Before going on to the exercises, review the terms below and refer to the previous section if you have any questions. Pronunciations are provided for certain terms. Sometimes information about where the word came from is included after the term. These etymologies (word histories) are for your information only. You do not need to memorize them.

Term	Definition
agglutination [ă-glū-tĭ-NĀ-shŭn] gluten, glue	Clumping of cells and particles in blood.
agglutinogen [ă-glū-TĬN-ō-jĕn]	Substance that causes agglutination.
agranulocyte [ā-GRĂN-yū-lō-sĭt]	Leukocyte with nongranular cytoplasm.
albumin [ăl-BYŪ-mĭn] Latin *albumen*, egg white	Simple protein found in plasma.
basophil [BĀ-sō-fĭl] baso-, base + -phil, attraction	Leukocyte containing heparin and histamine.
blood [blŭd] Old English *blod*	Fluid (containing plasma, red blood cells, white blood cells, and platelets) circulated throughout the arteries, veins, capillaries, and heart.
blood types or groups	Classification of blood according to its antigen and antibody qualities.
coagulation [kō-ăg-yū-LĀ-shŭn]	Changing of a liquid, especially blood, into a semi-solid.
electrophoresis [ē-lĕk-trō-FŌR-ē-sĭs] electro-, electricity + phoresis, carrying	Process of separating particles in a solution by passing electricity through the liquid.
eosinophil [ē-ō-SĬN-ō-fĭl] eosino-, fluorescent dye + -phil	Type of granulocyte.
erythrocyte [ĕ-RĬTH-rō-sīt] erythro-, red + -cyte (blood) cell	Mature red blood cell.
erythropoietin [ĕ-rĭth-rō-PŎY-ĕ-tĭn] erythro(cyte) + -poiesis, making	Hormone released by the kidneys to stimulate red blood cell production.
fibrin [FĪ-brĭn] **clot**	Clot-forming threads formed at the site of an injury during coagulation where platelets clump together with various other substances.
fibrinogen [fĭ-BRĬN-ō-jĕn] fibrino-, fibrin + -gen, producing	Protein in plasma that aids in clotting.

Term	Definition
gamma globulin [GĂ-mă GLŎB-yū-lĭn]	Globulin that arises in lymphatic tissue and functions as part of the immune system.
globin [GLŌ-bĭn] From Latin *globus*, ball	Protein molecule in the blood, a part of hemoglobin.
globulin [GLŎB-yū-lĭn] From Latin *globulus*, globule	Any of a family of proteins in blood plasma.
granulocyte [GRĂN-yū-lō-sīt] Latin *granulum*, granule + -cyte	Leukocyte with granular cytoplasm.
hematocrit [HĒ-mă-tō-krĭt, HĔM-ă-tō-krĭt] hemato- + Greek *krino*, to separate	Measure of the percentage of red blood cells in a blood sample.
hematocytoblast [HĒ-mă-tō-SĪ-tō-blăst] hemato-, blood + -cyto- cell + -blast, immature cell	Most immature blood cell.
heme [hēm] Greek *haima*, blood	Pigment containing iron in hemoglobin.
hemoglobin [hē-mō-GLŌ-bĭn] hemo-, blood + glob(ul)in	Protein in red blood cells essential to the transport of oxygen.
heparin [HĔP-ă-rĭn] From Greek *hepar*, liver	Substance in blood that prevents clotting.
histamine [HĬS-tă-mēn]	Substance released by basophils and eosinophils; involved in allergic reactions.
leukocyte [LŪ-kō-sīt] leuko-, white + -cyte	Mature white blood cell.
lymphocyte [LĬM-fō-sīt] lympho-, lymph + -cyte	Type of agranulocyte.
megakaryocyte [mĕg-ă-KĀR-ē-ō-sīt] mega-, large + karyo-, nucleus + -cyte	Large cells in red bone marrow that form platelets.
monocyte [MŎN-ō-sīt] mono-, one + -cyte	Type of agranulocyte.
neutrophil [NŪ-trō-fĭl] neutro-, neutral + -phil	Type of leukocyte; granulocyte.
plasma [PLĂZ-mă] Greek	Liquid portion of unclotted blood.
plasmapheresis [PLĂZ-mă-fĕ-RĒ-sĭs] plasma + -pheresis, removal	Process of removing blood from a person, centrifuging it, and returning only red blood cells to that person.
platelet [PLĀT-lĕt] plate + -let, small	Thrombocyte; part of a megakaryocyte that initiates clotting.
prothrombin [prō-THRŎM-bĭn]	Type of plasma protein that aids in clotting.
red blood cell	One of the solid parts of blood formed from stem cells and having hemoglobin within; erythrocyte.
red blood cell count	Measurement of red blood cells in a cubic millimeter of blood.
Rh factor rh(esus monkey)	Type of antigen in blood that can cause a transfusion reaction.
Rh-negative	Lacking Rh factor on surface of blood cells.
Rh-positive	Having Rh factor on surface of blood cells.

Term	Definition
serum [SĒR-ŭm] Latin, whey	The liquid left after blood has clotted.
stem cell	Immature cell formed in bone marrow that becomes differentiated into either a red or a white blood cell.
thrombin [THRŎMB-ĭn]	Enzyme that helps in clot formation.
thrombocyte [THRŎM-bō-sīt] thrombo-, blood clot + -cyte	Platelet; cell fragment that produces thrombin.
thromboplastin [thrŏm-bō-PLĂS-tĭn] thrombo- + Greek *plastos*, formed	Protein that aids in forming a fibrin clot.
transfusion [trăns-FYŪ-zhŭn] From Latin *transfundo*, to pour from one vessel to another	Injection of donor blood into a person needing blood.
white blood cell	One of the solid parts of blood from stem cells that plays a role in defense against disease; leukocyte.

STRUCTURE AND FUNCTION EXERCISES

Check Your Knowledge

After each of the following, write the letter of the component of blood that is most closely related to either a, b, or c.

    a. red blood cell   b. white blood cell   c. component of plasma

  1. albumin _____

  2. hemoglobin _____

  3. leukocyte _____

  4. eosinophils _____

  5. gamma globulin _____

  6. fibrinogen _____

  7. basophils _____

  8. beta globulin _____

  9. monocyte _____

 10. neutrophils _____

 11. histamine _____

 12. alpha globulin _____

 13. lymphocytes _____

Find the Type

Write the correct blood type, A, B, AB, or O, in the space following each phrase.

 14. Has A and B antigens _____

 15. Has neither A nor B antigens _____

 16. Has only B antigens _____

 17. Has only A antigens _____

 18. Has both anti-A and anti-B antibodies _____

 19. Has neither anti-A nor anti-B antibodies _____

 20. Has only anti-A antibodies _____

 21. Has only anti-B antibodies _____

Find a Match

Match the term in the left column with its correct definition in the right column.

 22. ____ coagulation   **a.** type of leukocyte

23. ____ heparin
24. ____ neutrophil
25. ____ albumin
26. ____ agglutination
27. ____ Rh factor
28. ____ erythrocyte
29. ____ platelet

b. a blood protein
c. clumping of incompatible blood cells
d. process of clotting
e. antigen
f. cell that activates clotting
g. an anticoagulant
h. red blood cell

CASE STUDY

Getting Treatment

John Maynard was admitted to the hospital on April 2, 2XXX, complaining of respiratory problems and left-sided lower abdominal pain. The doctor on call ordered blood tests, and Mr. Maynard was found to be anemic. Because of Mr. Maynard's multiple medical problems, a hematologist was called in to consult about the disease and treatment of this patient. The history as written in his medical record is as follows:

HISTORY OF PRESENT ILLNESS: John Maynard is an 83-year-old man who was admitted on April 2, 2XXX, with acute exacerbation of chronic obstructive pulmonary disease and left-sided lower abdominal pain. He has been admitted in the past with a similar kind of pain but on the right side. He was evaluated by Dr. Evans in the past, but no obvious additional problem was identified. During this present admission, he was also found to be anemic.

On direct interviewing: Mr. Maynard denies any acute blood loss. His stool and urine color are normal. He has a history of a stroke and has not been ambulatory. He lives with his nephew, who takes care of him. He denies any night sweats. He did not notice any new lumps or bruising anywhere. No new bone pain. He feels short of breath with minimal activity. He denies any chest pain or palpitations. He feels dizzy at times.

Critical Thinking

30. Blood tests can reveal problems almost anywhere in the body. Why are the elements in blood a good measure of many bodily functions?

31. Does Mr. Maynard's blood type (O positive) make him more susceptible to illnesses? Why or why not?

Combining Forms and Abbreviations

The lists below include combining forms and abbreviations that relate specifically to the blood system. Pronunciations are provided for the examples.

COMBINING FORM	MEANING	EXAMPLE
agglutin(o)	agglutinin	*agglutinogenic* [ă-GLŪ-tĭn-ō-JĔN-ĭk], causing the production of agglutinin
eosino	eosinophil	*eosinopenia* [Ē-ŏ-sĭn-ō-PĒ-nē-ă], abnormally low count of eosinophils

COMBINING FORM	MEANING	EXAMPLE
erythr(o)	red	*erythrocyte* [ĕ-RĬTH-rō-sīt], red blood cell
hemo, hemat(o)	blood	*hemodialysis* [HĒ-mō-dī-ĂL-ĭ-sĭs], external dialysis performed by separating solid substances and water from the blood
leuk(o)	white	*leukoblast* [LŪ-kō-blăst], immature white blood cell
phag(o)	eating, devouring	*phagocyte* [FĂG-ō-sīt], cell that consumes other substances, such as bacteria
thromb(o)	blood clot	*thrombocyte* [THRŎM-bō-sīt], cell involved in blood clotting

ABBREVIATION	MEANING	ABBREVIATION	MEANING
APTT	activated partial thromboplastin time	MCHC	mean corpuscular hemoglobin concentration
baso	basophil	MCV	mean corpuscular volume
BCP	biochemistry panel	mono	monocyte
BMT	bone marrow transplant	PCV	packed cell volume
CBC	complete blood count	PLT	platelet count
diff	differential blood count	PMN, poly	polymorphonuclear neutrophil
eos	eosinophils	PT	prothrombin time
ESR	erythrocyte sedimentation rate	PTT	partial thromboplastin time
G-CSF	granulocyte colony-stimulating factor	RBC	red blood cell count
GM-CSF	granulocyte macrophage colony-stimulating factor	SR, sed. rate	sedimentation rate
HCT, Hct	hematocrit	seg	segmented mature white blood cells
HGB, Hgb, HB	hemoglobin	WBC	white blood cell count
MCH	mean corpuscular hemoglobin		

COMBINING FORMS AND ABBREVIATIONS EXERCISES

Find a Match

Match the terms on the left that contain blood system combining forms with the correct definition on the right. You will be using the combining forms, suffixes, or prefixes you have learned in this chapter and in Chapters 1, 2, and 3.

32. _____ leukocytolysis

33. _____ hemotoxin

34. _____ thrombogenic

a. development of white blood cells

b. instrument for counting red blood cells

c. destruction of a clot

35. ____ hemostasis
36. ____ eosinopenia
37. ____ erythrocytometer
38. ____ hemanalysis
39. ____ thrombolysis
40. ____ erythralgia
41. ____ leukopoiesis

d. painful skin redness
e. destruction of white blood cells
f. substance that causes blood poisoning
g. causing blood coagulation
h. stoppage of bleeding
i. blood analysis
j. low number of eosinophils

Build Your Medical Vocabulary

Define the following words using the list of blood system combining forms above and the prefixes, suffixes, and combining forms in Chapters 1, 2, and 3.

42. agglutinophilic
43. thrombectomy
44. erythroblast
45. hematopathology
46. eosinotaxis
47. lymphoblast
48. phagosome

49. polycythemia
50. cytology
51. leukocyte
52. leukemia
53. thrombocytopenia
54. hematoma
55. erythrocytosis

CASE STUDY

Interpreting Results

The laboratory data on Mr. Maynard's record is as follows.

April 2, 2XXX: PSA 1.8
April 2, 2XXX: BUN 6, creatinine .7, calcium 8.3, uric acid 8.7, SGOT 42, SGPT 38, alkaline phosphatase 86, total bilirubin 0.7.
April 2, 2XXX: White blood cell count 5.8, hemoglobin 10.4, HCT 31.1, platelet count 275,000.
December 4, 2XXX: vitamin B12 1,230, folate 16.1.
December 6, 2XXX: HCT 38.9.
December 10, 2XXX: HCT 32.3.

Critical Thinking

56. What procedure is used to obtain the blood samples needed in Mr. Maynard's case? Is it safe to take several blood samples at once? Why or why not?
57. What is the difference between an RBC and a WBC?

Diagnostic, Procedural, and Laboratory Terms

Phlebotomy or **venipuncture,** the withdrawal of blood for examination, is probably the most frequently used diagnostic tool in medicine (Figure 12-7). Various measurements provide a clue as to someone's general health and aid in diagnosing specific conditions. Table 12-3 lists common blood analyses, and Figure 12-8 shows laboratory results for specific blood tests.

Elyse Armadian, M.D. 3 South Windsor Street Fairfield, MN 00219 300-546-7890	Laboratory Report Sunview Diagnostics 6712 Adams Drive Fairfield, MN 00220 300-546-7000	

Patient: Janine Josephs Date Collected: 09/30/XXXX Date Received: 09/30/XXXX	Patient ID: 099-00-1200 Time Collected: 16:05 Date Reported: 10/06/XXXX	Date of Birth: 08/07/43 Total Volume: 2000

Test	Result	Flag	Reference
Complete Blood Count			
WBC	4.0		3.9-11.1
RBC	4.11		3.80-5.20
HCT	39.7		34.0-47.0
MCV	96.5		80.0-98.0
MCH	32.9		27.1-34.0
MCHC	34.0		32.0-36.0
MPV	8.6		7.5-11.5
NEUTROPHILS %	45.6		38.0-80.0
NEUTROPHILS ABS.	1.82		1.70-8.50
LYMPHOCYTES %	36.1		15.0-49.0
LYMPHOCYTES ABS.	1.44		1.00-3.50
EOSINOPHILS %	4.5		0.0-8.0
EOSINOPHILS ABS.	0.18		0.03-0.55
BASOPHILS %	0.7		0.0-2.0
BASOPHILS ABS.	0.03		0.000-0.185
PLATELET COUNT	229		150-400
Automated Chemistries			
GLUCOSE	80		65-109
UREA NITROGEN	17		6-30
CREATININE (SERUM)	0.6		0.5-1.3
UREA NITROGEN/CREATININE	28		10-29
SODIUM	140		135-145
POTASSIUM	4.4		3.5-5.3
CHLORIDE	106		96-109
CO_2	28		20-31
ANION GAP	6		3-19
CALCIUM	9.8		8.6-10.4
PHOSPHORUS	3.6		2.2-4.6
AST (SGOT)	28		0-30
ALT (SGPT)	19		0-34
BILIRUBIN, TOTAL	0.5		0.2-1.2
PROTEIN, TOTAL	7.8		6.2-8.2
ALBUMIN	4.3		3.5-5.0
GLOBULIN	3.5		2.1-3.8
URIC ACID	2.4		2.0-7.5
CHOLESTEROL	232	*	120-199
TRIGLYCERIDES	68		40-199
IRON	85		30-150
HDL CHOLESTEROL	73	*	35-59
CHOLESTEROL/HDL RATIO	3.2		3.2-5.7
LDL, CALCULATED	148	*	70-129
T3, UPTAKE	32		24-37
T4, TOTAL	6.9		4.5-12.8

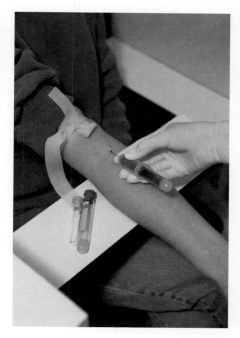

FIGURE 12-7 Venipuncture is used in most regular medical examinations to extract blood for analysis.

FIGURE 12-8 A laboratory report showing a number of tests and the expected range of results for each type of test.

Most of the blood tests described in Table 12-3 are performed in a laboratory. Names of tests may vary according to the region of the country or the practice of a particular doctor. For example, a biochemistry panel is sometimes called a **chemistry profile,** and a blood chemistry is sometimes

TABLE 12-3 Common Blood Analyses (see Appendix D for Normal Laboratory Values)

Test or Procedure	Purpose of Test	Common Diseases/Disorders That May Be Indicated
complete blood count (CBC)	common screen for basic medical checkup (Figure 12-8)	iron-deficiency anemia bacterial or viral infection internal bleeding dehydration aplastic anemia impaired renal function liver disease circulatory disorder
blood chemistry	test of plasma for presence of most substances, such as glucose, cholesterol, uric acid, and electrolytes	diabetes hyperlipidemia gout circulatory disorders impaired renal function liver diseases general metabolic disorder
biochemistry panel	group of automated tests for various common diseases or disorders	same as blood chemistry
blood indices	measurement of size, volume, and content of red blood cells	classification of anemias
blood culture	test of a blood specimen in a culture in which microorganisms are observed; test for infections	septicemia bacterial infections
erythrocyte sedimentation rate (ESR); sedimentation rate (SR)	test for rate at which red blood cells fall through plasma; indicator of inflammation and/or tissue injury	infections joint inflammation sickle cell anemia liver and kidney disorders
white blood cell differential and red blood cell morphology	test for number of types of leukocytes and shape of red blood cells	infection anemia leukemia poikilocytosis anisocytosis
platelet count (PLT)	test for number of thrombocytes in a blood sample	hemorrhage infections malignancy hypersplenism aplastic anemia thrombocytopenia
partial thromboplastin time (PTT)	test for coagulation defects	vitamin K deficiency hepatic disease hemophilia hemorrhagic disorders
prothrombin time (PT)	test for coagulation defects	vitamin K deficiency hepatic disease hemorrhagic disorders hemophilia

TABLE 12-3 **Common Blood Analyses (see Appendix D for Normal Laboratory Values) (cont.)**

Test or Procedure	Purpose of Test	Common Diseases/Disorders That May Be Indicated
antiglobulin test; *Coombs' test*	test for antibodies on red blood cells	Rh factor and anemia
white blood count (WBC)	number of white blood cells in a sample (usually done as part of complete blood count)	bacterial or viral infection aplastic anemia leukemia leukocytosis
red blood count (RBC)	number of red blood cells in a sample (usually done as part of complete blood count)	polycythemia dehydration iron-deficiency anemia blood loss erythropoiesis
hemoglobin (HGB, Hgb)	level of hemoglobin in blood (usually done as part of complete blood count)	polycythemia dehydration anemia sickle cell anemia recent hemorrhage
hematocrit (HCT, Hct)	measure of packed red blood cells in a sample (usually done as part of complete blood count). This shows the percent of red blood cells.	polycythemia dehydration blood loss anemia
mean corpuscular volume (MCV)	volume of individual cells (usually part of blood indices)	microcytic or macrocytic anemia
mean corpuscular hemoglobin (MCH)	weight of hemoglobin in average red blood cell (usually part of blood indices)	classification of anemia
mean corpuscular hemoglobin concentration (MCHC)	concentration of hemoglobin in a red blood cell (usually part of blood indices)	hyperchromic or hypochromic anemia

known as an **SMA (sequential multiple analyzer),** the name of the first machine used to analyze blood chemistries.

VOCABULARY REVIEW

In the previous section, you learned diagnostic, procedural, and laboratory terms. Before going on to the exercises, review the terms below and refer to the previous section if you have any questions. Pronunciations are provided for certain terms. Sometimes information about where the word came from is included after the term. These etymologies (word histories) are for your information only. You do not need to memorize them.

Term	Definition
antiglobulin [ĂN-tē-GLŎB-yū-lĭn] **test** anti(body) + globulin	Test for antibodies on red blood cells.
biochemistry panel	Common group of automated tests run on one blood sample.

Term	Definition
blood chemistry	Test of plasma for presence of a particular substance such as glucose.
blood culture	Test of a blood specimen in a culture medium to observe for particular microorganisms.
blood indices [ĬN-dĭ-sēz]	Measurement of the characteristics of red blood cells.
chemistry profile	*See* blood chemistry.
complete blood count (CBC)	Most common blood test for a number of factors.
erythrocyte sedimentation rate (ESR)	Test for rate at which red blood cells fall through plasma.
partial thromboplastin time (PTT)	Test for ability of blood to coagulate.
phlebotomy [flĕ-BŎT-ō-mē] phlebo-, vein + -tomy, a cutting	*See* venipuncture.
platelet count (PLT)	Measurement of number of platelets in a blood sample.
prothrombin time (PT)	Test for ability of blood to coagulate.
red blood cell morphology	Observation of shape of red blood cells.
sedimentation rate (SR)	*See* erythrocyte sedimentation rate.
SMA (sequential multiple analyzer)	Original blood chemistry machine; now a synonym for blood chemistry.
venipuncture [VĔN-ĭ-pŭnk-chŭr, VĒ-nĭ-pŭnk-chŭr] veni-, vein + puncture	Insertion of a needle into a vein, usually for the purpose of extracting a blood sample.

CASE STUDY

Evaluating the Tests

Mr. Maynard's record has the following notes from the hematologist's evaluation.

ASSESSMENT: Mr. Maynard has multiple medical problems. He has recently been admitted with abdominal discomfort, the etiology of which is unclear at this point. He was also found to have anemia. A review of his laboratory data shows that his hematocrit has been fluctuating between 27 and 38. His hematocrit on December 6 was 38.9, but within four days it dropped to 32.3. Since then there have also been several incidences in which his hematocrit dropped further, but then improved. This variation in the hematocrit is suggestive of some ongoing blood loss.

Critical Thinking

58. Other than blood loss, name at least two other conditions the HCT results might indicate.
59. What is the name of a test for leukocytes?

Match the Test

Match the name of the test in the column on the left to its correct description in the column on the right.

60. ____ blood culture

61. ____ hematocrit

62. ____ sedimentation rate

63. ____ white blood count

64. ____ antiglobulin test

65. ____ mean corpuscular hemoglobin concentration

66. ____ mean corpuscular volume

67. ____ complete blood count

68. ____ prothrombin time

69. ____ biochemistry panel

a. average red blood cell volume

b. antibodies on red blood cells

c. rate at which red blood cells fall

d. group of automated tests

e. most common blood test

f. clotting factors test

g. number of white blood cells

h. measure of packed red blood cells

i. concentration of hemoglobin in red blood cells

j. growing of microorganisms in a culture

Find the Value

Give the expected (normal) range for each of the following laboratory measurements.

70. cholesterol _____

71. sodium _____

72. iron _____

73. thyroid (T4) _____

74. MCV _____

75. PLT _____

76. HCT _____

77. RBC _____

78. WBC _____

79. MCHC _____

Pathological Terms

Many diseases and disorders have some effect on the blood, but they are really diseases of other body systems. For example, diabetes is a disorder of the endocrine system, but its diagnosis includes an analysis of blood glucose levels.

Actual diseases of the blood are characterized by changes in the supply or characteristics of blood cells, presence of microorganisms affecting the blood, or presence or lack of certain substances in the blood. **Dyscrasia** is a general term for any disease of the blood with abnormal material present.

Anemia is a general term for a condition in which the red blood cells do not transport enough oxygen to the tissues due to a deficiency in number or quality of red blood cells. The most common types of anemia include:

- *Iron-deficiency anemia*, a lack of enough iron in the blood that affects the production of hemoglobin
- *Aplastic anemia*, a failure of the bone marrow to produce enough red blood cells
- *Pernicious anemia*, a condition in which the shape and number of the red blood cells changes due to a lack of sufficient vitamin B_{12}

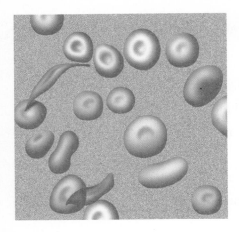

FIGURE 12-9 Characteristics of blood cells in certain anemias.

The Anemia Institute (www .anemiainstitute.org) provides detailed information about many types of anemia.

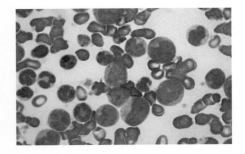

FIGURE 12-10 A blood smear showing chronic myelogenous leukemia (CML).

The Leukemia and Lymphoma Society's Web site (www.leukemia-lymphoma .org) has up-to-date information about various kinds of leukemia.

- *Sickle cell anemia*, a hereditary condition (usually in persons of African-American ancestry) characterized by sickle-shaped red blood cells and a breakdown in red blood cell membranes
- *Hemolytic anemia*, a disorder characterized by destruction of red blood cells
- *Posthemorrhagic anemia*, a disorder resulting from a sudden, dramatic loss of blood
- **Thalassemia,** an inherited disorder (usually in people of Mediterranean origin) resulting in an inability to produce sufficient hemoglobin (the most severe form of which is *Cooley's anemia*).

Figure 12-9 shows blood cell characteristics for some anemias.

Von Willebrand's disease is a hemorrhagic disorder in which there is a greater tendency to bleed due to the lack of a clotting factor called *Factor VIII*. Common symptoms are bruising and nosebleeds. Two other disorders of the blood that involve excessive bleeding are **hemophilia** and **thrombocytopenia.** Hemophilia is a hereditary lack of clotting Factor VIII (or, in 15 percent of the cases, a different clotting factor, Factor IX). Hemophiliacs can be treated with medications and transfusions. Thrombocytopenia is a bleeding disorder with insufficient platelets to aid in the clotting process. Thrombocytopenia is present in **purpura,** a condition with multiple tiny hemorrhages under the skin (Figure 12-10).

Small, flat, red spots called *petechiae* may indicate a deficiency in the number of platelets. There are a number of disorders of the blood cells or related substances in the blood. **Pancytopenia** is a condition with a low number of all blood cell components (red blood cells, white blood cells, and thrombocytes). The blood must be supplemented with transfusions. **Erythropenia** (also called *erythrocytopenia*) is a disorder with an abnormally low number of red blood cells. **Hemochromatosis** is a hereditary disorder leading to excessive buildup of iron in the blood. Because excessive iron in the blood can ultimately cause heart failure, people with this disorder have to limit their iron intake.

Polycythemia is a disease that causes an abnormal increase in red blood cells and hemoglobin. Various forms of the disease are associated with conditions such as hypertension and emphysema. **Anisocytosis** is characterized by red blood cells of differing sizes and shapes, a characteristic that prevents them from functioning normally. **Macrocytosis** is a disorder with abnormally large red blood cells present, and **microcytosis** is a disorder with abnormally small red blood cells present. **Poikilocytosis** is a disorder with irregularly-shaped red blood cells present. **Reticulocytosis** is a disorder with an abnormal number of immature erythrocytes present. **Hemolysis** is a disorder with breakdowns in the red blood cell membrane.

There are also disorders of white blood cells. The major disease involving white blood cells is **leukemia.** Leukemia is a general term for a disorder with an excessive increase in white blood cells in the bone marrow and bloodstream. People with leukemia may experience *remissions* (disappearances of the disease) and *relapses* (recurrences of the disease). Some leukemias (acute lymphocytic leukemia and chronic lymphocytic leukemia) occur in the lymph system.

The two most common leukemias of the bone marrow and bloodstream are AML and CML. *Acute myelogenous leukemia (AML)* is a disorder in which immature granulocytes (or **myeloblasts**) invade the bone marrow. *Chronic* *myelogenous leukemia (CML)* or chronic granulocytic leukemia is a disorder in which mature and immature myeloblasts are present in the bloodstream and marrow. It is usually a slowly developing illness with a reasonably good prognosis. *Acute lymphocytic leukemia (ALL)* is a disorder with an abnormal number of immature lymphocytes. It is usually a disease of childhood and adolescence. The prognosis for recovery is very good. *Chronic lymphocytic leukemia (CLL)* appears mainly in adults and includes an abnormal number of mature lymphocytes.

Another disorder of the white blood cells is **granulocytosis,** an abnormal increase in granulocytes in the bloodstream, such as neutrophils during infection. Granulocytosis can also occur in combination with allergic conditions or certain infections, in which case it is called **eosinophilia,** an abnormal increase in eosinophilic granuloctyes. **Basophilia** is an increase in basophilic granuloctyes that is found in some types of leukemia. *Neutropenia* is a disorder with an abnormally low number of neutrophils in the bloodstream. *Neutrophilia* is a disorder with an abnormal increase in neutrophils.

Erythroblastosis fetalis, or Rh factor incompatibility between the mother and a fetus, can cause death to the fetus or a type of fetal anemia. A blood transfusion or treatment with medication can sometimes save the fetus.

Multiple myeloma is a malignant tumor of the bone marrow. It involves overproduction of certain white blood cells that produce immunoglobulins. The myeloma cells then migrate to different areas of the body where they cause tumors and destroy bony structures.

> At www.multiplemyeloma.org, you can learn about the treatment options for multiple myeloma.

VOCABULARY REVIEW

In the previous section, you learned terms relating to pathology. Before going on to the exercises, review the terms below and refer to the previous section if you have any questions. Pronunciations are provided for certain terms. Sometimes information about where the word came from is included after the term. These etymologies (word histories) are for your information only. You do not need to memorize them.

Term	Definition
anemia [ă-NĒ-mē-ă] Greek *anaimia* from an-, without + *haima*, blood	Condition in which red blood cells do not transport enough oxygen to the tissues.
anisocytosis [ăn-Ī-sō-sĭ-TŌ-sĭs] aniso-, unequal + cyt-, cell + -osis, condition	Condition with abnormal variation in the size of red blood cells.
basophilia [bā-sō-FĬL-ē-ă]	Condition with an increased number of basophils in the blood.
dyscrasia [dĭs-KRĀ-zhē-ă] Greek, bad temperament	Any disease with abnormal particles in the blood.
eosinophilia [Ē-ō-sĭn-ō-FĬL-ē-ă]	Condition with an abnormal number of eosinophils in the blood.
erythroblastosis fetalis [ĕ-RĬTH-rō-blăs-TŌ-sĭs fē-TĂL-ĭs]	Incompatibility disorder between a mother with Rh negative and a fetus with Rh positive.

Term	Definition
erythropenia [ĕ-rĭth-rō-PĒ-nē-ă] erythro-, red blood cells + -penia, deficiency	Disorder with abnormally low number of red blood cells.
granulocytosis [GRĂN-yū-lō-sĭ-TŌ-sĭs] granulocyt(e) + -osis, condition	Condition with an abnormal number of granulocytes in the bloodstream.
hemochromatosis [HĔ-mō-krō-mă-TŌ-sĭs] hemo-, blood + chromat-, color + -osis	Hereditary condition with excessive iron buildup in the blood.
hemolysis [hē-MŎL-ĭ-sĭs] hemo-, blood + -lysis, destruction of	Disorder with breakdown of red blood cell membranes.
hemophilia [hē-mō-FĬL-ē-ă] hemo-, blood + -philia, attraction	Hereditary disorder with lack of clotting factor in the blood.
leukemia [lū-KĒ-mē-ă] leuk-, white + -emia, blood	General term for a number of disorders with excessive white blood cells in the bloodstream and bone marrow.
macrocytosis [MĂK-rō-sĭ-TŌ-sĭs] macro-, large + cyt- + -osis	Disorder with abnormally large red blood cells.
microcytosis [MĬK-rō-sĭ-TŌ-sĭs] micro-, small + cyt- + -osis	Disorder with abnormally small red blood cells.
multiple myeloma [mī-ĕ-LŌ-mă]	Malignant tumor of the bone marrow.
myeloblast [MĬ-ĕ-lō-blăst] myelo-, marrow + -blast, immature cell	Immature granulocytes.
pancytopenia [PĂN-sī-tō-PĒ-nē-ă] pan-, all + cyto- + -penia	Condition with a low number of blood components.
poikilocytosis [PŎY-kĭ-lō-sī-TŌ-sĭs] poikilo-, irregular + cyt- + -osis	Disorder with irregularly shaped red blood cells.
polycythemia [PŎL-ē-sī-THĒ-mē-ă] poly-, many + cyt- + -emia	Disorder with an abnormal increase in red blood cells and hemoglobin.
purpura [PŬR-pū-ră] Latin, purple	Condition with multiple tiny hemorrhages under the skin.
reticulocytosis [rĕ-TĬK-yū-lō-sī-TŌ-sĭs] recticulo-, fine network + cyt- + -osis	Disorder with an abnormal number of immature erythrocytes.
thalassemia [thăl-ă-SĒ-mē-ă] Greek *thalassa*, sea + -emia	Hereditary disorder characterized by inability to produce sufficient hemoglobin.
thrombocytopenia [THRŎM-bō-sī-tō-PĒ-nē-ă] thrombocyt(e) + -penia	Bleeding condition with insufficient production of platelets.
von Willebrand's [vŏn WĬL-lĕ-brăndz] **disease** After E. A. von Willebrand (1870–1949), Finnish physician	Hemorrhagic disorder with tendency to bleed from mucous membranes.

CASE STUDY

Reading the X-Rays

Next, the radiology report is added to Mr. Maynard's record, and the hematologist adds notes.

Critical Thinking

80. Does a CBC provide enough information for a diagnosis of anemia or chronic blood loss?

81. Is Rh factor important for an 83-year-old man? Why or why not?

RADIOLOGY: Abdomen: Adynamic ileus.

April 2, 2XXX: Chest; bibasilar changes compatible with a small pleural effusion. Increased density in the right lung and small localized density because of rotation.

December 4, 2XXX: Abdominal ultrasound; normal biliary examination. Bilateral multiple renal cysts. Liver; fatty texture.

In summary, I have initiated more workup for anemia. The possibilities include anemia of chronic disease, myelo-dysplasia, or chronic blood loss. If his workup is inconclusive, then he might require bone marrow aspiration and biopsy to establish the diagnosis.

PATHOLOGICAL TERMS EXERCISES

Spell It Correctly

The following terms are either spelled correctly or incorrectly. Put C in the space following correctly spelled words. Put the correct spelling in the space following incorrectly spelled words.

82. hemphilia _____

83. pancypenia _____

84. macrocytosis _____

85. anemia _____

86. alplastic anemia _____

87. eosinphilia _____

88. pupura _____

89. reticulocytosis _____

90. thrombocytenia _____

91. poikilocytosis _____

Check Your Knowledge

Circle T for true or F for false.

92. Sickle cell anemia is found primarily in people of Mediterranean origin. T F

93. All red blood cell disorders are inherited. T F

94. A sudden loss of blood can cause anemia. T F

95. Multiple myeloma is a form of cancer. T F

96. Rh factor incompatibility can cause hemochromatosis. T F

97. Pernicious anemia may result from a deficiency of vitamin B_{12}. T F

98. Leukemia and anemia are types of cancer. T F

99. Too many red blood cells can be a symptom of a disorder. T F

Find the Meaning

Describe the cause of each of the following forms of anemia.

100. aplastic anemia

101. iron-deficiency anemia

102. pernicious anemia

103. thalassemia

104. sickle cell anemia

CASE STUDY

Getting Confirmation

In addition to his other problems, Mr. Maynard has prostate cancer. His PSA has remained normal for a few years, so the cancer is thought to be in remission. However, the cause of the anemia was not confirmed. His diagnosis is also not confirmed, so a bone marrow biopsy is ordered. The bone marrow biopsy confirms aplastic anemia.

Critical Thinking

105. Describe the abnormality that the bone marrow biopsy reveals.

106. Does Mr. Maynard's condition require treatment before he has any surgery?

Surgical Terms

Surgery is not generally performed on the blood system. Sometimes venipuncture is considered a minor surgical procedure. (In this text, we have classified it as a diagnostic procedure.) The exceptions are **bone marrow biopsy** and **bone marrow transplant.**

A bone marrow biopsy is used in the diagnosis of various blood disorders, such as anemia and leukemia. A needle is introduced into the bone marrow cavity and marrow is extracted for examination.

A bone marrow transplant is performed for serious ailments, such as leukemia and cancer. In this procedure, a donor's marrow is introduced into the bone marrow of the patient. First, all the diseased cells are killed through extensive radiation and chemotherapy. After the donor's marrow is introduced, successful transplants result in healthy cells taking over the patient's marrow. Unsuccessful transplants may result in rejection of the marrow or a recurrence of the disease.

The National Marrow Donor Program (www.marrow.org) tells you how to become a bone marrow donor.

VOCABULARY REVIEW

In the previous section, you learned terms relating to surgery. Before going to the exercises, review the terms below and refer to the previous section if you have any questions. Pronunciations are provided for certain terms. Sometimes information about where the word came from is included after the term. These etymologies (word histories) are for your information only. You do not need to memorize them.

Term	Definition
bone marrow biopsy	Extraction of bone marrow, by means of a needle, for observation.
bone marrow transplant	Injection of donor bone marrow into a patient whose diseased cells have been killed through radiation and chemotherapy.

Pharmacological Terms

Medications that directly affect the work of the blood system are **anticoagulants** (to prevent blood clotting); **thrombolytics** (to dissolve blood clots); **coagulants** or clotting agents (to aid in blood clotting); and **hemostatics** (to stop bleeding, such as vitamin K). Anticoagulants are administered before most types of surgeries to prevent emboli. Blood flow is affected by vasoconstrictors and vasodilators, two medications given for cardiovascular problems.

Chemotherapy, therapy that uses drugs, is used to cause a **remission** (disappearance of the disease) in leukemia. Sometimes more treatment is needed when a **relapse** (recurrence of the disease) occurs. Table 12-4 lists common pharmaceutical agents used in treating blood disorders.

TABLE 12-4 Some Pharmaceutical Agents Used to Treat Blood Disorders

Drug Class	Purpose	Generic	Trade Name
anticoagulant	dissolves blood clots	warfarin	Coumadin
		heparin	various
		dipyrimadole	Persantine
		enoxaparin	Lovenox
clotting agent; coagulant	aids in clotting blood	phytonadione,	Mephyton
		vitamin K	
hemostatic	stops bleeding	aminocaproic acid	Amicar
		recombinant factor VIIa	NovoSeven
thrombolytic	dissolves blood clots	streptokinase	Streptase
		urokinase	Abbokinase
		alteplace	Activase

VOCABULARY REVIEW

In the previous section, you learned terms relating to pharmacology. Before going on to the exercises, review the terms below and refer to the previous section if you have any questions. Pronunciations are provided for certain terms. Sometimes information about where the word came from is included after the term. These etymologies (word histories) are for your information only. You do not need to memorize them.

Term	Definition
anticoagulant [ĂN-tē-kō-ĂG-yū-lĕnt] anti-, against + coagulant	Agent that prevents formation of blood clots.
coagulant [kō-ĂG-yū-lĕnt] Latin *coagulo*, to curdle	Clotting agent.
hemostatic [hē-mō-STĂT-ĭk] hemo-, blood + -static, maintaining a state	Agent that stops bleeding.
relapse [RĒ-lăps] From Latin *relabor*, to slide back	Recurrence of a disease.
remission [rē-MĬSH-ŭn] Latin *remissio*, a relaxation	Disappearance of a disease for a time.
thrombolytic [thrŏm-bō-LĬT-ĭk] thrombo-, thrombus + -lytic, a loosening	Agent that dissolves blood clots.

CASE STUDY

Coordinating Prescription Medication

Mr. Maynard's medication list at admission is:

Cardura 4 mg. p.o. q.h.s.
Ventolin unit does t.i.d.
Atrovent unit does t.i.d.
Ceftin 250 mg. b.i.d. prior to admission.
Magnesium citrate b.i.d.
Lactulose 30 cc p.o. b.i.d.

Cardura is for his high blood pressure and prostate problems. Ventolin and Atrovent are prescribed for his respiratory symptoms. Ceftin is an antibiotic for a urinary tract infection. Magnesium citrate and lactulose are laxatives.

Critical Thinking

107. Aspirin is known to promote some bleeding. Should Mr. Maynard use aspirin for pain?

108. What vitamin might improve Mr. Maynard's condition?

PHARMACOLOGICAL TERMS EXERCISES

Check Your Knowledge

Fill in the blanks.

109. Hemophiliacs require _____ and _____ to control bleeding.

110. A prescription for someone with coronary artery disease might include a(n) _____.

111. If medication is not taken regularly, a(n) _____ of a disease might occur.

112. Sometimes the temporary disappearance of a disease, called a(n) _____, is unexplained.

CHALLENGE SECTION

The form shown in Figure 12-8 gives results for a patient and expected ranges for lab tests done in a large lab service.

Critical Thinking

113. What tests, if any, are abnormal?

114. The laboratory was instructed to do a T3 and T4 uptake test. What was the patient's physician trying to determine?

TERMINOLOGY IN ACTION

Alicia Minot is a 21-year-old student who is prone to migraine headaches. Her latest visit to her family doctor included a general physical and a CBC as well as a urinalysis. All test results were normal except for a low hemoglobin count. Alicia complains that Tylenol does not relieve her headaches and she wants to use her mother's aspirin. Do you think the doctor will recommend aspirin? Why or why not? What are some steps Alicia can take in her daily life to raise her hemoglobin count?

USING THE INTERNET

Go to the Web site of the Aplastic Anemia Association (www.aplastic.org). Choose one of their online articles and write a paragraph summarizing its content.

CHAPTER REVIEW

The material that follows is to help you review all the material in this chapter.

Matching

Write the letter of the meaning of the term in the space provided.

115. _____ erythropoietin

116. _____ fibrinogen

117. _____ gamma globulin

118. _____ histamine

119. _____ plasmapheresis

120. _____ thromboplastin

a. Protein in the plasma that aids in clotting.

b. Substance released by basophils and eosinophils; involved in allergic reactions.

c. Protein that aids in forming a fibrin clot.

d. Hormone released by the kidneys to stimulate red blood cell production.

e. A protein that arises in lymphatic tissue and functions as part of the immune system.

f. Process of removing blood from a person, centrifuging it, and returning only red blood cells to that person.

Complete the Sentence

Circle the term that best describes the *italicized* description of the correct answer

121. Mrs. Sommers is *lacking the Rh factor on the surface of her red blood cells*, therefore she is (Rh-negative, Rh-neutral, Rh-positive).

122. Mr. Martinez has *an increase in his platelet count* or (thrombocytes, granulocytes, megakaryocytes).

123. *The liquid portion of unclotted blood* is called (serum, plasma, albumin).

124. The physician informed Mrs. Larkin that *the protein in the red cells essential to the transport of oxygen* was low. He was referring to her (red blood cell, hematocrit, hemoglobin) level.

125. *Basophils, eosinophils and neutrophils* are all considered (granulocytes, agranulocytes, hematocystoblasts).

126. The process of *infusing donor blood into a person needing blood* is known as: (plasmapheresis, agglutination, transfusion).

Root Out the Meaning

Separate the following terms into word parts; define each word part.

127. eosinophilic_____

128. hemolysis _____

129. hemocytometer_____

130. pancytopenia_____

131. phlebitis _____

132. phlebotomy_____

133. phlebectomy_____

134. hematoma_____

135. anisocytosis_____

136. thrombophlebitis _____

137. hemostatic _____

138. venospasm _____

139. hemogram _____

140. hemolytic _____

141. anemia _____

142. phlebography _____

143. phlebectasia _____

144. hemorrhage _____

145. hemopathy _____

146. hematopoiesis _____

147. hematology _____

148. plasmapheresis _____

149. sideropenia _____

150. basophil _____

Complete the Sentence

Circle the term that best describes the *italicized* description of the correct answer.

151. A disorder in which there are *excessive red blood cells* is known as: (eyrthrocytopenia, polycythemia, leukemia).

152. This test measures the amount of *protein essential to the transport of oxygen.* (hematocrit, hemogram, hemoglobin).

153. A *blood disorder with a tendency to hemorrhage* is known as (hemophilia, anemia, dyscrasia).

154. The test results indicated a *fragmentation of red blood cells* or (eosinosis, erythroclasis, erytholysis).

155. The term *hemocytoblasts* refers to (red cells, stem cells, white cells).

156. The *largest of the white blood cells* is called a (neutrophil, basophil, monocyte).

157. These cells *break off from larger cells in the red bone marrow* and assist in blood clotting (megakaryocytes, agranulocytes, proerythoblasts).

158. A MCV test can indicate (microcytic or macrocytic, hyperchromic or hypochromic) anemia.

Building Your Medical Vocabulary

Construct a word with each of the following meanings. Some of the word parts you need to use are in Chapters 1 and 2.

159. An immature white blood cell _____

160. Dissolution of red blood cells _____

161. The study of the structure of red blood cells _____

162. A normal (red) blood cell _____

163. A cell that ingests bacteria and other particles _____

164. Irregularly shaped red blood cells _____

165. A spherical red blood cell _____

166. White blood cell cancer _____

167. Removal of white blood cells from drawn blood _____

168. Forming new blood cells _____

Matching

Indicate whether the abbreviation refers to red cells, white cells or platelets.

 R = red cells
W = white cells
 P = platelets

169. ____ APTT

170. ____ seg

171. ____ SR

172. ____ PLT

173. ____ HCT

174. ____ ESR

175. ____ diff

176. ____ mono

177. ____ MCHC

178. ____ PMN, poly

Matching

Place the letter of the pharmaceutical agents used to treat blood disorders to the left in the blank and then state the drugs purpose in the blank after the drug class.

179. Thrombolytic: _____

180. Coagulant: _____

181. Hemostatic: _____

182. Anticoagulant: _____

a. heparin

b. streptokinase

c. vitamin K

d. aminocaproic acid

True or False

Indicate in the blank whether the statement is true or false.

183. The disappearance of a disease for a time is known as submission _____.

184. A bone marrow transplant is the extraction of bone marrow, by means of a needle, for observation _____.

185. A malignant tumor of the bone marrow is referred to as multiple myeloma _____.

186. Erythroblastosis fetalis is the a condition in which a fetus forms new red blood cells _____.

187. Purpura is a condition in which multiple tiny hemorrhages form under the skin _____.

188. Aplastic anemia is the failure of the bone marrow to produce enough red blood cells _____.

189. Hemodialysis is the internal dialysis performed by separating solid substances and water from the blood _____.

190. Agglutination is the clumping of cells and particles in the blood _____.

191. Plasma is the liquid portion of clotted blood _____.

192. A hereditary condition with excessive iron buildup in the blood is known as sickle cell anemia _____.

Check Your Spelling

If the word is spelled correctly place a C in the blank. If the term is not spelled correctly, place the correct spelling in the blank.

193. miloblast _____

194. hematoglobin _____

195. neutralphil _____

196. granulocytosis _____

197. histamean _____

198. antiglobulin _____

199. remission _____

200. thalassemia _____

201. anesocytosis _____

202. reticulocitosis _____

203. venapuncture _____

204. phlebodomy _____

DEFINITIONS

Define the following terms and combining forms. Review the chapter before starting. Make sure you know how to pronounce each term as you define it. The blue words in curly brackets are references to the Spanish Glossary available online at www.mhhe.com/medterm3e.

WORD

205. agglutin(o)

206. agglutination [ă-glū-tǐ-NĀ-shŭn] {aglutinación}

207. agglutinogen [ă-glū-TǏN-ō-jĕn] {aglutinógeno}

208. agranulocyte [ă-GRĂN-yū-lō-sǐt] {agranulocito}

209. albumin [ăl-BYŪ-mǐn] {albúmina}

210. anemia [ă-NĒ-mē-ă] {anemia}

211. anisocytosis [ăn-Ī-sō-sǐ-TŌ-sǐs] {anisocitosis}

212. anticoagulant [ĂN-tē-kō-ĂG-yū-lĕnt]

213. antiglobulin [ĂN-tē-GLŎB-yū-lǐn] test

214. basophil [BĀ-sō-fǐl] {basófilo}

215. basophilia [bā-sō-FǏL-ē-ă] {basofilia}

216. biochemistry panel

217. blood [blŭd] {sangre}

218. blood chemistry

219. blood culture

220. blood indices [ǏN-dǐ-sēz]

221. blood types or groups

222. bone marrow biopsy

223. bone marrow transplant

224. chemistry profile

225. coagulant [ko-ĂG-yŭ-lĕnt]

226. coagulation [kō-ăg-yū-LĀ-shŭn] {coagulación}

227. complete blood count (CBC)

228. dyscrasia [dǐs-KRĀ-zhē-ă] {discrasia}

229. electrophoresis [ē-lĕk-trō-FŌR-ē-sǐs] {electroforesis}

230. eosino

231. eosinophil [ē-ō-SǏN-ō-fǐl] {eosinófilo}

232. eosinophilia [Ē-ō-sǐn-ō-FǏL-ē-ă] {eosinofilia}

233. erythr(o)

234. erythroblastosis fetalis [ĕ-RǏTH-rō-blăs-TŌ-sǐs fē-TĂL-ǐs]

235. erythrocyte [ĕ-RǏTH-rō-sīt] {eritrocito}

236. erythrocyte sedimentation rate (ESR)

237. erythropenia [ĕ-rǐth-rō-PĒ-nē-ă] {eritropenia}

238. erythropoietin [ĕ-rǐth-rō-PŎY-ĕ-tǐn] {eritropoyetina}

239. fibrin [FǏ-brǐn] clot

240. fibrinogen [fǐ-BRǏN-ō-jĕn] {fibrinógeno}

241. gamma globulin [GĂ-mă GLŎB-yū-lǐn]

242. globin [GLŌ-bǐn] {globina}

243. globulin [GLŎB-yū-lǐn] {globulina}

244. granulocyte [GRĂN-yū-lō-sǐt]

245. granulocytosis [GRĂN-yū-lō-sǐ-TŌ-sǐs] {granulocitosis}

246. hematocrit [HĒ-mă-tō-krǐt, HĔM-ă-tō-krǐt] {hematócrito}

247. hematocytoblast [HĒ-mă-tō-SǏ-tō-blăst] {hematocitoblasto}

248. heme [hēm]

249. hemo, hemat(o)

250. hemochromatosis [HĒ-mō-krō-mă-TŌ-sǐs]

251. hemoglobin [hē-mō-GLŌ-bǐn] {hemoglobina}

252. hemolysis [he-MŎL-ǐ-sǐs] {hemólisis}

253. hemophilia [hē-mō-FǏL-ē-ă] {hemofilia}

254. hemostatic [hē-mō-STĂT-ǐk]

255. heparin [HĔP-ă-rǐn] {heparina}

256. histamine [HǏS-tă-mēn] {histamine}

257. leuk(o)

258. leukocyte [LŪ-kō-sǐt] {leucocito}

259. leukemia [lū-KĒ-mē-ă] {leucemia}

260. lymphocyte [LĬM-fō-sīt] {linfocito}

261. macrocytosis [MĂK-rō-sī-TŌ-sĭs] {macrocitosis}

262. megakaryocyte [měg-ă-KĀR-ē-ō-sīt] {megacariocito}

263. microcytosis [MĪK-rō-sī-TŌ-sĭs] {microcitosis}

264. monocyte [MŎN-ō-sīt] {monocito}

265. multiple myeloma [mī-ĕ-LŌ-mă]

266. myeloblast [MĪ-ĕ-lŏ-blăst] {mieloblasto}

267. neutrophil [NŪ-trō-fĭl] {neutrófilo}

268. pancytopenia [PĂN-sī-tō-PĒ-nē-ă] {pancitopenia}

269. partial thromboplastin time (PTT)

270. phag(o)

271. phlebotomy [flĕ-BŎT-ō-mē] {flebotomía}

272. plasma [PLĂZ-mă] {plasma}

273. plasmapheresis [PLĂZ-mă-fĕ-RĒ-sĭs] {plasmaféresis}

274. platelet [PLĀT-lĕt] {plaqueta}

275. platelet count (PLT)

276. poikilocytosis [PŎY-kĭ-lō-sī-TŌ-sĭs] {poiquilocitosis}

277. polycythemia [PŎL-ē-sī-THĒ-mē-ă] {policetemia}

278. prothrombin [prō-THRŎM-bĭn] {protrombina}

279. prothrombin time (PT)

280. purpura [PŬR-pū-ră] {púrpura}

281. red blood cell

282. red blood cell count

283. red blood cell morphology

284. relapse [RĒ-lăps]

285. remission [rē-MĬSH-ŭn]

286. reticulocytosis [rē-TĬK-yū-lō-sī-TŌ-sĭs] {reticulocitosis}

287. Rh factor

288. Rh-negative

289. Rh-positive

290. sedimentation rate (SR)

291. serum [SĒR-ŭm] {suero}

292. SMA (sequential multiple analyzer)

293. stem cell

294. thalassemia [thăl-ă-SĒ-mē-ă] {talasemia}

295. thromb(o)

296. thrombin [THRŎMB-ĭn] {trombina}

297. thrombocyte [THRŎM-bō-sīt] {trombocito}

298. thrombocytopenia [THRŎM-bō-sī-tō-PĒ-nē-ă]

299. thrombolytic [thrŏm-bō-LĬT-ĭk]

300. thromboplastin [thrŏm-bō-PLĂS-tĭn]

301. transfusion [trăns-FYŪ-zhŭn] {transfusión}

302. venipuncture [VĔN-ĭ-pŭnk-chŭr, VĒ-nĭ-pŭnk-chŭr] {venipuntura}

303. von Willebrand's [vŏn WĬL-lĕ-brăndz] disease

304. white blood cell

Abbreviations

Write the full meaning of each abbreviation.

305. APTT

306. baso

307. BCP

308. BMT

309. CBC

310. diff

311. eos

312. ESR

313. G-CSF

314. GM-CSF

315. HCT, Hct

316. HGB, Hgb, HB

317. MCH

318. MCHC

319. MCV

320. mono

321. PCV

322. PLT

323. PMN, poly

324. PT

325. PTT

326. RBC

327. SR, sed. rate

328. seg

329. WBC

Answers to Chapter Exercises

1. c
2. a
3. b
4. b
5. c
6. c
7. b
8. c
9. b
10. b
11. b
12. c
13. b
14. AB
15. O
16. B
17. A
18. O
19. AB
20. B
21. A
22. d
23. g
24. a
25. b
26. c
27. e
28. h
29. f
30. Blood circulates throughout the body and exchanges substances with most of the body's cells.
31. No; blood type does not make one more susceptible.
32. e
33. f
34. g
35. h
36. j
37. b
38. i
39. c
40. d
41. a
42. tending to clump together
43. removal of a thrombus
44. immature red blood cell
45. study of diseases of the blood
46. movement of eosinophils
47. immature white blood cell
48. part of the cell that aids a cell in digesting unwanted particles

49. disease with increased red blood cells
50. study of cells
51. white blood cell
52. disease (type of cancer) with abnormal number of white blood cells
53. abnormally small amount of platelets in the blood
54. blood-filled mass
55. disease with increased red blood cell counts
56. Venipuncture; Yes; small amounts of blood are replaced within a day or so.
57. RBC measures red blood cells and WBC measures white blood cells.
58. anemia; dehydration; polycythemia
59. white blood count (WBC)
60. j
61. h
62. c
63. g
64. b
65. i
66. a
67. e
68. f
69. d
70. 120–199
71. 135–145
72. 30–150
73. 4.5–12.8
74. 80.0–98.0
75. 150–400
76. 34.0–47.0
77. 3.80–5.20
78. 3.9–11.1
79. 32.0–36.0
80. Yes. Anemia and chronic blood loss are indicated by the percentage of red blood cells noted in a CBC.
81. Yes; it is important for everybody who might need a transfusion.
82. hemophilia
83. pancytopenia
84. C
85. C
86. aplastic anemia

87. eosinophilia
88. purpura
89. C
90. thrombocytopenia
91. C
92. F
93. F
94. T
95. T
96. F
97. T
98. T
99. T
100. failure in production of red blood cells
101. lack of enough iron either in diet or absorption, which causes insufficient production of hemoglobin
102. insufficient vitamin B_{12}, which causes abnormal red blood cell shape
103. hereditary blood disorder with insufficient hemoglobin production
104. hereditary red blood cell disorder with misshapen cells and breakdown in cell membranes that creates problems with carrying oxygen to the tissues
105. aplastic anemia, a failure of the bone marrow to produce enough red blood cells
106. Yes; anemia is a complication that should be dealt with first because of the probability of further blood loss during surgery.
107. No. He cannot afford to lose more blood.
108. Vitamin B_{12}
109. coagulants; hemostatics
110. anticoagulant
111. relapse
112. remission
113. cholesterol; HDL; LDL;
114. thyroid function
115. d
116. a
117. e
118. b
119. f
120. c

121. Rh-negative
122. thrombocytes
123. plasma
124. hemoglobin
125. granulocytes
126. transfusion
127. eosin(o), red (stain) + phil(o), affinity for + -ic, pertaining to
128. hem(o), blood + -lysis, destruction
129. hem(o), blood + cyt(o), cell + -meter, instrument used to measure
130. pan-, all + cyt(o), cells + -penia, deficiency
131. phleb(o), vein + -itis, inflammation
132. phleb(o), vein + -otomy, incision into
133. phleb(o), vein + -ectomy, excision
134. hemat(o), blood + -oma, tumor
135. an-, without + is(o), equal + cyt(o), cell + -osis, condition
136. thromb(o), clot + phleb(o), vein + -itis, inflammation
137. hem(o), blood + -static, stopping, maintaining
138. ven(o), vein + -spasm, contraction
139. hem(o), blood (tests) + -gram, a record
140. hem(o), blood + -lytic, destroying
141. an- without + -emia, blood
142. phleb(o), vein + -graphy, process of recording

143. phleb(o), vein + -ectasia, dilation
144. hem(o), blood + -rrhage, heavy discharge
145. hem(o), blood + -pathy, disease
146. hemat(o), blood + -poiesis, formation
147. hem(o), blood + -ology, study of
148. plasma, fluid part of blood + -pheresis, removal
149. sider(o), iron + penia, deficiency
150. bas(o), base (blue dye) + -phil, affinity for
151. polycythemia
152. hemoglobin
153. hemophilia
154. erythroclasis
155. stem cells
156. monocyte
157. megakaryocytes
158. microcytic or macrocytic
159. leukoblast
160. lysemia
161. red cell morphology
162. normocyte
163. phagocyte
164. poikilocytes
165. spherocyte
166. leukemia
167. leukopheresis
168. hemoplastic
169. P
170. W
171. W
172. P
173. R
174. R
175. W

176. W
177. R
178. W
179. b; dissolves blood clots
180. c; aids in clotting blood
181. d; stops bleeding
182. a; dissolves blood clots
183. F
184. F
185. T
186. F
187. T
188. T
189. F
190. T
191. F
192. F
193. myeloblast
194. hemoglobin
195. neutrophil
196. C
197. histamine
198. C
199. C
200. C
201. anisocytosis
202. reticulocytosis
203. venipuncture
204. phlebotomy
205–329. Answers are available in the vocabulary reviews in this chapter.

CHAPTER
13

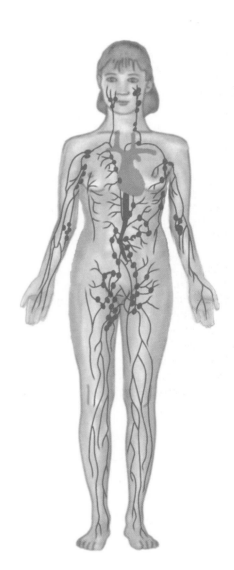

The Lymphatic and Immune Systems

▶ IMMUNOLOGY

After studying this chapter, you will be able to:

13.1   Name the parts of the lymphatic and immune systems and discuss the function of each part

13.2   Define combining forms used in building words that relate to the lymphatic and immune system

13.3   Identify the meaning of related abbreviations

13.4   Name the common diagnoses, clinical procedures, and laboratory tests used in treating disorders of the lymphatic and immune systems

13.5   List and define the major pathological conditions of the lymphatic and immune systems

13.6   Explain the meaning of surgical terms related to the lymphatic and immune systems

13.7   List common pharmacological agents used in treating disorders of the lymphatic and immune systems

Structure and Function

The lymphatic and immune systems share some of the same structures and functions. Neither system is an easily defined system as the digestive or endocrine systems are. The immune system utilizes other systems to maintain its functions. Both the lymphatic and immune systems contain the lymph nodes, spleen, thymus gland, and some of the disease-fighting immune cells. The lymphatic system provides the location to gather and concentrate foreign substances present in the body so that lymphocytes circulating through the lymphatic organs and vessels are able to destroy and remove them from the body.

The lymphatic system has the following functions:

- It reduces tissue edema by removing fluid from capillary beds.
- It returns the proteins from the fluids to the blood.
- It traps and filters cellular debris including cancer cells, microbes, etc. with the help of cells called macrophages.
- It recycles body fluid to various parts of the body.
- It circulates lymphocytes to assist with the immune response.
- It moves fats from the GI tract to the blood.

The immune system has the following functions:

- The immune system protects the body against foreign body invasion.
- In normal function, the immune system coordinates activities in the blood, body tissues, and the lymphatic system to protect the body from invasion.

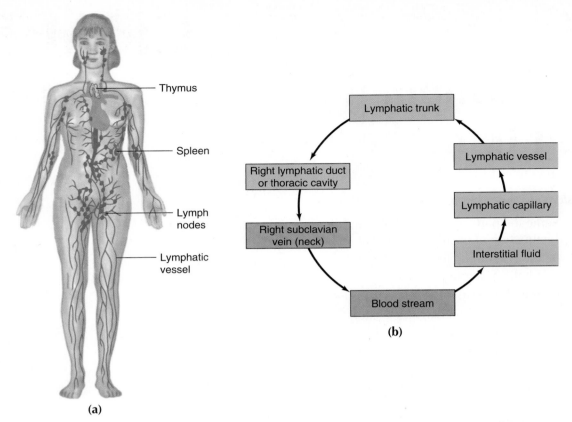

Thymus

Spleen

Lymph nodes

Lymphatic vessel

(a)

Lymphatic trunk

Lymphatic vessel

Right lymphatic duct or thoracic cavity

Lymphatic capillary

Right subclavian vein (neck)

Interstitial fluid

Blood stream

(b)

FIGURE 13-1 **(a)** The lymphatic and immune systems are the body's major defense against foreign substances; **(b)** flowchart of the path of lymph through the body.

- It fights off infections and protects against future infections by producing a variety of immune responses.
- It produces antibodies (immunoglobulins).

Figure 13-1a shows the lymphatic and immune systems. Figure 13-1b shows how lymph circulates throughout the body.

Lymphatic Organs and Structures

The lymphatic system is similar to both the cardiovascular and blood systems in that it involves a network of vessels that transports fluid around the body. The liquid part of the blood, plasma, has the ability to leave the blood capillaries and enter the cellular areas of the body. Once plasma leaves the vascular system, it is known as interstitial fluid. This interstitial fluid provides nutrients and performs other functions in the exchange of fluids to and from the cells. The lymphatic system serves as a drainage system to remove fluid from the cellular areas. It concentrates foreign substances to assist the immune system.

The lymphatic system consists of the following parts:

1. The *lymphatic pathways* are the vessels that transport **lymph** (the fluid of the lymphatic system) around the body. The smallest part of these pathways are the *microscopic capillaries* located in the capillary beds of the body. The capillary beds are thin-walled vessels that receive fluid and debris from the bloodstream. Once inside the beds, the fluid is known as lymph. The lymph travels throughout the lymphatic vessels in one direction only—back toward the heart. Lymphatic vessels

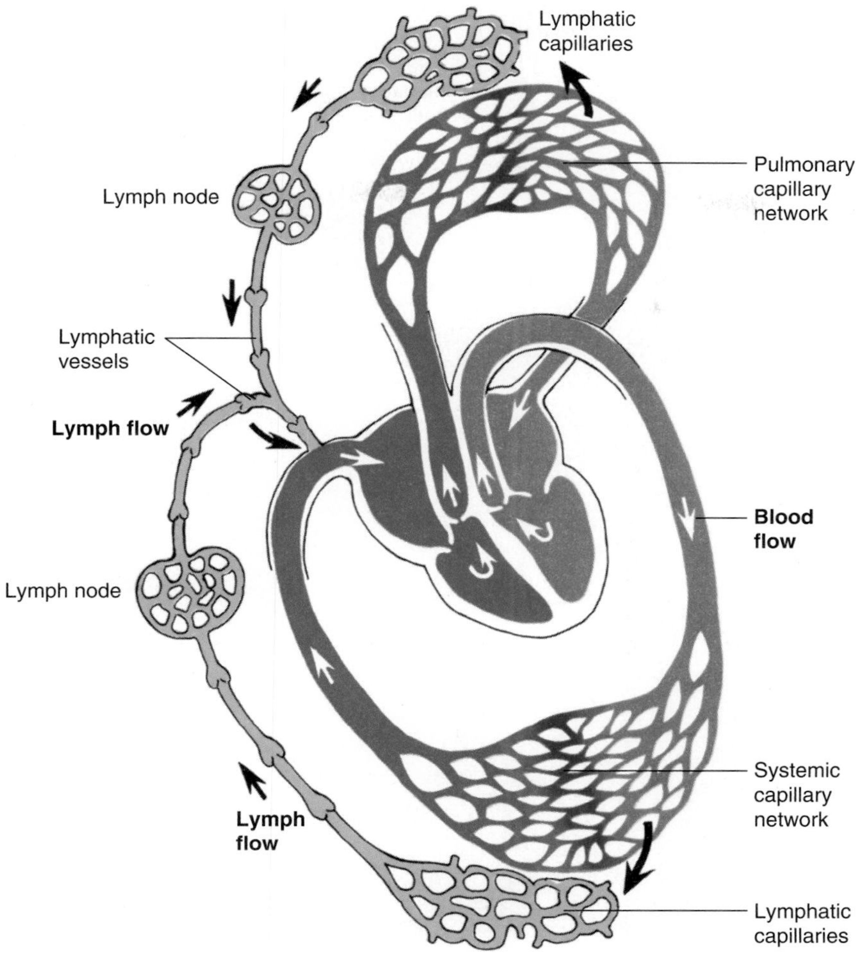

Lymphatic capillaries

Lymph node

Lymphatic vessels

Lymph flow

Lymph node

Lymph flow

Pulmonary capillary network

Blood flow

Systemic capillary network

Lymphatic capillaries

FIGURE 13-2 Lymphatic capillaries gather the lymph from the space between tissues.

contain valves that prevent backflow of lymph. As the vessels approach the heart, they carry more fluid and are larger in size. Figure 13-2 illustrates the flow of lymph through the body.

2. Located along the lymphatic vessels are the **lymph nodes** (Figure 13-3), small lumps of lymphatic tissue that serve as a collecting point to filter the lymph. The lymph passes through many lymph nodes for filtering so that it is ready for transferring back to the vascular system. By the time the fluid reaches the thoracic cavity, it has been filtered many times. The lymph nodes contain special cells (macrophages) that devour foreign substances. Lymph nodes become swollen with *lymphocytes* (lymph cells) and macrophages. Lymph nodes are located throughout the body except in the central nervous system. They are quite numerous near the joints of the body. The major groups of lymph nodes are located in the throat (the tonsils and adenoids are actually lymph tissue), neck, axilla (armpit), mediastinum, and groin.

3. The largest lymphatic organ, the **spleen,** is located in the upper left portion of the abdominal cavity, where unfortunately it can easily be injured and ruptured. In such cases, it must be repaired or removed (its functions are taken over by the lymph nodes, liver, and bone marrow). The function of the spleen is to filter foreign material from the blood, to store blood, to remove damaged or old red blood cells, and to activate lymphocytes that destroy some of the foreign substances filtered from the blood (Figure 13-4). The spleen is important not only

FIGURE 13-3 Lymph nodes contain cells (lymphocytes and macrophages) that ingest foreign substances.

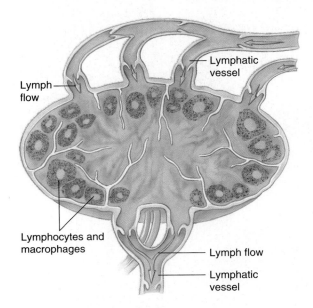

Lymphatic vessel

Lymph flow

Lymphocytes and macrophages

Lymph flow

Lymphatic vessel

FIGURE 13-4 The spleen, like the lymph nodes, contains cells that destroy foreign substances.

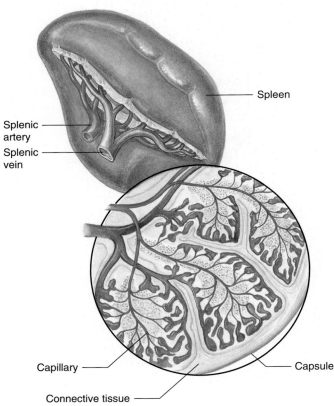

Spleen

Splenic artery

Splenic vein

Capillary

Connective tissue

Capsule

to the lymphatic system but also to the circulatory system; its association with the circulatory system is similar to the association of the lymph node to the lymphatic system. The spleen is also a major site for immunoglobulin production by *B lymphocytes* that have differentiated into antibody-producing plasma cells.

4. The **thymus gland** is a two-lobed, soft gland located in the thoracic cavity (Figure 13-5). It is large during infancy and early childhood when immunity is most crucial, but gradually shrinks until it becomes connective tissue in adulthood (when the body has acquired other types of immunities). The thymus gland contains a high number of **T lymphocytes**

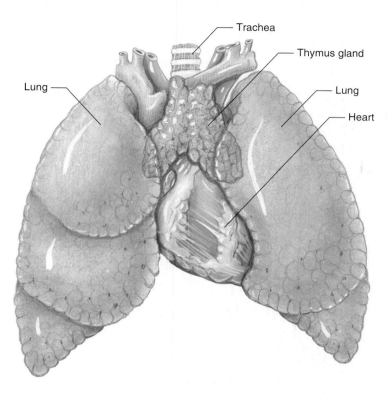

Trachea

Thymus gland

Lung

Lung

Heart

FIGURE 13-5   The thymus gland is located between the lungs.

(**T cells**) and a decreased number of **B lymphocytes** (**B cells**). After being produced in the bone marrow, some of the lymphocytes (immature T cells) migrate through the thymus gland where they acquire the marker that identifies them as T lymphocytes. Other lymphocytes become B cells. T cells provide immunity after they leave the thymus. Their movement is aided by **thymosin,** a hormone secreted by the thymus.

The Immune System

The immune system relies on several other systems to accomplish its duties. The *reticuloendothelial system* (RES), *hematopoietic system, mononuclear phagocytic system* (or *phagocytic system*), and *lymphoid system* are significant in the functions of the immune system. The hematopoietic system is responsible for the production of the blood cells in the bone marrow. The blood cells include the erythrocytes (red blood cells), leukocytes (white blood cells), and thrombocytes (platelets). The leukocytes include **lymphocytes,** monocytes, and granulocytes (*polymorphonucleated cells* or PMN). The RES and phagocytic systems provide the phagocytes of the tissues and the phagocytes of the blood that are called **macrophages** and **microphages.** Phagocytes remove foreign particles from the body by the process of **phagocytosis,** the internalization or "eating" of the particles and the digestion of the particles for presentation to the appropriate cells of the immune system. The immune response is divided into two kinds: the *cellular response* and the *humoral* or *immunoglobulin (antibody) response*.

Lymphocytes are one kind of leukocytes that are intimately involved in the immune system. Included in the classification of lymphocytes are the T lymphocytes (T cells) and the B lymphocytes (B cells). T cells are involved in both types of the immune response. In the cellular response the T cells accept information about the invading particle (antigen) and produce chemical substances called *lymphokines* to destroy the antigen. The B cells are responsible for the production of **antibodies** (also called immunoglobulins), i.e., the humoral response. The humoral response, or the antibody production, requires the assistance of the T cells through their production of other chemical substances that act as signals to the B cells to begin antibody production.

The immune system shares several parts with the lymphatic system (lymph nodes, spleen, and thymus gland). These parts serve as defense mechanisms protecting the body. Parts of other systems, such as the skin, also play an important role in protecting the body from disease. The immune system of the body consists of all the processes that perform a series of defenses to protect from and respond to disease.

Mechanical and Chemical Defenses

The human body includes a number of mechanical, chemical, and other defenses against disease. When disease-causing agents, **pathogens,** try to enter the body, they are often stopped by the skin, the cilia in the nostrils, and by various mucous membranes—all of which are mechanical barriers to intrusion.

If some pathogens get past the mechanical defenses, they may be stopped by chemical barriers, such as gastric juices in the stomach. Pathogens in the bloodstream may be destroyed by phagocytosis, the ingesting of foreign substances by specialized cells like macrophages. In addition, humans are resistant to some diseases that affect other animals and vice versa. This natural resistance may occur because the pathogen finds the human's internal environment harmful to its survival.

On the other hand, some pathogens prefer the environment of the human body as opposed to that of other animals, so they affect humans but not animals. Some tick-borne diseases such as Lyme disease can have devastating consequences to humans but remain dormant in animals. Some bacteria are beneficial in humans because they help ward off disease. In the bloodstream, certain substances called **antigens** may provoke an immune response to certain diseases.

The Immune Process

Mechanical or chemical defenses work together to avert or attack disease. In addition, the body has specific defenses of the immune system called **immunity** that provide resistance to particular pathogens. There are three major types of immunity—natural immunity, acquired active immunity, and acquired passive immunity.

Natural Immunity

Natural immunity is the human body's natural resistance to certain diseases. This natural resistance varies for individuals, even to the extent that persons of certain racial backgrounds tend to have more or less resistance to certain diseases. Natural resistance depends on the individual's genetic characteristics and on some of the natural chemical defenses.

Acquired Active Immunity

The body develops **acquired active immunity** either by having a disease and producing natural antibodies to it or by being vaccinated against the disease. **Immunization** or **vaccination** is the injection of an **antigen,** a substance that provokes an immune response, from a different organism that causes active immunity via the production of antibodies. The substance is called a **vaccine.**

Acquired active immunity is further divided into two types. The first, **humoral immunity,** is immunity provided by **plasma cells,** which produce antibodies called **immunoglobulins.** There are five major types of immunoglobulins:

- *Immunoglobulin* G *(IgG)* is effective against bacteria, viruses, and toxins.
- *Immunoglobulin* A *(IgA)* is common in exocrine gland secretions, such as breast milk, tears, nasal fluid, gastric juice, and so on. IgA transfers immunity from mother to infant through breast milk.
- *Immunoglobulin* M *(IgM)* develops in the blood plasma in response to certain antigens within the body or from foreign sources. It is the first antibody to be produced after infection.
- *Immunoglobulin* D *(IgD)* is important in B cell activation, which helps immunity by transforming itself into a plasma cell in the presence of a specific type of antigen.
- *Immunoglobulin* E *(IgE)* appears in glandular secretions and is associated with allergic reactions.

The second type of acquired active immunity, or **cell-mediated immunity,** is provided by the action of T cells. The T cells respond to antigens by multiplying rapidly and producing proteins called *lymphokines* (for example, **interferons** and **interleukins**) that have antiviral properties or properties that affect the actions of other cells in the body. T cells also produce substances to stimulate B cells to differentiate into plasma cells and to produce antibodies.

Three types of other specialized T cells are:

- **Helper cells** or CD4 cells that stimulate the immune response.
- **Cytotoxic cells** or CD8 cells that help in the destruction of infected cells.
- **Suppressor cells** or T cells (mainly CD8 and some CD4) that suppress B cells and other immune cells.

Acquired Passive Immunity

Acquired passive immunity is immunity provided in the form of antibodies or antitoxins that have been developed in another person or another species. Acquired passive immunity is necessary in cases of snakebite and tetanus or any problem where immediate immunity is needed. In such cases, a dose of **antitoxin** (antibody directed against specific toxins) is given to provide antibodies. Passive immunity may also be administered to lessen the chance of catching a disease or to lessen the severity of the course of the disease. **Gamma globulin** is a preparation of collected antibodies given to prevent or lessen certain diseases, such as hepatitis A, varicella, and rabies.

MORE ABOUT . . .

Immunization

Most children are immunized against childhood diseases routinely and those vaccines are thought to be safe and effective. There is a very small incidence of bad reactions to vaccines that have harmed some children. Recently, some groups have studied what is thought to be the higher incidence of autism since the introduction of routine vaccinations. So far, the evidence is that there is no connection between autism and childhood immunization through vaccine. Also, the risk of getting some of the diseases which the vaccines prevent is thought to have the potential for much greater harm to children.

Vocabulary Review

In the previous section, you learned terms relating to the lymphatic and immune systems. Before going on to the exercises, review the terms below and refer to the previous section if you have any questions. Pronunciations are provided for certain terms. Sometimes information about where the word came from is included after the term. The etymologies (word histories) are for your information only. You do not need to memorize them.

Term	Definition
acquired active immunity	Resistance to a disease acquired naturally or developed by previous exposure or vaccination.
acquired passive immunity	Inoculation against disease or poison, using antitoxins or antibodies from or in another person or another species.
antibody [ĂN-tē-bŏd-ē] anti-, against + body	Specialized protein that fights disease; also called immunoglobulin.
antigen [ĂN-tĭ-jĕn] anti(body) + -gen, producing	Any substance that can provoke an immune response.
antitoxin [ăn-tē-TŎK-sĭn] anti-, against + toxin	Antibodies directed against a particular disease or poison.
B lymphocytes [LĬM-fō-sīts], **B cells**	A kind of lymphocyte that manufactures antibodies.
cell-mediated immunity	Resistance to disease mediated by T cells.
cytotoxic [sī-tō-TŎK-sĭk] **cell** cyto-, cell + toxic	T cell that helps in destruction of infected cells throughout the body.
gamma globulin [GĂ-mă GLŎB-yū-lĭn]	Antibodies given to prevent or lessen certain diseases.
helper cell	T cell that stimulates the immune response.
humoral [HYŪ-mōr-ăl] **immunity**	Resistance to disease provided by plasma cells and antibody production.
immunity [ĭ-MYŪ-nĭ-tē] Latin *immunitas*, freedom from service	Resistance to particular pathogens.
immunization [ĬM-yū-nĭ-ZĀ-shŭn]	Vaccination.
immunoglobulin [ĬM-yū-nō-GLŎB-yū-lĭn] immuno-, immunity + globulin	Antibody.
interferon [ĭn-tĕr-FĒR-ŏn]	Protein produced by T cells and other cells; destroys disease-causing cells with its antiviral properties.
interleukin [ĭn-tĕr-LŪ-kĭn] inter-, among + leuk(ocyte)	Protein produced by T cells; helps regulate immune system.
lymph [lĭmf] Latin *lympha*, clear spring water	Fluid that contains white blood cells and other substances and flows in the lymphatic vessels.
lymph node	Specialized organ that filters harmful substances from the tissues and assists in the immune response.

Term	Definition
lymphocytes [LĬM-fō-sīts] lympho-, lymph + -cyte, cell	White blood cells made in the bone marrow that are critical to the body's defense against disease and infection.
macrophage [MĂK-rō-fāj] macro-, large + -phage, eating	Special cell that devours foreign substances.
microphage [MĬK-rō-fāj] micro-, small + -phage, eating	Small phagocytic cell that devours foreign substances.
natural immunity	Inherent resistance to disease found in a species, race, family group, or certain individuals.
pathogen [PĂTH-ō-jĕn] patho-, disease + -gen, producing	Disease-causing agent.
phagocytosis [FĂG-ō-sī-TŌ-sĭs] phagocyt(e) + -osis, condition	Ingestion of foreign substances by specialized cells.
plasma [PLĂZ-mă] **cell**	Specialized lymphocyte that produces immunoglobulins.
spleen [splēn] Greek *splen*	Organ of lymph system that filters and stores blood, removes old red blood cells, and activates lymphocytes.
suppressor [sŭ-PRĔS-ōr] **cell**	T cell that suppresses B cells and other immune cells.
T cells	Specialized white blood cells that receive markers in the thymus, are responsible for cellular immunity, and assist with humoral immunity.
thymosin [THĪ-mō-sĭn]	Hormone secreted by the thymus gland that aids in distribution of thymocytes and lymphocytes.
thymus [THĪ-mŭs] **gland** Greek *thymos*, sweetbread	Soft gland with two lobes that is involved in immune responses; located in mediastinum.
T lymphocytes	*See* T cells.
vaccination [VĂK-sĭ-NĀ-shŭn] Latin *vaccinus*, relating to a cow	Injection of an antigen from a different organism to cause active immunity.
vaccine [văk-SĒN, VĂK-sēn]	Antigen developed from a different organism that causes active immunity in the recipient.

CASE STUDY

Researching a Cure

Some hospitals are part of large university complexes. These hospitals often do many kinds of research and offer tertiary care, medical care at a center that has a unit specializing in certain diseases. They may provide data on drug trials. They may work on improving diagnostic testing. Some research is focused on diseases that are infectious and for which there is not yet a cure. The goal of many studies is to produce a vaccine.

Critical Thinking

1. Why would researchers want to produce a vaccine?
2. What form of immunity would a vaccination provide?

Find a Match

Match the correct definition in the right-hand column with the terms in the left-hand column.

3. ____ T cell   **a.** T cell that helps destroy foreign cells or substances

4. ____ pathogen   **b.** T cell that regulates the amounts of antibody

5. ____ immunoglobulin E   **c.** T cell that stimulates antibody production

6. ____ IgD   **d.** antibody important in B-cell activation

7. ____ helper cell   **e.** agent given to prevent or lessen disease

8. ____ cytotoxic cell   **f.** lymphocyte associated with cellular immunity

9. ____ suppressor cell   **g.** helps produce resistance to a disease or a poison

10. ____ antitoxin   **h.** protein produced by B cells that fight foreign cells

11. ____ antibody   **i.** disease-causing agent

12. ____ gamma globulin   **j.** antibody associated with allergic reactions

Check Your Knowledge

Fill in the blanks

13. People are born with some _____ immunity.

14. Vaccinations give _____ _____ immunity.

15. Antitoxins give _____ _____ immunity.

16. The special cells that ingest foreign substances are called _____.

17. Lymph contains _____ blood cells.

18. The thymus gland provides markers for cells that become _____ _____.

19. Agents of T cells that destroy disease-causing cells are _____ and _____.

20. The fluid in the space between tissues is called _____ _____.

Combining Forms and Abbreviations

The lists below include combining forms and abbreviations that relate specifically to the lymphatic and immune systems. Pronunciations are provided for the examples.

COMBINING FORM	MEANING	EXAMPLE
aden(o)	gland	*adenocarcinoma* [ĂD-ē-nō-kăr-sĭ-NŌ-mă], glandular cancer
immun(o)	immunity	*immunosuppressor* [ĬM-yū-nō-sŭ- PRĔS-ōr], agent that suppresses the immune response
lymph(o)	lymph	*lymphocyte* [LĬM-fō-sīt], white blood cell associated with the immune response

COMBINING FORM	MEANING	EXAMPLE
lymphaden(o)	lymph nodes	*lymphadenopathy* [lĭm-făd-ĕ-NŎP-ă-thē], disease affecting the lymph nodes
lymphangi(o)	lymphatic vessels	*lymphangitis* [lĭm-făn-JĪ-tĭs], inflammation of the lymphatic vessels
splen(o)	spleen	*splenectomy* [splē-NĔK-tō-mē], removal of the spleen
thym(o)	thymus	*thymectomy* [thī-MĔK-tō-mē], removal of the thymus
tox(o), toxi, toxico	poison	*toxicosis* [tŏk-sĭ-KŌ-sĭs], systemic poisoning

ABBREVIATION	MEANING	ABBREVIATION	MEANING
AIDS	acquired immunodeficiency syndrome	CML	chronic myelogenous leukemia
ALL	acute lymphocytic leukemia	CMV	cytomegalovirus
AML	acute myelogenous leukemia	EBV	Epstein-Barr virus
AZT	Azidothymidine	EIA, ELISA	Enzyme-linked immunosorbent assay
CLL	chronic lymphocytic leukemia	HIV	human immunodeficiency virus
HSV	herpes simplex virus	IgM	immunoglobulin M
IgA	immunoglobulin A	PCP	Pneumocystis carinii pneumonia
IgD	immunoglobulin D	SLE	systemic lupus erythematosus
IgE	immunoglobulin E	ZDV	Zidovudine
IgG	immunoglobulin G		

CASE STUDY

Checking for Immunity

Jill, a three-year-old girl, was playing barefoot in her backyard when she stepped on a rusty nail. The nail punctured her skin and made her vulnerable to tetanus, a muscle disease (see Chapter 5). Jill is up to date on all her vaccinations. The most common early childhood vacinnation is DPT (diphtheria, pertussis, and tetanus). The vaccinations last for a number of years.

Critical Thinking

21. Is it likely that Jill will contract tetanus? Why or why not?
22. What type of immunity to tetanus does Jill have?

COMBINING FORMS AND ABBREVIATIONS EXERCISES

Build Your Medical Vocabulary

Fill in the missing word part.

23. Removal of lymph nodes: _____ectomy

24. Hemorrhage from a spleen: _____rrhagia

25. Tumor of the thymus: _____oma

26. Lacking in some immune function: _____deficient

27. Cell of a gland: _____cyte

28. Skin disease caused by a poison: _____derma

29. Dilation of the lymphatic vessels: _____ectasis

30. Resembling lymph: _____oid

Find a Match

Match the term on the left with the correct definition on the right.

31. _____ toxicologist

32. _____ splenomegaly

33. _____ lymphangiosarcoma

34. _____ splenomyelomalacia

35. _____ lymphocele

36. _____ lymphadenitis

37. _____ toxanemia

a. anemia resulting from a poison

b. malignancy in the lymphatic vessels

c. cystic mass containing lymph

d. inflammation of a lymph node

e. spleen enlargement

f. expert in the science of poisons

g. softening of the spleen and bone marrow

Diagnostic, Procedural, and Laboratory Terms

Abnormalities of lymph organs can be checked in a CAT scan. Several blood tests that indicate the number and condition of white blood cells are used in diagnosing lymph and immune systems diseases. HIV infection is diagnosed mainly with two blood serum tests, **enzyme-linked immunosorbent assay (EIA, ELISA)** and **Western blot.** ELISA tests blood for the antibody to the HIV virus (as well as antibodies to other specific viruses, such as hepatitis B), and the Western blot is a confirming test for the presence of HIV antibodies. A diagnosis of AIDS is made on the basis of the presence of opportunistic infections and T cell counts in specified ranges.

Allergy tests are performed by an allergist. Tests usually consist of some form of exposure to a small amount of the suspected allergen to see if a reaction occurs. Now there are even home allergy tests available that can detect allergies by testing a small amount of blood.

VOCABULARY REVIEW

In the previous section, you learned terms relating to diagnosis, clinical procedures, and laboratory tests. Before going on to the exercises, review the terms below and refer to the previous section if you have any questions. Pronunciations are provided for certain terms. Sometimes information about where the word came from is included after the term. The etymologies (word histories) are for your information only. You do not need to memorize them.

Term	Definition
enzyme-linked immunosorbent assay (EIA, ELISA [ĕ-LĪ-ză, ĕ-LĪ-să])	Test used to screen blood for the presence of antibodies to different viruses or bacteria.
Western blot	Test primarily used to check for antibodies to HIV in serum.

DIAGNOSTIC, PROCEDURAL, AND LABORATORY TERMS EXERCISES

Check Your Knowledge

Circle T for true or F for false.

38. The ELISA tests for HIV. T F

39. A Western blot determines if Hepatitis B is present. T F

40. An analysis of white blood cells can help in diagnosing lymph and immune system diseases. T F

CASE STUDY

Handling the Emergency

Kyle, a seven-year-old boy, came to the emergency room at the hospital in respiratory distress. His mother says that he often has respiratory allergies. He was taken to the imaging area for chest x-rays. His lungs show some restricted areas. He is also given a thorough medical exam to make sure that nothing other than an allergic reaction is causing the breathing difficulties. If the examination is normal, Kyle will be sent to an allergist to determine the cause of his allergic reaction. The resident performing the exam marks the patient's record as shown below.

Critical Thinking

41. Why did Kyle need a thorough physical exam?

42. Did the physical exam show any abnormalities other than respiratory allergies?

GENERAL: He is a well-developed, well-nourished male in moderate respiratory distress.

HEENT: Tympanic membranes unremarkable. Eyes, nose, mouth, and throat normal.

NECK: No masses. Supple.

LUNGS: Breath sounds clear bilaterally with somewhat decreased air exchange and diffuse expiratory wheeze. Work of breathing is mildly to moderately increased.

CARDIAC: No murmur or gallop. Pulses 2+ and symmetrical.

ABDOMEN: Soft and nontender without organomegaly or mass.

GU: Normal male.

EXTREMITIES: Unremarkable.

NEUROLOGIC: Alert and appropriate. Cranial nerves intact. Reflexes 2+ and symmetrical.

Pathological Terms

Diseases of the lymph and immune systems include diseases that attack lymph tissue itself; diseases that are spread through the lymphatic pathways; and diseases that flourish because of a suppression of the immune response. Disorders of the lymph and immune systems can be caused by an overly vigorous response to an immune system invader. This is the case with some diseases of other body systems, such as multiple sclerosis, in which the immune system attacks some of the nervous system's protective covering, myelin. It is also the case with **allergy,** an immune overresponse to a stimulus.

The most widespread virus that attacks the immune system is the **human immunodeficiency virus (HIV)**, a virus spread by sexual contact, exchange of bodily fluids, or intravenous exposure. A person may be *HIV positive*, meaning that the person carries the HIV virus but has not yet come down with HIV infections (diseases that tend to occur in HIV-positive people) or been given a diagnosis of AIDS. Many people are HIV positive without knowing it; only a test can make that diagnosis when there are no symptoms. Figure 13-6 shows an HIV virus.

AIDS

AIDS or **acquired immunodeficiency syndrome** is the most widespread **immunosuppressive disease,** a disease that suppresses the ability of the immune system to defend against infection. AIDS is a complex of symptoms and caused by the HIV virus. The HIV virus is a type of **retrovirus,** a ribonucleic acid (RNA) that causes reversal of normal cell copying. The retro- (reverse) is the opposite of the ordinary method of DNA copying itself onto RNA.

AIDS patients are subject to a number of **opportunistic infections,** infections that a healthy immune system can easily fight off but take hold because of the lowered immune response. Many of these infections are present in other body systems. Table 13-1 lists some opportunistic infections commonly present in AIDS patients and the parts of the body affected.

The CDC has a group called the Divisions of HIV/AIDS prevention (www.cdc.gov/hiv/dhap.htm) that provides up-to-date information on prevention, research, and testing.

FIGURE 13-6 A microscopic picture of an HIV virus.

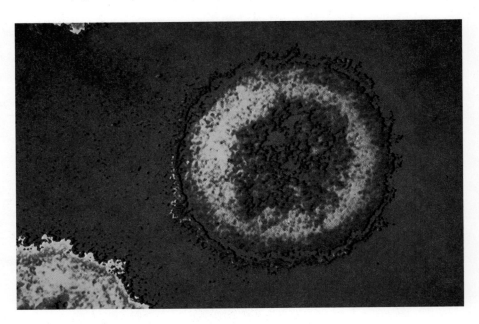

TABLE 13-1 Some Opportunistic Malignancies and Infections That Often Accompany AIDS

Opportunistic Infection	Type of Malignancy or Infection	Areas Affected
candidiasis	caused by fungus—Candida albicans	digestive tract, respiratory tract, skin, and some reproductive organs (particularly the vagina)
cytomegalovirus	Herpesviridae	can infect various cells or organs (like the eyes); causes swelling
Kaposi's sarcoma	malignancy arising from capillary linings	skin and lymph nodes
Mycobacterium avium-intracellulare (MAI)	caused by bacterium found in soil and water	systemic infection with fever, diarrhea, lung and blood disease, and wasting
Pneumocystis carinii pneumonia (PCP)	caused by parasite—Pneumocystis carinii	lungs—a particularly dangerous type of pneumonia

AIDS affects the entire body, with diseases such as herpes, candidiasis, and Kaposi's sarcoma appearing on the skin, and Pneumocystis carinii pneumonia (PCP) appearing in the lungs.

Other Immune System Disorders

Opportunistic infections also attack the immune systems of people with immunosuppressive disorders other than AIDS. Any recipient of an organ transplant must take immunosuppressive drugs to avoid organ rejection.

MORE ABOUT . . .

Contracting AIDS

When the AIDS epidemic began in the United States, many people feared that the HIV virus could be spread by casual contact. In fact, time has shown that there are very few specific ways it can be transmitted. These are the ways that AIDS is transmitted and how it is not transmitted.

How HIV Is Transmitted

Sexual contact, particularly vaginal, anal, and oral intercourse

Contaminated needles (intravenous drug use, accidental needle stick in medical setting)

During birth from an infected mother

Receiving infected blood or other tissue (rare; precautions usually prevent this)

How HIV Is NOT Transmitted

Casual contact (social kissing, hugging, handshakes)

Objects—toilet seats, deodorant sticks, doorknobs

Mosquitoes

Sneezing and coughing

Sharing food

Swimming in the same water as an infected person

These drugs leave the patient open to opportunistic infections. There are a number of other immunosuppressive disorders. Some are congenital and may be inherited. Others are a result of disease; for example, a severe case of diabetes can weaken the immune system.

Lymphoma, cancer of the lymph nodes, is a relatively common cancer with high cure rates. Some AIDS patients are especially susceptible to lymphomas because of their lowered immune systems. There are many different types of lymphomas. Two of the most common are **Hodgkin's lymphoma (Hodgkin's disease)**, a type of lymph cancer of uncertain origin that generally appears in early adulthood, and **non-Hodgkin's lymphoma,** a cancer of the lymph nodes with some cells resembling healthy cells and spreading in a diffuse pattern. It usually appears in mid-life. Depending on how far the disease has spread **(metastasis)**, both types can be arrested with chemotherapy and radiation. Surgery (bone marrow transplantation) is also useful in Hodgkin's lymphoma.

Malignant tumors appear in many places in the lymph system. A **thymoma** is a tumor of the thymus gland. Hodgkin's lymphoma is a malignancy of the lymph nodes and spleen. Enlarged lymph nodes, enlarged spleen **(splenomegaly),** and overactive spleen **(hypersplenism)** characterize this disease. Non-Hodgkin's lymphoma is a disease with malignant cells that resemble large lymphocytes **(lymphocytic lymphoma)** or large macrophages called *histiocytes* (hence the name **histiocytic lymphoma**).

Nonmalignant lesions on the lymph nodes, lungs, spleen, skin, and liver can indicate the presences of **sarcoidosis,** an inflammatory condition that can affect lung function. Swollen lymph nodes **(lymphadenopathy)** can also indicate the presence of **infectious mononucleosis,** an acute infectious disease caused by the Epstein-Barr virus. Infectious mononucleosis is often called the "kissing disease," because it is usually transmitted through mouth-to-mouth contact during kissing, sharing drinks, and sharing eating utensils. Rest is generally the only cure.

The Allergic Response

Allergies are a problem of the immune system that affect millions of people. They are due to the production of IgE antibodies against an **allergen,** an allergy-causing substance (Figure 13-7). Antibodies and some antigens cause a histamine to be released into the tissues. This histamine release is the cause of the symptoms of allergies.

Allergies vary for different people depending on time of year, amount of exposure to different allergens, and other immunological problems.

The Lymphoma Research Foundation (www.lymphoma.org) is dedicated to assisting people with lymphoma and related diseases and ultimately to eradicating the disease.

FIGURE 13-7 Some common allergens that provoke a response in many people.

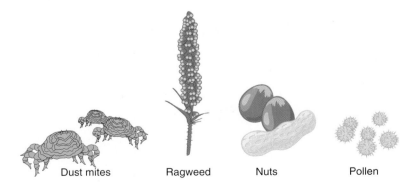

Dust mites   Ragweed   Nuts   Pollen

Hypersensitivity increases as exposure increases, sometimes resulting in **anaphylaxis** (or *anaphylactic reaction* or *shock*), a reaction so severe that it can be life-threatening by decreasing blood pressure, affecting breathing, and causing loss of consciousness. Some people are extremely allergic to peanuts. A person with a severe peanut allergy who ingests even a tiny amount of peanuts (as in a cookie) will immediately go into an anaphylactic reaction. Some people are allergic in the same way to other foods and to bee stings. Most severely allergic people carry a dose of epinephrine to slow the reaction.

The Food Allergy and Anaphylaxis Network (www.foodallergy.org) provides up-to-date information about foods that have been recalled due to undeclared potentially allergic products such as peanuts and milk hidden in them.

Autoimmune Disorders

The immune system can also turn against its own healthy tissue. **Autoimmune diseases,** such as rheumatoid arthritis, lupus, and scleroderma, result from the proliferation of T cells that react as though they were fighting a virus, but are actually destroying healthy cells. **Autoimmune responses** often result from the body's need to fight an actual infection, during which the immune system becomes overactive.

The American Autoimmune and Related Diseases Association (www.aarda.org) keeps track of autoimmune diseases and provides helpful patient information.

VOCABULARY REVIEW

In the previous section, you learned terms relating to pathology. Before going on to the exercises, review the terms below and refer to the previous section if you have any questions. Pronunciations are provided for certain terms. Sometimes information about where the word came from is included after the term. The etymologies (word histories) are for your information only. You do not need to memorize them.

Term	Definition
acquired immunodeficiency [ĬM-yū-nō-dē-FĬSH-ĕn-sē] **syndrome**	AIDS.
AIDS [ādz]	Most widespread immunosuppressive disease; caused by the HIV virus.
allergen [ĂL-ĕr-jĕn] allerg(y) + -gen, producing	Substance to which exposure causes an allergic response.
allergy [ĂL-ĕr-jē]	Production of IgE antibodies against an allergen.
anaphylaxis [ĂN-ă-fĭ-LĂK-sĭs]	Life-threatening allergic reaction.
autoimmune [ăw-tō-ĭ-MYŪN] **disease** auto-, self + immune	Any of a number of diseases, such as rheumatoid arthritis, lupus, and scleroderma, caused by an autoimmune response.
autoimmune response	Overactivity in the immune system against the body, causing destruction of one's own healthy cells.
histiocytic [HĬS-tē-ō-SĪT-ĭk] **lymphoma**	Lymphoma with malignant cells that resemble histiocytes.
Hodgkin's lymphoma, Hodgkin's disease After Thomas Hodgkin (1798–1866), British physician	Type of lymph cancer of uncertain origin that generally appears in early adulthood.

Term	Definition
human immunodeficiency [ĬM-yū-nō-dē-FĬSH-ĕn-sē] **virus (HIV)**	Virus that causes AIDS; spread by sexual contact, exchange of body fluids, and shared use of needles.
hypersensitivity [HĪ-pĕr-sĕn-sĭ-TĬV-ĭ-tē] hyper-, excessive + sensitivity	Abnormal reaction to an allergen.
hypersplenism [hĭ-pĕr-SPLĒN-ĭzm]	Overactive spleen.
immunosuppressive [ĬM-yū-nō-sŭ-PRĔS-ĭv] **disease**	Disease that flourishes because of lowered immune response.
infectious mononucleosis [MŎN-ō-nū-klē-Ō-sĭs] mono-, one + nucle(us) + -osis, condition	Acute infectious disease caused by the Epstein-Barr virus.
lymphadenopathy [lĭm-făd-ĕ-NŎP-ă-thē]	Swollen lymph nodes.
lymphocytic [lĭm-fō-SĬT-ĭk] **lymphoma**	Lymphoma with malignant cells that resemble large lymphocytes.
lymphoma [lĭm-FŌ-mă] lymph-, lymph + -oma, tumor	Cancer of the lymph nodes.
metastasis [mĕ-TĂS-tă-sĭs] Greek, a removing	Spread of a cancer from a localized area.
non-Hodgkin's lymphoma	Cancer of the lymph nodes with some cells resembling healthy cells and spreading in a diffuse pattern.
opportunistic [ŏp-pōr-tū-NĬS-tĭk] **infection**	Infection that takes hold because of lowered immune response.
retrovirus [rĕ-trō-VĪ-rŭs]	Type of virus that spreads by using the body's DNA to help it replicate its RNA.
sarcoidosis [săr-kŏy-DŌ-sĭs] sarcoid, former word for sarcoma + -osis	Inflammatory condition with lesions on the lymph nodes and other organs.
splenomegaly [splēn-ō-MĔG-ă-lē] spleno-, spleen + -megaly, enlargement	Enlarged spleen.
thymoma [thĭ-MŌ-mă] thym(us) + -oma, tumor	Tumor of the thymus gland.

CASE STUDY

Helping to Manage a Disease

University Hospital has an extensive oncology department involved in research. Jane Bryant is a 32-year-old woman with AIDS. Recently, Kaposi's sarcoma has appeared on her arms and back. She was referred to the oncology department for chemotherapy. In addition, her doctors prescribed a new medication that increases T cell count and the effectiveness of the immune response.

Critical Thinking

43. What might be the advantage for a chronically ill person to be treated in a research hospital?

44. Jane has AIDS, an immunosuppressive disease. Why is she being referred to the oncology department?

Spell It Correctly

Put a C after each word that is spelled correctly; if a word is incorrectly spelled, write it correctly.

45. retorvirus_____

46. immunosuppressive_____

47. imunodeficiency_____

48. sarcodosis_____

49. lumphoma_____

50. mononucleosis_____

51. anphylaxis_____

52. histocytic_____

53. metastasis_____

54. thimoma_____

Check Your Knowledge

For each of the following statements, write either lymph or immune in the blank to complete the sentence.

55. Allergies involve a(n) _____ response.

56. Splenomegaly is a symptom of _____ system disease.

57. Multiple sclerosis is a disease in which the _____ system attacks some of the body's cells.

58. Sarcoidosis is an inflammatory condition of the _____ system.

59. AIDS is a disease of the _____ system.

Surgical Terms

Cancers of the lymph system may require a **lymph node dissection,** removal of cancerous lymph nodes for microscopic examination. A **lymphadenectomy** is the removal of a lymph node, and a **lymphadenotomy** is an incision into a lymph node. A **splenectomy** is removal of the spleen, which is usually required if it is ruptured. Other organs of the body, such as the liver, will take over the functions of the spleen if it is removed. A **thymectomy** is removal of the thymus gland, which is very important to the maturation process but not as serious once a patient reaches adulthood.

MORE ABOUT . . .

Lymph Node Surgery

A person with a malignant neoplasm in the breast must have further tests to determine if the cancer has metastasized. In the past, biopsies included removal of many lymph nodes until one without cancer was found. Now, a procedure called sentinel node biopsy is commonly used. A contrast medium is injected into the area around the tumor. The first node it reaches is the sentinel node. It is checked for malignancy. If that node is clean, then no further biopsy is done on the other lymph nodes, and the patient is spared painful surgical side effects.

VOCABULARY REVIEW

In the previous section, you learned terms relating to surgery. Before going on to the exercises, review the terms below and refer to the previous section if you have any questions. Pronunciations are provided for certain terms.

Sometimes information about where the word came from is included after the term. The etymologies (word histories) are for your information only. You do not need to memorize them.

Term	Definition
lymphadenectomy [lǐm-făd-ě-NĚK-tō-mē] lymphaden-, lymph node + -ectomy, removal	Removal of a lymph node.
lymphadenotomy [lǐm-făd-ě-NŎ-tō-mē] lymphadeno-, lymph node + -tomy, a cutting	Incision into a lymph node.
lymph node dissection	Removal of a cancerous node for microscopic examination.
splenectomy [splē-NĚK-tō-mē] splen-, spleen + -ectomy	Removal of the spleen.
thymectomy [thī-MĚK-tō-mē] thym(us) + -ectomy	Removal of the thymus gland.

CASE STUDY

Getting an Examination

John Latella, a patient with AIDS, came to the hospital's clinic for his monthly T cell test and to review the medications he is taking. He seems to be feeling more energetic, so John believes his T cell test will show improvement. During the examination, however, the doctor notices an enlargement in John's lymph nodes. He sends John to the outpatient surgical unit for a biopsy.

Critical Thinking

60. If the node is malignant, what kind of surgery will most likely be performed?
61. A malignancy may have to be treated with radiation and/or chemotherapy, both of which destroy some healthy cells at the same time that they destroy malignant cells. Why would such treatment be especially risky for an AIDS patient?

SURGICAL TERMS EXERCISES

Build Your Medical Vocabulary

Write and define the lymph and immune system combining forms in the following words.

62. splenectomy
63. lymphadenotomy
64. thymectomy
65. lymphangioma

Pharmacological Terms

Diseases of the lymph and immune systems are often treated with relatively high doses of chemotherapy and/or radiation. Advances in AIDS research have made it possible to manage this disease (i.e., to prolong patient's life) once thought fatal. A "cocktail" of anti-HIV drugs, a potential HIV/AIDS vaccine, and other newer drug compounds are bringing hope for long-term vitality to people with AIDS. Other drug compounds have been developed to fight opportunistic infections. Table 13-2 lists some of the important immune system medications.

TABLE 13-2 Medications Used to Treat Disorders of the Lymphatic and Immune Systems

Drug Class	Purpose	Generic	Trade Name
antiviral used in AIDS	to block virus growth	zidovudine lopinavir and ritonavir didanosine stavudine, lamivudine, and nevirapine	Retrovir, AZT Kaletra Videx Triomune
antimicrorganism agent used in AIDS	to prevent PCP	pentamidine	Pentam 300
antihistamines		loratidine diphenhydramine fexofenadine	Claritin Benadryl Allegra

Genetic research is focusing on all the major chronic diseases. While diseases of the lymphatic and immune systems do not currently have specific genetic therapies, many researchers believe that advances in genetic therapies will bring relief for many of these diseases.

CASE STUDY

Getting Good News

John Latella's biopsy reveals that the node is not malignant. The swelling is thought to be an infection. Further blood tests show that it is. John already takes a number of prophylactic medications aimed at preventing infection. For this infection, he is put on a course of antibiotics.

Critical Thinking

66. Why does John find it difficult to fight infections?
67. What results are the antibiotics supposed to provide?

PHARMACOLOGICAL TERMS EXERCISES

Check Your Knowledge

Fill in the blanks.

68. AIDS patients often have to take many medications, including some to avoid _____ infections.
69. Lymphomas are generally treatable with _____ and _____.
70. One AIDS drug that blocks virus growth is _____.
71. One body substance manufactured and given in high doses in immune disorders is _____.

CHALLENGE SECTION

The clinic at University Hospital is treating a young woman with AIDS. She is monitored monthly at the clinic. Her latest blood test is shown on the next page.

Critical Thinking

72. Is this lab test a test for AIDS?
73. Which lab test results are indicative of opportunistic infection?

```
                            Laboratory Report
                            University Hospital
                               3 Center Drive
                            Westford, NH 11114
                               900-546-8000
```

Patient: Amy Carr	Patient ID: 099-00-1200	Date of Birth: 12/04/81
Date Collected: 04/30/XXXX	Time Collected: 16:05	Total Volume: 2000
Date Received: 04/30/XXXX	Date Reported: 5/06/XXXX	

Test	Result	Flag	Reference
Complete Blood Count			
WBC	13.2	*	3.9-11.1
RBC	4.11		3.80-5.20
HCT	39.7		34.0-47.0
MCV	96.5		80.0-98.0
MCH	32.9		27.1-34.0
MCHC	34.0		32.0-36.0
MPV	8.6		7.5-11.5
NEUTROPHILS %	45.6		38.0-80.0
NEUTROPHILS ABS.	1.82		1.70-8.50
LYMPHOCYTES %	36.1		15.0-49.0
LYMPHOCYTES ABS.	1.44		1.00-3.50
EOSINOPHILS %	4.5		0.0-8.0
EOSINOPHILS ABS.	0.18		0.03-0.55
BASOPHILS %	0.7		0.0-2.0
BASOPHILS ABS.	0.03		0.000-0.185
PLATELET COUNT	229		150-400
Automated Chemistries			
GLUCOSE	80		65-109
UREA NITROGEN	17		6-30
CREATININE (SERUM)	0.6		0.5-1.3
UREA NITROGEN/CREATININE	28		10-29
SODIUM	140		135-145
POTASSIUM	4.4		3.5-5.3
CHLORIDE	106		96-109
CO_2	28		20-31
ANION GAP	6		3-19
CALCIUM	9.8		8.6-10.4
PHOSPHORUS	3.6		2.2-4.6
AST (SGOT)	28		0-30
ALT (SGPT)	19		0-34
BILIRUBIN, TOTAL	0.5		0.2-1.2
PROTEIN, TOTAL	7.8		6.2-8.2
ALBUMIN	4.3		3.5-5.0
GLOBULIN	3.5		2.1-3.8
URIC ACID	2.4		2.0-7.5
CHOLESTEROL	172		120-199
TRIGLYCERIDES	68		40-199
IRON	85		30-150
HDL CHOLESTEROL	54		35-59
CHOLESTEROL/HDL RATIO	3.2		3.2-5.7
LDL, CALCULATED	80		70-129
T3, UPTAKE	32		24-37
T4, TOTAL	6.9		4.5-12.8

USING THE INTERNET

Go to the CDC's National Prevention Information Network (http://www.cdcnpin.org) and choose an article from one of their featured publications. Write a paragraph summarizing the content of the article.

CHAPTER REVIEW

The material that follows is to help you review this chapter.

Check Your Knowledge

Circle T for true and F for false

74. An antigen is a specialized protein that fights disease. T F

75. A T cell that helps in destruction of infected cells throughout the body is known as a cytotoxic cell. T F

76. Pathogens are prevented from entering the body by the skin, the cilia in the nostrils, and by various mucus membranes. T F

77. A person develops natural immunity by either having a disease or by being vaccinated against the disease. T F

78. Rheumatoid arthritis, lupus, and scleroderma are considered to be autoimmune diseases. T F

Find the Match

Write the letter of the definition for each term in the space provided.

79. ____ immunoglobulin G (IgG)

80. ____ immunoglobulin A (IgA)

81. ____ immunoglobulin M (IgM)

82. ____ immunoglobulin D (IgD)

83. ____ immunoglobulin E (IgE)

a. appears in glandular secretions

b. first antibody to be produced after infection

c. assists in B cell activity

d. effective against bacteria, viruses, and toxins

e. common in exocrine gland secretions

Find the Match

Write the letter of the definition for each term in the space provided.

84. ____ antigen

85. ____ antibody

86. ____ helper cells

87. ____ cytotoxic cells

88. ____ suppressor cells

a. CD4 cells that stimulate the immune response

b. T cells that suppress B cells and other immune cells

c. any substance that can provoke an immune response

d. specialized protein that fights disease

e. CD8 cells that help in the destruction of infected cells

Build Your Medical Vocabulary

Divide each of the following terms into words parts and then define the term.

89. lymphangiogram: _____

90. thymopathy: _____

91. lymphadenopathy: _____

92. splenomalacia: _____

93. splenorrhagia: _____

DEFINITIONS

Define and pronounce each of the following terms. The terms in the curly blue brackets refer to the Spanish glossary available online at www.mhhe.com/medterm3e.

WORD

94. acquired active immunity

95. acquired passive immunity

96. acquired immunodeficiency [ĬM-yū-nō-dē-FĬSH-ĕn-sē] syndrome

97. aden(o)

98. AIDS

99. allergen [ĂL-ĕr-jĕn] {alergeno}

100. allergy [ĂL-ĕr-jē] {alergia}

101. anaphylaxis [ĂN-ă-fĭ-LĂK-sĭs] {anafilaxia o anafilaxis}

102. antibody [ĂN-tē-bŏd-ē] {anticuerpo}

103. antigen [ĂN-tĭ-jĕn] {antígeno}

104. antitoxin [ăn-tē-TŎK-sĭn] {antitoxina}

105. autoimmune [ăw-tō-ĭ-MYŪN] disease

106. autoimmune response

107. B lymphocytes [LĬM-fō-sīts], B cells

108. cell-mediated immunity

109. cytotoxic [sī-tō-TŎK-sĭk] cell

110. enzyme-linked immunosorbent assay (EIA, ELISA)

111. gamma globulin [GĂ-mă GLŎB-yū-lĭn]

112. helper cell

113. histiocytic [HĬS-tē-ō-SĬT-ĭk] lymphoma

114. Hodgkin's lymphoma, Hodgkin's disease

115. human immunodeficiency [ĬM-yū-nō-dē-FĬSH-ĕn-sē] virus (HIV)

116. humoral [HYŪ-mōr-ăl] immunity

117. hypersensitivity [HĪ-pĕr-sĕn-sĭ-TĬV-ĭ-tē] {hipersensibilidad}

118. hypersplenism [hī-pĕr-SPLĒN-izm]

119. immun(o)

120. immunity [ĭ-MYŪ-nĭ-tē] {inmunidad}

121. immunization [ĬM-yū-nĭ-ZĀ-shŭn]

122. immunoglobulin [ĬM-yū-nō-GLŎB-yū-lĭn] {inmunoglobina}

123. immunosuppressive [ĬM-yū-nō-sŭ-PRĔS-ĭv] disease

124. infectious mononucleosis [MŎN-ō-nū-klē-Ō-sĭs]

125. interferon [ĭn-tĕr-FĒR-ŏn]

126. interleukin [ĭn-tĕr-LŪ-kĭn] {interleucina}

127. lymph [lĭmf] {linfa}

128. lymph(o)

129. lymphaden(o)

130. lymphadenectomy [lĭm-făd-ĕ-NĔK-tō-mē] {linfadenectomía}

131. lymphadenopathy [lĭm-făd-ĕ-NŎP-ă-thē] {linfadenopatía}

132. lymphadenotomy [lĭm-făd-ĕ-NŎ-tō-mē]

133. lymphangi(o)

134. lymph node

135. lymph node dissection

136. lymphocytes [LĬM-fō-sīts] {linfocitos}

137. lymphocytic [lĭm-fō-SĬT-ĭk] lymphoma

138. lymphoma [lĭm-FŌ-mă] {linfoma}

139. macrophage [MĂK-rō-fāj] {macrófago}

140. metastasis [mĕ-TĂS-tă-sĭs] {metastasis}

141. microphage [MĪK-rō-fāj] {micrófago}

142. natural immunity

143. non-Hodgkin's lymphoma

144. opportunistic [ŏp-pōr-tū-NĬS-tĭk] infection

145. pathogen [PĂTH-ō-jĕn] {patógeno}

146. phagocytosis [FĂG-ō-sī-TŌ-sĭs] {fagocitosis}

147. plasma [PLĂZ-mă] cell

148. retrovirus [rĕ-trō-VĪ-rŭs] {retrovirus}

149. sarcoidosis [săr-kŏy-DŌ-sĭs] {sarcoidosis}

150. spleen [splēn] {bazo}

151. splen(o)

152. splenectomy [splē-NĔK-tō-mē] {esplenectomía}

153. splenomegaly [splēn-ō-MĔG-ă-lē]

WORD

154. suppressor [sŭ-PRĔS-ōr] cell
155. T cells
156. thym(o)
157. thymectomy [thī-MĔK-tō-mē] {timectomía}

158. thymoma [thī-MŌ-mă] {timoma}
159. thymosin [THĪ-mō-sĭn] {timosina}
160. thymus [THĪ-mŭs] gland
161. T lymphocytes

162. tox(o), toxi, toxico
163. vaccination [VĂK-sĭ-NĀ-shŭn] {vacunación}
164. vaccine [văk-SĒN, VĂK-sēn] {vacuna}
165. Western blot

Abbreviations

Write the full meaning of each abbreviation

ABBREVIATION

166. AIDS
167. ALL
168. AML
169. AZT
170. CLL
171. CML
172. CMV

173. EBV
174. EIA, ELISA
175. HIV
176. HSV
177. IgA
178. IgD
179. IgE

180. IgG
181. IgM
182. PCP
183. SLE
184. ZDV

Answers to Chapter Exercises

1. to lessen the progress of or to prevent disease
2. acquired active immunity
3. f
4. i
5. j
6. d
7. c
8. a
9. b
10. g
11. h
12. e
13. natural
14. acquired active
15. acquired passive
16. macrophages or microphages
17. white
18. T cells
19. interferon, interleukin
20. interstitial fluid
21. No, since she has already been vaccinated, tetanus should not develop.
22. acquired active immunity
23. lymphaden
24. spleno
25. thym
26. immuno
27. adeno
28. toxi
29. lymphangi
30. lymph
31. f
32. e
33. b
34. g
35. c
36. d
37. a
38. T

39. F
40. T
41. to see if his breathing problems are caused by something other than allergies
42. no, just the blocked breathing caused by allergies
43. The patient might be eligible to be part of a new drug testing program.
44. Jane has a type of cancer—Kaposi's sarcoma.
45. retrovirus
46. C
47. immunodeficiency
48. sarcoidosis
49. lymphoma
50. C
51. anaphylaxis
52. histiocytic
53. C
54. thymoma
55. immune
56. lymph
57. immune
58. lymph
59. immune
60. lymphadenectomy
61. AIDS patients already have compromised immune systems. Any destruction of healthy cells can be devastating to their immune system and may allow other infections to take hold.
62. splen-, spleen
63. lymphadeno-, lymph node
64. thym-, thymus gland
65. lymphangio-, lymphatic vessels
66. AIDS has resulted in a compromised immune system that does not provide sufficient immune response.

67. They should resolve the lymph node infection.
68. opportunistic
69. radiation, chemotherapy
70. AZT (or others shown in Table 13-2)
71. interferon
72. No. It is a blood profile.
73. WBC
74. F
75. T
76. T
77. F
78. T
79. d
80. e
81. b
82. c
83. a
84. c
85. d
86. a
87. e
88. b
89. lymphangio-, lymph vessels, -gram, a recording; imaging of lymph vessels
90. thymo-, thymus, -pathy, disease; disease of the thymus gland
91. lymphadeno-, lymph glands, -pathy, disease; disease of the lymph glands
92. spleno-, spleen, -malacia, softening; softening of the spleen
93. spleno-, spleen, -rrhagia, hemorrhage; bursting forth of the spleen
94–184. Answers are available in the vocabulary reviews of this chapter.

CHAPTER 14

The Digestive System

▶ **GASTROENTEROLOGY**

After studying this chapter, you will be able to:

14.1   Name the parts of the digestive system and discuss the function of each part

14.2   Define combining forms used in building words that relate to the digestive system

14.3   Identify the meaning of related abbreviations

14.4   Name the common diagnoses, clinical procedures, and laboratory tests used in treating disorders of the digestive system

14.5   List and define the major pathological conditions of the digestive system

14.6   Explain the meaning of surgical terms related to the digestive system

14.7   Recognize common pharmacological agents used in treating disorders of the digestive system

Structure and Function

The three basic functions of the digestive system are as follows:

1. **Digestion** is the process of breaking down foods into nutrients that can be absorbed by cells. *Mechanical digestion* takes place in the mouth by chewing and in the stomach by churning actions. *Chemical digestion* takes place in the mouth by the addition of the saliva and continues in the stomach with the addition of digestive juices to chemically break down the food into simpler elements.
2. **Absorption** is the passing of digested nutrients into the bloodstream. This primarily occurs in the small intestines.
3. **Elimination** is the conversion of any residual material from a liquid to a solid and removal of that material from the alimentary canal via defecation.

The digestive system consists of the **alimentary canal** (digestive tract or gastrointestinal tract) and several accessory organs. Food enters the alimentary canal through the **mouth,** passes through the **pharynx** and **esophagus** into the **stomach,** then into the **small intestine** and **large intestine** or **bowels,** and then into the **anal canal.** Figure 14-1a shows the digestive system, and Figure 14-1b diagrams the digestive process.

The alimentary canal is a tube that extends from the mouth to the **anus.** The wall of the alimentary canal has four layers that aid in the digestion of the food that passes through it.

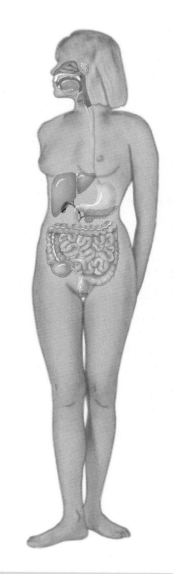

Colorado State University has a Web site (http://arbl.cvmbs.colostate.edu/hbooks/pathphys/digestion) that describes a voyage through the digestive tract.

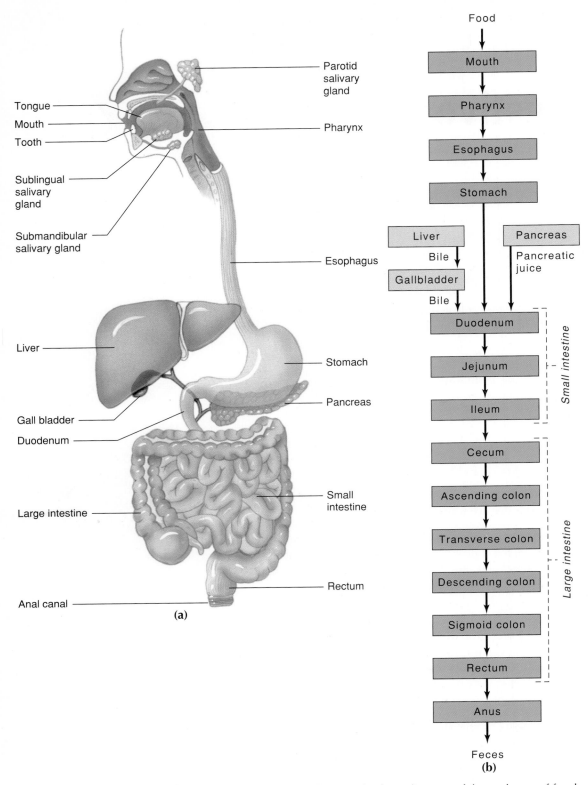

Food

Mouth

Pharynx

Esophagus

Stomach

Liver — Bile → Gallbladder — Bile →

Pancreas — Pancreatic juice →

Duodenum
Jejunum
Ileum
} Small intestine

Cecum
Ascending colon
Transverse colon
Descending colon
Sigmoid colon
Rectum
} Large intestine

Anus

Feces
(b)

Parotid salivary gland

Tongue
Mouth
Tooth

Pharynx

Sublingual salivary gland

Submandibular salivary gland

Esophagus

Liver

Stomach

Pancreas

Gall bladder

Duodenum

Small intestine

Large intestine

Rectum

Anal canal

(a)

FIGURE 14-1 **(a)** The process of digestion begins in the mouth. **(b)** A diagram of the pathway of food through the body.

- The outer covering is a serous (watery) layer of tissue that protects the canal and lubricates the outer surface so that organs within the abdominal cavity can slide freely near the canal.
- The next layer is the muscular layer, which contracts and expands in wavelike motions called **peristalsis,** to move food along the canal.
- The third layer is made of loose connective tissue that holds various vessels, glands, and nerves that both nourish and carry away waste from surrounding tissue.
- The innermost layer is a mucous membrane that secretes mucus and digestive enzymes while protecting the tissues within the canal.

Digestive **enzymes** convert complex proteins into **amino acids,** compounds that can be absorbed by the body. Complex sugars are reduced to **glucose** and other simpler sugars, and fat molecules are reduced to **fatty acids** and other substances through the action of the digestive enzymes.

Mouth

The **lips** sense the food that is about to enter the mouth. They sense the temperature and texture of the food and can thus protect the mouth from receiving food that is too hot or too rough on the surface. Once food is taken into the oral cavity (mouth), it is chewed with the help of the muscles of the **cheeks** (the walls of the oral cavity), and the **tongue** (which moves food during **mastication,** chewing). The last mechanical process that takes place in the mouth is **deglutition** (swallowing). The tongue has **papillae,** small raised areas that contain the taste buds (cells that provide the sensation of taste). The tongue is connected to the floor of the mouth by a mucous membrane called a **frenulum.** At the back of the tongue, **lingual tonsils** form two rounded mounds of lymphatic tissue that play an important role in the immune system (see Chapter 13).

The roof of the mouth is formed by the **hard palate,** the hard anterior part of the palate with irregular ridges of mucous membranes called **rugae,** and the **soft palate,** the soft posterior part of the palate. At the back of the soft palate is a downward cone-shaped projection called the **uvula.** During swallowing, the soft palate and the uvula direct food downward into the esophagus, thus preventing any food from entering the sinus area. On either side of the back of the mouth are rounded masses of lymphatic tissue called the **palatine tonsils.** The mouth also contains the **gums,** the fleshy sockets that hold the teeth. Chapter 21 discusses the teeth.

Digestion of food begins in the mouth with mastication. In addition, the three sets of **salivary glands** surrounding the oral cavity secrete **saliva,** a fluid containing enzymes (such as **amylase,** an enzyme that begins the digestion of carbohydrates) that aid in breaking down food. Each gland has ducts through which the saliva travels to the mouth. The three pairs of salivary glands are the *parotid glands*, located inferior to the cheekbone; the *submandibular glands*, located below the mandible; and the *sublingual glands*, located in the base of the mouth below the tongue (Figure 14-2).

Pharynx

From the mouth, food goes through the pharynx (**throat**). Both food and air share this passageway. The pharynx is a muscular tube (about 5 inches long in adults) that moves food into the esophagus. Air moves through the

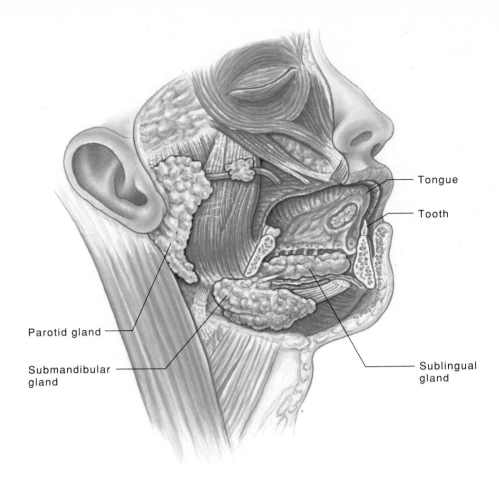

trachea (windpipe). When we eat and swallow food, a flap of tissue (the **epiglottis**) covers the trachea until the food is moved into the esophagus. The epiglottis prevents food from entering the larynx (the voice box). Food that happens to get into the larynx when we are eating causes choking.

Esophagus

The esophagus is a muscular tube (9 to 10 inches long in the average adult) that contracts rhythmically (peristalsis) to push food toward the stomach. At the bottom of the esophagus, just above the stomach, is a group of thickened muscles in the esophageal wall called the *lower esophageal sphincter* or

MORE ABOUT . . .

Choking

People have died of choking, even when efforts were made to save them. If an object such as a chicken bone became lodged in the windpipe, it was difficult to remove it while still allowing the person to breathe. A doctor, Harry J. Heimlich, discovered that a simple series of movements can prevent choking to death in most cases. The movements involve placing arms around the abdomen just below the diaphragm, grasping fists, and thrusting upward to dislodge the item. Testimony from around the world affirms that this maneuver is put to good use every day.

TABLE 14-1 **Major Components of Gastric Juice**

Component	Function
pepsin	digests almost all types of protein
hydrochloric acid	provides acidic environment for action of pepsin
mucus	provides alkaline protective layer on the inside of the stomach wall

cardiac sphincter. The cardiac sphincter is a group of muscles that regulates the opening and closing of the stomach entrance. As the swallowed food is advanced toward the stomach by the peristaltic wave, the cardiac sphincter will open briefly. Once the food is in the stomach, it will close. This prevents **reflux** (backflow) and **emesis** or **regurgitation** (vomiting). Every time more food comes through the esophagus to the stomach, the muscles relax and allow the food to pass.

Stomach

The stomach is a pouchlike organ in the left hypochondriac region of the abdominal cavity. The stomach receives food from the esophagus and mixes it with gastric juice. The enzyme **pepsin** in the gastric juice begins protein digestion. Table 14-1 shows the major components of gastric juice. Gastric juice is produced by the gastric glands, which are stimulated to produce this substance continuously but in varying amounts depending on the amount of food being absorbed.

The stomach has four regions (Figure 14-3).

- The *cardiac region*, the region closest to the heart, is where the cardiac sphincter allows food to enter the stomach and prevents regurgitation.

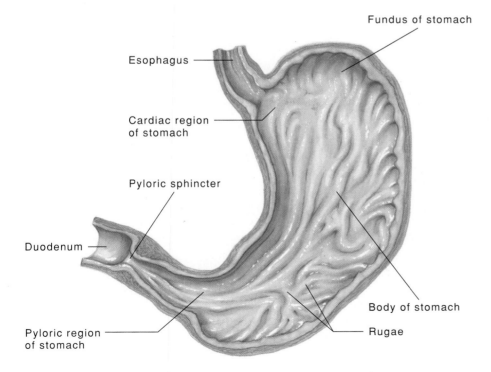

FIGURE 14-3 The stomach has four regions and rugae in its lining.

Esophagus

Fundus of stomach

Cardiac region of stomach

Pyloric sphincter

Duodenum

Pyloric region of stomach

Rugae

Body of stomach

If the cardiac sphincter does not close completely, or if it fails to remain closed, stomach juices can splash into the esophagus where there is no protective lining. This causes extreme burning known as *heartburn*.

- The **fundus** is the upper, rounded portion of the stomach.
- The **body** is the middle portion.
- The **pylorus,** the narrowed bottom part of the stomach, has a powerful, circular muscle at its base, the *pyloric sphincter*. This sphincter controls the emptying of the stomach's contents into the small intestine.

Stomach juices are extremely acidic in order for them to digest food. The lining of the stomach (and of the intestines) serves to protect the cells of the lining from being affected by the digestive juices in the stomach. The lining is relatively thick with many folds of mucous tissue called *rugae*. As the stomach fills up, the wall distends and the folds disappear.

After eating, the muscular movements of the stomach and the mixing of food with gastric juice forms a semifluid mass called **chyme.** Chyme may consist of food that has been in the stomach for several hours, or it may contain food that is broken down in as little as one hour. The type of food and the amounts eaten determine how long it takes for the stomach to release the chyme. The muscles of the stomach release the chyme in small batches at regular intervals into the small intestine, where further digestion takes place.

Small Intestine

The small intestine receives chyme from the stomach, bile from the liver, and pancreatic juice from the pancreas (Figure 14-4). The small intestine has the following three parts:

1. The **duodenum** is only about 10 inches long. In it, chyme mixes with bile to aid in fat digestion; with pancreatic juice to aid in digestion of starch, proteins, and fat; and with intestinal juice to aid in digesting sugars (glucose). Glands in the walls of the small intestine excrete intestinal

FIGURE 14-4 The small intestine connects the stomach to the large intestine.

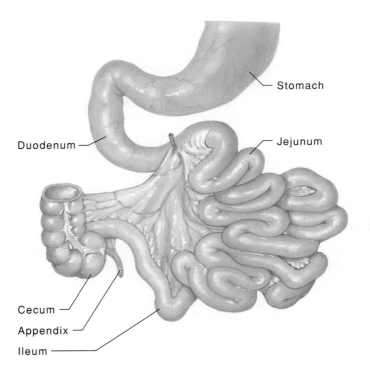

juice. The juices also help change starch (**glycogen**) into glucose. The entire small intestine is lubricated by secretions from mucous glands. The small intestine is lined with **villi** (singular, **villus**), tiny, one-cell-thick finger-like projections with capillaries through which digested nutrients are absorbed into the bloodstream and lymphatic system.

2. The **jejunum** is an eight-foot long section of the small intestine in which the digestive process continues.

3. The **ileum** connects the small intestine to the large intestine. Located at the bottom of the ileum is the *ileocecal sphincter muscle* that relaxes to allow undigested and unabsorbed food material into the large intestine in fairly regular waves. Other muscular contractions segment the ileum and prevent waste material in the large intestine from backing up into the small intestine.

Together, the three sections of the small intestine are about 20 feet long from the stomach to the large intestine. The small intestine lies within the abdominopelvic cavity, where it is held in place by the **mesentery,** a membranous tissue that attaches both the small and large intestines to the muscle wall at the dorsal part of the abdomen. Absorption (passage of material through the walls to the bloodstream) begins in the small intestines. Chyme takes from one to six hours to travel through the small intestine before it enters the large intestine. The length of time for digestion varies depending on the food being digested and the health of the digestive system.

Large Intestine

The large intestine (Figure 14-5), which is about five feet long, has the following four parts:

1. The **cecum** is a pouch attached to the bottom of the ileum of the small intestine. The cecum has three openings: one from the ileum into the cecum; one from the cecum into the colon; and another from the cecum into a wormlike pouch on the side, the **appendix** (also called the *vermiform appendix*). The appendix is filled with lymphatic tissue, but is considered an **appendage,** an accessory part of the body that has no central function, because it no longer has a role in the digestive process. The appendix can, however, become inflamed and may require surgical removal. Within the cecum, the process of turning waste material into semisolid waste (*feces*) begins, as water and certain necessary substances are absorbed back into the bloodstream. As the water is removed, a semisolid mass is formed and moved into the colon.

MORE ABOUT . . .

Intestinal Health

Intestinal health is often directly related to the amount of fiber in a person's diet. In 2005, the federal nutritional guidelines specifically recommended an increase in fibrous foods as a boost to general health and especially to digestive health. The most fibrous foods include vegetables, fruits, and whole grains. Nutritional labels on food give the amount of dietary fiber per serving. It is generally recommended that a person ingest 25 grams of fiber per day.

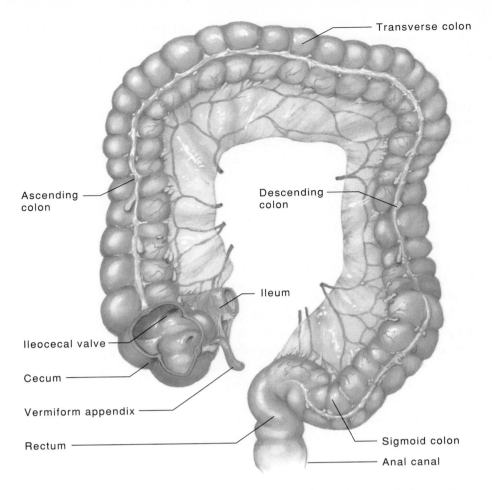

FIGURE 14-5 The large intestine leads from the small intestine to the anal canal.

Transverse colon

Ascending colon

Descending colon

Ileum

Ileocecal valve

Cecum

Vermiform appendix

Rectum

Sigmoid colon

Anal canal

2. The next section is the **colon.** The colon is further divided into three parts—the *ascending colon*, the *transverse colon*, and the *descending colon*. The ascending colon extends upward from the cecum to a place under the liver where it makes a right-angle bend known as the *hepatic flexure*. After the bend, the transverse colon continues across the abdomen from right to left where it makes a right-angle bend (the *splenic flexure*) toward the spleen. After the bend, the descending colon extends down to the rim of the pelvis where it connects to the sigmoid colon.

3. The **sigmoid colon** is an s-shaped body that goes across the pelvis to the middle of the sacrum, where it connects to the rectum.

4. The **rectum** attaches to the *anal canal.* **Feces (stool)** then pass from the anal canal into the anus. The anus and anal canal open during the release of feces from the body (**defecation**).

The entire large intestine forms a rectangle around the tightly packed small intestine. Undigestible waste products from digestion usually remain in the large intestine from 12 to 24 hours.

Liver

The **liver** is an important digestive organ located in the right, upper quadrant of the abdominal cavity. Although it is not within the digestive tract, it performs many digestive functions. The liver is a relatively large organ weighing about 3 pounds in the average adult. It is divided into two lobes, the right lobe and the left lobe (Figure 14-6).

The *hepatic portal system* is the group of blood vessels that transports blood and other substances to and from the liver. This system is particularly important in regard to the newly absorbed nutrients and other, possibly more harmful, substances that may have been ingested. The portal vein within this system directs all blood from the small intestines, with the newly absorbed substances from the villi, directly to the liver where there will be some filtration of harmful substances and some conversion of nutrients and medication into a form usable by the body.

Aside from changing food nutrients into usable substances, the liver also secretes **bile** (a yellowish-brown to greenish fluid), which is stored in the gallbladder for use in breaking down fats and other digestive functions. It stores glucose and certain vitamins for release when the body needs them. The liver also secretes **bilirubin,** a bile pigment that is combined with bile and excreted into the duodenum.

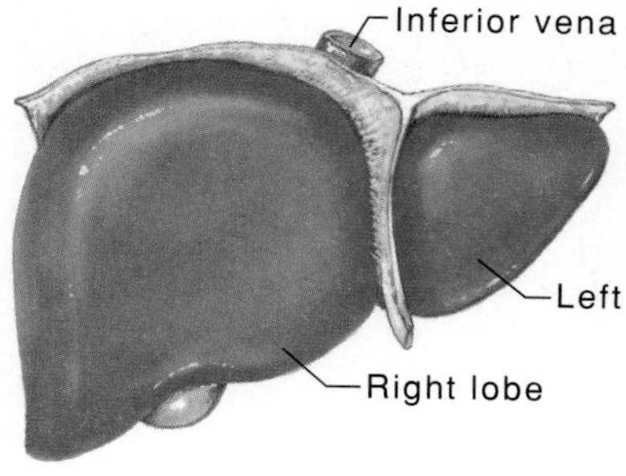

FIGURE 14-6 The liver secretes bile, a fluid that is important in digestion of fats.

Gallbladder

The bile released from the liver to the *hepatic duct* is then released into the *cystic duct*, which brings the substance into the **gallbladder.** The gallbladder performs two functions. It stores bile until it is needed for digestion and it concentrates bile by removing some of the water. Bile is thicker and richer in the gallbladder than it is in the liver, which is why gallstones form in the gallbladder. Then the bile is forced out of the cystic duct into the *common bile duct*.

At the entrance to the duodenum, bile mixes with pancreatic juices and enters the duodenum from the common bile duct. There the bile aids in **emulsification,** the breaking down of fats.

Pancreas

The chyme that empties into the small intestine mixes with secretions from the pancreas and liver. The **pancreas** is five to six inches long and lies across the posterior side of the stomach. The pancreas is a digestive organ in that it secretes digestive fluids into the small intestine through its system of ducts. The digestive fluid is called *pancreatic juice,* which includes various enzymes such as *amylase* and **lipase.** The pancreas is also an endocrine gland that regulates blood sugar through the release of insulin (a hormone) and, as such, is discussed in Chapter 15.

VOCABULARY REVIEW

In the previous section, you learned terms relating to the digestive system. Before going on to the exercises, review the terms below and refer to the previous section if you have any questions. Pronunciations are provided for certain terms. Sometimes information about where the word came from is included after the term. The etymologies (word histories) are for your information only. You do not need to memorize them.

Term	Meaning
absorption [ăb-SŎRP-shŭn] Latin *absorptio*, a swallowing	Passing of nutrients into the bloodstream.
alimentary [ăl-ĭ-MĔN-tĕr-ē] canal	Muscular tube from the mouth to the anus; digestive tract; gastrointestinal tract.

Term	Meaning
amino [ă-MĒ-nō] **acid**	Chemical compound that results from digestion of complex proteins.
amylase [ĂM-ĭl-ās]	Enzyme that is part of pancreatic juice and saliva and that begins the digestion of carbohydrates.
anal [Ā-năl] **canal**	Part of the digestive tract extending from the rectum to the anus.
anus [Ā-nŭs]	Place at which feces exit the body.
appendage [ă-PĔN-dĭj]	Any body part (inside or outside) either subordinate to a larger part or having no specific central function.
appendix [ă-PĔN-dĭks] Latin, appendage	Wormlike appendage to the cecum.
bile [bīl] Latin *bilis*	Yellowish-brown to greenish fluid secreted by the liver and stored in the gallbladder; aids in fat digestion.
bilirubin [bĭl-ĭ-RŪ-bĭn] bili-, bile + Latin *ruber*, red	Pigment contained in bile.
body	Middle section of the stomach.
bowel [bŏw-l] Latin *botulus*, sausage	Intestine.
cecum [SĒ-kŭm] Latin, blind	Pouch at the top of the large intestine connected to the bottom of the ileum.
cheeks	Walls of the oral cavity.
chyme [kīm] Greek *chymos*, juice	Semisolid mass of partially digested food and gastric juices that passes from the stomach to the small intestine.
colon [KŌ-lŏn] Greek *kolon*	Major portion of the large intestine.
defecation [dĕ-fĕ-KĀ-shŭn] Latin *defaeco*, to remove the dregs	Release of feces from the anus.
deglutition [dē-glŭ-TĬSH-ŭn] Latin *deglutio*, to swallow	Swallowing.
digestion [dī-JĔS-chŭn] Latin *digestio*	Conversion of food into nutrients for the body and into waste products for release from the body.
duodenum [dū-ō-DĒ-nŭm] Latin *duodeni*, twelve (about equal in size to the width of twelve fingers)	Top part of the small intestine where chyme mixes with bile, pancreatic juices, and intestinal juice to continue the digestive process.
elimination [ē-lĭm-ĭ-NĀ-shŭn]	The conversion of waste material from a liquid to a semisolid and removal of that material via defecation.
emesis [ĕ-MĒ-sĭs]	*See* regurgitation.
emulsification [ĕ-MŬL-sĭ-fĭ-KĀ-shŭn]	Breaking down of fats.
enzyme [ĔN-zīm]	Protein that causes chemical changes in substances in the digestive tract.

Term	Meaning
epiglottis [ĕ-pĭ-GLŎ-tĭs]	Movable flap of tissue that covers the trachea.
esophagus [ĕ-SŎF-ă-gŭs]	Part of alimentary canal from the pharynx to the stomach.
fatty acid	Acid derived from fat during the digestive process.
feces [FĒ-sēz] Latin *faeces*, dregs	Semisolid waste that moves through the large intestine to the anus, where it is released from the body.
frenulum [FRĔN-yū-lŭm] Latin, small bridle	Mucous membrane that attaches the tongue to the floor of the mouth.
fundus [FŬN-dŭs] Latin, bottom	Upper portion of the stomach.
gallbladder [GĂWL-blăd-ĕr]	Organ on lower surface of liver; stores bile.
glucose [GLŪ-kōs]	Sugar found in fruits and plants and stored in various parts of the body.
glycogen [GLĪ-kō-jĕn]	Starch that can be converted into glucose.
gums [gŭmz]	Fleshy sockets that hold the teeth.
hard palate [PĂL-ăt]	Hard anterior portion of the palate at the roof of the mouth.
ileum [ĬL-ē-ŭm]	Bottom part of the small intestine that connects to the large intestine.
jejunum [jĕ-JŪ-nŭm] Latin *jejunus*, empty	Middle section of the small intestine.
large intestine	Passageway in intestinal tract for waste received from small intestine to be excreted through the anus; also, place where water reabsorption takes place.
lingual tonsils [LĬNG-gwăl TŎN-sĭls]	Two mounds of lymph tissue at the back of the tongue.
lipase [LĬP-ās]	Enzyme contained in pancreatic juice.
lips Old English *lippa*	Two muscular folds formed around the outside boundary of the mouth.
liver [LĬV-ĕr] Old English *lifer*	Organ important in digestive and metabolic functions; secretes bile.
mastication [măs-tĭ-KĀ-shŭn] Latin *mastico*, to chew	Chewing.
mesentery [MĔS-ĕn-tĕr-ē, MĔZ-ĕn-tĕr-ē] Greek *mesenterion*	Membranous tissue that attaches small and large intestines to the muscular wall at the dorsal part of the abdomen.
mouth Old English *muth*	Cavity in the face in which food and water is ingested.
palatine [PĂL-ă-tĭn] **tonsils**	Mounds of lymphatic tissue on either side of the pharynx.
pancreas [PĂN-krē-ăs] Greek *pankreas*, sweetbreads	Digestive organ that secretes digestive fluids; endocrine gland that regulates blood sugar.
papilla (*pl.*, **papillae**) [pă-PĬL-ă (-ē)] Latin, nipple	Tiny projection on the superior surface of the tongue that contains taste buds.

Term	Meaning
pepsin [PĔP-sĭn] Greek *pepsis*, digestion	Digestive enzyme in gastric juice.
peristalsis [pĕr-ĭ-STĂL-sĭs] peri-, around + Greek *stalsis*, constriction	Coordinated, rhythmic contractions of smooth muscle that force food through the digestive tract.
pharynx [FĂR-ĭngks] Greek, throat	Tube through which food passes to the esophagus.
pylorus [pī-LŌR-ŭs] Latin, gatekeeper	Narrowed bottom part of the stomach.
rectum [RĔK-tŭm] Latin, straight	Bottom portion of large intestine; connected to anal canal.
reflux [RĒ-flŭks] re-, back + Latin *fluxus*, a flow	*See* regurgitation.
regurgitation [rē-GŬR-jĭ-TĀ-shŭn] re- + Latin *gurgito*, to flood	Backward flow from the normal direction.
rugae [RŪ-gē] Latin, wrinkles	Folds in stomach lining; irregular ridges of mucous membrane on the hard palate.
saliva [să-LĪ-vă] Latin	Fluid secreted by salivary glands; contains amylase.
salivary [SĂL-ĭ-vār-ē] **glands**	Glands in the mouth that secrete fluids that aid in breaking down food.
sigmoid [SĬG-mŏyd] **colon**	S-shaped part of large intestine connecting at the bottom to the rectum.
small intestine	Twenty-foot long tube that continues the process of digestion started in the stomach; place where most absorption takes place.
soft palate [PĂL-ăt]	Soft posterior part of the palate in the mouth.
stomach [STŎM-ăk] Latin *stomachus*	Large sac between the esophagus and small intestine; place where food is broken down.
stool [stūl] Old English *stol*, seat	Feces.
throat Old English *throtu*, throat	Pharynx.
tongue [tŭng] Old English *tunge*	Fleshy part of the mouth that moves food during mastication (and speech).
uvula [YŪ-vyū-lă] Latin, small grape	Cone-shaped projection hanging down from soft palate.
villus (*pl.*, villi) [VĬL-ŭs (-ī)] Latin, shaggy animal hair	Tiny, fingerlike projection on the lining of the small intestine with capillaries through which digested nutrients are absorbed into the bloodstream and lymphatic system.

STRUCTURE AND FUNCTION EXERCISES

Complete the Diagram

1. Label the digestive system parts in the illustration on the right.

   a. _____

   b. _____

   c. _____

   d. _____

   e. _____

e._____ _____

a._____

Pancreas

Gall bladder _____

Duodenum _____

c._____ _____ _____

b._____ _____

d._____

Anal canal _____

Check Your Knowledge

For each of the following words, write C in the space provided if the word is spelled correctly. If it is not, spell the word correctly.

2. papilae _____

3. frenelum _____

4. deglutition _____

5. chime _____

6. glycogen _____

7. villi _____

8. amylase _____

9. lypase _____

10. bilirubin _____

Fill in the Blanks

11. Food is moved along the alimentary canal by a process called _____.

12. The four areas of the stomach are _____, _____, _____, _____, and _____.

13. The three parts of the small intestine are the _____, _____, and _____.

14. The four parts of the large intestine are the _____, _____, _____, _____, and _____.

15. The longest intestine is the _____ intestine.

16. A group of blood vessels that transports blood and other substances to and from the liver is called the _____, _____, _____.

17. Two enzymes in pancreatic juice are _____ and _____.

18. Bile aids in the breaking down of fats, a process called _____.

CASE STUDY

Getting a Referral

Asmin Sahib reported burning chest pains to her general practitioner. Ms. Sahib feared that the pains indicated that she was having a heart attack. After a thorough examination, including an ECG, the physician found Ms. Sahib to have no cardiovascular pathology. The general practitioner referred Asmin to Dr. Mary Walker, a gastroenterologist (specialist in the digestive system).

Critical Thinking

19. Why might Asmin feel she is having a heart attack?

20. What parts of the body will the gastroenterologist treat?

Combining Forms and Abbreviations

The lists below include combining forms and abbreviations that relate specifically to the digestive system. Pronunciations are provided for the examples.

COMBINING FORM	MEANING	EXAMPLE
an(o)	anus	*anoplasty* [ā-nō-PLĂS-tē], surgical repair of the anus
append(o), appendic(o)	appendix	*appendicitis* [ă-pĕn-dĭ-SĪ-tĭs], inflammation of the appendix
bil(o), bili	bile	*biliverdin* [bĭl-ĭ-VĔR-dĭn], green bile pigment
bucc(o)	cheek	*buccogingival* [būk-ō-JĬN-jĭ-văl], pertaining to the cheeks and gums
cec(o)	cecum	*cecopexy* [SĒ-kō-pĕk-sē], surgical repair or fixing of the cecum to correct excessive mobility
celi(o)	abdomen	*celioma* [SĒ-lē-ō-mă], tumor in the abdomen
chol(e), cholo	bile	*choleic* [kō-LĒ-ĭk], pertaining to bile
cholangi(o)	bile vessel	*cholangiogram* [kō-LĂN-jē-ō-grăm], x-ray image of the bile vessels
cholecyst(o)	gallbladder	*cholecystectomy* [kō-lē-sĭs-TĔK-tō-mē], removal of the gallbladder
choledoch(o)	common bile duct	*choledochotomy* [kō-lĕd-ō-KŎT-ō-mē], incision into the common bile duct
col(o), colon(o)	colon	*colectomy* [kō-LĔK-tō-mē], removal of all or part of the colon
duoden(o)	duodenum	*duodenitis* [dū-ŏd-ĕ-NĪ-tĭs], inflammation of the duodenum

Combining Form	Meaning	Example
enter(o)	intestines	*enteropathy* [ĕn-tĕr-ŎP-ă-thē], any intestinal disease
esophag(o)	esophagus	*esophagoscopy* [ĕ-sŏf-ă-GŎS-kō-pē], examination of the interior of the esophagus
gastr(o)	stomach	*gastralgia* [găs-TRĂL-jē-ă], stomachache
gloss(o)	tongue	*glossopharyngeal* [GLŎS-ō-fă-RĬN-jē-ăl], of the tongue and pharynx
gluc(o)	glucose	*glucogenesis* [glū-kō-JĔN-ĕ-sĭs], formation of glucose
glyc(o)	sugar	*glycosuria* [glī-kō-SŪ-rē-ă], abnormal excretion of carbohydrates in urine
glycogen(o)	glycogen	*glycogenolysis* [GLĪ-kō-jĕ-NŎL-ĭ-sĭs], breakdown of glycogen to glucose
hepat(o)	liver	*hepatitis* [hĕp-ă-TĪ-tĭs], liver disease or inflammation
ile(o)	ileum	*ileitis* [ĭl-ē-Ī-tĭs], inflammation of the ileum
jejun(o)	jejunum	*jejunostomy* [jĕ-jū-NŎS-tō-mē], surgical opening to the outside of the body for the jejunum
labi(o)	lip	*labioplasty* [LĀ-bē-ō-plăs-tē], surgical repair of lips
lingu(o)	tongue	*linguodental* [lĭng-gwō-DĔN-tăl], pertaining to tongue and teeth
or(o)	mouth	*orofacial* [ōr-ō-FĀ-shăl], pertaining to mouth and face
pancreat(o)	pancreas	*pancreatitis* [păn-krē-ă-TĪ-tĭs], inflammation of the pancreas
periton(eo)	peritoneum	*peritonitis* [PĔR-ĭ-tō-NĪ-tĭs], inflammation of the peritoneum
pharyng(o)	pharynx	*pharyngotonsillitis* [fă-RĬN-jō-tŏn-sĭ-LĪ-tĭs], inflammation of tonsils and pharynx
proct(o)	anus, rectum	*proctologist* [prŏk-TŎL-ō-jĭst], specialist in study and treatment of diseases of the anus and rectum
pylor(o)	pylorus	*pylorospasm* [pī-LŌR-ō-spăzm], involuntary contraction of the pylorus
rect(o)	rectum	*rectoabdominal* [RĔK-tō-ăb-DŎM-ĭ-năl], of the rectum and abdomen
sial(o)	saliva, salivary gland	*sialism* [SĪ-ă-lĭzm], excessive secretion of saliva
sialaden(o)	salivary gland	*sialoadenitis* [SĪ-ă-lō-ă-dĕ-NĪ-tĭs], inflammation of the salivary glands
sigmoid(o)	sigmoid colon	*sigmoidoscopy* [SĬG-mŏy-DŎS-kō-pē], visual examination of the sigmoid colon

COMBINING FORM	MEANING	EXAMPLE
steat(o)	fats	*steatorrhea* [stē-ă-tō-RĒ-ă], greater than normal amounts of fat in the feces
stomat(o)	mouth	*stomatitis* [STŌ-mă-TĪ-tĭs], inflammation of the lining of the mouth

ABBREVIATION	MEANING	ABBREVIATION	MEANING
ALT, AT	alanine transaminase	IBD	inflammatory bowel disease
AST	aspartic acid transaminase	IBS	irritable bowel syndrome
BE	barium enema	NG	nasogastric
BM	bowel movement	NPO	nothing by mouth (Latin, *nul per os*)
EGD	esophagogastroduodenoscopy	SGOT	serum glutamic oxaloacetic transaminase
ERCP	endoscopic retrograde cholangiopancreatography	SGPT	serum glutamic pyruvic transaminase
GERD	gastroesophageal reflux disease	TPN	total parenteral nutrition
GI	gastrointestinal	UGI(S)	upper gastrointestinal (series)

CASE STUDY

Seeing a Specialist

Dr. Walker reviewed Asmin Sahib's family history. It showed that two members of her immediate family had died from cancer of the digestive tract. Her father had stomach cancer, and her sister had liver cancer. Since Asmin has always known the risks associated with digestive cancers, she has maintained a healthy diet and has had regular checkups to detect any signs of the kinds of cancer that have afflicted her family.

Critical Thinking

21. Why is family history important in evaluating a patient?
22. Before cancer was detected in her family members, they suffered from chronic stomach and liver inflammations. What are the medical names for these two conditions?

COMBINING FORMS AND ABBREVIATIONS EXERCISES

Build Your Medical Vocabulary

Use the following combining forms or roots along with suffixes you learned in Chapter 2 to give the missing term.
gastr(o) esophag(o) proct(o) chol(o) cholecyst(o) choledoch(o) hepat(o) pancreat(o) colon(o) duoden(o) rect(o)

23. Excision (removal) of the stomach: _____

24. Inflammation of the esophagus: _____

25. Prolapse of the rectum: _____

26. Pertaining to the duodenum: _____

27. Excision of a part of the common bile duct: _____

28. Inflammation of the pancreas: _____

29. Pain in the rectum: _____

30. Visual examination of the colon: _____

31. Enlargement of the liver: _____

32. Suture of the stomach: _____

33. Specialist in the study of diseases and treatment of the rectum and anus: _____

34. Inflammation of the gallbladder: _____

35. Liver tumor: _____

Find the Combining Forms

For the following terms, write the gastrointestinal combining form(s) in the space provided and define each term.

36. pyloroduodenal _____

37. perianal _____

38. enterocolostomy _____

39. ileocecal _____

40. sublingual _____

40. appendectomy _____

41. cecostomy _____

42. enteromycosis _____

43. gastrocolostomy _____

44. buccogingival _____

45. cholecystitis _____

46. labiodental _____

47. appendicolith _____

48. hepatomegaly _____

49. gastroenterology _____

50. esophagogastroduodenoscopy _____

51. proctitis _____

52. oropharynx _____

53. celiac _____

54. pancreatolysis _____

55. biliuria _____

56. enteroecstasis _____

57. ileopexy _____

58. hepatotoxic _____

59. peritonitis _____

60. pharyngitis _____

CASE STUDY

Treating the Symptoms

Dr. Walker finds Asmin to be a healthy 49-year-old except for the burning sensations in her chest. Dr. Walker has decided to have Asmin try a bland diet (avoidance of spicy food, alcohol, and caffeine) and sleeping with the head of the bed raised. She prescribes a mild antacid. Dr. Walker suggests a return visit in three weeks to see if the steps to avoid esophageal reflux are showing improvement.

After three weeks, Asmin has shown marked improvement. Dr. Walker tells her she can add some spicy foods back into her diet slowly, but to continue to avoid alcohol and caffeine. Asmin will need a checkup with Dr. Walker in six months.

Critical Thinking

61. What diagnostic test will Dr. Walker use to check Asmin's reflux condition in six months?

62. What other tests might Dr. Walker prescribe for someone with a family history of intestinal cancer?

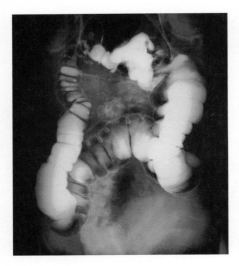

FIGURE 14-7 A scanned image of the intestinal tract.

Diagnostic, Procedural, and Laboratory Terms

The digestive or gastrointestinal system is examined in many different ways to diagnose a number of problems. Gastroenterologists (specialists in the digestive system) perform procedures to examine the internal health of various organs. They order blood tests to look for signs of infection or disease and also use some of the extensive number of imaging procedures available for this body system.

A stool specimen may be tested to identify disease-causing organisms such as parasites. This test is called a *stool culture*. A *stool culture and sensitivity test* (C & S) is used to try out different medications on *microorganisms* to check for effectiveness. A *chemical test of a stool specimen* (*hemoccult* test or *stool guaiac*) indicates whether there is bleeding in the digestive tract. Guaiac is a substance added to the stool sample that reacts with any occult (not visible) blood.

Various types of endoscopes are used to examine the digestive system, either through the mouth, the anus, or an opening into the abdominal cavity. An **esophagoscopy** is the use of an *esophagoscope* to illuminate the esophagus as it is passed through the mouth and into the esophagus. When ulcers are seen in the digestive system through the endoscope, a diagnosis of H. pylori (Helicobacter pylori), bacteria that cause ulcers, is given. This is usually treated with an antibiotic and dietary modification. A *gastroscope* is used to examine the stomach in **gastroscopy.** A **colonoscopy** is the use of an endoscope to examine the colon. A *proctoscope* is used to examine the rectum and anus in a **proctoscopy.** A *sigmoidoscope* is used to examine the sigmoid colon in **sigmoidoscopy.** *Endoscopic retrograde cholangiopancreatography* (ERCP) is a procedure used to examine the biliary ducts with x-ray, a contrast medium, and the use of an endoscope. **Peritoneoscopy** or *laparoscopy* is the examination of the abdominal cavity with an instrument called a *peritoneoscope* or a *laparoscope*.

X-rays and other imaging techniques are used extensively to search for abnormalities. An MRI shows the major organs of the digestive system. A CAT scan provides a visual image of the abdominal cavity and the digestive tract. To examine more specific areas, patients are usually given a contrast medium or other substance that stands out against the background of the x-ray produced. A *barium swallow* is the ingestion of a barium solution before an x-ray of the esophagus, which is generally used to locate foreign objects that have been swallowed (Figure 14-7). A *barium enema* is the administration of a barium solution through an enema before taking a series of x-rays of the colon called a *lower GI series*. An *upper GI series* (UGIS) provides x-rays of the esophagus, stomach, and duodenum, usually after the patient swallows a barium solution or other contrast medium. A *cholangiogram* is an image of the bile vessels taken in **cholangiography,** an x-ray of the bile ducts. A *cholecystogram* is an image of the gallbladder taken in **cholecystography,** an x-ray of the gallbladder taken after the patient swallows iodine. A liver scan, done after injection of radioactive material, can reveal abnormalities. Ultrasound is used to provide images of the entire abdominal area, as in *abdominal ultrasonography*.

Several serum tests indicate how the liver is functioning. A *serum glutamic oxaloacetic transaminase* (SGOT) or an *aspartate transaminase* (AST) measures the enzyme levels in serum that has leaked from damaged liver cells. Another serum test for liver function is the *serum glutamic pyruvic transaminase* (SGPT). This test is also known as an *alanine transaminase* (ALT, AT). A *serum bilirubin* measures bilirubin in the blood as an indicator of jaundice.

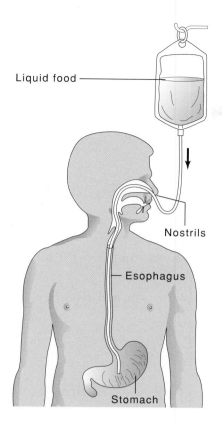

Liquid food

Nostrils

Esophagus

Stomach

FIGURE 14-8 Liquid nourishment can be provided through a nasogastric (NG) tube. This type of tube may also be used to relieve fluid buildup in the stomach or to take stomach content samples.

An *alkaline phosphatase* reveals levels of the enzyme alkaline phosphatase in serum as an indicator of liver disease, especially liver cancer.

A *nasogastric (NG) tube* is passed through the nose to the stomach to relieve fluid buildup or to take stomach content samples for analysis (Figure 14-8). This process is called *nasogastric intubation*.

VOCABULARY REVIEW

In the previous section, you learned terms relating to diagnosis, clinical procedures, and laboratory tests. Before going on to the exercises, review the terms below and refer to the previous section if you have any questions. Pronunciations are provided for certain terms. Sometimes information about where the word came from is included after the term. The etymologies (word histories) are for your information only. You do not need to memorize them.

Term	Meaning
cholangiography [kō-lăn-jē-ŎG-ră-fē] cholangio-, bile vessel + -graphy, a recording	X-ray of the bile ducts.
cholecystography [kō-lē-sĭs-TŎG-ră-fē] chole-, bile + cysto-, bladder + -graphy	X-ray of the gallbladder.
colonoscopy [kō-lŏn-ŎS-kō-pē] colono-, colon + -scopy, a viewing	Examination of the colon using an endoscope.
esophagoscopy [ĕ-sŏf-ă-GŎS-kō-pē] esophago-, esophagus + -scopy	Examination of the esophagus with an esophagoscope.
gastroscopy [găs-TRŎS-kō-pē] gastro-, stomach + -scopy	Examination of the stomach using an endoscope.

Term	Meaning
peritoneoscopy [PĔR-ĭ-tō-nē-ŎS-kō-pē] peritoneo-, peritoneum + -scopy	Examination of the abdominal cavity using a peritoneoscope.
proctoscopy [prŏk-TŎS-kō-pē] procto-, rectum +-scopy	Examination of the rectum and anus using a proctoscope.
sigmoidoscopy [SĬG-mŏy-DŎS-kō-pē] sigmoido-, sigmoid colon + -scopy	Examination of the sigmoid colon using a sigmoidoscope.

DIAGNOSTIC, PROCEDURAL, AND LABORATORY TERMS EXERCISES

Find a Match

Match the diagnostic test in the left-hand column with the definition or possible diagnosis resulting from the test in the right-hand column.

63. _____ serum bilirubin
64. _____ alkaline phosphatase
65. _____ upper GI series
66. _____ image of bile vessels
67. _____ testing of waste for disease-causing organisms
68. _____ tube to retrieve stomach contents for examination
69. _____ element in a solution used in x-rays
70. _____ test for liver function
71. _____ x-rays of the intestines and anal canal
72. _____ hemoccult test

a. x-ray of esophagus, stomach, and duodenum
b. barium
c. cholangiogram
d. nasogastric tube
e. SGOT
f. stool guaiac
g. jaundice
h. liver cancer
i. stool culture
j. lower GI series

CASE STUDY

Testing and Diagnosing

Dr. Walker has morning hours at a local hospital several days a week. Today, Jim Santarelli is scheduled for a colonoscopy. His medical record is shown below:

Critical Thinking

73. What might Dr. Walker be looking for in this procedure?
74. If the examination shows a clear colon, what lifestyle changes might Dr. Walker recommend?

PROCEDURE: colonoscopy

SURGEON: Dr. Walker

INDICATION: This man has a two-year history of increasing, intermittent, sudden bouts of diarrhea without mucus or blood. Antispasmodic treatment with Bentyl has failed. He had a negative barium enema 3 1/2 months ago. Stools have been hemoccult negative. There are no systemic symptoms. The frequency of the diarrhea is once every other day to twice a week.

With the patient turned onto his left side, he was monitored using continuous SAO2 pulse monitoring and intermittent blood pressure monitoring. An IV was started in the left forearm. Mr. Santarelli was given 50 mg of Demerol and 10 mg of Valium by slow intravenous injection. After adequate sedation was achieved, the colonoscopy was performed.

Pathological Terms

The digestive system is both the site and the source of many diseases and disorders. What we take into our mouths determines the type of nutrition our body receives. Eating disorders can be the catalyst for disease processes to start.

Eating Disorders

Anorexia is a loss of appetite. In its most severe form, **anorexia nervosa,** it is a morbid refusal to eat because the person wishes to be dangerously thin. **Bulimia** is a disease wherein bingeing on food and then purposely purging or vomiting is also a quest for abnormal weight loss. Both anorexia nervosa and bulimia can produce many health problems and symptoms, such as hair loss, amenorrhea, and heart damage. Figure 14-9 shows the overlap of starving, bingeing, and purging that can be present in both anorexia nervosa and bulimia. **Obesity** is often the result of overeating, although recent gene studies indicate a possible hereditary defect in many obese people. Obesity can be one of the factors in many health problems, such as heart disease and diabetes. Many eating disorders can be treated with psychological counseling; some, such as anorexia nervosa, may result in death if the patient is not treated at an eating disorder unit or clinic.

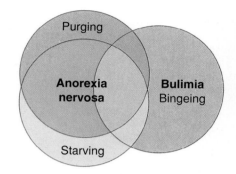

FIGURE 14-9 Starving, bingeing, and purging are symptoms that can overlap in both anorexia nervosa and bulimia.

The National Association of Anorexia Nervosa and Related Disorders (www .anad.org) offers support for eating disorders at their Web site.

Disorders of the Mouth, Pharynx, and Esophagus

Areas in the mouth can become inflamed from an infection, allergy, injury, or internal disorder. **Cheilitis** occurs on the lips; **glossitis** occurs on the tongue; **sialoadenitis** occurs in the salivary glands; and **parotitis** or **parotiditis** occurs in the parotid glands. Various other dental disorders may similarly cause inflammation (see Chapter 20). **Halitosis** is unusually foul mouth odor, which may be caused by poor dental hygiene, gum disease, certain foods, or by an internal disorder such as a sinus infection. **Ankyloglossia** is a condition in which the tongue is partially or completely attached to the floor of the mouth, thereby preventing normal movement. Normal swallowing is an important part of maintaining good nutrition. People with swallowing disorders usually have to have their diet supplemented via a tube. **Aphagia** is an inability to swallow; **dysphagia** is difficulty in swallowing.

Diseases of the pharynx are discussed in Chapter 7 as part of the respiratory system. Food travels into the mouth, through the pharynx, and into the esophagus. *Esophageal varices* are twisted veins in the esophagus that are prone to hemorrhage and ulcers. **Esophagitis** is any inflammation of the esophagus. *Gastroesophageal reflux disease* (GERD) or *esophageal reflux* involves malfunctioning of the sphincter muscle at the bottom of the esophagus. It opens at the wrong time to allow backflow of stomach contents into the esophagus, causing irritation of the esophageal lining. **Achalasia** is the failure of the same esophageal sphincter to relax during swallowing and allow food to pass easily from the esophagus into the stomach to continue the digestive process. This disorder interferes with the intake of normal amounts of nutrients.

Stomach Disorders

The stomach is also the site of many disorders. Some people are sensitive to various foods (such as very spicy dishes) or have allergies to others (as milk products). **Achlorhydria** is the lack of hydrochloric acid in the stomach, a chemical necessary for digestion. **Dyspepsia** is difficulty in digesting food, particularly in the stomach. **Gastritis** is any stomach inflammation. **Gastroenteritis** is an inflammation of both the stomach and small intestine. **Flatulence** is an accumulation of gas in the stomach or intestines. **Eructation** (belching) may release some of this gas. **Nausea** is a sick feeling in the stomach caused by illness or the ingestion of spoiled food. Nausea may also be felt in certain situations such as early pregnancy or when repetitive motion causes discomfort as in car sickness, sea sickness, and so on. **Hematemesis** is the vomiting of blood from the stomach, usually a sign of a severe disorder. *Stomach ulcers* or gastric ulcers are a type of **peptic ulcer,** a sore on the mucous membrane of any part of the gastrointestinal system. A **hiatal hernia** is a protrusion of the stomach through an opening in the diaphragm called the hiatal opening. The pyloric sphincter can become abnormally narrow and cause the condition known as *pyloric stenosis.*

Disorders of the Liver, Pancreas, and Gallbladder

Secretions of the liver, pancreas, and gallbladder mix with the stomach contents that move into the duodenum. The liver can be the site of **jaundice** or **icterus,** when excessive bilirubin in the blood (**hyperbilirubinemia**) causes a yellow discoloration of the skin. Newborn jaundice may be a result of liver disease or many other factors. It is sometimes treated with exposure to artificial lights or sunlight. **Hepatomegaly** is an enlarged liver. **Hepatopathy** is a general term for liver disease, and **hepatitis** is a term for several types of contagious diseases, some of which are sexually transmitted (see Chapter 10). **Cirrhosis** is a chronic liver disease usually caused by poor nutrition and excessive alcohol consumption. **Pancreatitis** is an inflammation of the pancreas. (Other pancreatic diseases are discussed in Chapter 15.)

The gallbladder can be the site of calculi (**gallstones** or **cholelithiasis**) that block the bile from leaving the gallbladder. The presence of gallstones in the common bile duct is called *choledocholithiasis*. **Cholangitis** is any inflammation of the bile ducts. **Cholecystitis** is any inflammation of the gallbladder, either acute or chronic. The duodenum can be the site of **duodenal ulcers.** Duodenal ulcers are a type of peptic ulcer and are thought to be bacterial (H. pylori) in origin. This discovery has lead to the widespread use of antibiotics to treat many types of ulcers. On the side of the duodenum lies the appendix, which can become inflamed if gastric substances leak into it from the duodenum. This condition is called **appendicitis,** which usually requires surgery to prevent the appendix from bursting.

Intestinal Disorders

The small and large intestines can have ulcers, obstructions, irritations, inflammations, abnormalities, and cancer. An **ileus** is an intestinal blockage, which may be caused by lack of sufficient moisture to move waste material through the system or by an internal disorder. **Enteritis** and **colitis** are general terms for inflammations in the small intestine. **Ulcerative colitis** is a chronic type of *irritable bowel disease* (IBD) or *inflammatory bowel disease* with recurring ulcers and inflammations. Other symptoms may include cramping, abdominal pain, and diarrhea. IBDs are often associated with stress. **Crohn's**

The American Liver Foundation (www.liverfoundation.org) supports research into the causes and cure of liver disease.

disease is another type of IBD with symptoms similar to ulcerative colitis but lacking ulcers and sometimes having **fistulas,** abnormal passages or openings in tissue walls. **Colic** is a condition (usually in infants) of gastrointestinal distress due to allergies, an underdeveloped digestive tract, or other conditions that prevent easy digestion of food. In infants, colic usually resolves itself within a few months as the infant matures. **Diverticulosis** is a condition in which **diverticula,** small pouches in the intestinal wall, trap food or bacteria. **Diverticulitis** is an inflammation of the diverticula. **Ileitis** is an inflammation of the ileum. **Dysentery** is a general term for irritation of the intestinal tract with loose stools and other symptoms, such as abdominal pain and weakness. It is often caused by bacteria such as those found in many underdeveloped countries. **Polyposis** is a general term for a condition in which polyps develop in the intestinal tract. Polyps can become cancerous so they are often checked or removed to detect any abnormalities at an early stage. *Colonic polyposis* is polyps in the colon, which have a high likelihood of changing to *colorectal cancer.*

A **volvulus,** an intestinal blockage caused by twisting of the intestine on itself, requires emergency surgery (Figure 14-10). An **intussusception** is the telescoping of the intestine. One section prolapses (collapses) into a neighboring part (Figure 14-11). The abdominal and peritoneal regions surrounding the intestinal tract can become filled with fluid (**ascites**) or inflamed (**peritonitis**).

The Rectum and Anus

The rectum, anus, and stool may play a role in some disorders. **Proctitis** is an inflammation of the rectum and anus. **Constipation** is a condition with infrequent or difficult release of bowel movements, sometimes the result of insufficient moisture to soften and move stools. **Diarrhea** is loose, watery stools that may be the result of insufficient roughage or of an internal disorder. **Flatus** is the release of gas through the anus.

The analysis of stool for blood, bacteria, and other elements can provide a clue to various ailments. **Melena** is a condition in which blood that is not fresh appears in the stool as a black, tarry mass. **Hematochezia** is bright red blood in the stool. **Steatorrhea** is fat in the stool.

A small opening in the anal canal is called an **anal fistula.** Waste material can enter the abdominal cavity through a fistula. The anus may be the site of **hemorrhoids,** swollen, twisted veins that can cause great discomfort.

Hernias

A *hernia* is any loop or twist of an intestine or other organ not positioned correctly in the abdomen. There are many types of hernias. Some common ones are as follows:

- A *hiatal* hernia is the protrusion of the stomach through the esophageal hiatus of the diaphragm.
- An *inguinal hernia* is a protrusion of the intestine through a weakness in the abdominal wall (Figure 14-12).
- A *strangulated hernia* is one in which blood flow is restricted or absent.
- A *femoral hernia* is a protrusion of a loop of intestine into the femoral canal.

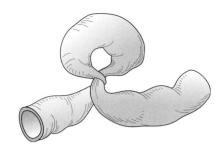

FIGURE 14-10 A volvulus is a twisting of the intestine that causes a blockage and requires surgery.

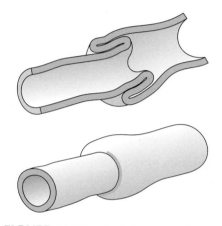

FIGURE 14-11 An intussusception occurs most often in children and requires surgical correction.

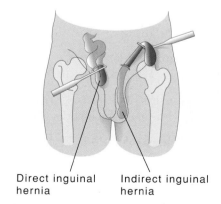

Direct inguinal hernia   Indirect inguinal hernia

FIGURE 14-12 An inguinal hernia usually requires surgery.

- An *umbilical hernia* is a protrusion of part of the intestine into the umbilicus.
- An *incarcerated hernia* is one in which movement of bowel is restricted or obstructed.

VOCABULARY REVIEW

In the previous section, you learned terms relating to pathology. Before going on to the exercises, review the terms below and refer to the previous section if you have any questions. Pronunciations are provided for certain terms. Sometimes information about where the word came from is included after the term. The etymologies (word histories) are for your information only. You do not need to memorize them.

Term	Definition
achalasia [ăk-ă-LĀ-zhē-ă] a-, without + Greek *chalasis*, a relaxing	Inability of a muscle, particularly the cardiac sphincter, to relax.
achlorhydria [ā-klōr-HĪ-drē-ă]	Lack of hydrochloric acid in the stomach.
anal fistula [Ā-năl FĬS-tyū-lă]	Small opening in the anal canal through which waste matter can leak into the abdominal cavity.
ankyloglossia [ĂNG-kĭ-lō-GLŎS-ē-ă] Greek *ankylos*, bent + *glossus*, tongue	Condition of the tongue being partially or completely attached to the bottom of the mouth.
anorexia nervosa [ăn-ō-RĔK-sē-ă nĕr-VŌ-să] an-, without + Greek *orexis*, appetite	Eating disorder with extreme weight loss.
aphagia [ă-FĀ-jē-ă] a-, without + -phagia, eating	Inability to swallow.
appendicitis [ă-pĕn-dĭ-SĪ-tĭs] appendic-, appendix + -itis, inflammation	Inflammation of the appendix.
ascites [ă-SĪ-tēs] Latin, bags	Fluid buildup in the abdominal and peritoneal cavities.
bulimia [bū-LĒM-ē-ă] Greek *boux*, ox + *limos*, hunger	Eating disorder with bingeing and purging.
cheilitis [kī-LĪ-tĭs] Greek *cheilos*, lip + -itis	Inflammation of the lips.
cholangitis [kō-lăn-JĪ-tĭs] cholangi-, bile vessel + -itis	Inflammation of the bile ducts.
cholecystitis [KŌ-lē-sĭs-TĪ-tĭs] chole-, bile + cyst-, bladder + -itis	Inflammation of the gallbladder.
cholelithiasis [KŌ-lē-lĭ-THĪ-ă-sĭs] chole- + Greek *lithos*, stone + -iasis, condition	Gallstones in the gallbladder.
cirrhosis [sĭr-RŌ-sĭs] Greek *kirrhos*, yellow + -osis, condition	Liver disease, often caused by alcoholism.
colic [KŎL-ĭk] Greek *kolikos*, of the colon	Gastrointestinal distress, especially of infants.

Term	Definition
colitis [kō-LĪ-tǐs] col-, colon + -itis	Inflammation of the colon.
constipation [kǒn-stǐ-PĀ-shǔn] Latin *constipo*, to press together	Difficult or infrequent defecation.
Crohn's [krōnz] **disease** After Burrill Crohn (1884–1983), U. S. gastroenterologist	Type of irritable bowel disease with no ulcers.
diarrhea [dī-ă-RĒ-ă] Greek *diarrhoia*, a flowing through	Loose, watery stool.
diverticula [dī-věr-TĬK-yū-lă] Latin *diverticulum*, a side road	Small pouches in the intestinal walls.
diverticulitis [DĪ-věr-tǐk-yū-LĪ-tǐs] diverticul(a) + -itis	Inflammation of the diverticula.
diverticulosis [DĪ-věr-tǐk-yū-LŌ-sǐs] diverticul(a) + -osis	Condition in which diverticula trap food or bacteria.
duodenal [DŪ-ō-DĒ-năl] **ulcer**	Ulcer in the duodenum.
dysentery [DĬS-ěn-těr-ē] Greek *dysenteria*, bad bowels	Irritation of the intestinal tract with loose stools.
dyspepsia [dǐs-PĔP-sē-ă] dys-, bad + -pepsia, digestion	Indigestion.
dysphagia [dǐs-FĀ-jē-ă] dys- + -phagia, eating	Difficulty in swallowing.
enteritis [ěn-těr-Ī-tǐs] enter-, intestine + -itis	Inflammation of the small intestine.
eructation [ē-rŭk-TĀ-shǔn] Latin *eructo*, to belch	Belching.
esophagitis [ě-sǒf-ă-JĪ-tǐs] esophag-, esophagus + -itis	Inflammation of the esophagus.
fistula [FĬS-tyū-lă] Latin, a pipe	Abnormal opening in tissue.
flatulence [FLĂT-yū-lěns]	Gas in the stomach or intestines.
flatus [FLĂ-tŭs] Latin, a blowing	Gas in the lower intestinal tract that can be released through the anus.
gallstones	Calculi in the gallbladder.
gastritis [gǎs-TRĪ-tǐs] gastr-, stomach + -itis	Inflammation of the stomach.
gastroenteritis [GĂS-trō-ěn-těr-Ī-tǐs] gastro- + enter- + -itis	Inflammation of the stomach and small intestine.
glossitis [glǒ-SĪ-tǐs] gloss-, tongue + -itis	Inflammation of the tongue.

Term	Definition
halitosis [hăl-ĭ-TŌ-sĭs] Latin *halitus*, breath + -osis	Foul mouth odor.
hematemesis [hē-mă-TĔM-ē-sĭs] hemat-, blood + emesis	Blood in vomit.
hematochezia [HĒ-mă-tō-KĒ-zhē-ă] hemato-, blood + Greek *chezo*, to defecate	Red blood in stool.
hemorrhoids [HĔM-ō-rŏydz]	Swollen, twisted veins in the anus.
hepatitis [hĕp-ă-TĪ-tĭs] hepat-, liver + -itis	Inflammation or disease of the liver.
hepatomegaly [HĔP-ă-tō-MĔG-ă-lē] hepato-, liver + -megaly, enlargement	Enlarged liver.
hepatopathy [hĕp-ă-TŎP-ă-thē] hepato- + -pathy, disease	Liver disease.
hiatal hernia [hī-Ā-tăl HĔR-nē-ă]	Protrusion of the stomach through an opening in the diaphragm.
hyperbilirubinemia [HĪ-pĕr-BĬL-ĭ-rū-bĭ-NĒ-mē-ă] hyper-, excessive + bilirubin + -emia, blood	Excessive bilirubin in the blood.
icterus [ĬK-tĕr-ŭs] Greek *ikteros*	Jaundice.
ileitis [ĬL-ē-Ī-tĭs] ile-, ileum + -itis	Inflammation of the ileum.
ileus [ĬL-ē-ŭs] Latin, a twisting	Intestinal blockage.
intussusception [ĬN-tŭs-sŭ-SĔP-shŭn] Latin *intus*, within + *suscipio*, to take up	Prolapse or collapse of an intestinal part into a neighboring part. One section collapses into another like a telescope.
jaundice [JĂWN-dĭs]	Excessive bilirubin in the blood causing yellowing of the skin.
melena [mĕ-LĒ-nă] Greek *melaina*, black	Old blood in the stool.
nausea [NĂW-zhē-ă] Latin, seasickness	Sick feeling in the stomach.
obesity [ō-BĒS-ĭ-tē] Latin *obesus*, fat	Abnormal accumulation of fat in the body.
pancreatitis [PĂN-krē-ă-TĪ-tĭs] pancreat-, pancreas + -itis	Inflammation of the pancreas.
parotitis, parotiditis [păr-ō-TĪ-tĭs, pă-rŏt-ĭ-DĪ-tĭs] parot(id gland) + -itis	Inflammation of the parotid gland.
peptic ulcer	Sore on the mucous membrane of the digestive system; stomach ulcer or gastric ulcer.

Term	Definition
peritonitis [PĔR-ĭ-tō-NĪ-tĭs] periton-, peritoneum + -itis	Inflammation of the peritoneum.
polyposis [PŎL-ĭ-PŌ-sĭs] polyp + -osis	Condition with polyps, as in the intestines.
proctitis [prŏk-TĪ-tĭs] proct-, rectum + -itis	Inflammation of the rectum and anus.
sialoadenitis [SĪ-ă-lō-ăd-ĕ-NĪ-tĭs] sialoaden-, salivary gland + -itis	Inflammation of the salivary glands.
steatorrhea [STĒ-ă-tō-RĒ-ă] steato-, fat + -rrhea, a flowing	Fat in the blood.
ulcerative colitis [kō-LĪ-tĭs]	Inflammation of the colon with ulcers.
volvulus [VŎL-vyū-lŭs] Latin *volvo*, to roll	Intestinal blockage caused by the intestine twisting on itself.

PATHOLOGICAL TERMS EXERCISES

Find a Match

Match the terms in the left-hand column with the correct definition in the right-hand column.

75. ____ bulimia
76. ____ colitis
77. ____ diverticula
78. ____ eructation
79. ____ hematochezia
80. ____ intussusception
81. ____ jaundice
82. ____ peritonitis
83. ____ steatorrhea
84. ____ volvulus

a. intestinal blockage caused by the intestine twisting on itself
b. red blood in the stool
c. prolapse of an intestinal part into a neighboring part
d. eating disorder with bingeing and purging
e. inflammation of the colon
f. inflammation of the peritoneum
g. fat in the stool
h. small pouches in the intestinal wall
i. icterus
j. belching

Check Your Knowledge

Circle the correct term that completes the sentence.

85. Jane's parents have brought her to see an internist. Jane is 5′10″ and weighs 105 pounds. Jane thinks she is fat. The doctor suspects Jane's problem is _____. (obesity, anorexia, aphagia)

86. John was seen in the emergency room. He complained of abdominal pain with cramping and diarrhea. He was concerned that he might have _____. (constipation, irritable bowel disease, hemorrhoids)

87. Jean has been complaining of severe pain in the RUQ following the ingestion of food, especially foods like nuts and ice cream. She believes she might have _____. (pancreatitis, appendicitis, cholecystitis)

88. Dora is feeling sluggish and unwell. She complains to her doctor that she has been unable to have a bowel movement for the past 5 days. She is diagnosed with _____. (diarrhea, hematochezia, constipation)

89. Many people cannot lie flat after eating because of a burning sensation in the chest and throat. The pain makes the person feel that he or she is having a heart attack. This condition, seen frequently in the emergency room, is called _____. (inguinal hernia, dysentery, gastroesophageal reflux)

Spell It Correctly

For each of the following words, write C if the spelling is correct. If it is not, write the correct spelling.

90. dypepsia _____

91. hyperbilirubinemia _____

92. diverticuli _____

93. hematochazia _____

94. inginal hernia _____

95. iliitis _____

96. polyposis _____

97. cirrosis _____

98. hietal hernia _____

99. achlorhydria _____

100. flatusence _____

CASE STUDY

Performing Surgery

Dr. Walker has another patient scheduled for a colonoscopy. Laura Martinez had an earlier colonoscopy, which was negative. Since then, she has experienced some rectal bleeding. This time her colonoscopy shows several suspicious-looking polyps near the rectum. Dr. Walker biopsies several of them. The result is positive for cancer, but the area of malignancy that needs to be removed is limited.

Critical Thinking

101. What operation will likely be performed?

102. Why might the operation include a colostomy?

Surgical Terms

Treating the digestive tract often includes biopsies, surgeries, and observation using endoscopes. The following is a list of some of the surgical procedures performed on the digestive system.

- **Abdominocentesis** or **paracentesis** is a surgical puncture to remove fluid or relieve pressure in the abdomal cavity, as in ascites.
- **Cholelithotomy** is an incision for the removal of stones. **Choledocholithotomy** is an incision for removal of stones in the common bile duct. **Cholelithotripsy** is the crushing of gallstones using sound waves or other techniques.
- Surgical repair of the digestive tract includes **cheiloplasty** (lip repair); **glossorrhaphy** (tongue suturing); **esophagoplasty** (esophagus repair); and **proctoplasty** (repair of the rectum and anus).
- Some parts of the digestive tract may require partial or complete removal because of malignancies or chronic inflammation. A **glossectomy** is removal of the tongue. A **polypectomy** is the removal of polyps, particularly in areas such as the colon, which are susceptible to cancer. An **appendectomy** is the removal of a diseased appendix

that is in danger of rupturing. A **cholecystectomy** is the removal of the gallbladder, particularly one that is constantly inflamed and susceptible to painful bouts of gallstones. A **diverticulectomy** is removal of diverticula. A **gastrectomy** is removal of some or all of the stomach. It may be followed by a gastric resection, to repair the remaining part of the stomach. A **gastric resection** or **gastric bypass** removes a portion of the stomach to limit overeating as a treatment for obesity. A simpler procedure called *gastric lap band surgery* is also used as a treatment for obesity. A **colectomy** is the removal of some or all of the colon. This may be a temporary operation that is followed by a surgical reconnection of parts of the colon or it may require the use of a colostomy bag. A **pancreatectomy** is removal of the pancreas usually only in cases with malignancy. A **hemorrhoidectomy** is the removal of hemorrhoids, which are sometimes treated by laser cauterization. A **hepatic lobectomy** is removal of one or more lobes of the liver. It is usually preceded by a **liver biopsy** to determine the type and extent of disease. People can live with only part of a liver. However, if a person with a completely diseased liver does not receive an organ transplant, he or she will usually die. An anal fistula is removed in an **anal fistulectomy. Billroth's I** and **Billroth's II** are two types of operations. The first is the excision of the pylorus, and the second is the resectioning of the pylorus with the stomach.

- An **anastomosis,** a surgical union of two hollow tubes, is sometimes used to bypass parts of the intestines as in the case of removal of a section of the intestines. There are many types of anastomoses used in various body systems. There are a number of ways that anastomoses can correct digestive disorders. An *ileorectal anastomosis* is the connection of the ileum and the rectum after a total colectomy. An *end-to-side anastomosis* is a connection of the end of one vessel to the side of a larger one.

Look at the following website for information concerning gastric bypass and gastric lap band surgery. http://www.webmd.com/video/lap-band-after-gastric-bypass

MORE ABOUT . . .

Gastric Lap Band Surgery

This surgical procedure is one of the newer method for weight loss surgery that places a silicone band device around the stomach. Unlike gastric bypass surgery, which removes part of the stomach, this procedure surgically implants a band at the upper part of the stomach, forming a small pouch that can hold only a small amount of food. The surgery only involves cutting into the abdomen for the placement of the band. No cutting is done on the stomach itself. Patients must be willing to make major changes in their eating habits and lifestyles just as they would with other weight loss practices. To be eligible, other nonsurgical weight loss methods have not been successful and a person must have a Body Mass Index (BMI) of at least 40 and with one or more comorbidities.

Research suggests that although weight loss is usually not as extreme, gastric lap band surgery can be as beneficial in sending diabetes into remission as gastric bypass surgery. Linking research on the disease processes that are exacerbated by obesity is an important association when making advances in our ability to reduce the effects of the over weight condition of our population's health.

For more information, go to http://www.fda.org and http://nlm.nih.gov/medlineplus.

- Openings may have to be made in the gastrointestinal tract. Sometimes they are temporary to allow evacuation of waste material. In some cases, they are permanent as when intestinal parts cannot be reconnected. An **ileostomy** is the creation of an opening in the abdomen, which is attached to the ileum to allow fecal matter to discharge into a bag outside the body. A **colostomy** is an opening in the colon to the abdominal wall to create a place for waste to exit the body other than through the anus. A colostomy is sometimes required in the case of diseases such as cancer and ulcerative colitis.

VOCABULARY REVIEW

In the previous section, you learned terms relating to surgery. Before going on to the exercises, review the terms below and refer to the previous section if you have any questions. Pronunciations are provided for certain terms. Sometimes information about where the word came from is included after the term. The etymologies (word histories) are for your information only. You do not need to memorize them.

Term	Definition
abdominocentesis [ăb-DŎM-ĭ-nō-sĕn-TĒ-sĭs] Latin *abdominis*, abdomen + -centesis, puncture	Incision into the abdomen to remove fluid or relieve pressure.
anal fistulectomy [Ā-năl fĭs-tyū-LĔK-tō-mē]	Removal of an anal fistula.
anastomosis [ă-NĂS-tō-MŌ-sĭs] Greek *anastomoo*, to furnish with a mouth	Surgical union of two hollow structures.
appendectomy [ăp-pĕn-DĔK-tō-mē] append-, appendix + -ectomy, removal	Removal of the appendix.
Billroth's [BĬLL-rŏths] **I** After C. A. Billroth (1829–1894), Austrian surgeon	Excision of the pylorus.
Billroth's II	Resection of the pylorus with the stomach.
cheiloplasty [KĪ-lō-plăs-tē] Greek *cheilos*, lip + -plasty, repair	Repair of the lips.
cholecystectomy [KŌ-lē-sĭs-TĔK-tō-mē] cholecyst-, gallbladder + -ectomy	Removal of the gallbladder.
choledocholithotomy [kō-LĔD-ō-kō-lĭ-THŎT-ō-mē] choledocho-, common bile duct + Greek *lithos*, stone + -tomy, a cutting	Removal of stones from the common bile duct.
cholelithotomy [KŌ-lē-lĭ-THŎT-ō-mē] chole-, bile + Greek *lithos*, stone + -tomy	Removal of gallstones.
cholelithotripsy [kō-lē-LĬTH-ō-trĭp-sē] chole- + Greek *lithos*, stone + *tripsis*, a rubbing	Breaking up or crushing of stones in the body, especially gallstones.
colectomy [kō-LĔK-tō-mē] col-, colon + -ectomy	Removal of the colon.

Term	Definition
colostomy [kō-LŎS-tō-mē] colo-, colon + -stomy, mouth, opening	Creation of an opening from the colon into the abdominal wall.
diverticulectomy [dĭ-vĕr-tĭk-ū-LĔK-tō-mē]	Removal of diverticula.
esophagoplasty [ĕ-SŎF-ă-gō-plăs-tē] esophago-, esophagus + -plasty	Repair of the esophagus.
gastrectomy [găs-TRĔK-tō-mē] gastr-, stomach + -ectomy	Removal of part or all of the stomach.
gastric resection or gastric bypass	Removal of part of the stomach and repair of the remaining part.
glossectomy [glŏ-SĔK-tō-mē] gloss-, tongue + -ectomy	Removal of the tongue.
glossorrhaphy [glŏ-SŌR-ă-fē] glosso-, tongue + -rrhapy, suturing	Suture of the tongue.
hemorrhoidectomy [HĔM-ō-rŏy-DĔK-tō-mē] hemorrhoid(s) + -ectomy	Removal of hemorrhoids.
hepatic lobectomy [hĕ-PĂT-ĭk lō-BĔK-tō-mē]	Removal of one or more lobes of the liver.
ileostomy [ĬL-ē-ŎS-tō-mē] ileo-, ileum + -stomy	Creation of an opening into the ileum.
liver biopsy	Removal of a small amount of liver tissue to examine for disease.
pancreatectomy [PĂN-krē-ă-TĔK-tō-mē] pancreat-, pancreas + -tomy	Removal of the pancreas.
paracentesis [PĂR-ă-sĕn-TĒ-sĭs] Greek *parakentesis*, a tapping for edema	Incision into the abdominal cavity to remove fluid or relieve pressure.
polypectomy [pŏl-ĭ-PĔK-tō-mē] polyp + -ectomy	Removal of polyps.
proctoplasty [PRŎK-tō-plăs-tē] procto-, rectum + -plasty	Repair of the rectum and anus.

SURGICAL TERMS EXERCISES

Fill in the Blanks

103. Removal of a liver lobe is a(n) _____ _____.

104. Repair of a part of the stomach is a(n) _____ _____.

105. Two openings that allow waste to exit the body other than through the anus are a(n) _____ and a(n) _____.

106. The crushing of gallstones is called _____.

107. Incision into the intestinal tract to remove fluid is _____ or _____.

Resolving a Complaint

Dora, a patient complaining of constipation, was given a laxative to regulate her bowel movements. Doctors found that Dora avoided foods high in roughage because of an acid condition in her stomach.

Critical Thinking

108. Why is it important that Dora eat foods with high roughage content?

109. What other medication might the doctor prescribe to make it easier for her to digest such foods?

Pharmacological Terms

Aside from treatments for cancer, medications for the digestive tract counteract situations that occur in various parts of the tract. **Antacids** neutralize stomach acid. Many antacids are taken before meals to prevent the building up of excess stomach acids. Others are taken after symptoms appear. **Antiemetics** prevent vomiting. **Antispasmodics** relieve spasms in the gastrointestinal tract. A **laxative** stimulates movement of bowels. A **cathartic** induces vomiting. An **antidiarrheal** helps to control loose, watery stools. Table 14-2 lists some common medications used to treat the intestinal tract.

Many antacids are a good source of calcium.

TABLE 14-2 Medications Used to Treat Digestive Disorders

Drug Class	Purpose	Generic	Trade Name
antacid and anti-gastric reflux agents	to neutralize stomach acid	cimetidine aluminum & magnesium hydroxide famotodine magaldrate ranitidine esomeprazole	Tagamet Maalox, Mylanta, Di-Gel Pepcid Riopan Zantac Nexium
antidiarrheal	to control loose stools	bismuth subsalicylate loperamide attapulgite	Pepto-Bismol Imodium Kaopectate, Diasorb
antiemetic	to prevent regurgitation	dimenhydrinate meclizine	Dramamine Bonine, Antivert
antispasmodic	to calm spasms in the intestinal tract	dicyclomine hyoscyamine	Antispas, Bentyl Anaspaz, Cystospaz
cathartic	to cause vomiting (after ingestion of poison)	ipecac syrup	none
laxative	to relieve constipation	psyllium bisacodyl senna docusate	Metamucil Dulcolax, Theralax Senokot Therevac

VOCABULARY REVIEW

In the previous section, you learned terms relating to pharmacology. Before going on to the exercises, review the terms below and refer to the previous section if you have any questions. Pronunciations are provided for certain terms. Sometimes information about where the word came from is included after the term. The etymologies (word histories) are for your information only. You do not need to memorize them.

Term	Definition
antacid [ănt-ĂS-ĭd] ant-, against + acid	Agent that neutralizes stomach acid.
antidiarrheal [ăn-tē-dī-ă-RĒ-ăl] anti-, against + diarrhea	Agent that controls loose, watery stools.
antiemetic [ĂN-tē-ĕ-MĔT-ĭk] anti- + emetic, related to vomiting	Agent that prevents vomiting.
antispasmodic [ăn-tē-spăz-MŎD-ĭk] anti- + spasmodic	Agent that controls intestinal tract spasms.
cathartic [kă-THĂR-tĭk] Greek *katharsis*, purification	Agent that induces vomiting; also a strong laxative for emptying the bowels.
laxative [LĂX-ă-tĭv] Latin *laxativus*	Agent that induces bowels to move in order to relieve constipation.

PHARMACOLOGICAL TERMS EXERCISES

Find a Match

Match the pharmacological agent in the left-hand column with its use in the right-hand column.

110. _____ antacid

111. _____ antidiarrheal

112. _____ antiemetic

113. _____ antispasmodic

114. _____ cathartic

115. _____ laxative

a. causes vomiting

b. calms spasms

c. prevents regurgitation

d. relieves constipation

e. controls loose, watery stools

f. relieves burning sensation in digestive disorder

CHALLENGE SECTION

The record for Dr. Walker's patient, Holly Berger, shows a history of gastrointestinal problems. Dr. Walker performed a procedure that allowed a full examination and biopsies of certain sections of Holly's intestinal tract. The procedure was performed in the hospital, and the patient was able to leave after a few hours in the recovery room.

Critical Thinking

116. Why did Dr. Walker take biopsies of various intestinal tract areas?

117. From his examination of the stomach and duodenum, Dr. Walker able to rule out Crohn's disease. What indication was most likely in the record that made this possible?

TERMINOLOGY IN ACTION

The patient record for Manny Ramos lists two procedures and four diagnostic terms. Define all six terms and break them down into their word parts.

MEDICAL RECORD	PROGRESS NOTES
DATE 6/28/XX	Patient complains of intermittent stomach pains, some rectal bleeding, heartburn. Schedule tests on two successive days in three weeks.
7/22/XX	8:00 Colonoscopy. Four polyps removed and biopsied. Otherwise normal. J Phelps, M.D.
7/23/XX	8:00 Esophagoscopy. Numerous lesions present. J. Phelps, M.D.
7/23/XX	Colonoscopy shows precancerous polyps. Recommend 6-month follow-up. Gastric reflux present—treat with Nexium; Stomach ulcers, give 4-week course of treatment and list of dietary restrictions. Recheck stool in 6 weeks. Recommend dental visit for persistent halitosis.

PATIENT'S IDENTIFICATION (For typed or written entries give: Name—last, first, middle; grade; rank; hospital or medical facility)

Manny Ramos
000-33-5555

REGISTER NO.

WARD NO.
4B

PROGRESS NOTES
STANDARD FORM 509

USING THE INTERNET

Go to the American Gastroenterological Association site (http://www.gastro.org), click the public section, then click the digestive health resource center, and then choose a gastroenterological disease site. Write a brief one-paragraph summary of some of the information you gather about the disease.

CHAPTER REVIEW

The material that follows is to help you review this chapter.

Root Out the Meaning

Separate the following terms into word parts and define each word part

118. buccal
119. cecotomy
120. cecopexy
121. cecal
122. celiorrhaphy
123. celiotomy
124. celiscopy
125. celiocentesis
126. cholelith
127. cholemesis
128. cholelithotomy
129. cholepoiesis
130. cholestatis
131. cholelithotripsy
132. cholangiocarcinoma
133. cholangiectasis
134. cholangiostomy
135. cholangiogram
136. cholangiography
137. cholangioma
138. cholangiopancreatography
139. cholangioscope
140. cholecystectomy
141. cholecyst
142. cholecystocolostomy

143. cholecystoduodenostomy
144. cholecystopexy
145. cholecystogram
146. cholecystorrhaphy
147. cholecystosonography
148. cholecystostomy
149. cholecystotomy
150. choledocholithiasis
151. colitis
152. colorectitis
153. colostomy
154. duodenectomy
155. enteritis
156. enterocolitis
157. esophagocele
158. gastrocolitis
159. gastroenteritis
160. glossitis
161. hepatoscopy
162. ileostomy
163. jejunectomy
164. labiogingival
165. pancreatopathy
166. pharyngectomy

Complete the Sentence

Circle the term that best describes the *italicized* description of the correct answer

167. *Creation of an opening* from the *colon* (colonostomy, colectomy, colostomy) into the abdominal wall.

168. A(n) (fistula, anastomosis, icterus), *a surgical union of two hollow tubes,* is sometimes used to bypass parts of the intestines as in the case of removal of a section of the intestines.

169. A gastric bypass or (gastrotomy, gastric resection, gastric ascites) *removes a portion of the stomach* to limit overeating as a treatment for obesity.

170. Mrs. Abernathy has been experiencing an uncomfortable *burning in her upper chest area* after eating. The doctor suspects (UGIS, GERD, EGD).

171. The *coordinated, rhythmic contractions of smooth muscle* that force food through the digestive tract are known as: (peritoneal, peristatic, peritalsis).

Build Your Medical Vocabulary

Build a word that means the same as each of the phrases below.

172. Abnormal condition of fungus in the mouth _____

173. Fatty inflammation of the liver _____

174. Excessive secreting of saliva _____

175. Pertaining to the rectum and abdomen _____

176. Surgical fixation of the liver _____

177. Herniation of the liver _____

178. Surgically created opening in the stomach _____

179. Surgical repair of the stomach and the intestines _____

180. Incision into the esophagus _____

181. Pertaining to the intestines _____

182. Observation of the duodenum: _____

183. Any intestinal disease _____

184. Discharge of abnormal amounts of sugar _____

185. The study of the intestines _____

186. Surgical fixation of the intestines _____

187. Pertaining to the ileum and cecum _____

188. A stone or calculus in the stomach _____

189. An x-ray examination of the liver _____

190. Surgical suturing of the common bile duct _____

191. Pathological condition or state of stones in the gallbladder _____

192. Fibrous condition of the bile ducts _____

193. Inflammation of the abdomen _____

194. Production of bile _____

195. Inflammation of the common bile duct _____

196. A heavy (unusual) discharge from the colon _____

197. Presence of a gallstone _____

198. Disease of the gallbladder _____

199. Dilation of the bile ducts _____

Matching

Match each of the following medical conditions with its description.

200. ____ intestinal blockage caused by the intestine twisting on itself   **a.** anorexia nervosa

201. ____ condition of having polyps, as in the intestines

202. ____ foul mouth odor

203. ____ gas in the stomach or intestines

204. ____ inability to swallow

205. ____ eating disorder with binging and purging

206. ____ old blood in the stool

207. ____ blood in vomit

208. ____ eating disorder with extreme weight loss

209. ____ belching

210. ____ small pouches in the intestinal walls

211. ____ liver disease, often caused by alcoholism

212. ____ indigestion

213. ____ irritation of the intestinal tract with loose stools

214. ____ gastrointestinal distress, especially in infants

215. ____ fluid buildup in the abdominal and peritoneal cavities

216. ____ abnormal opening in tissue

217. ____ prolapse or collapse of an intestinal part into a neighboring part

218. ____ jaundice

219. ____ protrusion of the stomach through an opening in the diaphragm

b. eructation

c. colic

d. polyposis

e. halitosis

f. aphagia

g. bulimia

h. icterus

i. volvulus

j. melena

k. diverticula

l. dyspepsia

m. fistula

n. intussusception

o. hiatal hernia

p. cirrhosis

q. dysentery

r. hematemesis

s. flatulence

t. ascites

True or False

Indicate in the blank whether the statement is true (T) or false (F).

220. Reflux is another name for regurgitation. T F

221. Crohn's disease is a type of IBD. T F

222. An inguinal hernia is the protrusion of the intestine through a weakness in the stomach wall. T F

223. The medical term for red blood in the stool is *hematochezia*. T F

224. *Cheil(o)* and *labi(o)* are both word parts for the lip(s). T F

225. A cathartic is a medication used to stop diarrhea. T F

226. The definition of dysphagia is inability to speak. T F

227. A strangulated hernia is one in which movement of bowel is restricted or obstructed. T F

228. Another name for the digestive tract is the alimentary canal. T F

229. The upper portion of the stomach is known as the frenulum. T F

Check Your Spelling

Write the correct spelling in the blank to the right of each word. If the word is already spelled correctly, place a C in the blank.

230. rectoskope _____

231. esophagomalacia _____

232. coalopexy _____

233. cheilorrhaphy _____

234. enzime _____

235. mastacation _____

236. paracentesis _____

237. antidirrheal _____

238. emasis _____

239. rugay _____

DEFINITIONS

Define the following terms and combining forms. Review the chapter before starting. Make sure you know how to pronounce each term as you define it. The blue words in curly brackets refer to the Spanish glossary available online at www.mhhe.com/medterm3e.

WORD

240. abdominocentesis [ăb-DŎM-ĭ-nō-sĕn-TĒ-sĭs]

241. absorption [ăb-SŎRP-shŭn] {absorción}

242. achalasia [ăk-ă-LĀ-zhē-ă] {acalasia}

243. achlorhydria [ā-klōr-HĪ-drē-ă]

244. alimentary [ăl-ĭ-MĔN-tĕr-ē] canal

245. amino [ă-MĒ-nō] acid {aminoácido}

246. amylase [ĂM-ĭl-ās] {amilasa}

247. anal [Ā-năl] canal

248. anal fistula [FĬS-tyū-lă]

249. anal fistulectomy [fĭs-tyū-LĔK-tō-mē]

250. anastomosis [ă-NĂS-tō-MŌ-sĭs] {anastomosis}

251. ankyloglossia [ĂNG-kĭ-lō-GLŎS-ē-ă] {anquiloglosia}

252. an(o)

253. anorexia nervosa [ăn-ō-RĔK-sē-ă nĕr-VŌ-să]

254. antacid [ănt-ĂS-ĭd]

255. antidiarrheal [ăn-tē-dī-ă-RĒ-ăl]

256. antiemetic [ĂN-tē-ĕ-MĔT-ĭk]

257. antispasmodic [ăn-tē-spăz-MŎD-ĭk]

258. anus [Ā-nŭs] {ano}

259. aphagia [ă-FĀ-jē-ă] {afagia}

260. append(o), appendic(o)

261. appendage [ă-PĔN-dĭj] {apéndice}

262. appendectomy [ăp-pĕn-DĔK-tō-mē] {apendectomía}

263. appendicitis [ă-pĕn-dĭ-SĪ-tĭs] {appendicitis}

264. appendix [ă-PĔN-dĭks] {apéndice}

265. ascites [ă-SĪ-tēs] {ascitis}

266. bil(o), bili

267. bile [bīl] {bilis}

268. bilirubin [bĭl-ĭ-RŪ-bĭn] {bilirrubina}

269. Billroth's [BĬLL-rŏths] I

270. Billroth's II

271. body {cuerpo}

272. bowel [bŏw-l] {intestine}

273. bucc(o)

274. bulimia [bū-LĒM-ē-ă]

275. cathartic [kă-THĂR-tĭk]

276. cec(o)

277. cecum [SĒ-kŭm] {ciego}

278. celi(o)

279. cheeks {carrillos}

280. cheilitis [kī-LĪ-tĭs] {queilitis}

281. cheiloplasty [KĪ-lō-plăs-tē]

282. chol(e), cholo

283. cholangi(o)

284. cholangiography [kō-lăn-jē-ŎG-ră-fē]

285. cholangitis [kō-lăn-JĪ-tĭs] {colangitis}

286. cholecyst(o)

287. cholecystectomy [KŌ-lē-sĭs-TĔK-tō-mē]

288. cholecystitis [KŌ-lē-sĭs-TĪ-tĭs] {colecistitis}

289. cholecystography [kō-lē-sĭs-TŎG-ră-fē] {colecistografía}

290. choledoch(o)

291. choledocholithotomy [kō-LĔD-ō-kō-lĭ-THŎT-ō-mē]

292. cholelithiasis [KŌ-lē-lĭ-THĪ-ă-sĭs]

293. cholelithotomy [KŌ-lē-lĭ-THŎT-ō-mē]

294. cholelithotripsy [kō-lē-LĪTH-ō-trĭp-sē]

295. chyme [kīm] {quimo}

296. cirrhosis [sĭr-RŌ-sĭs] {cirrosis}

297. col(o), colon(o)

298. colectomy [kō-LĔK-tō-mē] {colectomía}

299. colic [KŎL-ĭk] {cólico}

300. colitis [kō-LĪ-tĭs] {colitis}

301. colon [KŌ-lŏn] {colon}

302. colonoscopy [kō-lŏn-ŎS-kō-pē] {colonoscopia}

303. colostomy [kō-LŎS-tō-mē] {colostomía}

304. constipation [kŏn-stĭ-PĀ-shŭn] {constipación}

305. Crohn's [krōnz] disease

306. defecation [dĕ-fĕ-KĀ-shŭn] {defecación}

307. deglutition [dē-glū-TĬSH-ŭn] {deglución}

308. diarrhea [dĭ-ā-RĒ-ă] {diarrea}

309. digestion [dĭ-JĔS-chŭn] {digestión}

310. diverticula [dĭ-vĕr-TĬK-yū-lă]

311. diverticulectomy [dĭ-vĕr-tĭk-ū-LĔK-tō-mē]

312. diverticulitis [DĪ-vĕr-tĭk-yū-LĪ-tĭs] {diverticulitis}

313. diverticulosis [DĪ-vĕr-tĭk-yū-LŌ-sĭs] {diverticulosis}

314. duoden(o)

315. duodenal [DŪ-ō-DĒ-năl] ulcer

316. duodenum [dū-ō-DĒ-nŭm] {duodeno}

317. dysentery [DĬS-ĕn-tĕr-ē] {disentería}

318. dyspepsia [dĭs-PĔP-sē-ă] {dyspepsia}

319. dysphagia [dĭs-FĀ-jē-ă] {disfagia}

320. elimination [ē-lĭm-ĭ-NĀ-shŭn]

321. emesis [ĕ-MĒ-sĭs] {emesis}

322. emulsification [ĕ-MŬL-sĭ-fĭ-KĀ-shŭn]

323. enter(o)

324. enteritis [ĕn-tĕr-Ī-tĭs] {enteritis}

325. enzyme [ĔN-zīm] {enzima}

326. epiglottis [ĕp-ĭ-GLŎ-tĭs] {epiglotis}

327. eructation [ē-rŭk-TĀ-shŭn] {eructación}

328. esophag(o)

329. esophagitis [ĕ-sŏf-ă-JĪ-tĭs] {esofagitis}

330. esophagoplasty [ĕ-SŎF-ă-gō-plăs-tē] {esofagoplastia}

331. esophagoscopy [ĕ-sŏf-ă-GŎS-kō-pē] {esofagoscopia}

332. esophagus [ĕ-SŎF-ă-gŭs] {esófago}

333. fatty acid

334. feces [FĒ-sēz] {heces}

335. fistula [FĬS-tyū-lă] {fistula}

336. flatulence [FLĂT-yū-lĕns] {flatulencia}

337. flatus [FLĂ-tŭs] {flato}

338. frenulum [FRĔN-yū-lŭm] {frenillo}

339. fundus [FŬN-dŭs] {fondo}

340. gallbladder [GĂWL-blăd-ĕr] {vesícula biliar}

341. gallstone {cálculo biliar}

342. gastrectomy [găs-TRĔK-tŏ-mē] {gastrectomía}

343. gastric bypass

344. gastric resection

345. gastritis [găs-TRĪ-tĭs] {gastritis}

346. gastr(o)

347. gastroenteritis [GĂS-trō-ĕn-tĕr-Ī-tĭs] {gastroenteritis}

348. gastroscopy [găs-TRŎS-kō-pē] {gastroscopia}

349. gloss(o)

350. glossectomy [glŏ-SĔK-tō-mē]

351. glossitis [glŏ-SĪ-tĭs] {glositis}

352. glossorrhaphy [glō-SŌR-ă-fē]

353. gluc(o)

354. glucose [GLŪ-kōs] {glucosa}

355. glyc(o)

356. glycogen(o)

357. glycogen [GLĪ-kō-jĕn] {glucógeno}

358. gums [gŭmz] {encía}

359. halitosis [hăl-ĭ-TŌ-sĭs] {halitosis}

360. hard palate [PĂL-ăt]

361. hematemesis [hē-mă-TĔM-ē-sĭs] {hematemesis}

362. hematochezia [HĒ-mă-tō-KĒ-zhē-ă]

363. hemorrhoidectomy [HĔM-ō-rŏy-DĔK-tō-mē] {hemorroidectomía}

364. hemorrhoids [HĔM-ō-rŏydz] {hemorroides}

365. hepat(o)

366. hepatic lobectomy [hĕ-PĂT-ĭk lō-BĔK-tō-mē]

367. hepatitis [hĕp-ă-TĪ-tĭs] {hepatitis}

368. hepatomegaly [HĔP-ă-tō-MĔG-ă-lē] {hepatomegalia}

369. hepatopathy [hĕp-ă-TŎP-ă-thē] {hepatopatía}

370. hiatal hernia [hĭ-Ā-tăl HĔR-nē-ă]

371. hyperbilirubinemia [HĪ-pĕr-BĬL-ĭ-rū-bĭ-NĒ-mē-ă]

372. icterus [ĬK-tĕr-ŭs] {icterus}

373. ile(o)

374. ileitis [ĬL-ē-Ī-tĭs] {ileitis}

375. ileostomy [ĬL-ē-ŎS-tō-mē] {ileostomía}

376. ileum [ĬL-ē-ŭm] {íleon}

377. ileus [ĬL-ē-ŭs] {íleo}

378. intussusception [ĬN-tŭs-sŭ-SĔP-shŭn]

379. jaundice [JĂWN-dĭs] {ictericia}

380. jejun(o)

381. jejunum [jĕ-JŪ-nŭm] {yeyuno}

382. labi(o)

383. large intestine

384. laxative [LĂX-ă-tĭv]

385. lingu(o)

386. lingual tonsils [LĬNG-gwăl TŎN-sĭls]

387. lipase [LĬP-ās] {lipasa}

388. lips {labio}

389. liver [LĬV-ĕr] {hígado}

390. liver biopsy

391. mastication [măs-tĭ-KĀ-shŭn] {masticación}

392. melena [mĕ-LĒ-nă] {melena}

393. mesentery [MĔS-ĕn-tĕr-ē, MĒZ-ĕn-tĕr-ē] {mesenterio}

394. mouth {boca}

395. nausea [NĂW-zhē-ă] {náusea}

396. obesity [ō-BĒS-ĭ-tē] {obesidad}

397. or(o)

398. palatine [PĂL-ă-tĭn] tonsils

399. pancreas [PĂN-krē-ăs] {páncreas}

400. pancreat(o)

401. pancreatectomy [PĂN-krē-ă-TĔK-tō-mē] {pancreatectomía}

402. pancreatitis [PĂN-krē-ă-TĪ-tĭs] {pancreatitis}

403. papilla (pl., papillae) [pă-PĬL-ă (-ē)] {papilas}

404. paracentesis [PĂR-ă-sĕn-TĒ-sĭs]

405. parotitis, parotiditis [păr-ō-TĪ-tĭs, pă-rŏt-ĭ-DĪ-tĭs]

406. pepsin [PĔP-sĭn] {pepsina}

407. peptic ulcer

408. peristalsis [pĕr-ĭ-STĂL-sĭs] {peristaltismo}

409. periton(eo)

410. peritoneoscopy [PĔR-ĭ-tō-nē-ŎS-kō-pē] {peritoneoscopia}

411. peritonitis [PĔR-ĭ-tō-NĪ-tĭs] {peritonitis}

412. pharyng(o)

413. pharynx [FĂR-ĭngks] {faringe}

414. polypectomy [pŏl-ĭ-PĔK-tō-mē] {polipectomía}

415. polyposis [PŎL-ĭ-PŌ-sĭs] {poliposis}

416. proct(o)

417. proctitis [prŏk-TĪ-tĭs] {proctitis}

418. proctoplasty [PRŎK-tō-plăs-tē]

419. proctoscopy [prŏk-TŎS-kō-pē]

420. pylor(o)

421. pylorus [pī-LŌR-ŭs] {píloro}

422. rect(o)

423. rectum [RĔK-tŭm] {recto}

424. reflux [RĒ-flŭks] {reflujo}

425. regurgitation [rē-GŬR-jĭ-TĀ-shŭn] {regurgitación}

426. rugae [RŪ-gē] {rugae}

427. saliva [să-LĪ-vă] {saliva}

428. salivary [SĂL-ĭ-vār-ē] glands

429. sial(o)

430. sialaden(o)

431. sialoadenitis [SĪ-ă-lō-ăd-ĕ-NĪ-tĭs]

432. sigmoid(o)

433. sigmoid [SĬG-mŏyd] colon

434. sigmoidoscopy [SĬG-mŏy-DŎS-kō-pē]

435. small intestine

436. soft palate [PĂL-ăt]

437. steat(o)

438. steatorrhea [STĒ-ă-tō-RĒ-ă] {esteatorrea}

439. stomat(o)

440. stomach [STŎM-ăk] {estómago}

441. stool [stūl] {heces}

442. throat [thrōwt] {garganta}

443. tongue [tŭng] {lengua}

444. ulcerative colitis [ŬL-sĕr-ă-tĭv kō-LĪ-tĭs]

445. uvula [YŪ-vyū-lă] {uvula}

446. villus (pl., villi) [VĬL-ŭs (-ī)] {vellosidad}

447. volvulus [VŎL-vyū-lŭs] {vólvulo}

Abbreviations

Write the full meaning for each abbreviation.

448. ALT, AT

449. AST

450. BE

451. BM

452. EGD

453. ERCP

454. GERD

455. GI

456. IBD

457. IBS

458. NG

459. NPO

460. SGOT

461. SGPT

462. TPN

463. UGI(S)

Answers to Chapter Exercises

1. a. stomach; b. small intestine; c. large intestine; d. rectum; e. liver
2. papillae
3. frenulum
4. C
5. chyme
6. C
7. C
8. C
10. lipase
11. C
12. peristalsis
13. cardiac region, fundus, body, pylorus
14. duodenum, jejunum, ileum
15. cecum, colon, sigmoid colon, rectum
16. small
17. hepatic portal system
18. amylase, lipase
19. emulsification
20. Burning chest pains may also be a sign of a heart attack.
21. Esophagus and stomach, because the burning sensation is probably related to backflow from the stomach to the esophagus.
21. Many diseases are either directly hereditary or may be the result of a hereditary tendency. Early detection may enable better treatment.
22. gastritis and hepatitis
23. gastrectomy
24. esophagitis
25. rectocele
26. duodenal
27. choledochectomy
28. pancreatitis
29. rectodynia, rectalgia
30. colonoscopy
31. hepatomegaly
32. gastrorrhaphy
33. proctologist
34. cholecystitis
35. hepatoma
36. pyloro, duoden, of the pylorus and duodenum
37. an-, around the anus
38. entero, colo-, opening between the small intestine and colon

39. ileo-, cec-, of the ileum and cecum
40. lingu-, under the tongue
40. append(o)-, appendix + -ectomy, surgical removal
41. cec(o)-, cecum + -stomy, surgically created opening
42. enter(o), intestines + myc(o), fungus + -osis abnormal condition of
43. gastr(o), stomach + col(o), colon + -stomy, surgically created opening
44. bucc(o)-, cheek + gingivo-, gums, + -al, pertaining to
45. cholecyst(o)-, gallbladder + -it is, inflammation
46. labi(o), lip + dent(o), teeth + -al, pertaining to
47. appendic(o)-, appendix + -lith, stone
48. hepat(o), liver + -megaly, enlargement of
49. gastr(o), stomach + enter(o), intestines + -logy, study or practice of
50. esophag(o), esophagus + gastr(o), stomach + duoden(o), duodenum + -scopy, use of an instrument for observing
51. proct(o), rectum + -itis, inflammation
52. or(o), mouth + -pharynx, throat
53. celi(o), abdomen + -ac, pertaining to
54. pancreat(o), pancreas + -lysis, destruction of
55. bili-, bile + -uria, urine
56. enter(o), intestines + -ectasis, expanding, dilating
57. ilei(o), ileum + -pexy, surgical fixation of
58. hepat(o), liver + tox(o), toxic, poison + -ic, pertaining to
59. periton(eo), peritoneum + -itis, inflammation of the
60. pharyng(o), pharynx, throat + -itis, inflammation of
61. gastroscopy
62. biopsies for cancer, blood tests for liver function

63. g
64. h
65. a
66. c
67. i
68. d
69. b
70. e
71. j
72. f
73. colitis, colon cancer, or other colon disorders
74. bland diet, avoiding alcohol and caffeine
75. d
76. e
77. h
78. j
79. b
80. c
81. i
82. f
83. g
84. a
85. anorexia
86. irritable bowel disease
87. cholecystitis
88. constipation
89. gastroesophageal reflux
90. dyspepsia
91. C
92. diverticula
93. hematochezia
94. inguinal hernia
95. ileitis
96. C
97. cirrhosis
98. hiatal hernia
99. C
100. flatulence
101. colectomy
102. At least until reconstructive surgery is done, an alternative waste excretion site will be needed.
103. hepatic lobectomy
104. gastric resection
105. ileostomy, colostomy
106. cholelithotripsy
107. abdominocentesis or paracentesis
108. A diet high in roughage may eliminate constipation.

109. antacid
110. f
111. e
112. c
113. b
114. a
115. d
116. to check for cancer
117. There were ulcerations.
118. bucc(o), cheek + -al, pertaining to
119. cec(o)-, cecum + -tomy, incision into
120. cec(o)-, cecum + -pexy, surgical attachment
121. cec(o)-, cecum + -al, pertaining to
122. celi(o)-, abdomen + -ac pertaining to
123. celi(o), abdomen + -tomy, incision into
124. celi(o), abdomen + -scopy, use of an instrument for observing
125. celi(o)-, abdomen + -centesis, puncture
126. chol(e)-, abdomen + -lith, stone
127. chol(e)-, bile + -emesis, vomiting
128. chol(e)-, bile + lith(o)-, stone + -tomy, incision into
129. chol(e)-, bile + -poiesis, formation of
130. chol(e)-, bile + -stasis, stopping (of the flow of)
131. chol(e)-, bile + litho, stone + -tripsy, surgical crushing
132. cholangi(o), bile vessel or duct + carcin(o), cancer + -oma, tumor
133. cholangi(o), bile vessel or duct + -ectasis, dilation of the
134. cholangi(o), bile vessel or duct + -stomy, opening into
135. cholangi(o), bile vessel or duct + -gram, a record of
136. cholangi(o), bile vessel or duct + -graphy, process of recording
137. cholangi(o), bile vessel or duct + -oma, tumor
138. cholangi(o), bile vessel or duct + pancreat(o), pancreas + -graphy, process of recording

139. cholangi(o), bile vessel or duct + -scopy, instrument used for observing
140. cholecyst(o)-, gallbladder + -ectomy, removal
141. chol(e)-,gall + -cyst, bladder
142. cholecyst(o)-, gallbladder + col(o), colon + -stomy, surgically created opening
143. cholecyst(o)-, gallbladder + duoden(o), duodenum + -ostomy, surgically created opening
144. cholecyst(o)-, gallbladder + -pexy, surgical attachment
145. cholecyst(o)-, gallbladder + -gram, arecord
146. cholecyst(o)-, gallbladder + -rrhaphy, surgical suturing
147. cholecyst(o)-, gallbladder + son(o), sound + -graphy, process of recording
148. cholecyst(o)-, gallbladder + -stomy, surgically created opening
149. cholecyst(o)-, gallbladder + -tomy, incision into
150. choledoch(o), common bile duct + lith(o), stone(s) + -iasis, pathological condition or state
151. col(o), colon + -itis, inflammation
152. col(o), colon + rect(o), rectum + -itis, inflammation
153. col(o), colon + -stomy, surgically created opening
154. duoden(o), duodenum + -ectomy, surgical removal
155. enter(o), intestines + -itis, inflammation
156. enter(o), intestines + col(o), colon + -itis, inflammation
157. esophag(o), esophagus + -cele, herniation of
158. gastr(o), stomach + col(o), colon + -itis, inflammation
159. gastr(o), stomach + enter(o), intestines + -itis, inflammation
160. gloss(o), tongue + -itis, inflammation of
161. hepat(o), liver + -scopy, use of an instrument for observing
162. ilei(o), ileum + -stomy, surgically created opening

163. jejun(o), jejunum + -ectomy, removal of
164. labi(o), lip + gingiv(o), gums + -al, pertaining to
165. pancreat(o), pancreas + -pathy, disease of the
166. pharyng(o), pharynx, throat + -ectomy, surgical removal of
167. colostomy
168. anastomosis
169. gastric resection
170. GERD
171. peritalsis
172. stomatomycosis
173. steatohepatitis
174. sialism
175. rectoabdominal
176. hepatopexy
177. hepatocele
178. gastrostomy
179. gastroenteroplasty
180. esophagotomy
181. enteric
182. duodenoscopy
183. enteropathy
184. glycorrhea
185. enterology
186. enteropexy
187. ileocecal
188. gastrolith
189. hepatography
190. choledochorrhaphy
191. cholecystolithiasis
192. cholangilfibrosis
193. colitis
194. biligenesis
195. choledochitis
196. colorrhagia
197. cholecystolithiasis
198. cholecystopathy
199. cholangioectasis
200. i
201. d
202. e
203. s
204. f
205. g
206. j
207. r
208. a
209. b
210. k
211. p
212. l
213. q

214. c
215. t
216. m
217. n
218. h
219. o
220. T
221. T
222. F
223. T

224. T
225. F
226. F
227. F
228. T
229. F
230. rectoscope
231. C
232. colopexy
233. C

234. enzyme
235. mastication
236. C
237. antidiarrheal
238. emesis
239. rugae
240–463. Answers are available in the vocabulary reviews in this chapter.

CHAPTER 15

The Endocrine System

▶ ENDOCRINOLOGIST

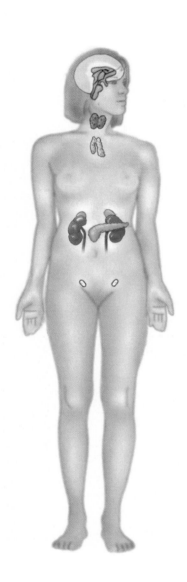

After studying this chapter, you will be able to:

15.1 Name the parts of the endocrine system and discuss the function of each part

15.2 Define combining forms used in building words that relate to the endocrine system

15.3 Identify the meaning of related abbreviations

15.4 Name the common diagnoses, clinical procedures, and laboratory tests used in treating disorders of the endocrine system

15.6 List and define the major pathological conditions of the endocrine system

15.7 Define surgical terms related to the endocrine system

15.8 Recognize common pharmacological agents used in treating disorders of the endocrine system

Structure and Function

The endocrine system is a group of glands that act as the body's master regulator (Figure 15-1a). It regulates many bodily functions as diagrammed in Figure 15-1b. It helps to maintain homeostasis by regulating the production of chemicals that affect most functions of the body. It secretes substances that aid the nervous system in reacting to stress, and it is an important regulator of growth and development. The endocrine system is made up of various **glands** and other tissue that secrete **hormones,** specialized chemicals, into the bloodstream to be circulated throughout the body. The hormones are effective only in specific **target cells,** cells that have **receptors** that recognize a compatible hormone. A group of such cells forms *target tissue.* Minute amounts of hormones can initiate a strong reaction in some target cells.

Unlike **exocrine glands,** which secrete substances into ducts directed toward a specific location, **endocrine glands** secrete hormones into the bloodstream and are also known as **ductless glands.** Some endocrine glands are also exocrine glands. For example, as an endocrine gland, the pancreas secretes insulin, and as an exocrine gland, it releases digestive juices through ducts to the small intestine.

The hormones that are secreted by the endocrine glands go directly into *intercellular* spaces. From there, the hormones diffuse directly into the blood and are carried throughout the body. Each hormone may then bind to a cell that has specific receptors for that hormone, triggering a reaction in the cell. Such a cell is called a *target organ cell.* Hormones are the main regulators of

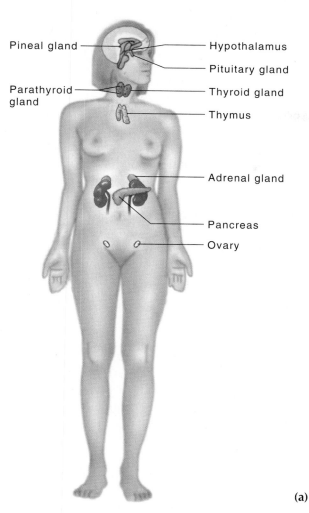

Pineal gland — Hypothalamus

— Pituitary gland

Parathyroid gland — Thyroid gland

— Thymus

— Adrenal gland

— Pancreas

— Ovary

(a)

FIGURE 15-1 **(a)** The endocrine system secretes hormones that affect all parts of the body. **(b)** The bodily functions affected by the endocrine hormones.

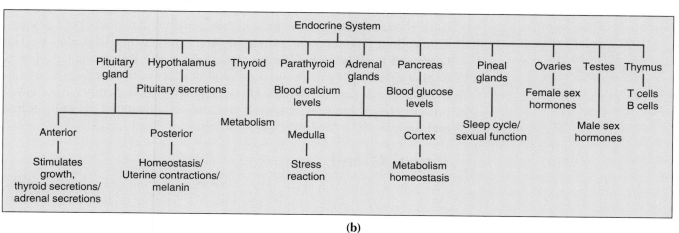

(b)

metabolism growth and development, reproduction, and many other body activities. Hormones make the difference between normalcy and many kinds of abnormalities such as dwarfism, gigantism, and sterility. They are important not only for the healthy survival of each one of us but also for the survival of the human species. Each type of hormone is transported differently throughout the body according to its chemical properties. Hormone release is triggered

To see pictures of endocrine glands, go to a special Web site run by the University of Delaware (http://www.udel.edu/Biology/Wags/histopage/colorpage/cen/cen.htm). Note: Use uppercase letters where indicated.

by various factors including age and various diseases of the endocrine glands. Tumors or other abnormalities frequently cause a gland to secrete too much or too little hormone. Production of too much hormone by a diseased gland is called *hypersecretion*. If too little hormone is produced, the condition is called *hyposecretion*. Hormones are removed from the bloodstream by kidney functions (which is why urine can be tested for trace hormones).

Prostaglandins (PGs) or tissue hormones are important and extremely powerful substances found in a wide variety of tissues. They play an important role in communication and the control of many body functions but do not meet the definition of a typical hormone. The term *tissue hormone* is appropriate because in many instances a prostaglandin is produced in a tissue and then travels only a short distance to act on cells within that tissue. Typical hormones influence and control activities of widely separated organs; typical prostaglandins influence activities of closely neighboring cells. The prostaglandins in the body are divided into several groups, although the best known include *prostaglandin A (PGA)*, *prostaglandin E (PGE)*, and *prostaglandin F (PGF)*. They have profound effects on many body functions. They influence respiration, blood pressure, the reproductive systems, and gastrointestinal secretions.

Hypothalamus

The **hypothalamus,** located in the brain superior to the pituitary gland, is a part of the nervous system that also serves as an endocrine gland because it analyzes the body's condition and directs the release of hormones that regulate pituitary hormones. The two hormones produced by the hypothalamus are ADH (antidiuretic hormone) and oxytocin. These hormones are then released by the pituitary gland. In addition to ADH and oxytocin, the hypothalamus also produces substances called *releasing hormones* (allowing the secretion of other hormones to take place) or *inhibiting hormones* (preventing the secretion of other hormones). These substances are produced in the hypothalamus and then travel directly through a specialized blood capillary system to the anterior section of the pituitary gland, where they cause the release of anterior pituitary hormones or, in a number of instances, inhibit their production and their release into the general circulation. The combined nervous and endocrine functions of the hypothalamus allow it to play a dominant role in the regulation of many body functions related to homeostasis. Examples include the regulation of body temperature, blood pressure, heartbeat, metabolism of fats and carbohydrates, appetite, thirst, and sugar levels in the blood.

Pineal Gland

The **pineal gland** is a small, pine-cone shaped gland near the roof of the third ventricle of the brain. It produces a number of hormones in very small quantities, with **melatonin** being the most significant. Melatonin is a hormone that inhibits the hormones that affect the ovaries, and it is thought to be involved in regulating the onset of puberty and the menstrual cycle in women. Because the pineal gland receives and responds to sensory information from the optic nerves, it is sometimes called the *third eye*. The pineal gland uses information regarding changing light levels to adjust its output of melatonin; melatonin levels increase during the night and decrease during the day. This is why the pineal gland is also believed to affect sleep.

Pituitary Gland

The **pituitary gland,** is a small but mighty structure. Although no larger than a pea, it is really two endocrine glands. One is called the *anterior pituitary gland* or **adenohypophysis,** and the other is called the *posterior pituitary gland* or **neurohypophysis.** Differences between the two glands are suggested by their names—*adeno-* means "gland," and *neuro-* means "nervous." The adenohypophysis has the structure of an endocrine gland, where as the neurohypophysis has the structure of nervous tissue. The hormones secreted from these two glands serve very different functions from each other. The pituitary gland is located deep in the cranial cavity at the base of the brain in an area called the *sella turcica.* The protected location of this dual gland suggests its importance to the functioning of the human body. A stemlike structure, the *pituitary stalk,* attaches the gland to the undersurface of the brain. More specifically, the stalk attaches the pituitary body to the hypothalamus. The pituitary is considered the body's master gland regulating or aiding in the secretion of essential hormones. Table 15-1 describes the functions of all parts of the endocrine system.

Thyroid Gland

The **thyroid gland** lies in the neck just below the larynx and consists of a left lobe and a right lobe sitting on either side of the trachea. The two lobes are connected by the **isthmus,** a narrow strip of tissue on the ventral surface of the trachea. Above the thyroid gland sits the *thyroid cartilage,* a large piece of cartilage that covers the larynx and produces the protrusion on the neck known as the **Adam's apple.** The thyroid gland secretes two thyroid hormones, **thyroxine** or **T4** and **triiodothyronine** or **T3.** It also secretes the hormone calcitonin. Of the two thyroid hormones, T4 is the more abundant; however, T3 is the more potent and is considered by physiologists to be the principal thyroid hormone. Thyroid secretions control **metabolism** (the chemical changes in cells that provide energy for vital processes and activities and through which new material is assimilated) and blood calcium concentrations. Of the thyroid hormones, T_4

MORE ABOUT . . .

Biological Rhythms

All living things have biological cycles determined by nature. Humans are considered to have three basic biological rhythms or *biorhythms*—*ultradian, infradian,* and *circadian.* Ultradian rhythms are those cycles (heartbeat, respiration) that are shorter than 24 hours. Infradian rhythms are those cycles (menstrual, ovulation) that are longer than 24 hours. Circadian rhythms occur in the 24-hour sleep-wake periods. Most of these cycles are affected by two things—factors outside the body and factors inside the body. Factors outside the body can include almost any environmental changes, such as light and dark, weather, physical activity, stress, and so on. Factors inside the body are affected mostly by hormones released from the endocrine system. People with rhythm disorders (like insomnia) are sometimes treated with hormone supplements. In addition, some health care practitioners believe that understanding and regulating the body's biorhythms may be a key to maintaining health. There are many Internet sites that promote personal software for mapping your own biorhythms. Many of these are not based on scientific understanding of body rhythms.

TABLE 15-1 Endocrine Glands, Their Secretions, and Their Functions

Endocrine Gland or Tissue	Hormone	Function
hypothalamus	pituitary-regulating hormones	either stimulate or inhibit pituitary secretions
neurohypophysis (pituitary gland—posterior)	**antidiuretic hormone (ADH), vasopressin** oxytocin	increase water reabsorption
adenohypophysis (pituitary gland—anterior)	**growth hormone (GH), somatotrophic hormone (STH)**	stimulate bone and muscle growth; regulate some metabolic functions, such as the rate that cells utilize carbohydrates and fats
	thyroid-stimulating hormone (TSH) adrenocorticotropic hormone (ACTH)	stimulates thyroid gland to secrete hormones stimulates secretion of adrenal cortex hormones
	follicle-stimulating hormone (FSH), luteinizing hormone (LH)	stimulate development of ova and production of female hormones; stimulates maturing of ova; secretion of estrogen, triggers ovulation; stimulates the production of melanin; in males, stimulates the secretion of testosterone; in the male stimulate testes to grow and secrete sperm
	prolactin	stimulates breast development and milk production stimulates uterine contractions and lactation
	melanocyte-stimulating hormone (MSH)	stimulates the production of melanin
thyroid	thyroxine (T4); triiodothyronine (T3) calcitonin	regulates metabolism; stimulates growth lowers blood calcium as necessary to maintain homeostasis
parathyroid	**parathormone, parathyroid hormone (PTH)**	increase blood calcium as necessary to maintain homeostasis
adrenal medulla	**epinephrine (adrenaline), norepinephrine** (*noradrenaline*)	work with the sympathetic nervous system to react to stress
adrenal cortex	**glucocorticoids (cortisol, corticosteroids,** *corticosterone*), **mineralocorticoids (aldosterone),** gonadocorticoids (androgens)	affect metabolism, growth, and aid in electrolyte and fluid balances
pancreas (in islets of Langerhans)	insulin, glucagon	maintain homeostasis in blood glucose concentration
pineal gland	melatonin	affects sexual functions and wake-sleep cycles; aids in developing skin pigment
ovaries	estrogen (estradiol, the most powerful estrogen), progesterone	promote development of female sex characteristics, menstrual cycle, reproductive functions
testes	androgen, testosterone	promote development of male sex characteristics, sperm production; also stimulate female sex drive
thymus gland	thymosin, thymic humoral factor (THF), factor thymic serum (FTS)	aid in development of T cells and some B cells; function not well understood

contains four atoms of iodine, and one molecule of T_3, as its name suggests, contains three iodine atoms. For T_4 to be produced in adequate amounts, the diet must contain sufficient iodine. Most endocrine glands do not store their hormones but secrete them directly into the blood as they are produced. The thyroid gland is different in that it stores considerable amounts of the thyroid hormones in the form of a material that is stored in the follicles of the gland, and when the thyroid hormones are needed, they are released directly into the blood. T4 and T3 influence every one of the trillions of cells in the human body. They make the cells speed up their release of energy from foods and even normal mental and physical growth and development is dependant on normal thyroid functioning. The third thyroid hormone, **calcitonin,** is secreted from the outside surface of thyroid cells and it decreases the concentration of calcium in the blood by first acting on bone to inhibit calcium breakdown there. It is a hormone that helps maintain homeostasis of blood calcium by preventing a harmful excess of calcium in the blood from accumulating, a condition called *hypercalcemia*.

Parathyroid Glands

The **parathyroid glands** are four oval-shaped glands located on the dorsal (back) side of the thyroid gland. The parathyroids help regulate calcium and phosphate levels, two elements also necessary to maintain homeostasis. The parathyroid glands secrete **parathyroid hormone (PTH).** Parathyroid hormone increases the concentration of calcium in the blood, the opposite effect of the thyroid gland's calcitonin. This is a matter of life-and-death importance because our cells are extremely sensitive to changing amounts of blood calcium. For example, if there is too much blood calcium, brain cells and heart cells soon do not function normally; a person becomes mentally disturbed and the heart may even stop. However, with too little blood calcium, nerve cells become overactive, sometimes to such a degree that they overstimulate the production of electrical impulses to the muscles causing the muscles to go into spasms.

Thymus Gland

The **thymus gland** is considered an endocrine gland because it secretes a hormone and is ductless; however, it is also an essential part of the immune system. It is located in the mediastinum (behind the sternum and between the two lungs), and in infants it may extend up into the neck as far as the lower edge of the thyroid gland. It secretes the hormone *thymosin*, which causes the production of certain white blood cells called T lymphocytes. These T cells protect the body against foreign microorganisms, thus helping to fight infections. The thymus gland is extremely important to the development of an immune response. (Chapter 13 discusses the immune system.)

Adrenal Glands

The **adrenal glands** (or **suprarenal glands**) are a pair of glands. Each of the glands sits atop a kidney. Each gland consists of two parts—the **adrenal cortex** (the outer portion) and the **adrenal medulla** (the inner portion). The adrenal cortex makes up the bulk of the adrenal gland. Its cells are organized into three layers, each secreting and essential hormone. Hormones secreted from the adrenal cortex include *aldosterone*, which regulates sodium reabsorption and potassium excretion by the kidneys; *cortisol*, also known as *hydrocortisone*, which helps the body during stressful situations and helps maintain the proper glucose concentration in the blood between meals as well as helps reduce the inflammatory response causing swelling; and *androgens*, sex hormones which stimulate the development of male sexual characteristics and in adult women, stimulate the female sex drive.

The **adrenal medulla,** or inner portion of the adrenal gland, secretes a class of hormones called **catecholamines,** specifically *epinephrine* and *norepinephrine*. These hormones help the body resist stress. They prolong and intensify changes in body function brought about by the stimulation of the sympathetic subdivision of the autonomic nervous system. The adrenal glands are **sympathomimetic,** imitative of the sympathetic nervous system. In Chapter 8, The Nervous System, a unique reaction called the *"fight or flight"* response is discussed.

Pancreas

The **pancreas** has a dual role in that it is part of the digestive system where its cells produce digestive enzymes known as *pancreatic juice,* and it is also part of the endocrine system where its *pancreatic islets* (also known as the *islets of Langerhans*) produce the hormones **insulin** and **glucagon.** These hormones help in maintaining a proper level of blood glucose. Within the pancreas, the **islets of Langerhans,** specialized hormone-producing cells, secrete insulin to lower blood sugar when blood sugar levels are high and glucagon to raise blood sugar levels when they are low. Insulin is produced by **beta cells** in the islets of Langerhans, and glucagon is produced by **alpha cells** in the islets. When blood sugar levels get too high in the body, the beta cells release insulin into the bloodstream. Insulin allows the glucose in the blood to be transformed in the liver into *glycogen,* which is stored animal starch. The glucose is also moved into the muscle cells and adipose tissue. When blood glucose levels fall, such as between meals or during the night, the secretion of insulin decreases. If levels fall too low, alpha cells secrete glucagon which stimulates the liver to convert the stored glycogen into glucose, thus raising blood glucose levels. Figure 15-2 shows the glucagon/glucose production process.

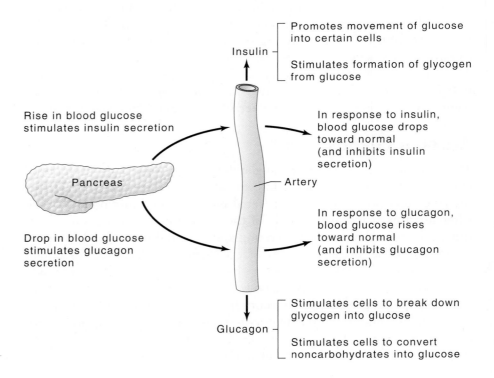

FIGURE 15-2 Glucagon and insulin help to maintain stable blood glucose levels in the body.

The pancreas is both an endocrine and an exocrine gland. The islets of Langerhans serve its endocrine functions, and the remaining cells its exocrine ones (as discussed in the digestive system in Chapter 14).

Ovaries

The **ovaries,** or female gonads, are paired glands about the size of unshelled almonds and are found in the female pelvic region, one on either side of the uterus at the top of each fallopian tube. (Chapter 10 describes the female reproductive system.) These organs produce eggs, or ova, as exocrine glands and as endocrine glands produce the female sex hormones estrogen and progesterone. Estrogen causes the development of the female reproductive structures: the fallopian tubes, uterus, and vagina. It also causes the development of the breasts, fat deposits on the hips and thighs, bone development resulting in broad hips, a higher pitched voice, and onset of the menstrual cycle.

Testes

The **testes (testicles)** or male gonads, are paired oval glands located in the scrotum, a sac on the outside of the male body. Externally, it appears as a single pouch of skin, but is actually separated into two sacs internally by a septum. Each sac contains a single testis. As an exocrine gland, the testes produce spermatozoa, which fertilize ova. As an endocrine gland, the testes produce male sex hormones called **androgens,** the most important of which is testosterone. Testosterone is the "*masculinizing hormone*" and is responsible for the development of the male reproductive structures, and at puberty, the enlargement of the testes and penis. It also promotes external male characteristics such as beard and chest hair growth, deepening of the voice, muscular development, bone growth resulting broad shoulders and narrow hips. It promotes the development of the male sexual drive and aggressiveness. (Chapter 11 describes the male reproductive system.)

VOCABULARY REVIEW

In the previous section you learned terms related to the endocrine system. Before going on to the exercises, review the terms below and refer to the previous section if you have any questions. Pronunciations are provided for certain terms. Sometimes information about where the word came from is included after the term. The etymologies (word histories) are for your information only. You do not need to memorize them.

Term	Meaning
Adam's apple	Protrusion in the neck caused by a fold of thyroid cartilage.
adenohypophysis [ĂD-ĕ-nō-hī-PŎF-ĭ-sĭs] adeno-, gland + hypophysis	Anterior lobe of the pituitary gland.
adrenal cortex [ă-DRĒ-năl KŎR-tĕks]	Outer portion of the adrenal gland; helps control metabolism, inflammations, sodium and potassium retention, and effects of stress.
adrenal gland	One of two glands, each of which is situated on top of each kidney.

Term	Meaning
adrenaline [ă-DRĔ-nă-lĭn]	Epinephrine; secreted by adrenal medulla.
adrenal medulla [mĕ-DŪL-lă]	Inner portion of adrenal glands; releases large quantities of hormones during stress.
adrenocorticotropic [ă-DRĒ-nō-KŌR-tĭ-kō-TRŌ-pĭk] **hormone (ACTH)** adreno-, adrenal glands + cortico(steroid) + -tropic, turning	Hormone secreted by anterior pituitary; involved in the control of the adrenal cortex.
aldosterone [ăl-DŎS-tēr-ōn]	Hormone secreted by adrenal cortex; mineralocorticoid.
alpha [ĂL-fă] **cells**	Specialized cells that produce glucagon in the pancreas.
androgen [ĂN-drō-jĕn] andro-, man + -gen, producing	Any male hormone, such as testosterone.
antidiuretic [ĂN-tē-dī-yū-RĔT-ĭk] **hormone (ADH)** anti-, against + diuretic	Posterior pituitary hormone that increases water reabsorption.
beta [BĀ-tă] **cells**	Specialized cells that produce insulin in the pancreas.
calcitonin [kăl-sĕ-TŌ-nĭn] calci-, calcium + Greek *tonos*, a stretching	Hormone secreted by the thyroid gland and other endocrine glands; helps control blood calcium levels.
catecholamines [kăt-ĕ-KŌL-ă-mĕnz]	Hormones, such as epinephrine, released in response to stress.
corticosteroids [KŎR-tĭ-kō-STĒR-ŏydz]	Steroids produced by the adrenal cortex.
cortisol [KŎR-tĭ-sōl]	Hydrocortisone.
ductless gland	Endocrine gland.
electrolyte [ē-LĔK-trō-līt]	Any substance that conducts electricity and is decomposed by it.
endocrine [ĔN-dō-krĭn] **gland** endo-, within + -crine, secreting	Gland that secretes substances into the bloodstream instead of into ducts.
epinephrine [ĔP-ĭ-NĔF-rĭn] epi-, upon + nephr-, kidney + -ine, chemical compound	Hormone released by the adrenal medulla in response to stress; adrenaline.
exocrine [ĔK-sō-krĭn] **gland** exo-, external + -crine	Any gland that releases substances through ducts to a specific location.
follicle-stimulating hormone (FSH)	Hormone released by the anterior pituitary to aid in production of ova and sperm.
gland Latin *glans*, acorn	Any organized mass of tissue secreting or excreting substances.
glucagon [GLŪ-kă-gŏn]	Hormone released by the pancreas to increase blood sugar.
glucocorticoids [glū-kō-KŌR-tĭ-kŏydz] gluco- + corticoid	Hormones released by the adrenal cortex.

Term	Meaning
glycogen [GLĪ-kō-jĕn] glyco-, glycogen + -gen	Converted glucose stored in the liver for future use.
growth hormone (GH)	Hormone released by the anterior pituitary for stimulating growth.
hormone [HŌR-mōn] Greek *hormon*, rousing	Substance secreted by glands and carried in the bloodstream to various parts of the body.
hypophysis [hī-PŎF-ĭ-sĭs] Greek, undergrowth	Pituitary gland.
hypothalamus [HĪ-pō-THĂL-ă-mŭs] hypo-, beneath + thalamus	Gland in the nervous system that releases hormones to aid in regulating pituitary hormones.
inhibiting factor	Substance in a hormone that prevents the secretion of other hormones.
insulin [ĬN-sū-lĭn] Latin *insula*, island	Substance released by the pancreas to lower blood sugar.
islets of Langerhans [LĂN-gĕr-hănz] After Paul Langerhans (1847–1888), German anatomist	Specialized cells in the pancreas that release insulin and glucagon.
isthmus [ĬS-mŭs] Greek *isthmos*, narrow band	Narrow band of tissue connecting the two lobes of the thyroid gland.
luteinizing [LŪ-tē-ĭn-ĪZ-ĭng] **hormone (LH)**	Hormone released to aid in maturation of ova and ovulation in the female; and aids in the secretion of testosterone in males.
melanocyte-stimulating [mĕ-LĂN-ō-sīt, MĔL-ă-nō-sīt] **hormone (MSH)**	Hormone released by the pituitary gland; aids in development of melanin pigment of the skin.
melatonin [mĕl-ă-TŌN-ĭn] Greek *melas*, dark + *tonos*, a stretching	Hormone released by the pineal gland; affects sexual function and sleep patterns.
metabolism [mĕ-TĂB-ō-lĭzm]	The chemical changes in cells that provide energy for vital processes and activities and through which new material is assimilated.
mineralocorticoid [MĬN-ĕr-ăl-ō-KŌR-tĭ-kŏyd] mineral + corticoid, steroid secretion	Steroid secreted by adrenal cortex.
neurohypophysis [NŪR-ō-hī-PŎF-ĭ-sĭs] neuro-, nerve + hypophysis	Posterior lobe of pituitary gland.
norepinephrine [NŌR-ĕp-ĭ-NĔF-rĭn]	Hormone secreted by adrenal medulla.
ovary [Ō-văr-ē] Latin *ovum*, egg	One of two female reproductive glands that secrete hormones in the endocrine system.
oxytocin [ŏk-sĭ-TŌ-sĭn] Greek *oxytokos*, swift birth	Hormone released by the posterior pituitary gland to aid in uterine contractions and lactation.
pancreas [PĂN-krē-ăs] Greek *pankreas*, sweetbread	Gland of both the endocrine system (blood sugar control) and the digestive system (as an exocrine gland).

Term	Meaning
parathormone [păr-ă-THŌR-mŏn] **(PTH)** parath(yroid) + (h)ormone	Parathyroid hormone.
parathyroid [păr-ă-THĪ-rŏyd] **gland** para-, adjacent + thyroid	One of four glands located adjacent to the thyroid gland on its dorsal surface that help maintain levels of blood calcium.
parathyroid hormone (PTH)	Hormone released by parathyroid glands to help raise blood calcium levels.
pineal [PĬN-ē-ăl] **gland** Latin *pineus*, relating to pine	Gland located above pituitary gland; secretes melatonin.
pituitary [pĭ-TŪ-ĭ-tār-ē] **gland** Latin *pituita*	Major endocrine gland; secretes hormones essential to metabolic functions.
receptor [rē-SĔP-tōr] Latin, receiver	Part of a target cell with properties compatible with a particular substance (hormone).
releasing factor	Substance in a hormone that allows secretion of other hormones.
somatotrophic [SŌ-mă-tō-TRŌF-ĭk] **hormone (STH)** somato-, sleep + -trophic, nutritional	Hormone secreted by anterior pituitary gland; important in growth and development.
suprarenal [SŪ-pră-RĒ-năl] **gland** supra-, above + renal	Adrenal gland.
sympathomimetic [SĬM-pă-thō-mĭ-MĔT-ĭk] sympath(etic) + Greek *mimikos*, imitating	Mimicking functions of the sympathetic nervous system.
target cell	Cell with receptors that are compatible with specific hormones.
testis (*pl.,* **testes**) [TĔS-tĭs (TĔS-tēz)], **testicle** [TĔS-tĭ-kl] Latin	One of two male organs that secrete hormones in the endocrine system.
thymus [THĪ-mŭs] **gland** Greek *thymos*, sweetbread	Gland that is part of the immune system as well as part of the endocrine system; aids in the maturation of T and B cells.
thyroid [THĪ-rŏyd] **gland** Greek *thyreos*, oblong shield	Gland with two lobes located on either side of the trachea; helps control blood calcium levels and metabolic functions.
thyroid-stimulating hormone (TSH)	Hormone secreted by anterior pituitary gland; stimulates release of thyroid hormones.
thyroxine [thĭ-RŎK-sēn, -sĭn] **(T_4)**	Compound found in or manufactured for thyroid gland; helps regulate metabolism.
triiodothyronine [trī-Ī-ō-dō-THĪ-rō-nēn] **(T_3)**	Thyroid hormone that stimulates growth.
vasopressin [vā-sō-PRĔS-ĭn]	Hormone secreted by pituitary gland; raises blood pressure.

CASE STUDY

Checking the Symptoms

Gail Woods is a 45-year-old woman who has noticed some disturbing symptoms, such as unusual fatigue, since her last checkup. She called her physician, Dr. Tyler, for an appointment. Dr. Tyler examined her and sent her to a lab for several tests.

Critical Thinking

1. Dr. Tyler ordered a urinalysis and blood tests. Why?
2. If Dr. Tyler is able to limit the symptoms to one body system, is he likely to send Gail to a specialist?

STRUCTURE AND FUNCTION EXERCISES

Find a Match

Match each hormone with its function by writing the name of the hormone on the appropriate line.

ADH prolactin insulin aldosterone oxytocin thyroxine testosterone thymosin melatonin epinephrine

3. may affect sleep habits: _____

4. reacts to stress: _____

5. decreases urine output: _____

6. stimulates uterine contractions and lactation: _____

7. helps transport glucose to cells and decreases blood sugar: _____

8. stimulates breast development and lactation: _____

9. affects electrolyte and fluid balances: _____

10. regulates rate of cellular metabolism: _____

11. promotes growth and maintenance of male sex characteristics and sperm production: _____

12. aids in development of the immune system: _____

Check Your Knowledge

For each of the following words, write C if the spelling is correct. If it is not, write the correct spelling.

13. adenohypophysis _____

14. adenal _____

15. hypophisis _____

16. suparenal _____

17. sympathomimetic _____

18. pituatary _____

19. lutinizing _____

20. triiodothyronine _____

CASE STUDY

Getting the Results

Gail's tests came back with abnormally high blood sugar. Her lab results are shown at right:

Critical Thinking

21. Were any other tests abnormal?
22. What body system is the likely origin of Gail's abnormal tests?

John Colter, M.D.
3 Windsor Street
Nome, AK 66660
777-546-7890

Laboratory Report
Grandview Diagnostics
12 Settlers Drive
Nome, AK 66661
777-546-7000

Patient: Gail Woods	Patient ID: 099-00-1200	Date of Birth: 06/10/59
Date Collected: 04/27/XXXX	Time Collected: 16:05	Total Volume: 2000
Date Received: 04/27/XXXX	Date Reported: 10/06/XXXX	

Test	Result	Flag	Reference
Complete Blood Count			
WBC	4.0		3.9-11.1
RBC	4.11		3.80-5.20
HCT	39.7		34.0-47.0
MCV	96.5		80.0-98.0
MCH	32.9		27.1-34.0
MCHC	34.0		32.0-36.0
MPV	8.6		7.5-11.5
NEUTROPHILS %	45.6		38.0-80.0
NEUTROPHILS ABS.	1.82		1.70-8.50
LYMPHOCYTES %	36.1		15.0-49.0
LYMPHOCYTES ABS.	1.44		1.00-3.50
EOSINOPHILS %	4.5		0.0-8.0
EOSINOPHILS ABS.	0.18		0.03-0.55
BASOPHILS %	0.7		0.0-2.0
BASOPHILS ABS.	0.03		0.000-0.185
PLATELET COUNT	229		150-400
Automated Chemistries			
GLUCOSE	275		65-109
UREA NITROGEN	17		6-30
CREATININE (SERUM)	0.6		0.5-1.3
UREA NITROGEN/CREATININE	28		10-29
SODIUM	152		135-145
POTASSIUM	4.4		3.5-5.3
CHLORIDE	106		96-109
CO_2	28		20-31
ANION GAP	6		3-19
CALCIUM	9.8		8.6-10.4
PHOSPHORUS	3.6		2.2-4.6
AST (SGOT)	28		0-30
ALT (SGPT)	19		0-34
BILIRUBIN, TOTAL	0.5		0.2-1.2
PROTEIN, TOTAL	7.8		6.2-8.2
ALBUMIN	4.3		3.5-5.0
GLOBULIN	3.5		2.1-3.8
URIC ACID	2.4		2.0-7.5
CHOLESTEROL	195		120-199
TRIGLYCERIDES	68		40-199
IRON	85		30-150
HDL CHOLESTEROL	73		35-59
CHOLESTEROL/HDL RATIO	3.2		3.2-5.7
LDL, CALCULATED	126		70-129
T3, UPTAKE	32		24-37
T4, TOTAL	6.9		4.5-12.8

Combining Forms and Abbreviations

The lists below include combining forms and abbreviations that relate specifically to the endocrine system. Pronunciations are provided for the examples.

COMBINING FORM	MEANING	EXAMPLE
aden(o)	gland	*adenopathy* [ă-dĕ-NŎP-ă-thē], glandular or lymph node disease
adren(o), adrenal(o)	adrenal glands	*adrenomegaly* [ă-drē-nō-MĔG-ă-lē], enlargement of the adrenal glands
gluc(o)	glucose	*glucogenesis* [glū-kō-JĔN-ĕ-sĭs], production of glucose
glyc(o)	glycogen	*glycolysis* [glī-KŎL-ĭ-sĭs], conversion of glycogen to glucose
gonad(o)	sex glands	*gonadotropin* [gō-NĂD-ō-trō-pĭn], hormone that aids in growth of gonads
pancreat(o)	pancreas	*pancreatitis* [păn-krē-ă-TĪ-tĭs], inflammation of the pancreas
parathyroid(o)	parathyroid	*parathyroidectomy* [pă-ră-thī-rŏy-DĔK-tō-mē], excision of the parathyroid glands
thyr(o), thyroid(o)	thyroid gland	*thyrotoxic* [thī-rō-TŎK-sĭk], having excessive amounts of thyroid hormones

ABBREVIATION	MEANING	ABBREVIATION	MEANING
ACTH	adrenocorticotropic hormone	IDDM	insulin-dependent diabetes mellitus
ADH	antidiuretic hormone	LH	luteinizing hormone
CRH	corticotropin-releasing hormone	MSH	melanocyte-stimulating hormone
DM	diabetes mellitus	NIDDM	noninsulin-dependent diabetes mellitus
OT	oxytoxin	PG	prostaglandins
FSH	follicle-stimulating hormone	PRL	prolactin
GH	growth hormone	PTH	parathyroid hormone, parathormone
GTT	glucose tolerance test	STH	somatotropin hormone
HCG	human chorionic gonadotropin	TSH	thyroid-stimulating hormone

COMBINING FORMS AND ABBREVIATIONS EXERCISES

Build Your Medical Vocabulary

Using the combining forms learned in this chapter, construct five words about the endocrine system that fit the definitions provided.

23. inflammation of a gland: _____

24. disease of the pancreas: _____

25. production of glycogen: _____

26. enlargement of the thyroid gland: _____

27. beneficial thyroid function: _____

Know the Meaning

Write the definitions for the following terms.

28. adrenalectomy: _____

29. pancreatectomy: _____

30. adenoma: _____

31. gonadotropin: _____

32. thyromegaly: _____

Diagnostic, Procedural, and Laboratory Terms

A thorough assessment can help to identify an endocrine disorder. The patient with such a disorder, or disease, commonly reports fatigue, weakness, weight changes, mental status changes, polyuria, polydipsia, and abnormalities of sexual maturity and function. A detailed family history can also help uncover a familial tendency toward endocrine disease. The only endocrine glands that can be physically examined (palpated) are the thyroid gland and testes. In many patients, the thyroid gland isn't palpable. Enlargement or atrophy of these glands can be felt. Severe enlargement can also be seen.

The results of various diagnostic tests can be used to suggest, confirm, or rule out an endocrine disease. Endocrine function can be tested by direct, indirect, and radiographic studies. Direct testing, the most common method of measuring endocrine function, involves measuring the hormone levels in blood or urine. The most often performed tests include those measuring levels of cortisol, PTH, GH, T4 and T3, FSH, LH, oral glucose tolerance testing (GTT), calcium, potassium, phosphorus, glycosolated hemoglobin, and electrolyte studies. A **fasting blood sugar** test and a **glucose tolerance test** are both started after a 10 to 12-hour period where the individual has absolutely nothing by mouth. This includes chewing gum, coffee, cigarettes, bottled water, or even toothpaste. This time of fasting is written by the physician as "**NPO**" meaning, "*non per os*"—Latin for "*nothing by mouth.*" The glucose tolerance test is repeated every hour for 3 to 6 hours, according to the physician's orders, after the patient ingests a glucose solution. Results of this test analyze how efficiently the body handles sugars and carbohydrates and well it is able to balance itself after ingesting these substances. Diabetic patients often check **blood sugar** or **blood glucose** levels several times a day themselves to track fluctuations in blood sugar and/or to determine the correct amount of insulin to take. A **postprandial blood sugar** is a test usually taken 2 hours after a meal to determine whether blood sugar levels can return to normal ranges following a meal. A urine test, also called a urinalysis, can be performed to detect the presence of ketones (proteins) and/or types of sugar in the urine, both of which may indicate diabetes. For people already diagnosed with diabetes, a **glycosylated hemoglobin** (A1c or Hemoglobin A1c) test can track the effectiveness of a patient's insulin treatment by detecting the amount of glucose present on the surface of the blood's red cells after a period of 2–3 months. The lower the levels of glycosolated red cells present, the more balanced the patient's blood sugar levels have been.

Computed tomography scanning (CT), regular x-rays, ultrasounds, or magnetic resonance imaging (MRI) may help locate tumors, lesions, cysts, gland atrophy, or abnormal increased size, bone density or frailty in diagnosing an endocrine disorder, Overall endocrine system functioning is evaluated by using the serum or plasma from human blood. Many hormones and electrolytes are present in serum. Endocrine function can be tested in the plasma by using a **radioactive immunoassay,** a test using radioactive iodine to locate various substances in the plasma such as GH (Growth Hormone). Thyroid functioning can be tested in a **thyroid function test,** a blood test for various hormones secreted by the thyroid. A complete blood count (CBC) is used to analyze the overall composition of the entire blood to include the red cells, white cells, and platelets. A basic metabolic profile/panel (BMP) would report the levels of electrolytes and other chemical compounds found in the blood. A **radioactive iodine uptake** is a measure of how quickly ingested iodine is taken into the thyroid gland. A **thyroid scan** is a test for cancer or other abnormality using radionuclide imaging. In diabetics, an ophthalmologic examination may show diabetic retinopathy, a common eye disease in insulin dependent diabetics.

Vocabulary Review

In the previous section you learned terms related to diagnosis, clinical procedures, and laboratory tests. Before going on to the exercises, review the terms below and refer to the previous section if you have any questions. Pronunciations are provided for certain terms. Sometimes information about where the word came from is included after the term. The etymologies (word histories) are for your information only. You do not need to memorize them.

Term	Meaning
blood sugar, blood glucose	Test for glucose in blood.
fasting blood sugar	Test for glucose in blood following a fast of 12 hours.
glucose tolerance test (GTT)	Blood test for body's ability to metabolize carbohydrates; taken after a 10–12-hour fast, then repeated every hour for 4 to 6 hours after ingestion of a sugar solution.
glycosylated [GLĪ-kŎ-sil-ā-tĕd] hemoglobin A1C	Blood test for an average of glucose levels over the previous 2–3 months.
postprandial [pōst-PRĂN-dē-ăl] blood sugar	Test for glucose in blood, two hours after a meal.

Term	Meaning
radioactive immunoassay (RIA)	Test for measuring hormone levels in plasma; taken after radioactive solution is ingested.
radioactive iodine uptake	Test for how quickly the thyroid gland pulls in ingested iodine.
thyroid function test or study	Test for levels of TSH, T_3, and T_4 in blood plasma to determine thyroid function.
thyroid scan	Imaging test for thyroid abnormalities.
urine sugar	Test for diabetes; determined by presence of sugar in urine.

MORE ABOUT . . .

Diabetes and Diet

For many years, doctors prescribed a high-protein, low-carbohydrate diet for diabetics. In recent years, increased understanding of how food is metabolized by the body has led to changes in diets prescribed for diabetics. Most newly diagnosed diabetics are given a varied diet by a physician or a dietitian that is tailored to their specific needs—current weight, level of diabetes (mild, moderate, severe), and lifestyle. The American Dietetic Association and the American Diabetes Association provide the dietary information on which most diets for diabetics are based. A diabetic's personalized daily diet might include four fruit exchanges, three protein exchanges, three bread exchanges, and seven vegetable exchanges. Many suppliers of processed food, particularly those foods aimed at the health-conscious consumer, now list exchanges as part of their nutrition labels as shown here.

Nutrition Facts
Serving Size 1 cup (246g)
Servings Per Container about 2

Amount Per Serving

Calories 100	Calories from Fat 5
	% Daily Value*
Total Fat 0.5g	1%
Saturated Fat 0g	0%
Cholesterol 0mg	0%
Sodium 430mg	18%
Total Carbohydrate 23g	8%
Dietary Fiber 2g	8%
Sugars 1g	
Protein	4g
Vitamin A 30% • Vitamin C 15%	
Calcium 4% • Iron 6%	

* Percent Daily Values are based on a 2,000 calorie diet

DIETARY EXCHANGES PER SERVING:
1 Bread
1 Vegetable

Diet exchanges are based on Exchange Lists for Meal Planning, © 1989, the American Diabetes Assoc., Inc. and the American Dietetic Assoc.

CASE STUDY

Referring to a Specialist

Dr. Tyler reviewed Gail's symptoms and test results with her. She has lost 12 pounds rapidly over the last couple of months, is feeling abnormally tired, and is unusually thirsty. Dr. Tyler referred her to an endocrinologist.

Critical Thinking

33. What disease does Dr. Tyler think Gail has?

34. What test for blood glucose is taken after a meal?

DIAGNOSTIC, PROCEDURAL, AND LABORATORY TERMS EXERCISES

Match the Test

Match the test with the possible diagnosis. Write D if it is a test for diabetes or T if it is a test for thyroid function.

35. fasting blood sugar _____

36. radioactive iodine uptake _____

37. radioactive immunoassay _____

38. urine sugar _____

39. glucose tolerance test _____

Pathological Terms

Body activities, homeostasis, and the response to stress are controlled by two distinct but interconnected systems: the nervous system and the endocrine system. The nervous system (discussed in Chapter 8) creates an immediate but short-lived response. The endocrine system has a slightly slower onset and a longer duration of action, and uses highly specific and powerful hormones to control the body's response chemically. Certain endocrine glands are stimulated to secrete hormones in response to other hormones and therefore keep the body in balance or homeostasis. Diseases of the endocrine system commonly involve an abnormal increase or decrease in the secretion of hormones. Symptoms of disease vary with the degree of increase or decrease in hormonal secretion and the age of the patient. The remarkable work and importance of hormones is seen in their pathology. Sometimes a minute difference in the amount of hormone can make a huge difference in the seriousness of an illness. Changes in gland size that affect the gland's production and secretion of a hormone often result from trauma to the gland such as infection, surgical procedures, inflammation, and radiation. Most endocrine illnesses are the result of **hypersecretion** (oversecretion) or **hyposecretion** (undersecretion) of one or more hormones. Hypersecretion can be caused by excessive stimulation of a gland by a bacteria, virus, other microorganism or by a tumor affecting an endocrine gland. Diagnosing endocrine disorders requires correctly matching the patient's symptoms with a specific hormone dysfunction and confirming either the overproduction or underproduction of that specific hormone or group of hormones. After the endocrine problem has been identified and diagnosed, treatment is begun to either decrease the amount of hormone being released by subjecting the patient to radiation therapy, surgical removal of the gland, or reduction of the tumor or lesion stimulating the hypersecretion. In the case of hormone deficit or hyposecretion, hormone supplements or medications may be prescribed to stimulate a specific gland to produce and secrete more hormones or surgery may be necessary to remove the inhibiting factor causing the underproduction and secretion of the particular hormone.

Pituitary Disorders

Hyperpituitarism is a chronic, progressive disease caused by the excessive production and secretion of various pituitary hormones, such as human growth hormone (hGH). Excessive hGH produces two very distinct conditions, **acromegaly** and **gigantism. Acromegaly** (chronic hypersecretion of growth hormone (GH) beginning after puberty), causes abnormal overgrowth of the bones in the face, hands, and feet. It is often seen in patients between the ages of 30 and 40. **Gigantism** is caused by the hypersecretion of GH (somatotropin) before puberty and results in a proportional overgrowth of all body tissue. Symptoms usually appear over time and sexual and mental developments are often effected. Some patients may reach heights over 8 feet tall.

Hypopituitarism is a condition caused by a deficiency or complete absence of some, or any of the pituitary hormones, specifically those hormones produced by the anterior pituitary gland. Because the anterior pituitary gland is responsible for secretion of so many essential hormones, the condition may be very complex affecting several different areas of the body. Patients may experience stunted growth, sexual immaturity, and various metabolic problems. A decrease, or absence of pituitary hormones responsible for stimulating the production and secretion of other hormones in the endocrine system, can result in the *atrophy* or dysfunction of other endocrine glands. Hyposecretion of GH may result in a condition called **dwarfism** (Figure 15-3), which is the opposite of gigantism, and which normally occurs in children and results in the child being extremely short but with proportional body structure. The disease may be linked to mental retardation in the patient and other physical defects. Dwarfism may be congenital or the result of a cranial hemorrhage after birth. Head trauma, tumor, or infection may result in the undersecretion of the growth-hormone-releasing-hormone (GH-RH) which is produced by the hypothalamus. The age of the patient, the severity and type of deficiency, and the underlying cause of hypopituitarism will help determine the method of treatment. Treatment may include hormone supplements, including thyroxine, sex hormones, somatropin (hGH) or cortisone; and surgery to remove a tumor if this is the cause of the hormone inhibition.

The therapeutic use of human growth hormone was first shown in 1963. Since that time the number of approved and proposed uses of human growth hormone has grown from one to more than a dozen, and the number of patients being treated with it has increased from a handful to tens of thousands worldwide. The officially approved uses of human growth hormone vary from country to country, but it is commonly used for children with growth hormone deficiency or insufficiency, poor growth due to renal failure, and children born small for gestational age with poor growth past 2 years of age. In adults the approved uses include AIDS-related wasting and growth hormone deficiency (usually due to a pituitary tumor).

In addition to the generally accepted therapeutic uses of human growth hormone, many proposed uses have not been established. Human growth hormone is a potent hormone with a wide variety of effects. The

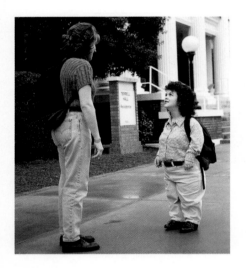

FIGURE 15-3 Dwarfism is a pituitary disorder.

anabolic actions of human growth hormone have made it attractive for people wishing to reverse the effects of ageing and to promote athletic abilities and muscles development. These last two potential uses have received the most attention as abuse of growth hormone. The classic form of "abuse" of human growth hormone are athletes or bodybuilders who use it as a way to gain an unfair advantage over their competitors. No good evidence or scientific research exists showing that human growth hormone actually works safely for this purpose. In addition to the lack of evidence for effectiveness of human growth hormone for these unsupported uses, it causes side effects such as diabetes, carpal tunnel syndrome, fluid retention, joint and muscle pain, and high blood pressure.

In addition to growth problems, hyposecretion of vasopressin or antidiuretic hormone (ADH) causes a condition know as **diabetes insipidus.** This is not the same as **diabetes mellitus** which is often treated with insulin injections but rather a disease caused by decreased levels of ADH by the posterior pituitary gland which results in extremely large amounts of diluted and colorless urine called **polyuria.** The patient will also experience excessive thirst known as **polydipsia** due to the dehydration caused by the polyuria. The disease may be inherited or the result of injury to the hypothalamus or pituitary gland and is more common in men than women. It can be treated with an antidiuretic medication, such as vasopressin nasal sprays, injections, or an oral medication. Hyposecretion of antidiuretic hormone also causes **syndrome of inappropriate ADH (SIADH),** which results in excessive water retention.

Thyroid Disorders

Thyroid diseases may also cause the oversecretion or undersecretion of the primary thyroid hormones, thyroxine (T4) and triiodothyronine (T3). The thyroid gland is the endocrine gland that most often produces disease and a **goiter** is often the first sign of thyroid disease. The term goiter refers to any enlargement of the thyroid gland. Most patients are asymptomatic until they notice a swollen mass appearing under the chin across the area where the thyroid gland is located. As this mass continues to grow, it may begin exerting pressure on the esophagus making the action of swallowing difficult. In extreme cases, the mass may become so large that it even presses on the trachea resulting in dyspnea or shortness of breath. Goiters can be the result of a shortage of iodine in the diet which results in the body not being able to metabolize and use T3 and T4; or inadequate levels of thyroid hormone which causes the anterior pituitary gland to increase secretion of thyrotropin (TSH). The release of TSH stimulates the thyroid gland to produce thyroid hormone but instead the thyroid gland begins to increase in size, thus creating the goiter.

Another hypothyroid condition occurs when the immune system attacks the thyroid gland in the form of an autoimmune disease called *Hashimoto's thyroiditis.* This is a chronic thyroiditis occurring in women eight times more often than men and is the leading cause of goiter and hypothyroidism. In addition to the symptoms of simple goiter, the patient may also develop weight gain, mental sluggishness, and extreme sensitivity to cold. While the true cause of Hashimoto's thyroiditis is unknown, a genetic factor is suspected and autoimmune factors have been documented through the discovery that antibodies appear to destroy thyroid tissue resulting in chronic inflammation of the thyroid gland and the production of scar tissue which enlarges the gland. Treatment for Hashimoto's is lifelong thyroid hormone replacement therapy. When the thyroid gland becomes overactive, causing **hyperthyroidism,** a condition known as **Graves' disease** will develop. Symptoms of Graves' disease are consistent with increased T3 and T4, which cause increased metabolic rate, weight loss, insomnia, sweating, rapid heartbeat and palpitations, nervousness, and excitability. **Exophthalmos,** bulging of the eyes, is also a sign that can occur in some instances of Graves' disease. General hyperactive behavior, loss of hair, and tremors are also seen A sudden exacerbation (flare up) of symptoms may be the first sign of **thyrotoxicosis** also called *"thyroid storm."* This is the result of extremely high levels of thyroid hormone and can be a life threatening situation. Treatment is focused on reducing the amount of thyroid hormone being released and is often accomplished by antithyroid medications. In severe cases, a thyroidectomy or radioactive iodine treatments may be necessary.

Hypothyroidism is a very common condition and refers to any state in which thyroid hormone production is below normal. Some symptoms may take years to develop and be noticed. The underactivity of the thyroid gland, causes sluggishness and slow pulse, often resulting in obesity. Patients may also exhibit cold sensitivity, constipation, dry and flaky skin conditions and extreme fatigue. There are several causes for hypothyroidism with hereditary factors at the top of the list. A simple blood test evaluating levels of TSH present in the body can determine whether this condition is present. In most cases, patients will be on lifelong medication such as *Synthroid* or *Levoxyl* as replacements or supplements to the low levels of hormone. Another form of hypothyroidism disease is cretinism or congenital hypothyroidism. This disease develops during infancy or early childhood, and is a congenital condition where the thyroid gland is completely absent at birth or the thyroid gland is unable to produce hormones. The child will develop with both mental and physical retardation. A lack of developing muscle will result in the child's inability to stand and walk. They will have very distinct physical features such as wide-set eyes, puffy eyelids, a protruding abdomen, dwarf-like height, expressionless face with a wide-open mouth and thick, protruding tongue, and dry skin. Early discovery and treatment may correct most of the physical deficiences but often does not help with the mental retardation. **Myxedema** is a severe type of hypothyroidism in older children and adults, usually female, with a range of symptoms depending on the age of the patient at onset of the disease. Symptoms may include puffiness in the extremities, slow muscular response, excessively dry skin, bloated face with thickened tongue, excessive fatigue, weight gain, loss of hair, slow or slurred speech, and menorrhagia in female patients. In severe cases, myxedema can progress into coma although this is a rare life-threatening form.

Thyroid cancer occurs in the thyroid gland and often does not cause symptoms until the disease is very advanced and often irreparable damage has occurred to the gland. Some patients may complain of hoarseness or difficulty swallowing. Patients with family history of thyroid cancer are ten times more likely to also develop thyroid cancer which indicates the disease may have a strong genetic link. Women are also three times more likely to develop thyroid cancer than men. The prognosis of patients with thyroid cancer greatly depends on the patient's age at diagnosis, the advancement of the cancer at diagnosis, and the size of the primary tumor. It is a condition caused by the overactivity of one or more of the four parathyroid glands and is usually caused by a tumor or excessive growth of one of the parathyroid glands (**adenoma**). Although some patients may have few symptoms, it may often result in such clinical symptoms as mental disturbances, fatigue, weakness, bone loss, and even in severe cases, kidney failure. **Hypoparathyroidism** (underactivity of the parathyroid glands) results from reduced levels of parathyroid hormone (PTH) and causes low blood calcium levels known as **hypocalcemia.** When levels of PTH are low, resulting in hypocalcemia, initial symptoms will include tingling of the nose, ears, fingertips or toes, followed by spasms, cramping, or twitching of the feet and hands. Severe, continual muscle contractions may then develop called **tetany.** The patient may experience emotional and mental status changes such as aggression, confusion, irritability, and memory loss. Left untreated, hypocalcemia will eventually progress into heart arrhythmias, spasms in the trachea leading to respiratory paralysis, respiratory arrest, and death. Calcium replacement therapy with vitamin D is effective in reducing hypocalcemia and this treatment is usually life-long unless the condition is discovered early enough in the patient's life to be completely treated.

Parathyroid Disorders

The parathyroid glands help control blood calcium levels, which contribute to bone growth and muscular health. **Hyperparathyroidism** is a condition caused by the overactivity of one or more of the four parathyroid glands and is usually caused by a tumor or excessive growth of one of the parathyroid glands (adenoma). Although some patients may have few symptoms, it often results in such clinical symptoms as mental disturbances, fatigue, weakness, bone loss, and even in severe cases, kidney failure.

Hypoparathyroidism (underactivity of the parathyroid glands) results from reduced levels of parathyroid hormone (PTH) and causes low blood calcium levels known as *hypocalcemia.* When levels of PTH are low, resulting in hypocalcemia, initial symptoms will include tingling of the nose, ears, fingertips or toes, followed by spasms, cramping, or twitching of the feet and hands. Severe, continual muscle contractions called *tetany* may then develop. The patient may experience emotional and mental status changes such as aggression, confusion, irritability, and memory loss. Left untreated, hypocalcemia will eventually progress into heart arrhythmias, spasms in the trachea leading to respiratory paralysis, respiratory arrest, and death. Calcium replacement therapy with vitamin D is effective in reducing hypocalcemia and this treatment is usually life-long unless the condition is discovered early enough in the patient's life to be completely reversed.

Adrenal Disorders

Like other endocrine glands, the adrenal glands may also become overactive (**hyperadrenalism**) or underactive (**hypoadrenalism**). Hyperadrenalism can be caused by an adrenal tumor, excessive secretion of corticotrophin (ACTH) from the pituitary gland, or the abnormal production of corticotrophin in another organ (occurs in the lung cancer). **Cushing's Syndrome** is a condition where there are excessive amounts of circulating cortisol levels in the blood. The patient presents with muscular weakness, fatigue, and physical changes in body appearance. Psychiatric problems are common in this disease and patients often develop diabetes mellitus. Prolonged use or large doses of glucocorticoids (steroids) to treat other conditions may result in Cushing's syndrome. Treatment of Cushing's depends on the cause of the hyperadrenal-ism and may include surgery to remove a tumor or radiation to reduce a tumor in the pituitary or adrenal gland. *Adrenogenital syndrome* results in symptoms of excessive androgens both in men and women, which, in turn, can result in **hirsutism,** abnormal hair growth. **Virilism** is also a condition caused by excessive androgen secretion. Virilism results in mature masculine features in children. Administration of steroids can keep the overactivity in balance.

Hypoadrenalism, or adrenal insufficiency, is also known as **Addison's disease** and is a partial or complete failure of adrenocortical function. It is characterized by weakness and fatigue, gastrointestinal disturbances, anorexia and weight loss, and a very distrinct bronze skin color. Reduced levels of aldosterone result in the body's inability to retain salt and water resulting in dehydration, hyperkalemia (excessive potassium blood levels), and other electrolyte imbalances. Hyperkalemia is a life-threatening condition requir-ing immediate emergency care. Treatment includes the replacement of natu-ral hormones and correction of salt and potassium levels. Perhaps the most famous Addison's patient was US President John F. Kennedy.

Pancreas Disorders

Sometimes, the pancreas may become inflamed, as in **pancreatitis** effecting the production and secretion of the hormone **insulin.** *Hyperinsulinsism* is the *over*secretion of insulin and may cause **hypoglycemia,** a dangerous lowering of blood sugar levels that deprives the body of needed glucose. Hypoglycemia can be successfully controlled with dietary changes and patient awareness of physical symptoms signaling the decline in blood glucose levels. Hyposecre-tion of insulin can cause **diabetes mellitus,** a widespread disease that affects about 4 percent of the U.S. population.

Diabetes or Failure of the Beta Cells

Diabetes occurs either as **Type I diabetes (insulin-dependent diabetes mel-litus or IDDM), Type II diabetes (noninsulin-dependent diabetes mellitus or NIDDM),** or **Type III diabetes (gestational diabetes or GDM).** Type I diabetes (formerly know as *juvenile onset diabetes*) usually occurs before the age of 30 and is the result of underproduction or complete absence of insu-lin production (hypoinsulinism) by the beta cells. A reduction in insulin deprives cells of the glucose fuel they need and they begin to metabolize proteins and fats as replacements. This activity causes metabolic waste products known as ketones to build up in the blood and spill over into the urine (ketonuria) and this leads to a very serious condition called *acidosis*. When excessive glucose accumulates in the blood and overflows into the urine a condition called **glucosuria (glycosuria)** develops. The goal of dia-betes treatment is to keep blood glucose levels as near to normal as possible. Type I diabetic may be treated with controlled doses of insulin along with consistent, moderate exercise and weight management. Type II diabetics (formerly known as *adult onset diabetes*) usually do not require insulin injec-tions but may need oral hypoglycemic medications and follow strict dietary guidelines, and exercise routines. Type II diabetes is the more common of the two diabetic forms and has a gradual onset in adults between the ages of 30 and 55. In Type II, pancreatic function of insulin production and secretion still remains but is insufficient for normal glucose metabolism. It is very common for overweight and obsess people whose responsiveness to insulin is abnormally low to develop Type II diabetes. This response is called *insulin resistance*.

Both Type I and Type II diabetes can lead to *insulin reaction* and/or *diabetic coma*. Insulin reaction or insulin shock, is a condition where excessive levels of insulin causes a rapid onset of symptoms such as tremors, tachycardia, hunger, dizziness, irritability, confusion, seizures, and loss of consciousness. Diabetic coma results from abnormally low levels of insulin, such as occurs when an insulin dose is skipped or excessive amounts of carbohydrates have been consumed by the patient. Diabetic coma has a slow onset and presents with such symptoms as excessive thirst, increased urination, nausea and vomiting, abdominal pain, flushed and dry skin, "fruity" breath odor, heavy respirations, dilated and fixed pupils, hyperglycemia, loss of consciousness, and coma. Left untreated, the patient could die.

Type III, or gestational, diabetes (GDM) is a condition where a female's body loses the ability to process carbohydrates and sugars during pregnancy. Affecting approximately four percent of pregnant women today, its onset usually occurs between weeks 24 to 28 of the pregnancy and may have most of the typical symptoms of the other forms of diabetes. During the pregnancy, the treatment of GDM is similar to the treatment of any diabetes, watching the mother and the fetus very closely due to the increased risk for complications. This condition usually disappears right after delivery of the baby with 30–40 percent of women with GDM developing Type II diabetes within 5 to 10 years after GDM.

Complications of diabetes cover a wide range of ailments from circulatory problems to infections to organ failure. **Diabetic nephropathy** is a kidney disease resulting from diabetes mellitus. Also called *glomerulosclerosis*, this condition can be expected to eventually develop in all Type I diabetic patients. Insufficient control of blood glucose levels and blood pressure by the diabetic patient will accelerate the destruction of the renal function. **Diabetic neuropathy** is loss of sensation in the extremities. This condition is compounded by hyperglycemia which delays healing and substantially reduces the diabetic's resistance to infection. Diabetics require close observation for the development of foot wounds and infections that may occur from circulatory difficulties common in diabetes, especially in the lower extremities. **Diabetic retinopathy** is a disease of the retinal blood vessels causing gradual visual loss leading to blindness. Diabetic retinopathy is a major cause of blindness and results from hemorrhages, abnormal dilation of retinal veins, the formation of abnormal new vessels, and damaging microaneurysms in the eyes. The body uses stored proteins and fats to replace glucose for energy, thereby causing **acidosis, ketoacidosis,** and **ketosis,** all of which are marked by the abnormal presence of ketone bodies in the blood and urine.

Before the discovery of insulin as a compound that affects blood sugar levels, people with diabetes usually died of some of the many complications of the disease. Although diabetes is still not curable, technology has given new solutions to diabetes care. Quick-acting and long-acting insulins provide more options for managing insulin-dependent diabetes. A wider range of oral drugs are available to treat Type II diabetes. New monitors make it easier and more comfortable for people to test and track their blood glucose. External insulin pumps can replace the discomfort of daily injections. Laser surgery can treat diabetic eye disease and prevent blindness. Successful kidney and pancreas transplantation procedures bring hope to people with organ failure. In addition, much has been learned about how to manage diabetes and prevent complications through weight reduction, blood glucose control, and exercise and there are more successful methods of managing diabetes during pregnancy today. Researchers have also identified lifestyle changes that can help prevent diabetes.

Cancers of the Endocrine System

Cancers occur commonly in the endocrine system. Many, such as thyroid cancer, can be treated with removal of the affected gland and supplementation with a synthetic version of the necessary hormones that are then missing from the body. In other endocrine cancers, such as pancreatic cancer, the prognosis is poor even after aggressive treatment. Cancer of the pancreas is the fourth-leading cause of cancer-related death in the United States. Surgical removal of the affected area of the pancreas is currently the only potential cure, however only 15–20 percent of diagnosed patients are candidates for surgery.

VOCABULARY REVIEW

In the previous section you learned terms related to pathology. Before going on to the exercises, review the terms below and refer to the previous section if you have any questions. Pronunciations are provided for certain terms. Sometimes information about where the word came from is included after the term. The etymologies (word histories) are for your information only. You do not need to memorize them.

Term	Meaning
acidosis [ăs-ĭ-DŌ-sĭs] acid + -osis, condition	Abnormal accumulation of ketones in the body.
acromegaly [ăk-rō-MĔG-ă-lē] acro-, extreme + -megaly, enlargement	Abnormally enlarged features resulting from a pituitary tumor and hypersecretion of growth hormone.
Addison's [ĂD-ĭ-sŏnz] **disease** After Thomas Addison (1793–1860), English physician	Underactivity of the adrenal glands.
Cushing's [KŪSH-ĭngs] **syndrome** After Harvey Cushing (1869–1939), U.S. neurosurgeon	Group of symptoms caused by overactivity of the adrenal glands.
diabetes [dī-ă-BĒ-tēz] Greek, a siphon	*See* Type I diabetes, Type II diabetes, Type III diabetes.
diabetes insipidus [ĭn-SĬP-ĭ-dŭs]	Condition caused by hyposecretion of antidiuretic hormone (ADH).

Term	Meaning
diabetes mellitus [MĔL-ĭ-tŭs, mĕ-LĪ-tŭs]	*See* Type I diabetes, Type II diabetes.
diabetic nephropathy [dī-ă-BĔT-ĭk nĕ-FRŎP-ă-thē]	Kidney disease due to diabetes.
diabetic neuropathy [nū-RŎP-ă-thē]	Loss of sensation in the extremities due to diabetes.
diabetic retinopathy [rĕt-ĭ-NŎP-ă-thē]	Gradual loss of vision due to diabetes.
dwarfism [DWŌRF-ĭzm] dwarf + -ism, state	Abnormally stunted growth caused by hyposecretion of growth hormone, congenital lack of a thyroid gland, or a genetic defect.
exophthalmos [ĕk-sŏf-THĂL-mŏs] ex-, out of + Greek *ophthalmos*, eye	Abnormal protrusion of the eyes typical of Graves' disease.
gigantism [JĪ-găn-tĭzm] Greek *gigas*, giant + -ism	Abnormally fast and large growth caused by hypersecretion of growth hormone.
glucosuria [glū-kō-SŪ-rē-ă] gluco-, glucose + -uria, urine	Glucose in the urine.
glycosuria [glī-kō-SŪ-rē-ă] glyco-, glycogen + -uria	Glucose in the urine.
goiter [GŎY-tĕr] Latin *guttur*, throat	Abnormal enlargement of the thyroid gland.
Graves' [grāvz] **disease** After Robert Graves (1796–1853), Irish physician	Overactivity of the thyroid gland.
hirsutism [HĔR-sū-tĭzm] hirsut(e), hairy + -ism	Abnormal hair growth due to an excess of androgens.
hyperadrenalism [HĪ-pĕr-ă-DRĒN-ă-lĭzm] hyper-, excessive + adrenal + -ism	Overactivity of the adrenal glands.
hyperparathyroidism [HĪ-pĕr-pă-ră-THĪ-rŏyd-ĭzm] hyper- + parathyroid + -ism	Overactivity of the parathyroid glands.
hypersecretion [HĪ-pĕr-sĕ-KRĒ-shŭn] hyper- + secretion	Abnormally high secretion, as from a gland.
hyperthyroidism [hī-pĕr-THĪ-rŏyd-ĭzm] hyper- + thyroid + -ism	Overactivity of the thyroid gland.
hypoadrenalism [HĪ-pō-ă-DRĒN-ă-lĭzm] hypo-, below normal + adrenal + -ism	Underactivity of the adrenal glands.
hypoglycemia [HĪ-pō-glī-SĒ-mē-ă] hypo- + glyc- + -emia	Abnormally low level of glucose in the blood.
hypoparathyroidism [HĪ-pō-pă-ră-THĪ-rŏyd-ĭzm] hypo- + parathyroid + -ism	Underactivity of the parathyroid glands.
hyposecretion [HĪ-pō-sĕ-KRĒ-shŭn] hypo- + secretion	Abnormally low secretion, as from a gland.
hypothyroidism [HĪ-pō-THĪ-rŏyd-ĭzm] hypo- + thyroid + -ism	Underactivity of the thyroid gland.

Term	Meaning
insulin-dependent diabetes mellitus (IDDM)	*See* Type I diabetes.
ketoacidosis [KĒ-tō-ă-sĭ-DŌ-sĭs] keto(ne) + acidosis	Condition of high acid levels caused by the abnormal accumulation of ketones in the body.
ketosis [kē-TŌ-sĭs] ket(one) + -osis, condition	Condition caused by the abnormal release of ketones in the body.
myxedema [mĭk-sĕ-DĒ-mă] Greek *myxa*, mucus + edema	Advanced adult hypothyroidism.
noninsulin-dependent diabetes mellitus (NIDDM)	*See* Type II diabetes.
pancreatitis [PĂN-krē-ă-TĪ-tĭs] pancreat-, pancreas + -itis, inflammation	Inflammation of the pancreas.
polydipsia [pŏl-ē-DĬP-sē-ă] poly-, much + Greek *dipsa*, thirst	Excessive thirst.
polyuria [pŏl-ē-YŪ-rē-ă] poly- + -uria	Excessive excretion of urine, resulting in frequent urination.
syndrome of inappropriate ADH (SIADH)	Excessive secretion of antidiuretic hormone.
tetany [TĔT-ă-nē] Greek *tetanos*, convulsive tension	Neurological syndrome, usually due to decreased serum levels of calcium in the blood.
thyrotoxicosis [THĪ-rō-tŏk-sĭ-KŌ-sĭs] thyro-, thyroid + toxic + -osis	State of dangerously high levels of thyroid hormone.
Type I diabetes	Endocrine disorder with abnormally low or completely absent levels of insulin; also known as insulin-dependent diabetes mellitus (IDDM).
Type II diabetes	Disease caused by failure of the body to recognize insulin that is present or by an abnormally low level of insulin; also known as noninsulin-dependent diabetes mellitus (NIDDM); usually adult onset.
virilism [VĬR-ĭ-lĭzm] Latin *virilis*, masculine	Condition with excessive androgen production, often resulting in the appearance of mature male characteristics in young.

CASE STUDY

Getting a Diagnosis

Gail decides to wait until after the holidays to make her appointment with the endocrinologist. She thinks that she will watch what she eats and then go to the doctor when she is less busy. For a few days, she moderates her eating and feels a little better. However, on the big holiday weekend, Gail goes to several parties, drinks, and overeats. When she wakes up in the morning, she feels dizzy, is in a cold sweat, and feels very hungry. Right away, she realizes that something is terribly wrong. Since it is a holiday weekend, she has a friend take her to the emergency room. Once there, her symptoms worsen. The emergency room doctor tests her blood sugar and finds it is very low. After she has eaten something, he tests it again. Because Gail is overweight, the doctor suspects that her body is not sensitive to insulin. Gail is sent to Dr. Malpas, an endocrinologist, the very next day.

Critical Thinking

40. What type of diabetes does Gail appear to have?
41. What might some recommendations be for Gail's diet?

PATHOLOGICAL TERMS EXERCISES

Write A for adrenal, PA for pancreas, PI for pituitary, and T for thyroid to indicate the gland from which each of the following diseases arises.

42. acromegaly: _____

43. diabetes mellitus: _____

44. exophthalmos: _____

45. gigantism: _____

46. goiter: _____

47. myxedema: _____

48. Cushing's syndrome: _____

49. Graves' disease: _____

50. Addison's disease: _____

51. dwarfism: _____

52. cretinism: _____

Surgical Terms

Certain endocrine glands that become diseased can be surgically removed and then synthetic versions of the hormones they formerly produced are given to the patients to help their bodies continue performing the necessary endocrine functions.

An **adenectomy** is the removal of any gland. An **adrenalectomy** is the removal of an adrenal gland. Adrenalectomy may be performed in two methods—an open procedure or a laparoscopic procedure. Open operations may be performed through the back (sometimes requiring partial removal of a rib), the flank, or the abdomen. Laparoscopic procedures use small telescopes and long instruments to remove the adrenal gland through a series of small incisions. Typically, patients having laparoscopic procedures have less pain and a rapid recovery.

Removal of the pituitary gland (also called hypophysis) is a **hypophysectomy.** It is most commonly performed to treat tumors and sometimes is used to treat Cushing's syndrome due to pituitary adenoma.

The pancreas is removed in a **pancreatectomy.** Operations on the pancreas typically require an abdominal incision with some dissection of the stomach and intestines to expose the pancreas located deep within the abdomen. Many tumors may be dissected out of the substance of the pancreas, but in some cases may require partial removal of the pancreas. Removal of the parathyroid gland is performed in a **parathyroidectomy.** An incision is made along the collar line. The surgeon will move the thyroid gland to one side, then the other, to allow inspection of the parathyroid glands, which are located behind or to the side of the thyroid, deep within the neck. The surgeon will remove one or more of the parathyroids, depending on the specific disorder. The muscles are then repaired and the skin incision is closed with sutures that will either absorb or be removed soon after the operation. Recently, there has been discussion of the acceptability of a minimally invasive, or "keyhole," surgery for this problem. This is sometimes feasible and is being investigated here in the United States very carefully. Although it is being performed in some areas of the world, there are concerns about the possibility of more complications and a lower success rate with this type of procedure. Therefore, it is not yet widely accepted as a standard operation. A **thymectomy** is an operation to remove the thymus gland, leading to remission. However, this remission may not be permanent. A thymectomy is mainly carried out in an adult. This is because the thymus loses most of its functional capacity after adolescence, but does retain a small portion of its function during adulthood. This is shown in the decreasing size of the thymus with increasing age after adolescence. A **thyroidectomy** is the removal of the entire thyroid gland. Surgery to remove only a portion of the thyroid is termed a partial, sub-total, or hemi-thyroidectomy. The metabolic functions of the thyroid are easily replaced with a well-tolerated oral medicine if surgery makes this necessary.

Some of these operations mentioned above may only require the removal of only the diseased part of a gland, leaving the remaining portion to continue its endocrine function. Other procedures that surgically remove the entire gland may require life-long hormone replacement or supplement therapy to replace the hormones once produced and secreted by the removed gland.

VOCABULARY REVIEW

In the previous section you learned terms related to surgery. Before going on to the exercises, review the terms below and refer to the previous section if you have any questions. Pronunciations are provided for certain terms. Sometimes information about where the word came from is included after the term. The etymologies (word histories) are for your information only. You do not need to memorize them.

Term	Meaning
adenectomy [ă-dĕ-NĔK-tō-mē] aden-, gland + -ectomy, removal	Removal of a gland.
adrenalectomy [ă-drē-năl-ĔK-tō-mē] adrenal + -ectomy	Removal of an adrenal gland.
hypophysectomy [hī-pŏf-ĭ-SĔK-tō-mē] hypophys(is) + -ectomy	Removal of the pituitary gland. Also called hypophysis.
pancreatectomy [PĂN-krē-ă-TĔK-tō-mē] pancreat-, pancreas + -ectomy	Removal of the pancreas.
parathyroidectomy [PĂ-ră-thī-rŏy-DĔK-tō-mē] parathyroid + -ectomy	Removal of one or more of the parathyroid glands.
thymectomy [thī-MĔK-tō-mē] thym(us) + -ectomy	Removal of the thymus gland.
thyroidectomy [thī-rŏy-DĔK-tō-mē] thyroid + -ectomy	Removal of the thyroid.

CASE STUDY

Controlling the Disease

After the emergency room incident, Gail goes to her appointment with the endocrinologist, where she is given medication to make her body more sensitive to insulin, and told to diet sensibly and exercise. When she returns three months later, Dr. Malpas is pleased to see that Gail is controlling her diabetes, losing weight slowly, and exercising regularly. Her outlook is favorable. Dr. Malpas has another patient, Will Burns, who has had an overactive thyroid since he was a child.

Lately, Will's hyperthyroidism has increased. Dr. Malpas biopsies Will's thyroid and tells Will it would be best to remove the thyroid.

Critical Thinking
53. What did Dr. Malpas probably find that necessitated thyroid removal?
54. What medications could Will be given after the operation?

SURGICAL TERMS EXERCISES

Build Your Medical Vocabulary

Supply the missing part of the term:

55. removal of a gland: _____ectomy

56. removal of the pituitary gland: _____ectomy

57. removal of an adrenal gland: _____ectomy

58. removal of the thymus gland: _____ectomy

59. removal of part of the pancreas: _____ectomy

60. removal of the thyroid gland: _____ectomy

61. removal of one or more of the parathyroid glands: _____ectomy

After completing the terms in items 55 through 61, use them to define the following treatments:

62. Treatment for Graves' disease: _____

63. Treatment for severe virilism: _____

64. Treatment for a cancerous gland: _____

65. Treatment for hyperparathyroidism: _____

66. Treatment for acromegaly: _____

Pharmacological Terms

Hormonal deficiencies are sometimes treated by **hormone replacement therapy (HRT)**. Common types of hormone therapy include synthetic thyroid, estrogen, and testosterone. Other medications include those that regulate levels of substances in the body, such as glucose levels in diabetics. An **antihypoglycemic** raises blood sugar. An **antihyperglycemic** or **hypoglycemic** lowers blood sugar. Instead of or in addition to using drugs to regulate blood sugar, many diabetics are now treated with medications that increase sensitivity to their own insulin. **Human growth hormone** (somatotropin) occurs naturally in the body. In some cases of dwarfism, a synthetic version of HGH is given to promote growth. **Steroids** are used in controlling various symptoms and treating many diseases within and outside the endocrine system. Steroids can also be abused for muscle growth as discussed in Chapter 5. Table 15-2 lists common pharmacological agents used in treating the endocrine system.

There are several new endocrine therapy drugs available for the replacement or supplemental treatment of hormone absence or deficiency. Tamoxifen is an orally estrogen which is used in the treatment of breast cancer and is currently the world's largest selling drug for that purpose. Anastrozole (trade name: Arimidex) is a drug indicated in the treatment of breast cancer in post-menopausal women. It is used both following surgery and in metastatic breast cancer. It has the effect of decreasing the amount of estrogens that the body makes. While officially indicated for women, this

Chapter 15   The Endocrine System   **511**

TABLE 15-2 Agents Used in Treating the Endocrine System

Drug Class	Purpose	Generic	Trade Name
antihyperglycemic	to lower blood sugar or increase sensitivity to insulin	insulin glyburide rosiglitazone pioglitazone chlorpropamide	Humulin, Novolin Diabeta, Micronase Avandia Actos Diabinese
antihypoglycemic	to prevent or relieve severe hypoglycemia or insulin reaction	glucagon	Glucagon Diagnostic Kit
human growth hormone	to increase height in cases of abnormal lack of growth	somatotropin	Humatrope, Nutropin
steroid	to increase growth; to relieve symptoms of various diseases	methylprednisolone prednisone desamethasone	Medrol Cortan, Deltasone Decadron, Cortastat

drug has proven effective in also reducing estrogens (in particular and more importantly, estradiol) in men. Excess estradiol in men can cause benign prostatic hyperplasia, gynecomastia, and symptoms of hypogonadism. Some athletes and body builders will also use anastrozole as a part of their steroid cycle to reduce and prevent symptoms of excess estrogens; in particular, gynecomastia and water retention. This drug is frequently used in the treatment of growth disorder affected children to stop or slow the onset of puberty. At the onset of puberty the bone growth plates begin to close. This can occur in children as young as 5 years old so for children severely behind in growth, the opportunity for increased growth is diminished. Arimidex is shown to slow or stop this process.

Carbimazole is used to treat hyperthyroidism by reducing the production of the thyroid hormones T3 and T4 thyroxine). Treatment is usually given for 12–18 months followed by a gradual withdrawal. Letrozole is approved by the United States Food and Drug Administration (FDA) for the treatment of local or metastatic breast cancer that is hormone receptor positive or has an unknown receptor status in postmenopausal women. Side effects include signs and symptoms of hypoestrogenism. Levothyroxine, a thyroid hormone, is used to treat hypothyroidism. When taken correctly, levothyroxine reverses the symptoms experienced with hypothyroidism. It is also used to treat congenital hypothyroidism (cretinism) and goiter (enlarged thyroid gland).

In 2002, studies on the effects of Hormone Replacement Therapy (HRT) for the treatment of menopause in women proclaimed HRT as a danger to women. The U.S. federal government halted the hormone trial of the Women's Health Initiative (WHI) early, a study Levothyroxine, a thyroid hormone, is used to treat hypothyroidism. When taken correctly, levothyroxine reverses the symptoms experienced with hypothyroidism. It is also used to treat congenital hypothyroidism (cretinism) and goiter (enlarged thyroid gland). But fast-forward to 2008 and the picture of hormone replacement therapy changed yet again. Because the 2002 WHI study included women from ages 50 to 79, the initial results were a combined tabulation of all age groups together. But when data was re-analyzed to focus on the youngest members alone, an entirely different risk-to-benefit ratio of HRT began to emerge. While the impact of HRT on the heart may seem less ominous today than in 2002, links to breast cancer are less clear—and some say less encouraging. Many experts say that in the years following the WHI announcement, women stopped taking hormones en masse and the incidence of breast cancer subsequently declined. While studies are still ongoing, and reanalysis of the original data continues to shape medical opinions, experts say there are a few lessons learned thus far that are not likely to change. Among them: That hormone replacement therapy is not a panacea for disease prevention, even in situations where it was found to be helpful, such as reduction in hip fractures. Moreover, if hormone replacement therapy must be used to control menopause symptoms, the lowest possible dose for the shortest possible duration is recommended. Today the emphasis rests on the importance of treating every woman individually, with decisions about hormone use made strictly on a case-by-case basis.

VOCABULARY REVIEW

In the previous section you learned terms related to pharmacology. Before going on to the exercises, review the terms below and refer to the previous section if you have any questions. Pronunciations are provided for certain terms. Sometimes information about where the word came from is included after the term. The etymologies (word histories) are for your information only. You do not need to memorize them.

Term	Meaning
antihyperglycemic [ĂN-tē-HĪ-pĕr-glī-SĒ-mĭk] anti-, against + hyperglycem(ia) + -ic, pertaining to	Agent that lowers blood glucose.
antihypoglycemic [ĂN-tē-HĪ-pō-glī-SĒ-mĭk] anti- + hyporglycem(ia) + -ic	Agent that raises blood glucose.
hormone replacement therapy (HRT)	Ingestion of hormones to replace missing (or increase low levels of needed) hormones.
human growth hormone	Naturally occurring substance in the body that promotes growth; synthesized substance that serves the same function.
hypoglycemic [HĪ-pō-glī-SĒ-mĭk] hypoglycem(ia) + -ic	Agent that lowers blood glucose.
radioactive iodine therapy	Use of radioactive iodine to eliminate thyroid tumors.
steroid [STĔR-ŏyd, STĒR-ŏyd] ster(ol), alcohol compound + -oid, like	A hormone or chemical substance released by several endocrine glands or manufactured in various medications.

CASE STUDY

Learning the Outcome

At the same time that Gail's diabetes is diagnosed, she is beginning to feel symptoms of menopause. Women in their late forties and throughout their fifties represent a large concentration of newly diagnosed diabetics. Will has had his thyroid removed. Both Gail and Will probably get hormone replacement therapy.

Critical Thinking

67. What hormones could be prescribed for Gail?

68. What hormones could be prescribed for Will?

PHARMACOLOGICAL TERMS EXERCISES

Build Your Medical Vocabulary

In the space provided, write the name of the gland from which a hormone is needed to relieve symptoms of the disease.

69. Addison's disease: _____

70. hyperglycemia: _____

71. diabetes insipidus: _____

72. myxedema: _____

73. panhypopituitarism: _____

CHALLENGE SECTION

The laboratory report shown here is for a woman on hormone replacement therapy who also takes thyroid medications.

Pathologist's Laboratory
West Lake Road
West Lake, CT 00008
555-678-8900

Patient Name: Sally Benedict **Age/Sex:** 50/F **Patient Number:** 41983

Requesting Physician: Jane Merdin, MD **D.O.B.:** 10/28/50

Source: 09/30/XXXX **Collected:** 03-27-XXXX 0826 **Reported:** 03-28-XXXX 1649

Comments: Fasting 12 hrs. **Operator:** _____
Thyroid & Hormone Meds. **Reviewed by:** _____

Test	Results	Normal Range	
		FEMALE (Adjusted For Age)	
CPK	66	24-170	IU/L
LDH	122	122-220	IU/L
SGOT (AST)	21	0-31	IU/L
SGPT (ALT)	28	0-31	IU/L
ALK PHOSPHATASE	54	39-117	IU/L
GGTP	21	7-33	IU/L
TOTAL BILIRUBIN	0.3	.0-1.0	MG/DL
URIC ACID	3.5	2.4-5.7	MG/DL
TRIGLYCERIDE	105	0-200	MG/DL
CHOLESTEROL	229	0-240	MG/DL

TRIG/CHOL RATIO	0.5		
GLUCOSE	103	70-105	MG/DL
BUN	14	5-23	MG/DL
CREATININE	1.0	.6-1.1	MG/DL
BUN/CREAT RATIO	14.0		
PHOSPHORUS	3.2	2.7-4.5	MG/DL
CALCIUM	8.1	8.7-10.4	MG/DL
TOTAL PROTEIN	6.7	6.5-8.0	GM/DL
ALBUMIN	4.2	3.5-5.5	GM/DL
GLOBULIN	2.5	2.2-4.2	GM/DL
A/G RATIO	1.7	1.2-2.2	
SODIUM	140	135-148	MEQ/L
POTASSIUM	4.0	3.5-5.3	MEQ/L
CHLORIDE	106	100-112	MEQ/L
IRON	79	40-145	UG/DL
**THYROID			
T UPTAKE	29.5	27.8-40.8	%
THYROXINE	7.5	4.5-13.0	UG/DL
F.T.I. (T7)	2.2	1.8-4.4	

Critical Thinking

From the results of the lab report, do you think the patient's thyroid medication is putting her thyroid in the normal range? Explain your answer.

TERMINOLOGY IN ACTION

Below is a lab report for a 55-year-old patient.

Claudia Dinavo, M.D. 20 Ridge Road Tuscaloosa, AL 99999 555-111-4444	Laboratory Report Lab Services University Square Tuscaloosa, AL 99999 555-111-2222	
Patient: Sam Oscar Date Collected: 03/28/XXXX Date Received: 03/28/XXXX	Patient ID: 099-00-1200 Time Collected: 09:10 Date Reported: 3/31/XXXX	Date of Birth: 4/3/XXXX Total Volume: 2000

Test	Result	Flag	Reference
Complete Blood Count			
WBC	5.2		3.9-11.1
RBC	4.11		3.80-5.20
HCT	39.7		34.0-47.0
MCV	96.5		80.0-98.0
MCH	32.9		27.1-34.0
MCHC	34.0		32.0-36.0
MPV	8.6		7.5-11.5
NEUTROPHILS %	45.6		38.0-80.0
NEUTROPHILS ABS.	3.4		1.70-8.50
LYMPHOCYTES %	36.1		15.0-49.0
LYMPHOCYTES ABS.	1.44		1.00-3.50
EOSINOPHILS %	4.5		0.0-8.0
EOSINOPHILS ABS.	0.18		0.03-0.55
BASOPHILS %	0.7		0.0-2.0
BASOPHILS ABS.	0.03		0.000-0.185
PLATELET COUNT	325		150-400
Automated Chemistries			
GLUCOSE	405	*	65-109

(continued)

Test	Result	Flag	Reference
UREA NITROGEN/CREATININE	28		10-29
SODIUM	152	*	135-145
POTASSIUM	4.4		3.5-5.3
CHLORIDE	106		96-109
CO$_2$	28		20-31
ANION GAP	6		3-19
CALCIUM	9.8		8.6-10.4
PHOSPHORUS	3.6		2.2-4.6
AST (SGOT)	28		0-30
ALT (SGPT)	19		0-34
BILIRUBIN, TOTAL	0.5		0.2-1.2
PROTEIN, TOTAL	7.8		6.2-8.2
ALBUMIN	4.3		3.5-5.0
GLOBULIN	3.5		2.1-3.8
URIC ACID	2.4		2.0-7.5
CHOLESTEROL	195		120-199
TRIGLYCERIDES	68		40-199
IRON	85		30-150
HDL CHOLESTEROL	73		35-59
CHOLESTEROL/HDL RATIO	3.2		3.2-5.7
LDL, CALCULATED	126		70-129
T3, UPTAKE	42	*	24-37
T4, TOTAL	13.6	*	4.5-12.8

Which items indicate abnormalities in the endocrine system?

_____

_____

USING THE INTERNET

Go to the site of The Endocrine Society (http://www.endo-society.org), click the news and fact section, then click the fact sheet, and click on an article about an endocrinological disease. Write a brief summary of the information you collect.

CHAPTER REVIEW

The material that follows is to help you review this chapter.

Match the Meaning

Match the following combining forms with the correct meanings. Some answers may be used more than once or not at all.

74. ____ dips(o)
75. ____ aden(o)
76. ____ thyr(o), thyroid(o)
77. ____ glyc(o)
78. ____ pancreat(o)
79. ____ acr(o)
80. ____ kal(i)
81. ____ calci(o)
82. ____ gluc(o)
83. ____ gonad(o)
84. ____ vag(o)
85. ____ cortic(o)
86. ____ endocrin(o)
87. ____ parathyroid(o)
88. ____ macr(o)
89. ____ oophor(o)
90. ____ orch(o), orchi(o), orchid(o)
91. ____ pachy(o)
92. ____ somat(o)
93. ____ thym(o)

a. large, long
b. gonads, sex glands
c. ovary
d. thymus gland
e. calcium
f. gland
g. extreme, extremity
h. thyroid gland
i. potassium
j. sugar, glyogen
k. body
l. vagus nerve
m. testis, testicle
n. uric acid
o. pancreas
p. glucose
q. cortex, outer layer of organs
r. endrocrine gland
s. parathyroid gland
t. thirst

Mix and Match

Match the following abbreviations with their correct meaning.

94. ____ ACTH
95. ____ HCG
96. ____ DM
97. ____ GH
98. ____ ADH
99. ____ GTT
100. ____ CRH
101. ____ FSH

a. somatotrophic hormone
b. glucose tolerance test
c. potassium
d. hormone Replacement Therapy
e. human chorionic gonadotropin
f. fasting blood sugar
g. insulin-dependant diabetes mellitus
h. thyroxine

102. ____ T3   i. triiodothyronine
103. ____ IDDM   j. rheumatoid arthritis
104. ____ HRT   k. parathyroid hormone, parathormone
105. ____ AODM   l. melanocyte-stimulating hormone
106. ____ T4   m. radioactive iodine uptake
107. ____ NIDDM   n. growth hormone
108. ____ PTH   o. corticotropin-releasing hormone
109. ____ STH   p. luteinizing hormone
110. ____ DI   q. antidiuretic hormone
111. ____ ERT   r. diabetes insipidus
112. ____ FBS   s. adult-onset diabetes mellitus
113. ____ K   t. adrenocorticotropic hormone
114. ____ RA   u. diabetes mellitus
115. ____ RAIU   v. non–insulin-dependant diabetes mellitus
116. ____ MSH   w. follicle-stimulating hormone
117. ____ LH   x. estrogen replacement therapy

Match the Suffix

Match the following suffixes commonly used with endocrine system terms with their correct meaning.

118. ____ -logy   a. study of
119. ____ -megaly   b. inflammation
120. ____ -emia   c. tumor, mass
121. ____ -ism   d. disease
122. ____ -oma   e. in the blood
123. ____ -ectomy   f. condition
124. ____ -itis   g. incision
125. ____ -osis   h. enlargement
126. ____ -otomy   i. state
127. ____ -pathy   j. excision

Match the Prefix

Match the following prefixes commonly used with endocrine system terms with their correct meaning.

128. ____ hypo-   a. excessive
129. ____ para-   b. deficient
130. ____ syn-   c. against, opposing
131. ____ poly-   d. all, entire
132. ____ pan-   e. good, well, normal
133. ____ hyper-   f. together, with, joined

134. ____ eu-

135. ____ anti-

g. alongside of, near

h. many, more than one

Word Building

Using word parts you have learned in this chapter, build the correct medical terms for the following definitions.

136. study of the endocrine system _____

137. not enough sugar in the blood _____

138. excessive potassium in the blood _____

139. disease of the adrenal glands _____

140. state of inadequate pituitary gland activity throughout _____

141. inflammation of the adrenal glands _____

142. excision of the thyroid gland _____

143. resembling the cortex _____

144. physician who studies endocrine disease _____

145. enlargement of the extremities _____

146. deficient calcium in the blood _____

147. excessive development of the adrenal cortex _____

148. inflammation of a gland _____

149. disease of the endocrine system _____

DEFINITIONS

Define and pronounce the following terms. The words in the curly blue brackets refer to the Spanish glossary available online at www.mhhe.com/medterm3e.

WORD

150. acidosis [ăs-ĭ-DŌ-sĭs] {acidosis}

151. acromegaly [ăk-rō-MĔG-ă-lē] {acromegalia}

152. Adam's apple

153. Addison's [ĂD-ĭ-sŏnz] disease

154. aden(o)

155. adenectomy [ă-dĕ-NĔK-tō-mē]

156. adenohypophysis [ĂD-ĕ-nō-hī-PŎF-ĭ-sĭs]

157. adren(o), adrenal(o)

158. adrenal cortex [ă-DRĒ-năl KŌR-tĕks]

159. adrenalectomy [ă-drē-năl-ĔK-tō-mē] {adrenalectomía}

160. adrenal {adrenal} gland

161. adrenaline [ă-DRĔ-nă-lĭn] {adrenalina}

162. adrenal medulla [mĕ-DŪL-lă]

163. adrenocorticotropic [ă-DRĒ-nō-KŌR-tĭ-kō-TRŌ-pĭk] hormone (ACTH)

164. aldosterone [ăl-DŎS-tēr-ōn] {aldosterina}

165. alpha [ĂL-fă] cells

166. androgen [ĂN-drō-jĕn] {andrógeno}

167. antidiuretic [ĂN-tē-dĭ-yū-RĔT-ĭk] hormone (ADH)

168. antihyperglycemic [ĂN-tē-HĪ-pĕr-glī-SĒ-mĭk]

169. antihypoglycemic [ĂN-tē-HĪ-pō-glī-SĒ-mĭk]

170. beta [BĀ-tă] cells

171. blood sugar, blood glucose

172. calcitonin [kăl-sĕ-TŌ-nĭn] {calcitonia}

173. catecholamines [kăt-ĕ-KŌL-ă-mēnz] {catecolaminas}

174. corticosteroids [KŎR-tǐ-kō-STĒR-ŏydz] {corticosteroides}

175. cortisol [KŎR-tǐ-sōl] {cortisol}

176. Cushing's [KŪSH-ĭngs] syndrome

177. diabetes [dī-ă-BĒ-tēz] {diabetes}

178. diabetes insipidus [ĭn-SĬP-ǐ-dŭs]

179. diabetes mellitus [MĔL-ĭ-tŭs, mě-LĪ-tŭs]

180. diabetic nephropathy [dī-ă-BĔT-ĭk ně-FRŎP-ă-thē]

181. diabetic neuropathy [nū-RŎP-ă-thē]

182. diabetic retinopathy [rět-ǐ-NŎP-ă-thē]

183. ductless gland

184. dwarfism [DWŎRF-ĭzm] {enanismo}

185. electrolyte [ē-LĔK-trō-līt] {electrólito}

186. endocrine [ĔN-dō-krĭn] gland {glándula endocrina}

187. epinephrine [ĔP-ǐ-NĔF-rĭn] {epinefrina}

188. exocrine [ĔK-sō-krĭn] gland {glándula exocrina}

189. exophthalmos [ěk-sŏf-THĂL-mŏs] {exoftalmía}

190. fasting blood sugar

191. follicle-stimulating hormone (FSH)

192. gigantism [JĪ-găn-tĭzm] {gigantismo}

193. gland {glándula}

194. gluc(o)

195. glucagon [GLŪ-kă-gŏn] {glucagon}

196. glucocorticoids [glū-kō-KŎR-tǐ-kŏydz]

197. glucose tolerance test (GTT)

198. glucosuria [glū-kō-SŪ-rē-ă]

199. glyc(o)

200. glycogen [GLĪ-kō-jěn] {glucógeno} glycated [GLĪ-kā-těd] hemoglobin

201. glycosuria [glǐ-kō-SŪ-rē-ă]

202. goiter [GŎY-těr] {bocio}

203. gonad(o)

204. Graves' [grāvz] disease

205. growth hormone (GH)

206. hirsutism [HĚR-sū-tǐzm] {hirsutismo}

207. hormone [HŌR-mōn] {hormona}

208. hormone replacement therapy (HRT)

209. human growth hormone

210. hyperadrenalism [HĪ-pěr-ă-DRĒN-ă-lĭzm]

211. hyperparathyroidism [HĪ-pěr-pă-ră-THĪ-rŏyd-ĭzm] {hiperparatiroidismo}

212. hypersecretion [HĪ-pěr-sě-KRĒ-shŭn]

213. hyperthyroidism [hī-pěr-THĪ-rŏyd-ĭzm] {hipertiroidismo}

214. hypoadrenalism [HĪ-pō-ă-DRĒN-ă-lĭzm] {hipoadrenalismo}

215. hypoglycemia [HĪ-pō-glǐ-SĒ-mē-ă] {hipoglucemia}

216. hypoglycemic [HĪ-pō-glǐ-SĒ-mǐk] {hipoglucémico}

217. hypoparathyroidism [HĪ-pō-pă-ră-THĪ-rŏyd-ĭzm] {hipoparatiroidismo}

218. hypophysectomy [hī-pŏf-ǐ-SĔK-tō-mē]

219. hypophysis [hī-PŎF-ǐ-sǐs] {hipófisis}

220. hyposecretion [HĪ-pō-sě-KRĒ-shŭn]

221. hypothalamus [HĪ-pō-THĂL-ă-mŭs] {hipotálamo}

222. hypothyroidism [HĪ-pō-THĪ-rŏyd-ĭzm] {hipotiroidismo}

223. inhibiting factor

224. insulin [ĬN-sū-lĭn] {insulina}

225. insulin-dependent diabetes mellitus (IDDM)

226. islets of Langerhans [LĂN-gěr-hănz]

227. isthmus [ĬS-mŭs] {istmo}

228. ketoacidosis [KĒ-tō-ă-sǐ-DŌ-sǐs] {cetoacidosis}

229. ketosis [kē-TŌ-sǐs] {cetosis}

230. luteinizing [LŪ-tē-ǐn-ĪZ-ǐng] hormone (LH)

231. melanocyte-stimulating [mě-LĂN-ō-sīt, MĔL-ă-nō-sīt] hormone (MSH)

232. melatonin [měl-ă-TŌN-ǐn]

233. metabolism [mě-TĂB-ō-lǐzm]

234. mineralocorticoid [MĬN-ěr-ăl-ō-KŌR-tǐ-kŏyd]

235. myxedema [mǐk-sě-DĒ-mă] {mixedema}

236. neurohypophysis [NŪR-ō-hǐ-PŎF-ǐ-sǐs]

237. noninsulin-dependent diabetes mellitus (NIDDM)

238. norepinephrine [NŌR-ěp-ǐ-NĔF-rǐn] {norepinefrina}

239. ovary [Ō-văr-ē] {ovario}

240. oxytocin [ŏk-sĭ-TŌ-sĭn] {oxitocina}

241. pancreas [PĂN-krē-ăs] {páncreas}

242. pancreat(o)

243. pancreatectomy [PĂN-krē-ă-TĔK-tō-mē]

244. pancreatitis [PĂN-krē-ă-TĪ-tĭs] {pancreatitis}

245. parathormone [păr-ă-THŌR-mōn] (PTH) {parathormona}

246. parathyroid(o)

247. parathyroidectomy [PĂ-ră-thĭ-rŏy-DĔK-tō-mē]

248. parathyroid [păr-ă-THĪ-rŏyd] gland {paratiroide}

249. parathyroid hormone (PTH)

250. pineal [PĬN-ē-ăl] gland

251. pituitary [pĭ-TŪ-ĭ-tār-ē] gland

252. polydipsia [pŏl-ē-DĬP-sē-ă] {polidipsa}

253. polyuria [pŏl-ē-YŪ-rē-ă] {poliuria}

254. postprandial [pōst-PRĂN-dē-ăl] blood sugar

255. radioactive immunoassay (RIA)

256. radioactive iodine therapy

257. radioactive iodine uptake

258. receptor [rē-SĔP-tōr] {receptor}

259. releasing factor

260. somatotrophic [SŌ-mă-tō-TRŌF-ĭk] hormone (STH)

261. steroid [STĔR-ŏyd, STĒR-ŏyd]

262. suprarenal [SŪ-pră-RĒ-năl] gland

263. sympathomimetic [SĬM-pă-thō-mĭ-MĔT-ĭk] {simpatomimético}

264. syndrome of inappropriate ADH (SIADH)

265. target cell

266. testis (pl., testes) [TĔS-tĭs (TĔS-tēz)], testicle [TĔS-tĭ-kl] {testículo}

267. tetany [TĔT-ă-nē] {tetania}

268. thymectomy [thĭ-MĔK-tō-mē] {timectomía}

269. thymus [THĪ-mŭs] gland

270. thyr(o), thyroid(o)

271. thyroidectomy [thĭ-rŏy-DĔK-tō-mē] {tiroidectomía}

272. thyroid function test

273. thyroid [THĪ-rŏyd] gland

274. thyroid scan

275. thyroid-stimulating hormone (TSH)

276. thyrotoxicosis [THĪ-rō-tŏk-sĭ-KŌ-sĭs]

277. thyroxine [thĭ-RŎK-sēn, -sĭn] (T$_4$)

278. triiodothyronine [trĭ-Ī-ō-dō-THĪ-rō-nēn] (T$_3$)

279. Type I diabetes

280. Type II diabetes

281. urine sugar

282. vasopressin [vā-sō-PRĔS-ĭn]

283. virilism [VĬR-ĭ-lĭzm] {virilismo}

Abbreviations

Write the full meaning of each abbreviation.

384. ACTH

385. ADH

286. CRH

287. DM

288. FSH

289. GH

290. GTT

291. HCG

292. IDDM

293. LH

294. MSH

295. NIDDM

296. PRL

297. PTH

298. STH

299. TSH

Answers to Chapter Exercises

1. to eliminate various diseases and to test for others
2. possibly yes, if her symptoms are serious enough
3. melatonin
4. epinephrine
5. ADH
6. oxytocin
7. insulin
8. prolactin
9. aldosterone
10. thyroxine
11. testosterone
12. thymosin
13. C
14. adrenal
15. hypophysis
16. suprarenal
17. C
18. pituitary
19. luteinizing
20. C
21. yes, sodium
22. endocrine
23. adenitis
24. pancreatopathy
25. glycogenesis
26. thyromegaly
27. euthyroid
28. removal of an adrenal gland
29. removal of part of the pancreas
30. glandular tumor
31. aid in sex cell development
32. abnormally large thyroid
33. diabetes
34. postprandial blood sugar
35. D
36. T
37. T
38. D
39. D
40. Type II diabetes
41. Gail has to pay attention to food quantities, as well as to the kinds of foods she should avoid.
42. PI
43. PA
44. T
45. PI
46. T
47. T
48. A

49. T
50. A
51. PI
52. T
53. cancer
54. thyroid hormones
55. adenectomy
56. hypophysectomy
57. adrenalectomy
58. thymectomy
59. pancreatectomy
60. thyroidectomy
61. parathyroidectomy
62. thyroidectomy
63. adrenalectomy
64. adenectomy
65. parathyroidectomy
66. hypophysectomy
67. estrogen, progesterone
68. thyroxine, triiodothyronine
69. adrenal
70. pancreas
71. pituitary
72. thyroid
73. pituitary
74. t
75. f
76. h
77. j
78. o
79. g
80. i
81. e
82. p
83. b
84. l
85. q
86. r
87. s
88. a
89. c
90. m
91. n
92. k
93. d
94. t
95. e
96. u
97. n
98. q
99. b
100. o

101. w
102. l
103. g
104. d
105. s
106. h
107. v
108. k
109. a
110. r
111. x
112. f
113. c
114. l
115. m
116. l
117. p
118. a
119. h
120. e
121. I
122. c
123. j
124. b
125. f
126. g
127. d
128. b
129. g
130. f
131. h
132. d
133. a
134. e
135. c
136. endocrinology
137. hypoglycemia
138. hyperkalemia
139. adrenopathy
140. panhypopituitarism
141. adrenalitis
142. thyroidectomy
143. corticoid
144. endocrinologist
145. acromegaly
146. hypocalcemia
147. adrenocoricohyperplasia
148. adenitis
149. endocrinopathy
150–299. Answers are available in the vocabulary reviews in this chapter.

The Sensory System

CHAPTER 16

▶ OPHTHALMOLOGY
▶ OTOLOGY

After studying this chapter, you will be able to:

16.1 Name the parts of the sensory system and discuss the function of each part

16.2 Define combining forms used in building words that relate to the sensory system

16.3 Identify the meaning of related abbreviations

16.4 Name the common diagnoses, clinical procedures, and laboratory tests used in treating disorders of the sensory system

16.5 List and define the major pathological conditions of the sensory system

16.6 Explain the meaning of surgical terms related to the sensory system

16.7 Recognize common pharmacological agents used in treating disorders of the sensory system

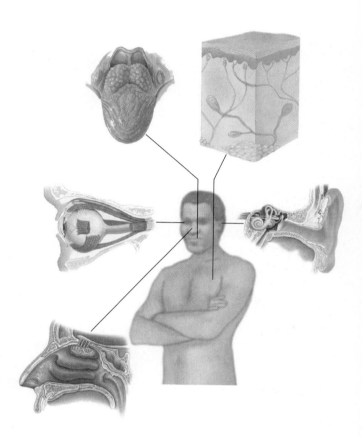

Structure and Function

The **sensory system** includes any organ or part involved in the perceiving and receiving of stimuli from the outside world and from within our bodies. Aristotle, a Greek philosopher who lived more than 2000 years ago, identified the five senses—**sight, touch, hearing, smell,** and **taste.** These senses are popularly thought of as the sensory system even though most of the senses are based on stimulation of nerves in the nervous system. The specialized nerve endings of each of the senses are neurons with specialized dendrites that respond to only one sensation. When stimulated, the electrochemical signal progresses to the brain for interpretation as with any afferent signal of the nervous system. For example, the rods and cones of the retina are stimulated by light.

While all five senses are the main structures for reacting to environmental stimuli, there are other ways in which our bodies "sense" and react to stimuli. For example, the islets of Langerhans sense high blood sugar and are stimulated to release insulin. This is but one example of a type of sense response in the body; however, the major parts of the sensory system relate specifically to

The Howard Hughes Medical Institute (http://www.hhmi.org/senses) has an informational Web site called "Seeing, Hearing, and Smelling the World."

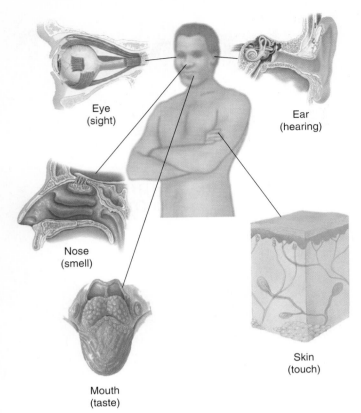

Eye
(sight)

Ear
(hearing)

Nose
(smell)

Skin
(touch)

Mouth
(taste)

FIGURE 16-1a   The sensory system includes organs of the five senses.

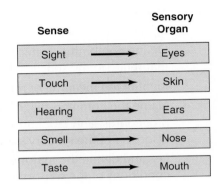

Sense		Sensory Organ
Sight	⟶	Eyes
Touch	⟶	Skin
Hearing	⟶	Ears
Smell	⟶	Nose
Taste	⟶	Mouth

FIGURE 16-1b   The locations where stimuli are sensed.

the organs of the five senses and related senses felt by those organs. Figure 16-1a shows the major organs of the sensory system. Figure 16-1b charts the location in the body where stimuli are sensed.

Sensory organs are also known as **sensory receptors.** All sensory receptors contain specialized receptor cells that are able to receive stimuli. They are designed to receive only certain stimuli (such as sound in the ear and light waves in the eye). Sensory receptor cells send impulses to the afferent (conductive) nerves in the central nervous system to interpret the stimuli.

Sight—the Eye

The **eyes,** organs of sight, contain about 70 percent of all the receptors in the human body. Each eye is made up of three layers—the sclera, the choroids, and the retinal layer.

The outer layer is a smooth, firm, white posterior section called the **sclera.** It is made of a thick, tough membrane. The sclera supports the eyeball. The **cornea** is the transparent, anterior section, which is the first place where light is bent or refracted as it enters the eye. This section has a greater curvature to capture and direct light into the eye. The sclera has blood vessels that nourish the cornea (which has no blood supply). The cornea is transparent, has no blood vessels, and bends (or refracts) light rays in a process called **refraction.** The outer layer is covered by the **eyelid.** The anterior surface of the eye and the posterior surface of the eyelid are lined with a mucous membrane (the **conjunctiva**).

The choroid or middle layer is the vascular layer of blood vessels, consisting of a thin posterior membrane, the **choroid.** Anteriorly, this is continuous with the **ciliary body,** which contains the ciliary muscles, used for focusing the eyes. Vision is the process that begins when light is refracted as it hits the cornea and again when it hits the *retina*. Light passes through the **pupil,** the black circular center of the eye, then passes through the **lens,** a colorless, flexible transparent body behind the **iris,** the colored part of the eye that expands and contracts in response to light, thereby opening and closing the pupil. From there it goes to the lens, which is suspended by ligaments that extend to the ciliary body. The ciliary body contracts to change the shape of the lens in a process called *accommodation*. Accommodation allows the eye to focus on objects at varying distances. This region of the eye which includes the iris, ciliary body, and choroid is known as the **uvea.**

The interior layer of the eye is called the *retinal layer*. It contains the **retina,** a light-sensitive membrane that can decode the light waves and send the information on to the brain, which interprets what we see. The retina itself has many layers. The thick layer of nervous tissue is called the **neuro-retina.** The neuro-retina consists of specialized nerve receptor cells called **rods,** sensors of black and white shades, and **cones,** sensors of color and the brightest light. There are three types of cones, one each for red, green, and blue. There are approximately 125 million rods and 7 million cones in each eye, along with other nerve cells, that convert the light images received to nerve impulses that are then transmitted through the **optic nerve** to the appropriate lobes of the brain.

The region where the retina connects to the optic nerve, where there are no rods or cones to receive images, is called the *optic disk* or *blind spot*. Light causes a chemical change in the rods and cones that allows them to convert the images to nerve impulses. The thin layer of the retina is made of pigmented epithelial tissue, which, along with the choroid, absorbs stray light that is not absorbed by the neuroretina and prevents reflections from the back of the retina. The center of the retina directly behind the lens has a small yellowish area called the **macula lutea,** which has a depression in the center called the **fovea centralis,** the area of sharpest vision.

The eyeball is divided into three cavities called *chambers*. The *anterior chamber* lies between the cornea and iris. The *posterior chamber* lies between the iris and the lens. Both the anterior and posterior chambers are filled with *aqueous humor,* a thin, watery liquid that provides nourishment to the lens and cornea and maintains a constant pressure within the eyeball. The tissue that holds the aqueous humor in until it exits the eye is made up of *trabeculae,* bundles of supportive fiber. The *vitreous chamber,* located posterior to the lens, occupies about 80 percent of the space in the eyeball. It is filled with *vitreous humor,* a gelatinous substance that nourishes parts of the eyes and maintains a supportive structure to keep the eye from collapsing.

MORE ABOUT . . .

Eye Color

Newborns with light skin are almost always born with blue eyes, even though their eyes may later turn brown or green. Eye color is determined by heredity. It takes several months for the melanocytes to be distributed to the anterior portion of the eye. Babies with darker skin normally have a higher concentration of melanocytes to begin with, and their eyes at birth are almost always dark. Albinos are born with no melanocytes in their body and they are, therefore, much more sensitive to light and have no pigment in the iris of their eyes.

FIGURE 16-2 The eye is the organ of sight.

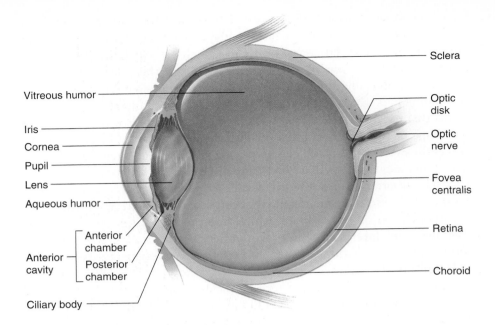

Several other structures are important to the eye. The eyelids close to protect the eyes or to allow rest and sleep. The **eyebrows** and **eyelashes** help keep foreign particles from entering the eye. The **lacrimal glands** secrete moisture into the *lacrimal ducts* or *tear ducts*. The resulting **tears** moisten the eyes, wash foreign particles off the eye, and distribute water and nutrients to parts of the eye. Tears may be secreted more heavily than necessary as a reaction to allergies, infections, or emotional upset. Figure 16-2 shows the eye.

Hearing and Equilibrium—the Ear

The **ear** is an organ of hearing and **equilibrium** (balance). The three major divisions of the ear are the *external ear*, the *middle ear*, and the *inner ear*.

The external ear begins on the outside of the head with a funnel-like structure called the **auricle** or **pinna.** This structure leads through part of the skull known as the *temporal bone* (which itself has a bony projection called the *mastoid process*) to an S-shaped tube called the *external auditory meatus*. The external auditory meatus contains glands that secrete *cerumen* or earwax, a brownish yellow, waxy substance.

The middle ear includes the *tympanic cavity*, in which sits the **eardrum (tympanic membrane)** and the **auditory ossicles,** three small, specially shaped bones. The eardrum is an oval, semitransparent membrane with skin on its outer surface and a mucous membrane on the inside. Sound waves change the pressure on the eardrum, which moves back and forth, thereby producing vibrations. The three ossicles are the **malleus** (hammer), **incus** (anvil), and **stapes** (stirrup). They are all attached to the tympanic cavity by tiny ligaments. The malleus is attached to the eardrum to help it maintain its oval and conic shape. Vibrations are carried from the eardrum through the malleus to the incus. The incus passes the movement onto the stapes, which is connected to the wall near the *oval window*, an opening leading to the inner ear. The middle ear is connected to the pharynx through the **eustachian tube** (*auditory tube*). This tube helps equalize air pressure on both sides of the eardrum, which is essential to hearing. The eustachian tube is connected to the nasal cavity. This explains why children are more susceptible to ear infections following a head cold.

The inner ear is a system of two tubes—the **osseus labyrinth** and the **membranous labyrinth.** The osseus labyrinth is a bony canal in the temporal bone. The membranous labyrinth is a tube within the osseus labyrinth and separated from it by **perilymph,** a liquid secreted by the walls of the osseus labyrinth. Inside the membranous labyrinth is another fluid, **endolymph.** The labyrinths include three **semicircular canals,** structures important to equilibrium, and a **cochlea,** a snail-shaped structure important to hearing. The cochlea is further divided into the *scala vestibuli*, which leads from the oval window to the apex of the cochlea, and the *scala tympani*, which leads from the apex of the cochlea to a covered opening in the inner ear called the *round window*. The cochlea has a membrane called the *basilar membrane* that has hairlike receptor cells located in the **organ of Corti** on the membrane's surface. The hairs move back and forth in response to sound waves and eventually send messages via neurotransmitters through the eighth cranial nerve and to the brain for interpretation. Table 16-1 shows various **decibel** (intensity of sound) levels that can be heard by a normal human ear. The scale of decibels (dB) gives the intensity of sound in progressions multiplied by 10. So 10dB is 10 times greater than the lowest perceptible decibel, 20dB is 100 times as great as 10dB, and so on. The easy availability of electronic equipment and the sound generated by modern machines have raised the decibel levels to which each successive generation is exposed.

The sense of equilibrium is the ability to maintain steady balance either when still, *static equilibrium*, or when moving, *dynamic equilibrium*. The bony chamber between the semicircular canal and the cochlea is called the **vestibule.** The vestibule contains a membranous labyrinth divided into two chambers, the *utricle* and *saccule*. Both of these chambers contain a **macula,** a structure with many hairlike sensory receptors that move forward, backward, or upward to move the gelatinous mass inside the inner ear. This mass contains **otoliths,** small calcifications that move to maintain gravitational balance. The semicircular canals also respond to movement and aid in maintaining balance. Figure 16-3 illustrates the structures of the ear.

Touch, Pain, and Temperature—the Skin

The skin's layers sense different intensities of touch. Light touch is felt in the top layer of skin, whereas touch with harder pressure is felt in the middle

TABLE 16-1 Decibel Levels

Decibel Level	Intensity of Sound	Effect on Hearing
40dB	10,000 times as great as 10dB	A whisper—perceptible to most people with normal hearing
60dB	1 million (1,000,000) times as great as 10dB	Regular conversational speech
80dB	100 million (100,000,000) times as great as 10dB	High noise such as in a crowded room or heavy traffic
130dB	10 trillion times as great as 10dB	Extremely loud rock concert; can cause ear damage.
140dB	100 trillion times as great as 10dB	Sound of a jet engine on takeoff. Hearing can be damaged.

FIGURE 16-3 The ear is the organ of hearing.

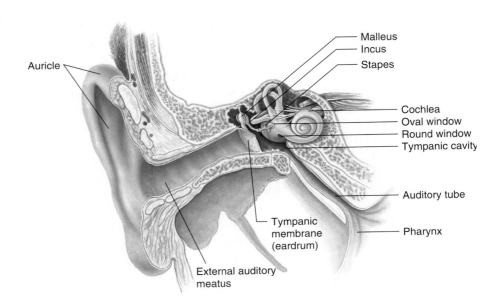

Auricle

Malleus
Incus
Stapes
Cochlea
Oval window
Round window
Tympanic cavity
Auditory tube
Pharynx
Tympanic membrane (eardrum)
External auditory meatus

MORE ABOUT...

Skin

One of the remarkable advances in genetic engineering is the ability to grow replacement skin. The new skin is grown from cells of skin from various parts of the body and can be used to replace burned or injured areas. If the skin is working once it is put in place, it will continue to grow and function like normal skin—helping to regulate body temperature, preventing foreign material from entering the body, and protecting inner organs from bruises.

or bottom layer. The skin's receptors can sense touch, pressure, pain, and hot and cold temperatures. Each type of receptor only senses one kind of sensation; for example, a heat receptor only senses heat; a pressure receptor only senses pressure. The skin also has pain receptors that sense any injury to skin tissue. Chapter 4 discusses the integumentary system, which is incorporated within the skin.

Smell—the Nose

The sense of smell or *olfactory stimulation* is activated by *olfactory receptors* located at the top of the nasal cavity. The olfactory receptors are neurons covered with cilia that send smell messages to the brain. The receptors are located within the **olfactory organs,** yellowish-brown masses along the top of the nasal cavity. For the sense of smell to sense an object, the object must be dissolved in a liquid in the olfactory organs. The sense of smell is closely related to the sense of taste.

Taste—the Tongue and Oral Cavity

Taste buds are organs that sense the taste of food. Most taste buds are on the surface of the tongue in small raised structures called **papillae,** but some also line the roof of the mouth and the walls of the pharynx. Each taste bud contains receptor cells, called **taste cells.** Nerve fibers wrapped around the taste cells transmit impulses to the brain. The taste buds are activated when the item being tasted dissolves in the watery fluid surrounding the taste buds. The salivary glands secrete this fluid. There are at least four types of taste buds to match the primary taste sensations—sweet, sour, salty, and bitter. Different sections of the tongue contain concentrations of receptors for each of the taste sensations. There are also receptors that sense the texture, odor, and temperature of food. In the case of food that is too hot, too spicy, or too cold, some pain receptors are activated. The combination of the primary taste sensations and the aroma of food will be interpreted in the brain as the specific flavor of food. This explains why someone with a head cold does not have a good appetite.

VOCABULARY REVIEW

In the previous section, you learned terms relating to the sensory system. Before going on to the exercises, review the terms below and refer to the previous section if you have any questions. Pronunciations are provided for certain terms. Sometimes information about where the word came from is included after the term. The etymologies (word histories) are for your information only. You do not need to memorize them.

Term	Meaning
auditory ossicles [ĂW-dĭ-tōr-ē ŎS-ĭ-klz]	Three specially shaped bones in the middle ear that anchor the eardrum to the tympanic cavity and that transmit vibrations to the inner ear.
auricle [ĂW-rĭ-kl] From Latin *auris*, ear	Funnel-like structure leading from the external ear to the external auditory meatus; also called pinna.
choroid [KŌ-rŏyd] Greek *chorioeides*, like a membrane	Thin posterior membrane in the middle layer of the eye.
ciliary [SĬL-ē-ăr-ē] **body**	Thick anterior membrane in the middle layer of the eye.
cochlea [KŎK-lē-ă] Latin, snail shell	Snail-shaped structure in the inner ear that contains the organ of Corti.
cones [kōnz]	Specialized receptor cells in the retina that perceive color and bright light.
conjunctiva (*pl.,* **conjunctivae**) [kŏn-JŬNK-tĭ-vă (kŏn-JŬNK-tĭ-vē)] From Latin *conjungo*, to join together	Mucous membrane lining the eyelid.
cornea [KŌR-nē-ă] Latin, like a horn	Transparent anterior section of the eyeball that bends light in a process called refraction.
decibel [DĔS-ĭ-bĕl] Latin *decimus*, tenth + *bel*, sound	Measure of the intensity of sound.
ear [ēr] Old English *eare*	Organ of hearing.
eardrum [ĒR-drŭm] ear + drum	Oval, semitransparent membrane that moves in response to sound waves and produces vibrations.
endolymph [ĔN-dō-lĭmf] endo-, within + lymph	Fluid inside the membranous labyrinth.

Term	Meaning
equilibrium [ē-kwǐ-LĬB-rē-ŭm] Latin *aequilibrium*, horizontal position	Sense of balance.
eustachian [yū-STĀ-shŭn, yū-STĀ-kē-ăn] **tube** After Bartolommeo Eustachio (1524–1574), Italian anatomist	Tube that connects the middle ear to the pharynx.
eye [ī] Old English *eage*	Organ of sight.
eyebrow [Ī-brŏw] eye + brow	Clump of hair, usually about a half an inch above the eye, that helps to keep foreign particles from entering the eye.
eyelashes [Ī-lăsh-ĕz] eye + lashes	Group of hairs protruding from the end of the eyelid; helps to keep foreign particles from entering the eye.
eyelid [Ī-lǐd] eye + lid	Moveable covering over the eye.
fovea centralis [FŌ-vē-ă sĕn-TRĂL-ĭs]	Depression in the center of the macula lutea; perceives sharpest images.
hearing	Ability to perceive sound.
incus [ĬN-kŭs] Latin, anvil	One of the three auditory ossicles; the anvil.
iris [Ī-rĭs] Greek, iris, rainbow	Colored part of the eye; contains muscles that expand and contract in response to light.
lacrimal [LĂK-rĭ-măl] **glands**	Glands that secrete liquid to moisten the eyes and produce tears.
lens [lĕnz] Latin, lentil	Colorless, flexible transparent body behind the iris.
macula [MĂK-yū-lă] Latin, spot	Inner ear structure containing hairlike sensors that move to maintain equilibrium.
macula lutea [lū-TĒ-ă]	Small, yellowish area located in the center of the retina, which has a depression called the fovea centralis.
malleus [MĂL-ē-ŭs] Latin, hammer	One of the three auditory ossicles; the hammer.
membranous labyrinth [LĂB-ǐ-rǐnth]	One of the two tubes that make up the semicircular canals.
neuroretina [nūr-ō-RĔT-ǐ-nă] neuro-, nerve + retina	Thick layer of nervous tissue in the retina.
olfactory [ōl-FĂK-tō-rē] **organs**	Organs at the top of the nasal cavity containing olfactory receptors.
optic nerve	Nerve that transmits nerve impulses from the eye to the brain.

Term	Meaning
organ of Corti [KŌR-tī]	Structure on the basilar membrane with hairlike receptors that receive and transmit sound waves.
osseus [ŎS-sē-ŭs] **labyrinth**	One of the two tubes that make up the semicircular canals.
otoliths [Ō-tō-lǐths] oto-, ear + -lith, stone	Small calcifications in the inner ear that help to maintain balance.
papillae [pă-PĬL-ē] Latin *papilla*, small pimple	Small, raised structures that contain the taste buds.
perilymph [PĔR-ǐ-lǐmf] peri-, around + lymph	Liquid secreted by the walls of the osseus labyrinth.
pinna [PĬN-ă] Latin, feather	Auricle.
pupil [PYŪ-pĭl] Latin *pupilla*	Black circular center of the eye; opens and closes when muscles in the iris expand and contract in response to light.
refraction [rē-FRĂK-shŭn] From Latin *refractus*, broken up	Process of bending light rays.
retina [RĔT-ǐ-nă]	Oval, light-sensitive membrane in the interior layer of the eye; decodes light waves and transmits information to the brain.
rods [rŏdz]	Specialized receptor cells in the retina that perceive black to white shades.
sclera (*pl.*, sclerae) [SKLĒR-ă (SKLĒR-ē)] Greek *skleros*, hard	Thick, tough membrane in the outer eye layer; supports eyeball structure.
semicircular canals	Structures in the inner ear important to equilibrium.
sensory receptors	Specialized tissue containing cells that can receive stimuli.
sensory system	Organs or tissue that perceive and receive stimuli from outside or within the body.
sight	Ability to see.
smell	Ability to perceive odors.
stapes (*pl.*, stapes, stapedes) [STĀ-pēz (STĀ-pĕ-dēz)]	One of the three auditory ossicles; the stirrup.
taste	Ability to perceive the qualities of ingested matter.
taste buds	Organs that sense the taste of food.
taste cells	Specialized receptor cells within the taste buds.
tears [tērz]	Moisture secreted from the lacrimal glands.
touch	Ability to perceive sensation on the skin.

Term	Meaning
tympanic [tĭm-PĂN-ĭk] membrane	Eardrum.
uvea [YŪ-vē-ă] Latin *uva*, grape	Region of the eye containing the iris, choroid membrane, and ciliary bodies.
vestibule [VĔS-tĭ-būl] Latin *vestibulum*, space	Bony chamber between the semicircular canal and the cochlea.

CASE STUDY

Checking Symptoms

John James, a 67-year-old male, presented at his family doctor's office very nervous and upset. His general health is excellent and, although he was widowed one year ago, he is proud of the way he has maintained his independence. His only complaint is diminished vision. He says his night vision is so bad that he has given up night driving. His family doctor gives him a general physical including laboratory tests. All of the test results prove normal. Mr. James is then referred to an ophthalmologist (eye specialist).

Critical Thinking
1. In addition to the general physical, why did the family doctor refer Mr. James to an ophthalmologist?
2. Why is a general physical necessary?

STRUCTURE AND FUNCTION EXERCISES

Find a Match

Match the terms in the left-hand column with the definitions in the right-hand column.

3. ____ iris
4. ____ sclera
5. ____ pupil
6. ____ optic disc
7. ____ eustachian
8. ____ incus
9. ____ malleus
10. ____ stapes
11. ____ tympanic membrane
12. ____ auricle
13. ____ cerumen

a. tough, white, outer coating of eyeball
b. dark opening of the eye, surrounded by the iris
c. earwax
d. hammer
e. eardrum
f. anvil
g. stirrup
h. auditory tube
i. pinna
j. blind spot of the eye
k. colored portion of the eye

Check Your Knowledge

Circle T for true or F for false.

14. The aqueous humor is a thick, gelatinous substance. T F
15. The sharpest images are perceived in the optic disk. T F

16. Rods and cones are receptor cells that sense light and color. T F
17. Olfactory receptors perceive light rays. T F
18. Semicircular canals in the ears are important to equilibrium. T F
19. Refraction is the focusing on distant objects. T F
20. The papillae house the taste buds. T F

Combining Forms and Abbreviations

The lists below include combining forms and abbreviations that relate specifically to the sensory system. Pronunciations are provided for the examples.

COMBINING FORM	MEANING	EXAMPLE
audi(o), audit(o)	hearing	*audiometer* [ăw-dē-ŎM-ĕ-tĕr], instrument for measuring hearing
aur(o), auricul(o)	hearing	*auriculocranial* [ăw-RĬK-yū-lō-KRĀ-nē-ăl], pertaining to the auricle of the ear and the cranium
blephar(o)	eyelid	*blepharitis* [blĕf-ă-RĪ-tĭs], inflammation of the eyelid
cerumin(o)	wax	*ceruminolytic* [sĕ-rū-mĭ-nō-LĬT-ĭk], agent for softening earwax
cochle(o)	cochlea	*cochleovestibular* [kōk-lē-ō-vĕs-TĬB-yū-lăr], pertaining to the cochlea and the vestibule of the ear
conjunctiv(o)	conjunctiva	*conjunctivoplasty* [kŏn-JŬNK-tĭ-vō-plăs-tē], plastic surgery on the conjunctiva
cor(o), core(o)	pupil	*coreoplasty* [KŌR-ē-ō-plăs-tē], surgical correction of the size and shape of a pupil
corne(o)	cornea	*corneoscleral* [kōr-nē-ō-SKLĔR-ăl], pertaining to the cornea and sclera
cycl(o)	ciliary body	*cyclodialysis* [sī-klō-dī-ĂL-ĭ-sĭs], method of relieving intraocular pressure in glaucoma
dacry(o)	tears	*dacryolith* [DĂK-rē-ō-lĭth], calculus in the tear duct
ir(o), irid(o)	iris	*iridoptosis* [ĭr-ĭ-dŏp-TŌ-sĭs], prolapse of the iris
kerat(o)	cornea	*keratoconus* [kĕr-ă-tō-KŌ-nŭs], abnormal protrusion of the cornea
lacrim(o)	tears	*lacrimotomy* [LĂK-rĭ-mŏ-tō-mē], incision into the lacrimal duct
mastoid(o)	mastoid process	*mastoiditis* [măs-tŏy-DĪ-tĭs], inflammation of the mastoid process

Combining Form	Meaning	Example
myring(o)	eardrum, middle ear	*myringitis* [mĭr-ĭn-JĪ-tĭs], inflammation of the tympanic membrane
nas(o)	nose	*nasosinusitis* [nās-zō-sĭ-nŭ-SĪ-tĭs], inflammation of the nasal and sinus cavities
ocul(o)	eye	*oculodynia* [ŏk-yū-lō-DĬN-ē-ă], pain in the eyeball
ophthalm(o)	eye	*ophthalmoscope* [ŏf-THĂL-mō-skōp], instrument for studying the interior of the eyeball
opt(o), optic(o)	eye	*optometer* [ŏp-TŎM-ĕ-tĕr], instrument for determining eye refraction
ossicul(o)	ossicle	*ossiculectomy* [ŎS-ĭ-kyū-LĔK-tō-mē], removal of one of the ossicles of the middle ear
phac(o), phak(o)	lens	*phacoma* [fā-KŌ-mă], tumor of the lens
pupill(o)	pupil	*pupillometer* [pyū-pĭ-LŎM-ĕ-tĕr], instrument for measuring the diameter of the pupil
retin(o)	retina	*retinitis* [rĕt-ĭ-NĪ-tĭs], inflammation of the retina
scler(o)	white of the eye	*sclerectasia* [sklĕr-ĕk-TĀ-zhē-ă], bulging of the sclera
scot(o)	darkness	*scotometer* [skō-TŎM-ĕ-tĕr], instrument for evaluating a scotoma or blind spot
tympan(o)	eardrum, middle ear	*tympanoplasty* [tĭm-pă-nō-PLĂS-tē], repair of a damaged middle ear
uve(o)	uvea	*uveitis* [yū-vē-Ī-tĭs], inflammation of the uvea

Abbreviation	Meaning	Abbreviation	Meaning
acc.	accommodation	D	diopter
AD	right ear	dB	decibel
ARMD	age-related macular degeneration	DVA	distance visual acuity
AS	left ear	ECCE	extracapsular cataract extraction
AU	both ears	EENT	eye, ear, nose, and throat
ENT	ear, nose, and throat	OU	each eye
ICCE	intracapsular cataract cryoextraction	PERRL, PERRLA	pupils equal, round, reactive to light (and accommodation)
IOL	intraocular lens	PE tube	polyethylene ventilating tube (placed in the eardrum)
IOP	intraocular pressure	SOM	serous otitis media
NVA	near visual acuity	VA	visual acuity

ABBREVIATION	MEANING	ABBREVIATION	MEANING
OD	right eye	VF	visual field
OM	otitis media	+	plus/convex
OS	left eye	−	minus/concave

CASE STUDY

Seeing a Specialist

Mr. James was next referred to an ophthalmologist who discovered that Mr. James had a cataract in his right eye that should be removed. He also had one in the left eye that did not need treatment at this time. During surgery, an IOL implant was placed in the right eye. After surgery, the ophthalmologist prescribed eyeglasses. The prescription form is used to instruct the optometrist or optician as to what corrective powers are necessary.

Critical Thinking

21. Through which eye can Mr. James see distant objects more clearly?
22. Did Mr. James need a corrective lens for his left eye?

Dr. Janet Maitland
3000 Blue Willow Lane
Forest Park, IL 99999
999-000-5555

NAME _John James_ DATE _2/3/XXXX_

R

	SPH.	CYL.	AXIS	PRISM	Remarks
R	-.75	+.75	180	20/20	1st Rx after cataract Sx OD
L	-2.00	+.75	005	20/50	

	ADD			P.D.	
R	+2.50		DIST 64	60	NEAR
L	+2.50				

☒ Janet Maitland, M.D.

EXPIRES _2/XXXX_ _Janet Maitland, M.D._
IL. LIC. NO. 7yytt8

COMBINING FORMS AND ABBREVIATIONS EXERCISES

Find the Roots

From the following list of combining forms and from the list of suffixes in Chapter 2, write the word that matches the definition.

audi(o) blephar(o) core(o) dacryocyst(o) irid(o) kerat(o) opt(o) ot(o) retin(o) scler(o)

23. _____ inflammation of the ear
24. _____ instrument for determining eye refraction
25. _____ study of the ear
26. _____ inflammation of the cornea
27. _____ instrument to examine the cornea
28. _____ disease of the iris
29. _____ pain in the tear sac

30. _____ repair of the pupil
31. _____ softening of the sclera
32. _____ inflammation of the sclera and cornea
33. _____ swelling in the eyelid
34. _____ pertaining to the retina
35. _____ paralysis of the iris
36. _____ earache

37. _____ study of hearing (disorders)

38. _____ inflammation of the eyelid

39. _____ hemorrhage from the ear

40. _____ instrument to measure hearing

Diagnostic, Procedural, and Laboratory Terms

Diagnosis of the sensory system usually includes testing of the sense in question and examination of the sensory structures. Loss of a sense can cause serious problems for an individual. In some cases, senses can be partially or totally restored through the use of prosthetic devices, transplants, or medication. In other cases, patients must adapt to the loss of a sense.

Diagnosing the Eye

An **ophthalmologist** (medical doctor who specializes in treatment and surgeries of the eye) and an **optometrist** (a trained nonmedical specialist who can examine patients for vision problems and prescribe lenses) both perform routine eye examinations. The most common diagnostic test of the eye is the visual acuity test, which measures the ability to see objects clearly at measured distances. The most common chart is the *Snellen Chart*. Perfect vision measures 20/20 on such a test. The first number, 20, is the distance (typically 20 feet) from which the person being tested reads a chart with black letters of different size. The second number is the distance from which the person being tested can read the size of the letters in relation to someone with normal vision. If the test shows that the subject can read only the letters on the 400 line, then the vision would be measured as 20/400. The 400 line means that someone with normal vision would be able to see from 400 feet away what the person being tested can see without corrective lenses at only 20 feet. A reading that shows less than 20/20 (for example 20/13) means that a person can read something at 20 feet that most people with 20/20 vision would only be able to read at 13 feet.

The next step in a routine eye examination is to examine peripheral vision, the area one is able to see to the side with the eyes looking straight ahead. This is usually done by telling a patient to follow a finger placed in front of their eyes while facing straight ahead. (In diagnosing some diseases, peripheral vision is tested in an examination called a *visual field examination*.) Depending on the patient's age, most routine eye examinations also include **tonometry,** a measurement of pressure within the eye (a test for glaucoma) and **ophthalmoscopy** (visual examination of the interior of the eye). If the patient needs corrective lenses, an **optician** (trained technician who makes and fits corrective lenses) can fill the prescription written by an ophthalmologist or an optometrist. Most optometrists and some ophthalmologists also fill prescriptions for lenses. A prescription includes the **diopter,** the unit of refracting power needed in a lens.

For further diagnosis of the eye, a *slit lamp ocular device* is used to view the interior of the eye magnified through a microscope (Figure 16-4). *Fluorescein angiography* is the injection of a contrast medium into the blood vessels to observe the movement of blood throughout the eye. This test is for people with diabetes and other diseases that may manifest lesions on various parts of the eye.

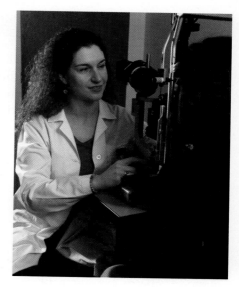

FIGURE 16-4   A slit lamp ocular device is a viewing device that uses a microscope to magnify the interior of the eye.

Diagnosing the Ear

Hearing tests are routinely given to young children to see if they have any hearing deficit. Later, hearing is checked when a person notices hearing loss or when that person's friends and family suspect it. An **otologist** is an ear specialist, and an **audiologist** is a nonmedical hearing specialist. **Otorhinolaryngologists** are specialists who practice *otorhinolaryngology*, the medical specialty covering the ear, nose, and throat. They all perform thorough examinations that include **otoscopy,** visual examination of the ear using an *otoscope*, a lighted viewing device (Figure 16-5). Such an examination might also include **audiometry,** the measurement of various acoustic frequencies to determine what frequencies the patient can or cannot hear. The device used is an *audiometer*, and the results of the test are plotted on a graph, an **audiogram.** The inside of the ear may be tested using a *pneumatic otoscope*, an otoscope that allows air to be blown into the ear to view the movement of the eardrum. A *tuning fork* compares the conduction of sound in one ear or between the two ears. The *Rinne test* and the *Weber test* are two tuning fork tests.

Hearing aids have improved both in the sound they provide and in the way they have been made so small as to be almost unnoticeable. Cochlear implants are another method of improving hearing.

Diagnosing Other Senses

The nose is usually observed as part of a general examination or, more specifically, a respiratory examination. Loss of the sense of smell is often the result of a disease process or of aging. The tongue and other parts of the mouth and the skin are also observed during a general examination. Loss of taste or touch may also be part of a disease process or of aging.

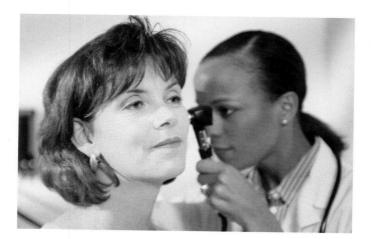

FIGURE 16-5   An otoscope is used to perform a visual examination of the ear. The family doctor here is examining a young patient with an earache.

VOCABULARY REVIEW

In the previous section, you learned diagnostic, procedural, and laboratory terms. Before going on to the exercises, review the terms below and refer to the previous section if you have any questions. Pronunciations are provided for certain terms. Sometimes information about where the word came from is included after the term. The etymologies (word histories) are for your information only. You do not need to memorize them.

Term	Meaning
audiogram [ĂW-dē-ō-grăm] audio- + -gram, a recording	Graph that plots the acoustic frequencies being tested.
audiologist [ăw-dē-ŎL-ō-jĭst] audio- + -logist, one who specializes	Specialist in evaluating hearing function.
audiometry [ăw-dē-ŎM-ĕ-trē] audio- + -metry, measurement	Measurement of acoustic frequencies using an audiometer.
diopter [dī-ŎP-tĕr] Greek *dioptra*, leveling instrument	Unit of refracting power of a lens.
ophthalmologist [ŏf-thăl-MŎL-ō-jĭst] ophthalmo-, eye + -logist	Medical specialist who diagnoses and treats eye disorders.
ophthalmoscopy [ŏf-thăl-MŎS-kō-pē] ophthalmo- + -scopy, viewing	Visual examination of the interior of the eye.
optician [ŏp-TĬSH-ŭn]	Technician who makes and fits corrective lenses.
optometrist [ŏp-TŎM-ĕ-trĭst] opto-, eye + Greek *metron*, measure	Nonmedical specialist who examines the eyes and prescribes lenses.
otologist [ō-TŎL-ō-jĭst] oto-, ear + -logist	Medical specialist in ear disorders.
otorhinolaryngologist [ō-tō-rī-nō-lăr-ĭng-GŎL-ō-jĭst] oto-, ear + rhino-, nose + laryngo-, throat + -ologist	Medical specialist who treats ear, nose, and throat disorders.
otoscopy [ō-TŎS-kō-pē] oto- + -scopy	Inspection of the ear using an otoscope.
tonometry [tō-NŎM-ĕ-trē] tono-, tension + -metry	Measurement of tension or pressure within the eye.

CASE STUDY

Another Problem Arises

Mr. James returned to the ophthalmologist in four months complaining of cloudy vision in his left eye. The ophthalmologist determined that it was time to remove the cataract in the left eye and replace it with an artificial lens or IOL. After a few weeks, Mr. James had regained night vision, even proclaiming that he could see better now than he had years before. His eyeglass prescription was changed. He only really needed his glasses for reading.

The ophthalmologist also recommended sunglasses for most outdoor daytime activities, because ultraviolet rays can harm the eyes.

Critical Thinking

41. An artificial lens replaces what part of the eye?
42. Does a lens implant change eye color?

DIAGNOSTIC, PROCEDURAL, AND LABORATORY TERMS EXERCISES

Know Your Senses

For each of the following diagnostic tests or devices, write A for eye, B for ear, or C for both eye and ear.

43. audiogram _____

44. otoscope _____

45. Rinne test _____

46. visual acuity _____

47. tuning fork _____

48. Snellen chart _____

49. tonometer _____

50. ophthalmoscope _____

Pathological Terms

Lost or damaged senses are illnesses in themselves. The disruption of losing or damaging a sense organ can lead to related illnesses. Much of the pathology of the sensory system results from age-related disorders or just age-related wear and tear on the sensory organs.

Eye Disorders

The most common eye disorders involve defects in the curvature of the cornea and/or lens or defects in the refractive ability of the eye due to an abnormally short or long eyeball. Such disorders are usually managed with corrective lenses. Corrective lenses may be placed in frames to be worn on the face or may be in the form of **contact lenses,** which are placed directly over the cornea of the eye centered on the pupil. Contact lenses come in a variety of types, including disposable, hard, soft, and long-term wear. The degree of correction of the lenses depends on the results of a visual acuity examination.

An eye examination may reveal an **astigmatism,** distortion of sight because light rays do not come to a single focus on the retina (Figure 16-6). It may also reveal **hyperopia (farsightedness)** or **myopia (nearsightedness).** All three are errors of refraction, the bending of light that causes light rays to fall at one point on the retina. Hyperopia is the focusing of light rays behind the retina, and myopia is the focusing of light rays in front of the retina. Figure 16-7 shows hyperopia and myopia. **Presbyopia** is loss of close reading vision due to lessened ability to focus and accommodate, a common disorder after age 40 and another refractive disorder.

Strabismus is eye misalignment (sometimes called "cross-eyed"). Two types of strabismus are **esotropia,** deviation of one eye inward, and **exotropia,** deviation of one eye outward. **Asthenopia** or **eyestrain** is a condition in

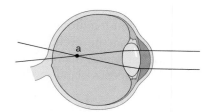

Astigmatism

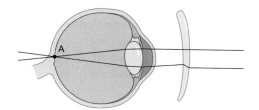

Correction

FIGURE 16-6 An astigmatism distorts light rays.

FIGURE 16-7 Hyperopia and myopia are errors of refraction.

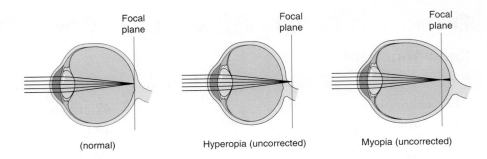

Focal plane

(normal)

Focal plane

Hyperopia (uncorrected)

Focal plane

Myopia (uncorrected)

which the eyes tire easily because of weakness of the ocular or ciliary muscles. Symptoms may include pain in or around the eyes, headache, dimness of vision, dizziness, and light nausea. **Diplopia** is double vision. **Photophobia** is extreme sensitivity to light, sometimes as a result of a disease.

Cataracts are cloudiness of the lens of the eye. They are usually a result of the aging process, but can be congenital or the result of a disease process or injury. Also, some types of medication may hasten the clouding of the lens. Removal of a cataract results in **aphakia,** absence of a lens. A **pseudophakia** is an implanted lens used to replace one that has been removed. A **scotoma** is a blind spot in vision.

Glaucoma is any disease caused by increased intraocular pressure of the aqueous humor. The pressure misaligns the lens and cornea and causes damage to the ciliary body. It can be treated in most cases by the use of special eye medications or surgical procedures (including laser treatments) to relieve the pressure. If not treatable, it can lead to **blindness,** loss of vision.

There are many other causes of blindness, such as congenital defects, trauma to the eyes, and **macular degeneration.** Macular degeneration is the breakdown of macular tissue, which leads to loss of central vision, the vision we use for reading, driving, and watching television. Some specific conditions within the eye may affect vision. One such is *papilledema* or *edema* of the optic disk. Diseases of other body systems can affect the senses. *Diabetic retinopathy* is a complication of diabetes mellitus that can result in vision loss. **Retinitis pigmentosa** is a progressive, inherited disorder, usually accompanied by scarring on the retina and **nyctalopia,** night blindness. The retina can tear or become detached and need surgical repair. Many of these conditions and other situations can lead to a form of partial blindness known as *legal blindness*. Legal blindness is a range of sight set by states. For example, someone whose vision can only be corrected to 20/400 may be considered legally blind.

The eyeball can protrude abnormally, as in **exophthalmus** or **exophthalmos,** usually caused by hyperthyroidism. **Lacrimation** or **epiphora** is excessive tearing, and **nystagmus** is excessive eyeball movement.

Inflammations and conditions of the eyelid include **blepharospasm,** involuntary eyelid movement causing excessive blinking; **blepharitis,** inflammation of the eyelid; **conjunctivitis** or **pinkeye,** a highly infectious inflammation of the conjunctiva; **blepharochalasis** or **dermatochalasis,** loss of elasticity of the eyelid; and **blepharoptosis,** paralysis of the eyelid causing drooping. A **chalazion** is a nodular inflammation that usually forms on the eyelid. **Trichiasis** is abnormal growth of eyelashes in a direction that causes them to rub on the eye. A **hordeolum** or **sty** is an infection of a sebaceous gland in the eyelid.

Inflammations of other parts of the eye include **dacryoadenitis,** inflammation of a lacrimal gland; **dacryocystitis,** inflammation of a tear duct; **iritis,** inflammation of the iris; **keratitis,** inflammation of the cornea; **retinitis,** inflammation of the retina; and **scleritis,** inflammation of the sclera.

Ear Disorders

The sense of hearing can be diminished or lost in a number of situations. **Anacusis** is total loss of hearing. **Paracusis** is impaired hearing. **Deafness** is either partial or total hearing loss. **Presbyacusis** or *presbycusis* is age-related hearing loss. *Conductive hearing loss* is caused by lessening of vibrations of the ear. *Sensorineural hearing loss* (also known as nerve deafness) is caused by lesions or dysfunction of those parts of the ear necessary to hearing. *Cerumen impaction*, abnormal wax buildup, can diminish hearing. **Otosclerosis** is the hardening of bone within the ear. **Tinnitus** is a constant ringing or buzzing in the ear. **Otalgia** or *earache* can interfere with hearing. **Otorrhagia,** bleeding in the ear, and **otorrhea,** purulent matter draining from the ear, can also impair hearing, usually temporarily. The sense of equilibrium is disturbed in **vertigo,** dizziness.

Various ear inflammations can diminish hearing or cause pain. **Otitis media** is inflammation of the middle ear. *Supperative otitis media* is bacterial in nature and is often found in children. *Serous otitis media* is fluid contained in the middle ear, preventing free movement of the tympanic membrane. **Otitis externa,** also known as *swimmer's ear,* is a fungal infection of the external ear canal often occurring in hot weather. **Labyrinthitis** is inflammation of the labyrinth. **Myringitis** or **tympanitis** is inflammation of the eardrum. **Mastoiditis** is inflammation of the mastoid process. Changes in atmospheric pressure, as in air travel, can result in **aerotitis media,** inflammation of the middle ear.

An *acoustic neuroma* is a benign tumor of the eighth cranial nerve that can affect hearing. A **cholesteatoma** is a fatty cyst within the middle ear. **Meniere's disease** is elevated fluid pressure within the cochlea, causing disturbances of the equilibrium and vertigo.

There are a number of organizations dedicated to fighting blindness or providing services for the blind. Prevent Blindness (www.preventblindness.org) is one example.

The Deafness Research Foundation (www.drf.org) provides research grants and disseminates information about deafness.

VOCABULARY REVIEW

In the previous section, you learned terms relating to pathology. Before going on to the exercises, review the terms below and refer to the previous section if you have any questions. Pronunciations are provided for certain terms. Sometimes information about where the word came from is included after the term. The etymologies (word histories) are for your information only. You do not need to memorize them.

TERM	MEANING
aerotitis media [ār-ō-TĪ-tĭs MĒ-dē-ă]	Inflammation of the middle ear caused by air pressure changes, as in air travel.
anacusis [ăn-ă-KŪ-sĭs] an-, without + Greek *akousis*, hearing	Loss of hearing.
aphakia [ă-FĀ-kē-ă] a-, without + Greek *phakos*, lentil-shaped	Absence of a lens.
asthenopia [ăs-thĕ-NŌ-pē-ă] Greek *astheneia*, weakness + ops, eye	Weakness of the ocular or ciliary muscles that causes the eyes to tire easily.

Term	Meaning
astigmatism [ă-STĬG-mă-tĭzm] a-, without + Greek *stigma*, point + -ism, state	Distortion of sight because of lack of focus of light rays at one point on the retina.
blepharitis [blĕf-ă-RĪ-tĭs] blephar-, eyelid + -itis, inflammation	Inflammation of the eyelid.
blepharochalasis [blĕf-ă-rō-KĂL-ă-sĭs] blepharo-, eyelid + Greek *chalasis*, a slackening	Loss of elasticity of the eyelid.
blepharoptosis [blĕf-ă-RŎP-tō-sĭs] blepharo- + Greek *ptosis*, a falling	Drooping of the eyelid.
blepharospasm [BLĔF-ă-rō-spăzm] blepharo- + spasm	Involuntary eyelid movement; excessive blinking.
blindness	Loss or absence of vision.
cataract [CĂT-ă-răkt] Latin *cataracta*	Cloudiness of the lens of the eye.
chalazion [kă-LĀ-zē-ŏn] Greek, little sty	Nodular inflammation that usually forms on the eyelid.
cholesteatoma [kō-lĕs-tē-ă-TŌ-mă] chole(sterol) + steato-, fat + -oma, tumor	Fatty cyst within the middle ear.
conjunctivitis [kŏn-jŭnk-tĭ-VĪ-tĭs] conjunctiv-, conjunctiva + -itis	Inflammation of the conjunctiva of the eyelid.
contact lenses	Corrective lenses worn on the surface of the eye.
dacryoadenitis [DĂK-rē-ō-ăd-ĕ-NĪ-tĭs] dacryo-, lacrimal gland + aden, gland + -itis	Inflammation of the lacrimal glands.
dacryocystitis [DĂK-rē-ō-sĭs-TĪ-tĭs] dacryo- + cyst + -itis	Inflammation of a tear duct.
deafness	Loss or absence of hearing.
dermatochalasis [DĔR-mă-tō-kă-LĀ-sĭs] dermato-, skin + Greek *chalasis*, a slackening	Loss of elasticity of the eyelid.
diplopia [dĭ-PLŌ-pē-ă] diplo-, double + -opia, vision	Double vision.
epiphora [ĕ-PĬF-ō-ră] Greek, a sudden flow	Excessive tearing.
esotropia [ĕs-ō-TRŌ-pē-ă] Greek *eso*, inward + -tropia, a turning	Deviation of one eye inward.
exophthalmos, exophthalmus [ĕk-sŏf-THĂL-mōs] ex-, out of + Greek *ophthalmos*, eye	Abnormal protrusion of the eyeballs.
exotropia [ĕk-sō-TRŌ-pē-ă] exo-, outward + -tropia	Deviation of one eye outward.
eyestrain eye + strain	Asthenopia.
farsightedness	Hyperopia.

TERM	MEANING
glaucoma [glăw-KŌ-mă] Greek *glaukoma*, opacity	Any of various diseases caused by abnormally high eye pressure.
hordeolum [hōr-DĒ-ō-lŭm]	Infection of a sebaceous gland of the eyelid; sty.
hyperopia [hī-pĕr-Ō-pē-ă] hyper-, excessive + -opia, vision	Focusing behind the retina causing vision distortion; farsightedness.
iritis [ī-RĪ-tĭs] ir-, iris + -itis	Inflammation of the iris.
keratitis [kĕr-ă-TĪ-tĭs] kerat-, cornea + -itis	Inflammation of the cornea.
labyrinthitis [LĂB-ĭ-rĭn-THĪ-tĭs] labyrinth + -itis	Inflammation of the labyrinth.
lacrimation [lăk-rĭ-MĀ-shŭn]	Secretion of tears, usually excessively.
macular [MĂK-yū-lăr] **degeneration**	Gradual loss of vision caused by degeneration of tissue in the macula.
mastoiditis [măs-tŏy-DĪ-tĭs] mastoid + -itis	Inflammation of the mastoid process.
Meniere's disease [mĕn-YĒRZ] After Prosper Meniere (1799–1862), French physician	Elevated pressure within the cochlea.
myopia [mī-Ō-pē-ă] Greek, from *my-*, muscle + -opia, vision	Focusing in front of the retina causing vision distortion; nearsightedness.
myringitis [mĭr-ĭn-JĪ-tĭs] myring-, eardrum + -itis	Inflammation of the eardrum.
nearsightedness	Myopia.
nyctalopia [nĭk-tă-LŌ-pē-ă] nyct-, night + Greek *alaos*, obscure + -opia, vision	Night blindness.
nystagmus [nĭs-STĂG-mŭs] Greek *nystagmos*, a nodding	Excessive involuntary eyeball movement.
otalgia [ō-TĂL-jē-ă] ot-, ear + -algia, pain	Pain in the ear.
otitis externa [ō-TĪ-tĭs ĕks-TĔR-nă]	Fungal infection of the external ear canal.
otitis media [MĒ-dē-ă]	Inflammation of the middle ear.
otorrhagia [ō-tō-RĀ-jē-ă] oto-, ear + -rrhagia, hemorrhage	Bleeding from the ear.
otorrhea [ō-tō-RĒ-ă] oto- + -rrhea, flow	Purulent discharge from the ear.
otosclerosis [ō-tō-sklĕ-RŌ-sĭs] oto- + sclerosis	Hardening of bones of the ear.
paracusis [PĂR-ă-KŪ-sĭs] para-, beyond + Greek *akousis*, hearing	Impaired hearing.

TERM	MEANING
photophobia [fō-tō-FŌ-bē-ă] photo-, light + -phobia, fear	Extreme sensitivity to light.
pinkeye	Conjunctivitis.
presbyacusis [prĕz-bē-ă-KŪ-sĭs] presby-, old age + Greek *akousis*, hearing	Age-related hearing loss.
presbyopia [prĕz-bē-Ō-pē-ă] presby- + -opia	Age-related diminished ability to focus or accommodate.
pseudophakia [sū-dō-FĀ-kē-ă] pseudo-, fake + Greek *phakos*, lentil	Eye with an implanted lens after cataract surgery.
retinitis [rĕt-ĭ-NĪ-tĭs] retin-, retina + -itis	Inflammation of the retina.
retinitis pigmentosa [pĭg-mĕn-TŌ-să]	Progressive, inherited disease with a pigmented spot on the retina and poor night vision.
scleritis [sklĕ-RĪ-tĭs]	Inflammation of the sclera.
scotoma [skō-TŌ-mă] Greek *skotoma*, vertigo	Blind spot in vision.
strabismus [stră-BĬZ-mŭs] Greek *strabismos*, a squinting	Eye misalignment.
sty, stye [stī] Old English *stigan*, to rise	Hordeolum.
tinnitus [tĭ-NĪ-tŭs, TĬ-nĭ-tŭs] Latin, a jingling	Constant ringing or buzzing in the ear.
trichiasis [trĭ-KĪ-ă-sĭs] trich-, hair + -iasis, condition	Abnormal growth of eyelashes in a direction that causes them to rub on the eye.
tympanitis [tĭm-pă-NĪ-tĭs] tympan-, eardrum + -itis	Inflammation of the eardrum.
vertigo [VĔR-tĭ-gō, vĕr-TĪ-gō] Latin	Dizziness.

CASE STUDY

Getting Treatment

After his 69th birthday, Mr. James noticed that his hearing had seriously diminished in the last year. His physician referred him to a specialist. It was found that Mr. James had a buildup of wax in his ear. After treatment, his hearing improved slightly, but not enough for Mr. James to feel comfortable.

Critical Thinking

51. What other condition might explain this patient's hearing loss?
52. What type of specialist should Mr. James be referred to?

PATHOLOGICAL TERMS EXERCISES

Sense the Diseases

For each of the diseases listed below, write A for eye, B for ear, or C for nose to indicate the organ associated with that disease.

53. conjunctivitis _____

54. cataract _____

55. nyctalopia _____

56. aerotitis media _____

57. presbyopia _____

58. allergic rhinitis _____

59. scotoma _____

60. nasosinusitis _____

61. Meniere's disease _____

Check Your Knowledge

Circle T for true or F for false.

62. A hordeolum is a sty. T F

63. The focusing of light rays behind the retina is myopia. T F

64. Myringitis is an inflammation of the tympanic membrane. T F

65. A chalazion is a nodular inflammation typically occurring in the nose. T F

66. Labyrinthitis occurs in the labyrinth of the eye. T F

Surgical Terms

Some of the sense organs require surgery at various times. Corneal transplants or **keratoplasty** may give or restore sight. Implantation of new sound wave devices may give or restore hearing. The eye, ear, and the nose are also the site of plastic surgery to correct congenital defects or the signs of aging. Microscopic laser surgery or microsurgery is often used to operate on the small, delicate sensory organs. Vision correction surgery is becoming quite common as advances in laser surgery make this possible.

Plastic surgery is used in **blepharoplasty,** eyelid repair; **otoplasty,** surgical repair of the outer ear; and **tympanoplasty,** eardrum repair. In some cases, removal of part of a sensory organ becomes necessary to treat a disorder or because a part has become damaged or cancerous.

Cataract extraction is the removal of a cloudy lens from the eye. It is usually followed by an *intraocular lens (IOL) implant,* during which an artificial lens is implanted to replace the natural lens of the eye that was removed. It is unusual for patients to be unable to tolerate the implant. When they do, however, special glasses are prescribed that allow the patient some, usually limited, sight. Ultrasound can be used to break up and remove cataracts in **phacoemulsification.** A **dacryocystectomy** is the removal of a lacrimal sac. **Enucleation** is the removal of an eyeball. **Iridectomy** is removal of part of the iris. A **trabeculectomy** is an incision into and removal of part of the trabeculae to allow aqueous humor to flow freely around the eye. An **iridotomy** is an incision into the iris to allow aqueous humor to flow from the posterior to the anterior chambers. Correction of nearsightedness is also available with a laser procedure that changes the curvature of the cornea by making spokelike incisions around it. A retina can tear or become detached due to a trauma. **Cryoretinopexy** or *cryopexy* is the use of extreme cold to repair the damage to the retina, which can also be repaired using laser surgery.

In the ear, hearing can sometimes be aided by a **stapedectomy,** removal of the stapes to correct otosclerosis and insertion of tissue to substitute for a damaged stapes. A **myringotomy** is the insertion of a small, polyethylene (PE or pressure-equalizing) tube to help drain fluid, thereby relieving some of the symptoms of otitis media. This operation is done frequently on infants and children with recurring ear infections. In addition, cochlear implants can now help deaf people hear and are used increasingly for deaf children.

VOCABULARY REVIEW

In the previous section, you learned terms relating to surgery. Before going on to the exercises, review the terms below and refer to the previous section if you have any questions. Pronunciations are provided for certain terms. Sometimes information about where the word came from is included after the term. The etymologies (word histories) are for your information only. You do not need to memorize them.

Term	Meaning
blepharoplasty [BLĔF-ă-rō-plăst-ē] blepharo-, eyelid + -plasty, repair	Surgical repair of the eyelid.
cryoretinopexy [krī-ō-rĕ-tĭn-nō-PĔKS-ē] cryo-, cold + retino-, retina + -pexy, a fixing	Fixing of a torn retina using extreme cold.
dacryocystectomy [dăk-rē-ō-sĭs-TĔK-tō-mē] dacryo-, lacrimal gland + cyst + -ectomy, removal	Removal of a lacrimal sac.
enucleation [ē-nū-klē-Ā-shŭn] From Latin *enucleo*, to remove the kernel	Removal of an eyeball.
iridectomy [ĭr-ĭ-DĔK-tō-mē] irid-, iris + -ectomy	Removal of part of the iris.
iridotomy [ĭr-ĭ-DŎT-ō-mē] irido-, iris + -tomy, a cutting	Incision into the iris to relieve pressure.
keratoplasty [KĔR-ă-tō-plăs-tē] kerato-, cornea + -plasty	Corneal transplant.
myringotomy [mĭr-ĭng-GŎT-ō-mē] myringo-, middle ear + -tomy	Insertion of a small tube to help drain fluid from the ears (particularly of children).
otoplasty [Ō-tō-plăs-tē] oto-, ear + -plasty	Surgical repair of the outer ear.
phacoemulsification [FĀ-kō-ē-mŭls-ĭ-fĭ-KĀ-shŭn] phaco-, lens + emulsification	Use of ultrasound to break up and remove cataracts.
stapedectomy [stā-pĕ-DĔK-tō-mē] stapes + -ectomy	Removal of the stapes to cure otosclerosis.
trabeculectomy [tră-BĔK-yū-LĔK-tō-mē] trabecul(um) + -ectomy	Removal of part of the trabeculum to allow aqueous humor to flow freely around the eye.
tympanoplasty [TĬM-pă-nō-plăs-tē] tympano- + -plasty	Repair of an eardrum.

Check Your Knowledge

Fill in the blanks.

67. A patient sustaining a third-degree burn to the pinna would likely require _____.

68. A stapedectomy would be performed to correct _____.

69. Cryoretinopexy would be performed to correct a _____ retina.

70. A corneal _____ may restore sight.

71. A child with chronic otitis media may need a _____.

CASE STUDY

Getting Help

Mr. James's great grandson came for a few days' visit with his mother. The two-year-old had had fairly frequent ear infections, but they seemed to have subsided for a month or two, so his mother decided to risk the overnight stay. The boy woke up screaming and clutching his ear. A local 24-hour clinic diagnosed severe otitis media and prescribed medication. When the boy returned home, his pediatrician wrote the note below in his medical record.

Critical Thinking

72. Is the child's otitis media infectious for Mr. James?

73. Why did the doctor suggest a myringotomy?

Patient name *Everett James*	Age *2*	Current Diagnosis _____
DATE/TIME 3/3/XXXX	*Notes: Frequent otitis media (7 times in the last 11 months). Suggest myringotomy. (Note: schedule during mother's work vacation 5/4–5/11.)*	
	J. Redpine, M.D.	

Pharmacological Terms

Eyes and ears can both be treated with the *instillation* of drops. *Antibiotic ophthalmic solution* is an antibacterial agent used to treat eye infections, such as conjunctivitis. A **mydriatic** solution dilates the pupil during an eye examination. A **miotic** solution causes the pupil to contract. The eye and the ear can both be *irrigated*, flushed with water or solution to remove foreign objects. *Ear irrigation* (*lavage*) is the irrigation of the ear canal to remove excessive cerumen buildup. Antibiotics, antihistamines, anti-inflammatories, and decongestants are used to relieve ear infections, allergies, inflammations, and congestion. Table 16-2 lists various medications used for disorders of the senses.

TABLE 16-2 Medications Used to Treat Disorders of the Senses

Drug Class	Purpose	Generic	Trade Name
antiseptic ear drops	to cleanse ears by dispelling earwax	isopropyl alcohol carbamide peroxide	Aqua Ear, Swim Ear Murine Ear Drops
anti-inflammatory ear drops	to reduce ear inflammation	hydrocortisone	Cortane-B, VoSol
eye drops	to reduce eye congestion	tetrahydrozoline	Murine, Visine
eye moisturizer	to moisten eyes	cyclosporine carboxymethylcellulose	Restasis Refresh Plus
miiotic	contraction of the pupil	carbachol	Isopto Carbachol, Miostat
mydriatic	dilation of the pupil	atropine tropicamide	Atropisol Mydriacil
nasal decongestant	to reduce nasal congestion	pseudoephredrine xylometazoline	Drixoral, Sudafed Otrivin

VOCABULARY REVIEW

In the previous section, you learned terms relating to pharmacology. Before going on to the exercises, review the terms below and refer to the previous section if you have any questions. Pronunciations are provided for certain terms. Sometimes information about where the word came from is included after the term. The etymologies (word histories) are for your information only. You do not need to memorize them.

Term	Meaning
miotic [mī-ŎT-ĭk] From Greek *meion*, less	Agent that causes the pupil to contract.
mydriatic [mĭ-drē-ĂT-ĭk] Greek *mydriasis*, excessive pupil dilation	Agent that causes the pupil to dilate.

CASE STUDY

Making Progress

When his great grandson came to visit the following year, Mr. James was hearing better with the help of a hearing aid. His eyesight was nearly perfect, and at age 70, he was happy to remain independent. His great-grandson's operation had proved effective. The boy had gone for about 10 months without any ear inflammations. On the second day of the visit, however, the boy started rubbing his eyes and complained of itching. His mother noticed a reddish area around the edge of his eyelid.

Critical Thinking

74. What was the likely cause of the child's itchy eyelids?
75. Is it surprising that Mr. James, who played with his great grandson frequently, developed the same condition five days later?

PHARMACOLOGICAL TERMS EXERCISES

Check Your Knowledge

Fill in the blanks.

76. What medication might be prescribed for conjunctivitis? _____

77. During an eye exam, what agent helps to open a part of the eye for better viewing? _____

78. What medication might be prescribed for otitis media? _____

CHALLENGE SECTION

Look at the letter below.

Critical Thinking

79. What eye conditions does this diabetic patient have?

80. What condition does he have that is probably not caused by diabetes?

Dr. Janet Maitland
3000 Blue Willow Lane
Forest Park, IL 99999
999-000-5555

5/6/XXXX

William Gonzalez, M.D.
7 Steele Drive
Forest Park, IL 99999
999-000-5444

Dear Dr. Gonzalez:

I was happy to evaluate our mutual patient, Joseph Consalvo, with regards to his recent Plaquenil prescription.

IMPRESSION: I do not see any evidence of Plaquenil toxicity on his examination, although there is a fair amount of macular disease due to previous diabetic retinopathy and subsequent laser therapy. He has recovered well from his cataract surgery, and his vision has returned to the expected level.

RECOMMENDATION: I think that I would continue to monitor him for problems every four to six months, both in regard to Plaquenil and with regard to his history of relatively severe nonproliferative diabetic retinopathy. We made an appointment for an examination after this period of time and he is to report any sudden changes in his vision to me directly.

I hope this information is helpful. Please let me know if I can be of any further help.

Sincerely,

Janet Maitland, M.D.

Janet Maitland, M.D.

JM/lrc

TERMINOLOGY IN ACTION

This prescription is for eyeglasses for a 55-year-old woman. What condition or conditions are being corrected?

Dr. Arif Namoun
North Street Eye Center
Greenville, OK 99999
999 000-5555

NAME _Susan Carver_   DATE _1/16/XXXX_

℞

	SPH.	CYL.	AXIS	PRISM	Remarks
R	300	-100	180	20/200	
L	-2.00	+.75	005	20/50	

	ADD
R	+2.50
L	+2.50

☒ Arif Namoun, M.D.

EXPIRES _6/XXXX_   _Arif Namoun, M.D._
IL. LIC. NO. 7yytt8

USING THE INTERNET

Go to the site of the American Society of Cataract and Refractive Surgery (http://www.ascrs.org). Write a brief description of any discussion of cataracts, including what type of surgery is available.

CHAPTER REVIEW

The material that follows is to help you review all the material in this chapter.

Build Your Medical Vocabulary

Divide each of the following terms into words parts and define them; then define the term. Use the information from Chapters 2 and 3 to help you.

81. corectopia: _____

82. keratoscope: _____

83. tympanitis: _____

84. blepharedema: _____

85. dacryolith: _____

86. optometry: _____

87. ossiculotomy: _____

88. scotoma: _____

89. auricular: _____

90. phacomalacia: _____

91. lacrimonasal: _____

92. cerumenosis: _____

93. cycloplegia: _____

94. uveoscleritis: _____

95. myringoplasty: _____

96. ophthalmalgia: _____

97. mastoidectomy: _____

98. retinopexy: _____

99. audiology: _____

100. iridopathy: _____

101. scleroconjunctival: _____

102. nasolacrimal: _____

103. cochleitis: _____

104. pupilloscope: _____

105. conjunctivitis: _____

106. iritis: _____

DEFINITIONS

Define and pronounce the following terms. The blue words in curly brackets are references to the Spanish glossary available online at www.mhhe.com/medterm3e.

WORD

107. aerotitis media [ār-ō-TĪ-tĭs MĒ-dē-ă]

108. anacusis [ăn-ă-KŪ-sĭs] {anacusia}

109. aphakia [ă-FĀ-kē-ă] {afaquia}

110. asthenopia [ăs-thĕ-NŌ-pē-ă] {astenopía}

111. astigmatism [ă-STĬG-mă-tĭzm] {astimagtismo}

112. audi(o), audit(o)

113. audiogram [ĂW-dē-ō-grăm] {audiograma}

114. audiologist [ăw-dē-ŎL-ō-jĭst] {audiólogo}

115. audiometry [ăw-dē-ŎM-ĕ-trē] {audiometría}

116. auditory ossicles [ĂW-dĭ-tōr-ē ŎS-ĭ-klz]

117. aur(o), auricul(o)

118. auricle [ĂW-rĭ-kl] {auricular}

119. blephar(o)

120. blepharitis [blĕf-ă-RĪ-tĭs] {blefaritis}

121. blepharochalasis [blĕf-ă-rō-KĂL-ă-sĭs]

122. blepharoplasty [BLĔF-ă-rō-plăst-ē]

123. blepharoptosis [blĕf-ă-RŎP-tō-sĭs]

124. blepharospasm [BLĔF-ă-rō-spăzm]

125. blindness {ceguera}

126. cataract [CĂT-ă-răkt] {catarata}

127. cerumin(o)

128. chalazion [kă-LĀ-zē-ŏn] {chalazión}

129. cholesteatoma [kō-lĕs-tē-ă-TŌ-mă]

130. choroid [KŌ-rŏyd] {coroides}

131. ciliary [SĬL-ē-ăr-ē] body

132. cochle(o)

133. cochlea [KŌK-lē-ă] {caracol}

134. cones [kōnz] {conos}

135. conjunctiv(o)

136. conjunctiva (pl., conjunctivae) [kŏn-JŬNK-tĭ-vă (-vē)] {conjuntiva}
137. conjunctivitis [kŏn-jŭnk-tĭ-VĪ-tĭs] {conjunctivitis}
138. contact lenses
139. cor(o), core(o)
140. corne(o)
141. cornea [KŌR-nē-ă] {cornea}
142. cryoretinopexy [krī-ō-rĕ-tĭn-nō-PĔKS-ē]
143. cycl(o)
144. dacry(o)
145. dacryoadenitis [DĂK-rē-ō-ăd-ĕ-NĪ-tĭs]
146. dacryocystectomy [dăk-rē-ō-sĭs-TĔK-tō-mē]
147. dacryocystitis [DĂK-rē-ō-sĭs-TĪ-tĭs]
148. deafness {sordera}
149. decibel [DĔS-ĭ-bĕl] {decibel}
150. dermatochalasis [DĔR-mă-tō-kă-LĀ-sĭs] {dermatocalasia}
151. diopter [dī-ŎP-tĕr]
152. diplopia [dĭ-PLŌ-pē-ă] {diplopía}
153. ear [ēr] {oreja, oído}
154. eardrum [ĒR-drŭm] {tambor de oído}
155. endolymph [ĔN-dō-lĭmf] {endolinfa}
156. enucleation [ē-nū-klē-Ā-shŭn] {enucleación}
157. epiphora [ĕ-PĬF-ō-ră] {epífora}
158. equilibrium [ē-kwĭ-LĬB-rē-ŭm] {equilibrio}
159. esotropia [ĕs-ō-TRŌ-pē-ă] {esotropía}
160. eustachian [yū-STĀ-shŭn, yū-STĀ-kē-ăn] tube
161. exophthalmos, exophthalmus [ĕk-sŏf-THĂL-mōs]
162. exotropia [ĕk-sō-TRŌ-pē-ă]

163. eye [ī] {ojo}
164. eyebrow [Ī-brŏw] {ceja}
165. eyelashes [Ī-lăsh-ĕz] {pestañas}
166. eyelid [Ī-lĭd] {párpado}
167. eyestrain {vista fatigada}
168. farsightedness {hiperopía}
169. fovea centralis [FŌ-vē-ă sĕn-TRĂL-ĭs]
170. glaucoma [glăw-KŌ-mă] {glaucoma}
171. hearing {audición}
172. hordeolum [hōr-DĒ-ō-lŭm] {orzuelo}
173. hyperopia [hī-pĕr-Ō-pē-ă]
174. incus [ĬN-kŭs] {incus}
175. ir(o), irid(o)
176. iridectomy [ĭr-ĭ-DĔK-tō-mē] {iridectomía}
177. iridotomy [ĭr-ĭ-DŎT-ō-mē]
178. iris [Ī-rĭs] {iris}
179. iritis [ī-RĪ-tĭs] {iritis}
180. kerat(o)
181. keratitis [kĕr-ă-TĪ-tĭs] {queratitis}
182. keratoplasty [KĔR-ă-tō-plăs-tē] {queratoplastia}
183. labyrinthitis [LĂB-ĭ-rĭn-THĪ-tĭs] {laberintitis}
184. lacrim(o)
185. lacrimal [LĂK-rĭ-măl] glands
186. lacrimation [lăk-rĭ-MĀ-shŭn] {lagrimeo}
187. lens [lĕnz] {lens, lente}
188. macula [MĂK-yū-lă] {macula}
189. macula lutea [lū-TĒ-ă]
190. macular [MĂK-yū-lăr] degeneration
191. malleus [MĂL-ē-ŭs] {malleus}
192. mastoid(o)
193. mastoiditis [măs-tŏy-DĪ-tĭs]
194. membranous labyrinth [LĂB-ĭ-rĭnth]

195. Meniere's [mĕn-YĒRZ] disease
196. miotic [mī-ŎT-ĭk]
197. mydriatic [mĭ-drē-ĂT-ĭk]
198. myopia [mī-Ō-pē-ă] {miopía}
199. myring(o)
200. myringitis [mĭr-ĭn-JĪ-tĭs] {miringitis}
201. myringotomy [mĭr-ĭng-GŎT-ŏ-mē]
202. nas(o)
203. nearsightedness {miopía}
204. neuroretina [nūr-ō-RĔT-ĭ-nă]
205. nyctalopia [nĭk-tă-LŌ-pē-ă] {nictalopía}
206. nystagmus [nĭs-STĂG-mŭs] {nistagmo}
207. ocul(o)
208. olfactory [ōl-FĂK-tō-rē] organs
209. ophthalm(o)
210. ophthalmologist [ŏf-thăl-MŎL-ō-jĭst] {oftalmólogo}
211. ophthalmoscopy [ŏf-thăl-MŎS-kō-pē] {oftalmoscopia}
212. opt(o), optic(o)
213. optician [ŏp-TĬSH-ŭn]
214. optic nerve
215. optometrist [ŏp-TŎM-ĕ-trĭst] {optometrista}
216. organ of Corti [KŌR-tī]
217. osseus [ŎS-sē-ŭs] labyrinth
218. ossicul(o)
219. otalgia [ō-TĂL-jē-ă] {otalgia}
220. otitis externa [ō-TĪ-tĭs ĕks-TĔR-nă] {otitis externa}
221. otitis media [MĒ-dē-ă] {otitis media}
222. otoliths [Ō-tō-lĭths] {otolitos}
223. otologist [ō-TŎL-ō-jĭst] {otólogo}
224. otoplasty [Ō-tō-plăs-tē] {otoplastia}

225. otorhinolaryngologist [ō-tō-rī-nō-lăr-ĭng-GŎL-ō-jĭst]

226. otorrhagia [ō-tō-RĀ-jē-ă] {otorragia}

227. otorrhea [ō-tō-RĒ-ă] {otorrea}

228. otosclerosis [ō-tō-sklĕ-RŌ-sĭs] {otosclerosis}

229. otoscopy [ō-TŎS-kō-pē] {otoscopia}

230. papillae [pă-PĬL-ē] {papilas}

231. paracusis [PĂR-ă-KŪ-sĭs] {paracusia}

232. perilymph [PĔR-ĭ-lĭmf]

233. phac(o), phak(o)

234. phacoemulsification [FĀ-kō-ē-mŭls-ĭ-fĭ-KĀ-shŭn]

235. photophobia [fō-tō-FŌ-bē-ă] {fotofobia}

236. pinkeye [PĬNK-Ī]

237. pinna [PĬN-ă]

238. presbyacusis [prĕz-bē-ă-KŪ-sĭs] {presbiacusia}

239. presbyopia [prĕz-bē-Ō-pē-ă] {presbiopía}

240. pseudophakia [sū-dō-FĀ-kē-ă] {seudofaquia}

241. pupil [PYŪ-pĭl] {pupila}

242. pupill(o)

243. refraction [rē-FRĂK-shŭn] {refracción}

244. retin(o)

245. retina [RĔT-ĭ-nă] {retina}

246. retinitis [rĕt-ĭ-NĪ-tĭs] {retinitis}

247. retinitis pigmentosa [pĭg-mĕn-TŌ-să]

248. rods [rŏdz] {bastoncillos}

249. scler(o)

250. sclera (pl., sclerae) [SKLĒR-ă (SKLĒR-ē)] {sclera}

251. scleritis [sklĕ-RĪ-tĭs] {escleritis}

252. scot(o)

253. scotoma [skō-TŌ-mă] {escotoma}

254. semicircular canals

255. sensory receptors

256. sensory system

257. sight {vista}

258. smell {olfacción, oler}

259. stapedectomy [stā-pē-DĔK-tō-mē]

260. stapes (pl., stapes, stapedes) [STĀ-pēz (STĀ-pē-dēz)] {estribo}

261. strabismus [stră-BĬZ-mŭs] {estrabismo}

262. sty, stye [stī] {orzuelo}

263. taste

264. taste buds

265. taste cells

266. tears [tērz] {lágrimas}

267. tinnitus [tĭ-NĪ-tŭs, TĬ-nĭ-tŭs] {tinnitus}

268. tonometry [tō-NŎM-ĕ-trē] {tonometría}

269. touch {tacto}

270. trabeculectomy [tră-BĔK-yū-LĔK-tō-mē]

271. trichiasis [tri-KĪ-ă-sĭs]

272. tympan(o)

273. tympanic [tĭm-PĂN-ĭk] membrane

274. tympanitis [tĭm-pă-NĪ-tĭs]

275. tympanoplasty [TĬM-pă-nō-plăs-tē]

276. uve(o)

277. uvea [YŪ-vē-ă] {úvea}

278. vertigo [VĔR-tĭ-gō, vĕr-TĪ-gō] {vértigo}

279. vestibule [VĔS-tĭ-būl] {vestíbulo}

Abbreviations

Write the full meaning of each abbreviation.

280. acc.

281. AD

282. ARMD

283. AS

284. AU

285. D

286. dB

287. DVA

288. ECCE

289. EENT

290. ENT

291. ICCE

292. IOL

293. IOP

294. NVA

295. OD

296. OM

297. OS

298. OU

299. PERRL, PERRLA

300. PE tube

301. SOM

302. VA

303. VF

304. +

305. −

Answers to Chapter Exercises

1. None of the general tests showed abnormal results so Mr. James's problem needs further investigation.
2. Eye disease can be part of a systemic problem.
3. k
4. a
5. b
6. j
7. h
8. f
9. d
10. g
11. e
12. i
13. c
14. F
15. F
16. T
17. F
18. T
19. F
20. T
21. right eye
22. yes
23. otitis
24. optometer
25. otology
26. keratitis
27. keratometer
28. iridopathy
29. dacryocystalgia
30. coreoplasty
31. scleromalacia
32. sclerokeratitis
33. blepharedema
34. retinal
35. iridoplegia
36. otalgia
37. otology/audiology
38. blepharitis
39. otorrhagia
40. otometer/ audiometer
41. lens
42. No, the lens is inside the eye; the iris determines eye color.
43. B
44. B
45. B
46. A

47. B
48. A
49. A
50. A
51. nerve deafness of old age or other systemic condition such as an infection
52. otologist
53. A
54. A
55. A
56. B
57. A
58. C
59. A
60. C
61. B
62. T
63. F
64. T
65. F
66. F
67. otoplasty
68. otosclerosis
69. detached
70. transplant
71. myringotomy
72. No—it is an inflammation of the middle ear.
73. to relieve the recurring ear infections
74. conjunctivitis (pinkeye)
75. No, it is highly infectious.
76. antibiotic ophthalmic solution
77. mydriatic
78. antibiotic
79. diabetic retinopathy, cataracts
80. cataracts
81. cor(e)-, pupil; ectopia, abnormal location—abnormal location of the pupil (not in the center of the eye
82. kerat(o)-, cornea; -scope, instrument for examining—instrument for examining the cornea
83. tympan(o)-, tympanum, eardrum; -itis, inflammation—inflammation of the eardrum.
84. blephar(o)-, eyelid; edema, swelling—swelling of the eyelid

85. dacry(o)-, lacrymal (tear) duct or sac, -lith, stone—calculus (stone) in the tear gland or sac
86. opt(o)-, vision; -metry, process or method of measuring something—the specialty of examining and diagnosing certain vision disorders and providing preventive care and corrective lenses
87. ossicul(o)-, the ossicle; -tomy, cutting operation—surgical incision into one of the ossicles of the ear
88. scot(o)-, darkness; -oma, tumor, neoplasm—an area of diminished vision
89. auricul(o)-, hearing; -ar, of or relating to—of or relating to the ear
90. phac(o)-, lens; -malacia, softening—a softening of the lens of an eye
91. lacrim(o)-, tear; nasal, of or referring to the nose—concerning the nose and tear gland, duct, and sac
92. cerumin(o)-, earwax; -osis, disorder, condition—the overproduction of earwax
93. cycl(o)-, ciliary body; -plegia, paralysis—paralysis of the ciliary muscle
94. uve(o)-, uvea (middle layer of the eye); scler(o)-, sclera (white of the eye); -itis, inflammation—inflammation of the sclera that initially developed in the uvea
95. myring(o)-, eardrum, middle ear; -plasty, surgical repair—surgical repair of the middle ear
96. ophthalm(o)-, eye; -algia, pain—pain in the eye
97. mastoid(o)-, mastoid process of the ear; -ectomy, surgical removal—surgical removal of part of the mastoid process
98. retin(o)-, retina; -pexy, surgical repair—surgical repair of a detached retina
99. audi(o)- hearing; -logy, study of—the study of hearing disorders

100. irid(o)-, iris; -pathy, disease—disease of the iris
101. scler(o)-, sclera; conjunctiv(o)-, conjunctiva; -al, or or relating to—of or relating to the sclera and the conjunctiva
102. nas(o)-, the nose; lacrimal, relating to the tear glands or ducts—of or relating to the nose and the tear glands or ducts
103. cochle(o)-, cochlea; -itis, inflammation of—inflammation of the inner ear
104. pupill(o)-, the pupil; -scope, instrument for examining—instrument for examining the pupil
105. conjunctiv(o)-, conjunctiva; -itis, inflammation of—inflammation of the conjunctiva
106. ir(o)-, iris; -itis, inflammation—inflammation of the iris
107–305. Answers are available in the vocabulary reviews in this chapter.

CHAPTER
17

Human Development

▶ PEDIATRICS
▶ GERONTOLOGY

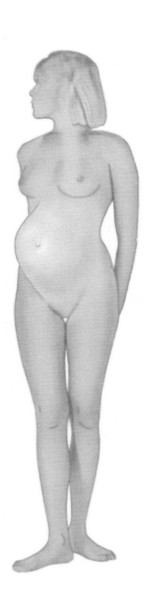

After studying this chapter, you will be able to

17.1 Describe each stage of human development

17.2 Name medical specialists that treat the disorders in each stage of the lifespan

17.3 List the diseases and disorders common to each stage of the lifespan

Stages of Development

The time between conception and death is the period of an individual's development. The average *lifespan* (length of life) varies from country to country. Each stage (see Table 17-1) is described in this chapter, as are the specialists who typically treat patients in a particular time in the lifespan. Pathology of the lifespan is also discussed.

Fertilization, Pregnancy, and Birth

Fertilization can occur as the result of sexual intercourse between a male and a female. It may also occur in a laboratory in cases of infertility. However it occurs, fertilization is the union of an egg cell (ovum) with a spermatozoon. (On occasion, more than one egg is fertilized by more than one sperm—producing fraternal twins or triplets—or a single egg divides into identical twins, triplets, quadruplets, and so on.) After traveling through the fallopian tube, the fertilized ovum (also called a *zygote)* is **implanted** or attached to the wall of the uterus. Once attached, the ovum (now called an **embryo** until it reaches 2 1/2 months or 10 weeks) remains *in utero,* or within the uterus, until development and birth. It takes an average of 40 weeks from the time that the ovum is fertilized until birth. This period of development is known as **gestation.** The embryo begins to change during the first 8 weeks of gestation. After 2 1/2 months, the embryo becomes a **fetus,** the developing product of conception prior to birth. For the mother, the 40-week period of gestation is the period known as *pregnancy.* Chapters 10 and 11 cover the female and male reproductive systems.

The birth process usually includes a period of **labor,** the process of expelling the fetus and the placenta from the uterus. Labor may end in a vaginal birth. If not, a **cesarean section,** removal of the fetus surgically through the abdomen, is performed. The reasons for performing a cesarean section vary widely, but may include fetal or maternal distress, complications (as in multiple births or premature birth), or extended labor without adequate dilation of the cervix. The fetus, in the majority of circumstances, is in a *cephalic* position

TABLE 17-1 Stages of Human Development

Lifespan Period	Average Time	Developmental Characteristics
fetus	period from 10 weeks of gestation to birth	development of all body systems that are present at birth
neonate	first 4 weeks of infancy	adjustment to life outside the uterus
infancy	first year of life	many physical and emotional developmental strides
toddler	ages 1 to 3	walking, talking, and becoming somewhat independent from caretakers
childhood	ages 3 to puberty	cognitive and physical development, usually including schooling
puberty	about ages 8 to 12	development of secondary sex characteristics
adolescence	period from puberty to full physical maturity	physical maturation and often psychological separation from the family leading to independence
young adulthood	ages 20–39	period of establishment of adult work and lifestyle situations
middle adulthood	ages 40–59	often stressful period of continued career and family development
old age	ages 60 on	period of diminishing physical and, sometimes, mental faculties
oldest old age	ages 90 on	period of late life, often with many physical and emotional difficulties
death	end of life	cessation of cardiovascular, respiratory, and nervous system functions

or head down in the birth canal. A fetus may be positioned in a **breech** position (infant in birth canal with feet or buttocks first) or may be *transverse,* sideways. *Obstetricians,* specialists in **obstetrics,** which includes fertility, pregnancy, and birth, assist in the vaginal birth of a breech baby, or turn a transverse baby so that it can be born vaginally. A breech or tranverse baby cannot exit the vagina without being harmed unless it is maneuvered into a position to allow it to come through the birth canal. Often, infants in such positions are at risk during the birth process and are much more likely to be born by cesarean section. Figure 17-1 shows cephalic and breech birth positions.

The period of time immediately after the birth (parturition) of the infant is known as *postpartum.* During this time, a woman may begin to experience a number of symptoms such as sadness, lack of energy, trouble concentrating, anxiety, and feelings of guilt and worthlessness. If these symptoms occur during anytime within the first year after childbirth, it is known as *postpartum depression.* The difference between postpartum depression and the baby blues is that postpartum depression often affects a woman's well-being and keeps her from functioning well for a longer period of time. Postpartum depression needs to be treated by a doctor. Counseling, support groups, and medicines are things that can help. *Postpartum psychosis* is rare. It occurs in 1 or 2 out of every 1000 births and usually begins in

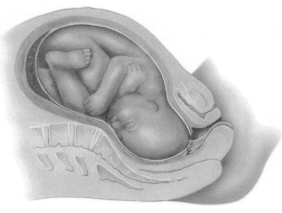 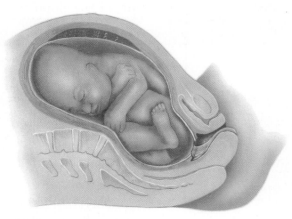

(a) Cephalic presentation

(b) Breech presentation

FIGURE 17-1   Birth position can determine whether a birth is vaginal or by caesarean section. Cephalic presentation **(a)** is usually vaginal. Breech presentation **(b)** is often by caesarean section.

the first 6 weeks postpartum. Women who have bipolar disorder or another psychiatric problem called schizoaffective disorder have a higher risk for developing postpartum psychosis.

Infancy

To read more about the Apgar score, go to www.childbirth.org.

A baby, also referred to as a newborn or *infant,* is born. At birth, personnel in the delivery room give the baby an **Apgar score,** a rating at both 1 and 5 minutes after birth for the following: A (activity); P (pulse); G (grimace or reflex); A (appearance of the skin); and R (respiration). The scoring is from 1 to 10. A total score of 7–10 is considered normal; below that, there may be need for special help from medical personnel.

For the first four weeks of life, the infant is referred to as a **neonate** (Figure 17-2). During the neonate period, body functions adjust to living outside the womb: temperature control, digestive system, respiratory system, sensory system, and the beginning of social development all start to change during this period. **Neonatology** is the medical specialty concerned with the care and treatment of neonates with severe health problems or who may have been born prematurely. *Neonatologists* are specialists in neonatology.

The remainder of the infancy period lasts the first year. During the next period, the child is often referred to as a *toddler.* The toddler is a young child who becomes competent at walking, begins to speak, and begins to handle some of the activities of daily living by himself or herself. This occurs in the period between the end of the first year and age three. **Pediatrics** is the specialty that treats children from the neonate stage through adolescence. *Pediatricians* are the practitioners of this specialty.

Childhood

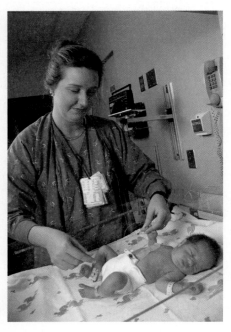

FIGURE 17-2   A neonate is an infant under 4 weeks old.

Childhood is the period of life from infancy to puberty. *Puberty* is a sequence of development of secondary sex characteristics beginning around ages 8 to 12. Childhood years vary because puberty may start very early or very late. Also, the onset of puberty is generally earlier in girls than in boys.

Adolescence

Adolescence is the period of physical maturation, usually between ages 13 and 19. During this time, the secondary sex characteristics fully develop (girls develop breasts, underarm hair, and pubic hair; boys develop facial hair, pubic hair, and underarm hair, and go through a voice change). It is the period when most people start to take the emotional steps that will lead them to be independent of their parents. Adolescents often experience the conflict of being more physically mature than emotionally ready to handle such things as pregnancy and parenthood.

Adulthood

Young adulthood comprises the period from ages 20 to 40. This is usually the period in which adults set up their first homes, become parents, and build their careers. Middle adulthood or *middle age* is the period from ages 40 to 60. Young adults may choose an internist or family practitioner as their primary physician. Many people start to look at alternative or preventive medicine at this stage of their lives (see Chapter 23). During middle adulthood, many physical changes (i.e., menopause, diminution of strength, reduction in hearing ability) occur. Middle adulthood is often the time that disorders are discovered and treatments are begun.

Old Age

Old age, also known as the **geriatric** period, begins at age 60 (or at age 65 depending on who is defining the age groups) and encompasses the years until death. The period of old age is sometimes further divided into *young old* (ages 60-74); *middle old* (75-84) and *oldest old* (ages 85 and older). The quality of life in old age usually reflects your family's genetic history, general health, and emotional attitudes. Some people live well into their 90s or early 100s independently and in good health. People who have such longevity, length of life beyond the average, are often referred to as the oldest old (Figure 17-3). Others may have heart attacks or other illnesses during middle age that lead to an old age that includes many periods of illness and may even include early death. **Gerontology** is the medical specialty that diagnoses and treats disorders present in old age. Gerontologists are specialists in treating ailments of the aging.

Death

Death, the end of life, occurs when the heart, respiratory system, and central nervous system cease functioning. This definition of death is being changed by life-support machines that are able to keep someone with respiratory or other body failure alive indefinitely. Because of the controversies surrounding the use of life-support machines near the end of life, several legal changes have been made in recent years. The actively dying body, without the aid of life support systems, will passes through predictable and symptoms and signs as the systems of the body decline. Palliative measures are comfort measures to provide pain relief comfort as this process progresses.

The practice of **euthanasia,** or assisted suicide, is allowed in certain countries in the world. In the United States, most states forbid this method

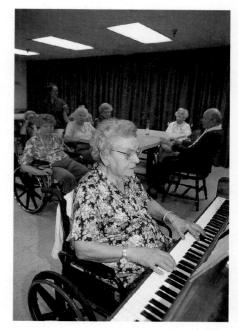

FIGURE 17-3 A 101-year-old woman playing piano in a nursing home.

of helping very sick people die comfortably. The field of *bioethics*, study of ethical medical treatment and research, has grown in the last part of the twentieth century.

Many people express their wishes regarding care at the end of life. Two legal documents called *advanced directives* state the patient's wishes about decisions for future health care. The first directive, a *living will*, is signed by a patient who prefers to be allowed to die rather than be kept alive by artificial means if there is no reasonable expectation of recovery. The second is a *durable power of attorney*, a document which appoints a *health care proxy*, a person to make decisions for the patient in case of disability. These directives may also include a *DNR* (do not resuscitate) order, which means that the patient is not to be resuscitated if breathing stops at a certain stage of illness. The movement toward *hospice*, a program of supportive care for dying patients in a nonhospital setting, has spread to all parts of the country. Hospice provides end-of-life pain relief (called *palliation*) and care (called *palliative care*), but does not try to artificially prolong life or resuscitate a patient who has stopped breathing.

VOCABULARY REVIEW

In the previous section, you learned terms about stages of development. Before going on to the exercises, review the terms below and refer to the previous section if you have any questions. Pronunciations are provided for certain terms. Sometimes information about where the word came from is included after the term. The etymologies (word histories) are for your information only. You do not need to memorize them.

Term	Definition
Apgar score After Virginia Apgar [ĂP-găr] (1909-1974), U.S. physician	A rating of a newborn's Activity, Pulse, Grimace, Appearance, and Respiration.
breech [brēch]	Birth canal position with feet or buttocks first.
cesarean [sĕ-ZĀ-rē-ăn] **section** From Latin *lex caesaria*, Roman law	Surgical removal of the fetus through the abdomen.
embryo [ĔM-brē-ō] Greek *embryon*	Fertilized ovum until about 10 weeks of gestation.
euthanasia [yū-thă-NĀ-zhē-ă] eu-, good + Greek *thanatos*, death	Assisting in the suicide of or putting a person with an incurable or painful disease to death.
fertilization [FĔR-tĭl-ĭ-ZĀ-shŭn]	Union of an egg cell(s) with sperm.
fetus [FĒ-tŭs]	Developing product of conception from 8 weeks to birth.
geriatric [JĔR-ē-Ă-trĭk]	Of or relating to old age.
gerontology [JĔR-ŏn-TŎL-ō-jē] geronto-, old age + -logy, study of	Medical specialty that diagnoses and treats disorders of old age.
gestation [jĕs-TĀ-shŭn] Latin *gestation*	Period of fetal development from fertilization until delivery.

Term	Definition
implant [ĭm-PLĂNT]	To attach to the lining of the uterus in the first stage of pregnancy.
labor [LĀ-bōr]	Process of expelling the fetus and placenta from the uterus.
neonate [NĒ-ō-nāt] neo-, new + Latin *natus*, born	Infant under 4 weeks old.
neonatology [NĒ-ō-nā-TŎL-ō-jē] neonat(e) + -logy	Medical specialty that diagnoses and treats disorders of neonates.
obstetrics [ŏb-STĔT-rĭks]	Medical specialty that guides women throughout fertilization, pregnancy, and birth.
pediatrics [PĒ-dē-ĂT-rĭks] From Greek *pais*, child + *iatrikos*, of medicine	Medical specialty that diagnoses and treats disorders in children from infancy through adolescence.

CASE STUDY

Spanning the Generations

Maria and Paul Adams were overjoyed upon discovering Maria's pregnancy at age 36. Maria's mother had had her children later in life. She was now turning 77, living alone since her husband died. Maria and Paul are part of what is called the "sandwich" generation—those people caring for their young children and their older parents at the same time. Maria's mother had a myocardial infarction a few years ago. She lives in the same town as Maria, who does her grocery shopping, takes her to doctors, and visits with her about four times a week. Maria also works as a systems analyst. Her paycheck is important to the couple, and Maria plans to go back to work after several months of pregnancy leave.

Critical Thinking

1. What stages of life will Maria and her child be going through simultaneously?
2. Will Paul and Maria need a neonatologist for their child?

STAGES OF DEVELOPMENT EXERCISES

Know the Lifespan

Write the stage of development of lifespan period(s) that best fits each description or profession.

3. In utero _____

4. Neonatologist _____

5. Secondary sex characteristics _____

6. First walking _____

7. Early schooling _____

8. Cessation of body functions _____

9. Establishment of adult work _____

10. Physical maturation _____

11. Two weeks old _____

12. Obstetrician _____

13. Gerontologist _____

Pathology of the Lifespan

The majority of diseases occur at the beginning (infancy) and at the end (old age) of life. Diseases or disorders may be determined or caused by genes (biological inheritance), environmental causes (as exposure to a virus or bacteria), or trauma (sudden, massive injury). A *geneticist* is a specialist in **genetics** (the science of biological inheritance) who can counsel people with genetic abnormalities who wish to have children. Some congenital diseases (severe spina bifida, anencephaly) are devastating. In some cases, geneticists can predict the odds of the newborn inheriting a gene. It is also possible to observe (via ultrasound) the fetus during its development. Fetuses are treated **in utero** (while in the uterus), either with medication or surgically, for a number of conditions. In addition, blood tests reveal genetic clues to disorders carried by the parents (Figure 17-4).

Table 17-2 lists some diseases common to the various stages of the lifespan. Some of these diseases appear at all stages of the lifespan, but occur most frequently in a particular stage.

TABLE 17-2   Pathology in Human Development

Lifespan Period	Average Time	Some Diseases Most Prevalent at Each Stage (See body systems chapters for further discussion of pathology)
fetus	during 40 weeks of gestation	hydrocephaly, spina bifida, Rh incompatibility (erythroblastosis fetalis)
neonate	first 4 weeks of infancy	jaundice, diarrhea, allergies, SIDS, hydrocephaly, spina bifida, premature birth, hyaline membrane disease, Down syndrome, Tay-Sach's disease, sickle cell anemia, pyloric stenosis
infancy	first year of life	Down syndrome, SIDS, otitis media, strep throat, allergies, diarrhea
toddler	ages 1 to 3	otitis media, strep throat, roseola, allergies, diarrhea
childhood	ages 3 to puberty	strep throat, otitis media, and if not vaccinated, measles, mumps, chicken pox, polio
puberty	about ages 8 to 12	same as during childhood
adolescence	period from puberty to full physical maturity	some childhood diseases, plus emotional problems (such as depression and anxiety)
young adulthood	ages 20-39	schizophrenia, multiple sclerosis, early cancers (prostate, cervical, uterine, and breast)
middle adulthood	ages 40-59	heart disease, stroke, cancer, Parkinson's disease, Alzheimer's disease, osteoporosis
old age	ages 60 on	same as middle adulthood plus senile dementia, depression
oldest old age	ages 90 on	same as old age
death	end of life	cessation of cardiovascular, respiratory, and nervous system functions

Diseases of Infancy and Childhood

Neonates born **prematurely,** after less than 37 weeks of gestation, often have underdeveloped lungs and other problems. Advances in neonatology save many premature infants. Birth after 40 weeks of gestation may also cause or indicate fetal problems, including high fetal weight.

Infants may die suddenly in an unknown manner (**sudden infant death syndrome** or **SIDS**), usually while sleeping. Safety measures that can prevent some suffocation deaths and/or respiratory problems are to place the infant on its back to sleep, avoid pillows or stuffed animals in the crib, and to avoid smoking in the house. Infants may also experience trauma (as in falls) or may contract infections (such as streptococcus or strep throat).

As children grow, they experience many of the diseases of the body systems covered in each of the body systems chapters in this book. Some childhood diseases help to strengthen the immune system for later life. For example, a childhood bout with chicken pox usually offers lifelong immunity against a disease that can have much more devastating effects in older people.

The March of Dimes (www.modimes. org) raises awareness about and raises money for research on birth defects.

Go to the American SIDS Institute's Web site (www.sids.org) and find out what current research has concluded about SIDS.

Diseases of Adulthood

Middle age is often the period during which the stress and wear and tear of daily life begin to take their toll. In this period, particularly, an unhealthy lifestyle can bring on major diseases. A high-fat diet can raise cholesterol, a major risk factor for coronary artery disease. Smoking increases the risk of heart disease and lung cancer. Lack of exercise can be a major factor in cardiovascular disease. Many diseases in this period can be prevented with systematic attention to lifestyle issues and to early warning tests, such as mammograms and PSA tests. The diseases of middle age usually worsen in the next stage of life.

Diseases of Old Age

Most of the pathology in life takes place in old age, with the wearing down of bone, the weakening of the musculoskeletal structure, and the diminishing of the central nervous system. Many doctors and patients focus on **preventive medicine,** a medical specialty concerned with preventing disease. Prevention may include lifestyle changes, medications (as tamoxifen for women with a family history of breast cancer), or frequent checkups (as for people with previous cancers). Newer drugs based on stem cells are helping to cure or manage some devastating diseases.

At the end of life, death is declared by a medical person. The exact definition of death varies but most states use the standards set forth in the federal Uniform Determination of Death Act that was proposed by a presidential commission. Most states have adopted two criteria for brain death—cessation of circulatory and respiratory functions, and irreversible cessation of brain function, including brain stem function. A physician checks for reflexes and responses before declaring brain death.

VOCABULARY REVIEW

In the previous section, you learned terms relating to the pathology of the lifespan. Before going on to the exercises, review the terms below and refer to the previous section if you have any questions. Pronunciations are provided for certain terms. Sometimes information about where the word came from is included after the term. The etymologies (word histories) are for your information only. You do not need to memorize them.

Term	Definition
genetics [jĕ-NĔT-ĭks] From Greek *genesis*, origin	Science of biological inheritance.
in utero [ĭn YŪ-tĕr-ō] Latin	Within the uterus; unborn.
premature [PRĒ-mă-chūr] Latin *praematurus*, too early	Born before 37 weeks of gestation.
preventive medicine	Medical specialty concerned with preventing disease.
sudden infant death syndrome (SIDS)	Death of an infant, usually while sleeping, of unknown cause.

CASE STUDY

Dealing with Complications

Maria's age prompted her obstetrician to ask whether she wanted amniocentesis, a test for fetal abnormalities. Maria decided to have the test. It came back normal. Meanwhile, Maria's mother had another heart attack. Maria and her mother decided to look for a living situation that would provide independence for her mother while providing care as necessary. They settled on an assisted living complex in the next town. This seemed to be ideal—Maria would have fewer tasks, and her mother would be around people all the time.

Around the beginning of Maria's seventh month of pregnancy, a routine visit to the doctor showed that her blood pressure had spiked to dangerous levels. Maria had a kidney infection and was dealing with a very stressful situation. She also had noticed some vague cramps. The kidney infection was treated, but, in addition, Maria was told to cut her work hours and spend more time resting in bed in preparation for the final stage of pregnancy. The cramps were a sign of possible early labor.

Critical Thinking

14. What is the danger to the fetus if Maria's obstetrician is not able to prevent early labor?
15. What are some of the abnormalities that might be seen on an ultrasound as opposed to those tested for in amniotic fluid?

PATHOLOGY OF THE LIFESPAN EXERCISES

Following the Stages of Life

Write the lifespan stage(s) during which each disease is most likely to occur. You may want to review Table 17-2 before proceeding with this exercise.

16. senile dementia _____
17. chicken pox _____
18. SIDS _____
19. Alzheimer's disease _____
20. erythroblastosis fetalis _____
21. Down syndrome _____
22. Parkinson's disease _____
23. spina bifida _____

TERMINOLOGY IN ACTION

For each of the following events, conditions, or diseases, put a number in the space to match the period of the lifespan (1 = birth to age 3; 2 = ages 3–12; 3 = ages 13–19; 4 = ages 20–40; 5 = ages 41 to 59; and 6 = 60 and older) in which it most often occurs. You may have to refer to earlier chapters on body systems if you do not know some of the answers.

24. osteoporosis _____

25. SIDS _____

26. menopause _____

27. acne _____

28. chicken pox _____

USING THE INTERNET

Go to the Hospice Foundation of America's Web site (http://www.hospicefoundation.org) and write a short paragraph on the goals of hospice.

CHAPTER REVIEW

The material that follows is to help you review this chapter.

Find a Match

Match the terms in the left-hand column with the correct definition in the right-hand column.

29. ____ preventive medicine

30. ____ neonatology

31. ____ pediatrics

32. ____ obstetrics

33. ____ gerontology

a. diagnoses and treats disorders of infants up to four weeks old

b. diagnoses and treats disorders of old age

c. guides women throughout fertilization, pregnancy and birth

d. diagnoses and treats disorders from infancy through adolescence

e. concerned with preventing disease

Know the Meaning

Write the definitions for each of the following terms.

34. bioethics: _____

35. advanced directives: _____

36. living will: _____

37. durable power of attorney: _____

38. health care proxy: _____

Check Your Knowledge

Circle T for true or F for false.

39. The birth process usually includes a period of implantation, the process of expelling the fetus and the placenta from the uterus. T F

40. At birth, a baby is rated using an Apgar score, which is assessed at 1 and 10 minutes after birth. T F

41. The practice of euthanasia, or assisted suicide, is allowed in certain countries of the world. T F

42. A neonate that is born after less than 37 weeks of gestation is considered premature. T F

43. A fetus presenting in a cephalic presentation must always be delivered by Caesarean section. T F

Find a Match

Match the terms in the left-hand column with the correct definition in the right-hand column.

44. ____ puberty

45. ____ oldest old age

46. ____ childhood

47. ____ death

48. ____ toddler

49. ____ adolescence

50. ____ neonate

a. first 4 weeks of infancy

b. end of life

c. ages 90 on

d. ages 1 to 3

e. period from puberty to full physical maturity

f. ages 3 to puberty

g. ages 8 to 12

DEFINITIONS

Define the following terms. Review the chapter before starting. Make sure you know how to pronounce each term as you define it.

WORD

51. Apgar score [ĂP-găr]

52. breech [brēch]

53. cesarean [sĕ-ZĀ-rē-ăn] section

54. embryo [ĔM-brē-ō]

55. euthanasia [yū-thă-NĀ-zhē-ă]

56. fertilization [FĔR-tĭl-ĭ-ZĀ-shŭn]

57. fetus [FĒ-tŭs]

58. genetics [jĕ-NĔT-ĭks]

59. geriatric [JĔR-ē-Ă-trĭk]

60. gerontology [JĔR-ŏn-TŎL-ō-jē]

61. gestation [jĕs-TĀ-shŭn]

62. implant [ĭm-PLĂNT]

63. in utero [ĭn YŪ-tĕr-ō]

64. labor [LĀ-bōr]

65. neonate [NĒ-ō-nāt]

66. neonatology [NĒ-ō-nā-TŎL-ō-jē]

67. obstetrics [ŏb-STĔT-rĭks]

68. pediatrics [PĒ-dē-ĂT-rĭks]

69. premature [PRĒ-mă-chūr]

70. preventive medicine

71. sudden infant death syndrome (SIDS)

Answers to Chapter Exercises

1. Maria will be in the young adulthood stage up to the time her child will finish the toddler stage. Then middle adulthood will coincide with the child's development through to young adulthood.
2. Not necessarily. Although Maria's age puts the fetus at higher risk for certain abnormalities, such as Down syndrome, only testing can determine if a fetus needs a specialist in neonatology.
3. fetus
4. neonate
5. puberty
6. toddler
7. childhood
8. death
9. young adulthood
10. adolescence
11. neonate
12. pregnancy
13. old age, oldest old age
14. Maria's baby might be born prematurely with physical problems due to underdevelopment.

15. limb abnormalities, spina bifida, hydrocephaly, and others that show up externally on the fetus
16. old age, oldest old age
17. childhood, puberty
18. infancy
19. middle adulthood, old age, oldest old age
20. fetus
21. neonate, infancy
22. middle adulthood, old age
23. fetus, neonate
24. 6
25. 1
26. 5
27. 3
28. 2
29. e
30. a
31. d
32. c
33. b
34. the study of the ethics of medical treatment and research
35. documents that state the patient's wishes about decisions of future health care

36. one of the advanced directive documents signed by the patient who prefers to be allowed to die than be kept alive by artificial means
37. a second advanced directive document which appoints a health care proxy
38. a person designated to make decisions for the patient in case of disability
39. F
40. F
41. T
42. T
43. F
44. g
45. c
46. f
47. b
48. d
49. e
50. a
51–71. Answers are available in the vocabulary reviews in this chapter.

Terms in Oncology— Cancer and Its Causes

After studying this chapter, you will be able to:

18.1 Name the types of cancers, discuss the major pathological conditions, and list some of their possible causes

18.2 Define the combining forms and suffixes used in building words that relate to oncology

18.3 Identify the meaning of related abbreviations

18.4 Name the laboratory tests and clinical procedures used in testing and treating cancer

18.5 Describe pathological terms related to cancer

18.6 Explain the meaning of surgical terms related to cancer

18.7 List common pharmacological agents used in treating cancer

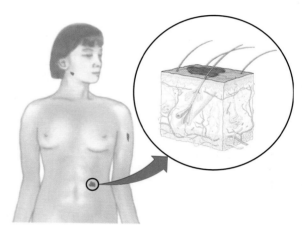

Tumors: Types and Causes

Tumors

Oncology is the study, diagnosis, and treatment of tumors. **Tumors** or **neoplasms** are growths made up of cells that reproduce abnormally. Cells in the body normally reproduce only at a rate to replace cells that have died. Cells also have a mechanism that signals them to die when they have passed a certain point of usefulness. Tumors are made up of cells that seem to be missing the mechanism that tells them either to stop reproducing or to die. The death of normal cells in a normal time cycle is called **apoptosis.**

Tumors can be **benign** (massed but containing cells that resemble the site of origin) or **malignant** (consisting of abnormal or mutated cells). Figure 18-1 shows a benign encapsulated tumor (a) and a malignant tumor (b). Tumors can be **encapsulated** (retained within a border of connective tissue) or they may reproduce in uncontrolled patterns. Most benign tumors are not life-threatening unless they grow in such a way that they damage essential organs. Malignant tumors can be life-threatening if they are not treated and they spread.

A *carcinoma*, the most common type of cancer, originates from epithelial tissue. Also called **solid tumors,** carcinomas make up about 90 percent of all tumors. Common sites are in the skin, lungs, breasts, colon, stomach, mouth, and uterus. Carcinomas spread by way of the lymphatic system.

A **sarcoma,** which is fairly rare, originates in muscle or connective tissue and lymph. A *mixed-tissue tumor* derives from tissue that is capable of

> The American Cancer Society (www.cancer.org) offers continually updated information about prevention, treatment, support, and volunteering opportunities.

569

FIGURE 18-1 **(a)** Benign tumors are not cancerous. In many cases, they do not have to be removed. **(b)** Malignancies have to be treated or they will spread.

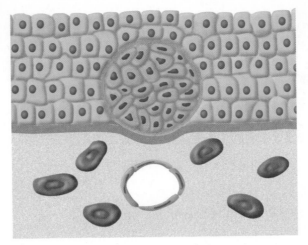

(a)

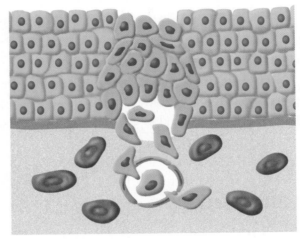

(b)

separating into either epithelial or connective tissue because it is composed of several types of cells. Such a tumor can be found in the kidneys, ovaries, or testes. Mixed-tissue tumors can be **teratomas,** growths containing bone, muscle, skin, and glandular tissue as well as other types of cells. There is also a class of cancers that arise from blood, lymph, or nervous system cells. Cancers such as leukemia fall into this category. As mentioned in Chapter 12, some leukemias are also sarcomas. Benign tumors are not life-threatening unless they impact organs (Figure 18-1a). They are made up of **differentiated** cells that reproduce abnormally but in an orderly fashion. Some benign tumors can cause pain from pressure exerted on an organ or tissue. Often, removal cures the problem.

Malignant tumors are **invasive,** extending beyond the tissue to infiltrate other organs (Figure 18-1b). Malignant tumors can be life-threatening. These tumors are made up of **dedifferentiated** cells, which lack the normal orderly arrangement of the cells from which they arise. *Undifferentiated* cells lack a defined mature cell structure. This loss of cell differentiation is called **anaplasia.**

Any abnormal tissue development is known as **dysplasia** or **heteroplasia.** The first stages of cancer development may be classified as dysplasia because they represent the beginning of abnormal tissue development. Detection of cancers at this early stage plays a vital role in treatment. The next stage may be a *carcinoma in situ,* a tumor in one place that affects all

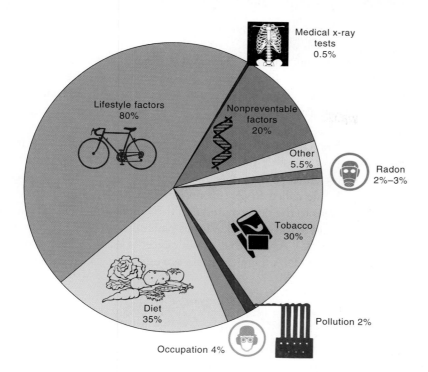

Medical x-ray
tests
0.5%

Lifestyle factors
80%

Nonpreventable
factors
20%

Other
5.5%

Radon
2%–3%

Tobacco
30%

Diet
35%

Pollution 2%

Occupation 4%

FIGURE 18-2 Many cancer deaths could be prevented by lifestyle and environmental changes.

layers of tissue. Finally, a *malignancy* occurs when the cells break loose and become invasive to surrounding tissue. The spread of a malignancy to other areas of the body is called **metastasis.** In earlier chapters, you learned about *homeostasis*, the maintaining of balance throughout the body. Metastasis is a state of imbalance, with cells spreading uncontrollably.

Causes of Cancer

Tumors appear under a number of different circumstances or combination of circumstances. One such is the exposure to *carcinogens,* cancer-causing agents. Carcinogens include environmental agents, such as chemicals, radiation, and viruses. Many chemicals, environmental factors, and viruses may be carcinogens, but they have not been tested thoroughly, and may not be for years. The process of proving a link between an agent and a resulting cancer is a long and tedious process. In some localities, cancer clusters (an unusually high number of cancers in a limited area) have led researchers to classify certain chemicals as carcinogens. Other agents, such as tobacco in any form, food additives, pharmaceutical agents, asbestos, insecticides, some dyes, and certain hormones, are also known carcinogens. Figure 18-2 is a chart giving the percentages of cancer deaths from preventable factors.

Another cause of cancer is from an inherited defect transmitted from parent(s) to child in the genetic material of the cell, *DNA (deoxyribonucleic acid)*. Figure 18-3 shows DNA in the nucleus of a cell. DNA contains coded material called genes that direct the growth of cells and the production of new proteins. When a cell divides into two cells in normal cell growth, exactly the same DNA appears in both cells. The body is constantly producing new cells. This process is called **mitosis.** Some genes in DNA may become defective in a process of change, called **mutation.** Most mutated cells either do not survive or are destroyed by the normal immune system. However, each new generation of malignant cells will increase the mutation of

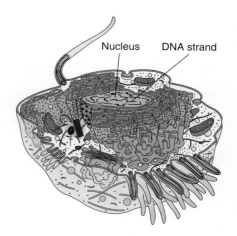

Nucleus   DNA strand

FIGURE 18-3 DNA strands contain genetic information in the cell.

the cell. The longer the malignancy has been established, the more mutated. A pathologist will assess this.

Mutations that do survive are then replicated over and over again and can lead to malignancies. Mutated DNA can predispose someone to cancer through heredity. Breast cancer and ovarian cancer are examples of largely inherited cancers. People with a family history of cancers are more likely to develop cancer. That does not mean, however, that people with no family history of a certain cancer (such as breast cancer) should ignore regular checkups. Nor does it mean that if your mother had breast cancer, you and your sisters are destined to have breast cancer. The other function of DNA is to copy its code onto another molecule called *RNA* (*ribonucleic acid*). RNA carries coded messages from the nucleus to the outer material of the cell, the **cytoplasm.** The messages signal what proteins are needed. Viruses heighten cancer risk (such as Kaposi's sarcoma from HIV). A virus that causes cancer is known as an *oncogenic* agent. An **oncogene** is a DNA fragment that converts normal cells into malignancies.

The National Cancer Institute (www.cancer.gov) is a governmental source for information about types of cancers, treatments, research, and many other cancer topics.

VOCABULARY REVIEW

In the previous section, you learned terms relating to oncology. Before going on to the exercises, review the terms below and refer to the previous section if you have questions. Pronunciations are provided for certain terms. Sometimes information about where the word came from is included after the term. These etymologies (word histories) are for your information only. You do not need to memorize them.

Term	Meaning
anaplasia [ăn-ă-PLĀ-zhē-ă] ana-, up + -plasia, formation	Loss of cell differentiation.
apoptosis [ă-pŏp-TŌ-sĭs] Greek, a dropping off	Normal death of cells.
benign [bĕ-NĪN] From Latin *benignus*, kind	Encapsulated; not malignant.
cytoplasm [SĪ-tō-plăzm] cyto-, cell + -plasm, formation	Outer portion of a cell surrounding the nucleus.
dedifferentiated [dē-DĬF-ĕr-ĕn-shē-Ā-tĕd] de-, away from + differentiated	Lacking in normal orderly cell arrangement.
differentiated [dĭf-ĕr-ĔN-shē-ā-tĕd]	Growing in an orderly fashion.
dysplasia [dĭs-PLĀ-zhē-ă] dys-, abnormal + -plasia	Abnormal tissue growth.
encapsulated [ĕn-KĂP-sū-lā-tĕd]	Held within a capsule; benign.
heteroplasia [HĔT-ĕr-ō-PLĀ-zē-ă] hetero-, different + -plasia	Dysplasia.
invasive [ĭn-VĀ-sĭv]	Infiltrating other organs; spreading.
malignant [mă-LĬG-nănt]	Growing uncontrollably.
metastasis [mĕ-TĂS-tă-sĭs] Greek: *meta-*, beyond + *stasis*, a standing still	Spread of malignant cells to other parts of the body.

Term	Meaning
mitosis [mī-TŌ-sĭs] From Greek *mitos*, thread	Cell division.
mutation [myū-TĀ-shŭn]	Alteration in DNA to produce defective cells.
neoplasm [NĒ-ō-plăzm] neo-, new + -plasm	Tumor; new growth.
oncogene [ŎNG-kō-jēn] onco-, tumor + gene	DNA fragment that causes malignancies.
sarcoma [săr-KŌ-mă] Greek *sarkoma*, fleshy growth	Relatively rare tumor that originates in muscle, connective tissue, and lymph.
solid tumor	Carcinoma; most common type of tumor.
teratoma [tĕr-ă-TŌ-mă] Greek *teras*, monster + -*oma*, tumor	Growth containing several types of tissue and various types of cells.
tumor [TŪ-mŏr] Latin, a swelling	Growth made up of cells that reproduce abnormally.

CASE STUDY

Finding a Symptom

Alicia Alvarez is fifty years old, has no family history of cancer, and is having her annual gynecological examination. Dr. Josiah Williams is a gynecologist specializing in the care of menopausal women. He notices a grayish area on the left side of Alicia's vulva. He recommends an immediate biopsy be taken in his office. Alicia expresses surprise and mentions that there is no cancer history in her family. Dr. Williams explains to Alicia that family history is just one factor in cancer of the female reproductive system. He also points out that a biopsy does not necessarily mean the tissue is cancerous; the discoloration may also be the result of an infection or irritation. Alicia agrees to have the biopsy.

Critical Thinking

1. The discoloration on Alicia's vulva is possibly a type of skin cancer appearing on a part of the female reproductive system. Skin discolorations are usually not cancer. If you have a biopsy and the results are negative, should you still examine the skin area every few months? Why?
2. Name two cancers of the female reproductive system.

TUMORS: TYPES AND CAUSES EXERCISES

Find a Match

Write the word from this list that matches each statement.

benign deoxyribonucleic acid anaplasia teratoma carcinogen metastasis differentiated malignant dedifferentiated invasive sarcoma oncogene

3. Lacking in normal orderly cell arrangement _____

4. Encapsulated, not malignant _____

5. Infiltrating other organs; spreading _____

6. Growing uncontrollably _____

7. Genetic material of a cell _____

8. DNA fragment that causes malignancies _____

9. Growth containing several types of tissue and various types of cells _____

10. Tumor that originates in muscle, connective tissue, and lymph; fairly rare _____

11. Spread of malignant cells _____

12. Cancer-causing agent _____

Spell It Correctly

For each of the following words, write C if the spelling is correct. If it is not correct, write the correct spelling.

13. mestastasis _____

14. apoptosis _____

15. carsinoma _____

16. dedifferentiated _____

17. deoxirebonuclaic _____

18. citoplasm _____

Match the Term

Write the letter of the meaning of the term in the space provided. These terms describe tumor appearance:

19. verrucous

20. polypoid

21. inflammatory

22. cystic

23. follicular

24. ulcerating

25. medullary

26. necrotic

a. filled with fluid

b. wartlike in appearance

c. containing glandular sacs

d. having open wounds

e. large and fleshy

f. containing dead tissue

g. containing polyps

h. having a red and swollen appearance

Combining Forms and Abbreviations

The lists below include combining forms, suffixes, and abbreviations that relate specifically to oncology. Pronunciations are provided for the examples.

COMBINING FORM	MEANING	EXAMPLE
blast(o)	immature cell	*blastoma* [blăs-TŌ-mă], tumor arising from an immature cell
carcin(o)	cancer	*carcinogen* [kăr-SĬN-ō-jĕn], cancer-causing agent
muta	genetic change	*mutation* [myū-TĀ-shŭn], process of genetic change
mutagen(o)	genetic change	*mutagenic* [myū-tă-JĔN-ĭk], causing genetic change
onc(o)	tumor	*oncology* [ŏn-KŎL-ō-jē], treatment and study of tumors
radi(o)	radiation, X rays	*radiation* [rā-dē-Ā-shŭn], process of exposure to or treatment with above-normal levels of radiation

SUFFIX	MEANING	EXAMPLE
-blast	immature cell	*leukoblast* [LŪ-kō-blăst], immature
-oma (*pl.*, -omata)	tumor	*fibroma* [fĭ-BRŌ-mă], benign tumor arising from connective tissue
-plasia	formation (as of cells)	*dysplasia* [dĭs-PLĀ-zhē-ă], abnormal tissue development
-plasm	formation (as of cells)	*neoplasm* [NĒ-ō-plăsm], abnormal tissue formed by abnormal cell growth
-plastic	formative	*neoplastic* [nē-ō-PLĂS-tĭk], growing abnormally (as a neoplasm)

ABBREVIATION	MEANING	ABBREVIATION	MEANING
ALL	acute lymphocytic leukemia	ER	estrogen receptor
AML	acute myelogenous leukemia	METS, mets	metastases
bx	biopsy	NHL	non-Hodgkin's lymphoma
CA	carcinoma	PSA	prostate-specific antigen
CEA	carcinogenic embryonic antigen	rad	radiation absorbed dose
chemo	chemotherapy	RNA	ribonucleic acid
CLL	chronic lymphocytic leukemia	RT	radiation therapy
CML	chronic myelogenous leukemia	TNM	tumor, nodes, metastasis
DES	diethylstilbestrol	Tx	treatment
DNA	deoxyribonucleic acid	XRT	x-ray or radiation therapy
DRE	digital rectal exam		

CASE STUDY

Being Careful

Frightened by Alicia's news of possible cancer, Peter Alvarez, her husband, went to Dr. John Chin, an internist, for a physical. He had not had a physical in the last five years, but felt now that he should. Peter is 50 years old and has no history of cancer. Dr. Chin had the nurse draw blood for various tests.

Dr. Chin explained that one of the tests that should be done on a yearly basis for males over the age of 45 is the PSA.

Critical Thinking

27. What part of the body does the PSA test evaluate?
28. Peter had not had a physical in five years. Why is it important to be checked on a yearly basis for certain types of cancer when you reach certain ages?

COMBINING FORMS AND ABBREVIATIONS EXERCISES

Build Your Medical Vocabulary

Using the combining forms and suffixes in this chapter and in Chapter 3, write a term for each definition.

29. therapy using radiation _____

30. bone tumor _____

31. immature red blood cell _____

32. fluid-filled glandular carcinoma _____

33. tumor of the meninges _____

34. cancer of the lymph system _____

Check Your Knowledge

For each of the following cancers, name the body part involved. Refer to Chapter 3 if you need to review combining forms for body parts.

35. adenoma _____

36. neuroblastoma _____

37. myoma _____

38. retinoblastoma _____

39. lymphocytoma _____

Find the Terms

Use the combining forms above to complete the following words.

40. tumor consisting of immature cells: _____ oma

41. treatment of tumors: _____ therapy

42. agent that promotes a genetic change: _____ gen

43. impenetrable by radiation: _____ opaque

44. destructive to cancer cells: _____ lytic

Root Out the Meaning

Divide each of the following words into word parts. Give the definition of the whole word and of each part.

45. androblastoma _____

46. carcinogenesis _____

47. mutagenesis _____

48. oncogene _____

49. radiotherapy _____

50. radionecrosis _____

51. hypernephroma _____

52. leiomyosarcoma _____

53. adenocarcinoma _____

54. oncologist _____

55. oncocyte _____

56. adenoma _____

57. astrocytoma _____

58. chondrosarcoma _____

59. liposarcoma _____

60. lymphoma _____

Diagnostic, Procedural, and Laboratory Terms

Cancer is a general term referring to any of various diseases with uncontrolled cell growth. Researchers have developed tests to detect many cancers and, in some cases, to detect cancer at its earliest stages. Survival rates have

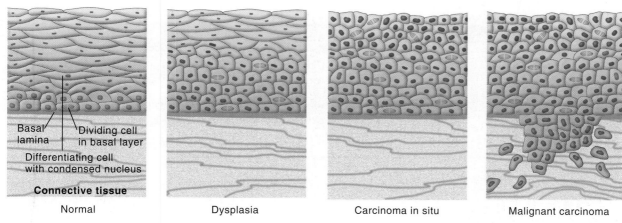

Basal lamina
Dividing cell in basal layer
Differentiating cell with condensed nucleus
Connective tissue

Normal   Dysplasia   Carcinoma in situ   Malignant carcinoma

FIGURE 18-4   A Pap smear is examined under a microscope to see if it is normal, has some dysplasia, if a carcinoma in situ is present, or if malignant carcinoma already exists.

improved because of diagnostic techniques. The sooner cell growth can be normalized, the greater the possibility of survival.

Routine medical checkups often include tests for cancer. Adult females usually have a *pap smear,* a test for cervical and uterine cancer (Figure 18-4), along with a breast examination, including palpation of the breasts for lumps. Adult males usually have a blood test called a *PSA (prostate-specific antigen)* that can detect prostate cancer. A *digital rectal exam (DRE)* is also a prostate cancer screening method. Doctors also check male testicles for any signs of tumors. Testicular cancer occurs fairly commonly.

Normal adult checkups usually include auscultation of the lungs, palpation of the abdomen, inspection of the rectum and an occult stool test (particularly if the patient has a family history of colon cancer or has some possible symptoms), and a discussion of any symptoms that may need further investigation. Some blood tests indicate a particular type of cancer. For example, patients with gastrointestinal tumors usually have *carcinoembryonic antigens (CEA)* in their bloodstream. An *alphafetoprotein test (AFP)* is given to detect the presence of liver or testicular cancer. *HCG* or *human chorionic gonadotropin* is usually present in the blood of patients with testicular cancer. *CA-125 (cancer antigen 125)* is a protein produced by ovarian cancer cells. Colorectal cancers can be detected by a colonoscopy.

With advances in understanding genetic markers for certain diseases, preventive measures can be offered to patients who have a genetic marker for a certain cancer. This has been used effectively, for example, in the prevention of breast cancer for people with Her-2nu genes, which indicate a high likelihood of developing breast cancer.

Imaging techniques now provide a detailed picture of various parts of the body. MRIs, CAT scans, mammograms, and the insertion of lighted instruments to view various body parts have advanced diagnostic techniques. Any tumors that are found are categorized by **grade,** the maturity of the tumor, and **stage,** the degree of spread or metastasis of the tumor. A common method for grading is the **TNM** (tumor, node, metastasis) **system,** which numbers the extent of the tumor, the extent of lymph nodes affected, and the degree of metastasis. This grading is most often done by examination under a microscope. Table 18-1 describes the grading used in the TNM system.

fification	Size Indicator	Meaning
mor)	0–4	0 means no tumor; 1–4 means progressively larger tumors.
(node)	0–4	0 means no lymph node involvement; 1–4 indicates extent to which cancer affects nodes.
M (metastasis)	0–3	0 means no metastasis. 1–3 are the stages of metastasis.

Tumors are also characterized by appearance under the microscope, and by observations made on visual examination. Some of the classifications of tumors are:

- **alveolar,** forming small sacs shaped like alveoli
- **anaplastic,** reverting to a more immature form
- **carcinoma in situ,** contained at a site without spreading
- **diffuse,** spreading evenly
- **dysplastic,** abnormal in cell appearance
- **epidermoid,** resembling epithelial cells
- **follicular,** containing glandlike sacs
- **hyperchromatic,** intensely colored
- **hyperplastic,** excessive in development (of cells)
- **hypoplastic,** underdeveloped as tissue
- **nodular,** formed in tight cell clusters
- **papillary,** having small papillae projecting from cells
- **pleomorphic,** having many types of cells
- **scirrhous,** made up of hard, densely packed cells
- **undifferentiated,** lacking a defined cell structure

Tumors are also described by their appearance during visual examination. Tumors can be described as:

- **cystic,** filled with fluid
- **fungating,** projecting from a surface in a mushroomlike pattern
- **inflammatory,** having an inflamed appearance (swollen and red)
- **medullary,** large and fleshy
- **necrotic,** containing dead tissue
- **polypoid,** containing polyps
- **ulcerating,** having open wounds
- **verrucous,** having wartlike, irregular growths

The Cancer Group Institute (www.cancergroup.com) is a commercial site that categorizes types of cancers.

Once a tumor is confirmed as malignant, doctor and patient discuss and agree on a **protocol,** a course of treatment. One of the possible treatments is **radiation,** the bombarding of the tumor with rays that damage the DNA of the tumor cells. Most radiation treatment is carefully pinpointed, but some surrounding cells usually suffer damage as well. Radiation can cause many unpleasant side effects, such as hair loss, nausea, and skin damage. Some cancerous tumors will respond to radiation better than others. A *radiosensitive tumor* will absorb the damaging radiation and respond by dying or shrinking. With a *radioresistant tumor,* the radiation has little effect on the growth of the tumor. The use of a drug called a *radiosensitizer* prior to the radiation treatments will increase the radiosensitivity of the tumor. Among the other possible treatments are the use of drugs and surgery.

VOCABULARY REVIEW

In the previous section, you learned terms relating to oncological diagnosis, clinical procedures, and laboratory tests. Before going on to the exercises, review the terms below and refer to the previous section if you have questions. Pronunciations are provided for certain terms. Sometimes information about where the word came from is included after the term. These etymologies (word histories) are for your information only. You do not need to memorize them.

Term	Meaning
alveolar [ăl-VĒ-ō-lăr]	Forming small sacs.
anaplastic [ăn-ă-PLĂS-tĭk] ana-, up + -plastic, forming	Reverting to a more immature form.
carcinoma in situ [kăr-sĭ-NŌ-mă ĭn SĬ-tū]	Contained at a site without spreading.
cystic [SĬS-tĭk]	Filled with fluid.
diffuse [dĭ-FYŪS]	Spreading evenly.
dysplastic [dĭs-PLĂS-tĭk] dys-, abnormal + -plastic	Abnormal in cell appearance.
epidermoid [ĕp-ĭ-DĔR-mŏyd] epiderm(us) + -oid, like	Resembling epithelial cells.
follicular [fŏl-LĬK-yū-lăr]	Containing glandular sacs.
fungating [FŬNG-āt-ĭng]	Growing in a mushroomlike pattern.
grade	Level of maturity of a tumor.
hyperchromatic [HĪ-pĕr-krō-MĂT-ĭk] hyper-, excessively + chromatic	Intensely colored.
hyperplastic [hī-pĕr-PLĂS-tĭk] hyper- + -plastic	Excessive in development (of cells).
hypoplastic [HĪ-pō-PLĂS-tĭk] hypo-, abnormally low + -plastic	Underdeveloped, as tissue.
inflammatory [ĭn-FLĂM-ă-tōr-ē]	Having an inflamed appearance (red and swollen).
medullary [MĔD-ū-lăr-ē]	Large and fleshy.
necrotic [nĕ-KRŎT-ĭk] Greek *nekrosis*, death	Containing dead tissue.
nodular [NŌD-yū-lăr]	Formed in tight clusters.
papillary [PĂP-ĭ-lār-ē]	Having papillae projecting from cells.
pleomorphic [plē-ō-MŌR-fĭk] pleo-, more + Greek *morphe*, form	Having many types of cells.
polypoid [PŎL-ĭ-pŏyd] poly(p) + -oid	Containing polyps.
protocol [PRŌ-tō-kŏl]	Course of treatment.

Term	Meaning
radiation [RĀ-dē-Ā-shŭn]	Bombarding of tumors with rays that damage the DNA of cells.
scirrhous [SKĬR-ŭs] Greek *skirrhos*, hard	Hard, densely packed.
stage	Degree of tumor spread.
TNM system	Tumor, node, metastasis system of categorizing tumors.
ulcerating [ŬL-sĕr-ā-tĭng]	Having open wounds.
undifferentiated [ŬN-dĭf-ĕr-ĔN-shē-ā-tĕd] un-, not + differentiated	Lacking a defined cell structure.
verrucous [vĕ-RŪ-kōs] Latin *verrucosus*	Wartlike in appearance.

CASE STUDY

Getting a Diagnosis

Dr. Williams sent Alicia's biopsy to Medical Center Pathologists. He received the following report.

Critical Thinking

61. Does the report cite any unusual growth of cells?

62. Have any of the cells invaded neighboring tissue?

> MICROSCOPIC: A single slide containing sections through the submitted material is reviewed. This biopsy of skin is centrally ulcerated. The area of ulceration is surrounded by keratinizing squamous epithelium, which exhibits a full-thickness dysplasia. This dysplastic change is characterized by cells that have a vertical growth pattern, somewhat hyperchromatic nuclei, and an increased mitotic rate. Mitoses do extend to the surface. The lesion does not appear to invade the underlying and associated stroma. Mild-to-moderate dysplastic changes are seen peripherally and do extend to the surgical margins.

DIAGNOSTIC, PROCEDURAL, AND LABORATORY TERMS EXERCISES

Find the Part

Write the body part(s) being tested for cancer by each of the following procedures:

63. mammogram: _____

64. DRE: _____

65. PSA: _____

66. pap smear: _____

Check Your Knowledge

Complete the sentences below by filling in the blanks.

67. A tumor filled with liquid is referred to as _____.

68. Some melanomas are _____, or intensely colored.

69. Chemotherapy is one _____ for treatment of cancer.

70. Tissue that is dead is referred to as _____.

71. Some cancers are _____, or wartlike in appearance.

Pathological Terms

Cancer is a pathological term. It can affect people from the fetal stage until old age. Many advances have been made in cancer prevention and treatment, but some cancers have had no increase in cure rates for many years, and others have increased within the population, which may be due in part to an increase in detection. Table 18-2 lists some common cancers. Figure 18-5 shows one of those cancers (Burkitt's lymphoma).

There are many websites with extensive information about cancer and its potential cures. Visit any of the following sites for information: www. cancer.gov/cancertopics/prevention-genetics-causes/genetics; www.nci.nih. gov/cancertopics/Genetic-Testing-for-Breast-and-Ovarian-Cancer-Risk; and www.cancer.org/docroot/home/index.asp.

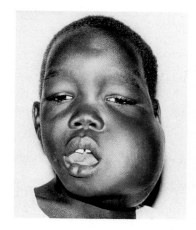

FIGURE 18-5 Burkitt's lymphoma in a child.

TABLE 18-2 Common Cancers

Type of Cancer	Where Cancer Starts	Common Sites in the Body	Specific Risk Groups (most cancers can affect anyone)	Prevention and Early Diagnosis
adenocarcinoma	gland	colon, stomach		high fiber diet; colonoscopy
adenoma	glandular epithelium	pituitary		
astrocytoma	neuroglia	brain		
basal cell carcinoma	skin	skin		avoiding sun exposure; examination of skin
Burkitt's lymphoma (Figure 18-5)	lymph			
carcinoma	epithelial tissue	glands, lungs, kidney, breast		avoidance of carcinogens such as tobacco, asbestos; early checkups
carcinoma in situ	encapsulated tumor	breast, cervix		self-examination; mammography
chondrosarcoma	cartilage			
Ewing's sarcoma	connective tissue			
fibrosarcoma	connective tissue			
glioblastoma	neurological tissue			
glioma	neurological	brain		

(continued)

TABLE 18-2 Common Cancers (cont.)

Type of Cancer	Where Cancer Starts	Common Sites in the Body	Specific Risk Groups (most cancers can affect anyone)	Prevention and Early Diagnosis
Hodgkin's disease	lymph system			
hypernephroma	kidneys			
Kaposi's sarcoma	first seen in skin of AIDS patient, then other organs		patients with HIV	preventative measures (such as safe sex)
leiomyosarcoma	smooth muscle			
leukemia	stem cells			
leukoplakia	tongue or cheeks			
liposarcoma	fat			
lymphoma	lymph system			
medulloblastoma	brain			
melanoma	skin			avoidance of sun; skin examination
nephrosarcoma	kidney			
neuroblastoma	adrenal glands	adrenal glands of infants and children		
non-Hodgkin's lymphoma	lymph tissue			
osteosarcoma	bone			
retinoblastoma	retina	eye		
rhabdomyosarcoma	striated muscle			
sarcoma	connective tissue			

CASE STUDY

Seeing a Specialist

Alicia's cancer is a carcinoma in situ. Dr. Williams refers Alicia to a surgical oncologist who performs the surgery to remove the tumor. The surgeon, Dr. Wilma Grant, examines surrounding tissue during the surgery and decides that Alicia does not need further treatment. The surgeon cautioned Alicia to make sure she has regular six-month checkups.

Critical Thinking

72. Why did the doctor recommend six-month checkups?

73. Dr. Grant did not recommend radiation or chemotherapy. Does that mean that Alicia's cancer has metastasized?

Find the Disease

Using Table 18-2, write at least one type of cancer for each location.

74. breast _____

75. colon _____

76. kidney _____

77. skin _____

78. brain _____

79. stem cells _____

80. lymph system _____

81. bone _____

82. fat _____

83. neurological tissue _____

84. neuroglia _____

Preventing and Detecting Cancers

Answer the following questions.

85. Using Table 18-2 as a guide, write a brief paragraph about how you can minimize the risk of contracting certain cancers.

   _____

   _____

   _____

86. What two types of cancer are detectable by self-examination at an early stage? _____
   and _____

Spell It Correctly

For each of the following words, write C if the spelling is correct. If it is not, write the correct spelling.

87. aveolar _____

88. follicular _____

89. displastic _____

90. medulary _____

91. pleomorphic _____

Surgical Terms

Many cancers can be diagnosed and treated with surgery. First, however, tissue is usually examined in a *biopsy*, the removal of a small amount of living tissue for diagnosis (under a microscope in most cases). There are many types of biopsies depending on the type of cancer suspected. Some common ones are:

- An **incisional biopsy** is the removal of a part of a tumor for examination.
- An **excisional biopsy** is one in which the tumor is removed and surrounding tissue is examined for spread of the tumor.
- A **brush biopsy** is the passing of a catheter with bristles on it into the ureter or other areas to remove cells for examination.

- A **needle biopsy** is any biopsy in which cells are aspirated through a needle.
- An **exfoliative biopsy** is one in which cells are scraped off of the skin for examination.

If a tumor is found to be malignant, the tumor is usually removed to an established *surgical margin* or to the point where it abuts normal tissue. A localized tumor can be removed in a **lumpectomy** or **tylectomy.** Some surgeries involve **resectioning,** removal of the tumor and a large amount of the surrounding tissue, including lymph nodes; others involve **exenteration,** removal of an organ, tumor, and surrounding tissue. Other surgical procedures are **cryosurgery,** destruction by freezing; **electrocauterization,** destruction by burning; or **fulguration,** destruction by high-frequency electrical current.

VOCABULARY REVIEW

In the previous section, you learned terms relating to surgery. Before going on to the exercises, review the terms below and refer to the previous section if you have questions. Pronunciations are provided for certain terms. Sometimes information about where the word came from is included after the term. These etymologies (word histories) are for your information only. You do not need to memorize them.

Term	Meaning
brush biopsy	The passing of a catheter with bristles into the ureter to gather cells for examination.
cryosurgery [krī-ō-SĔR-jĕr-ē] cryo-, cold + surgery	Destruction by freezing.
electrocauterization [ē-LĔK-trō-CĂW-tĕr-ĭ-ZĀ-shŭn] electro-, electrical + cauterization	Destruction by burning tissue.
excisional biopsy [ĕk-SĬZH-shŭn-l BĪ-ŏp-sē]	Removal of tumor and surrounding tissue for examination.
exenteration [ĕks-ĕn-tĕr-Ā-shŭn] ex-, out of + Greek *enteron*, bowel	Removal of an organ, tumor, and surrounding tissue.
exfoliative [ĕx-FŌ-lē-ā-tĭv] **biopsy**	The scraping of skin cells from the skin surface for examination.
fulguration [fŭl-gū-RĀ-shŭn]	Destruction by high-frequency current.
incisional [ĭn-SĬZH-ŭn-l] **biopsy**	Removal of a part of a tumor for examination.
lumpectomy [lŭm-PĔK-tō-mē] lump + -ectomy	Surgical removal of a localized tumor.
needle biopsy	Removal of cells for examination by aspirating them with a needle.
resectioning [rē-SĔK-shŭn-ĭng]	Removal of a tumor and a large amount of surrounding tissue.
tylectomy [tī-LĔK-tō-mē] Greek *tulos*, lump + -ectomy	Surgical removal of a localized tumor.

Find a Match

Match the correct term in the right-hand column with its definition in the left-hand column

92. _____ removal of part of a tumor for examination

93. _____ removal of a tumor and surrounding tissue for examination

94. _____ form of surgery using freezing

95. _____ form of surgery using burning

96. _____ form of surgery using high-frequency current

a. fulguration

b. cryosurgery

c. electrocauterization

d. incisional biopsy

e. excisional biopsy

CASE STUDY

Getting Information

Alicia was concerned about the possibility of a recurrence of cancer. She asked Dr. Williams for a copy of the pathologist's report. Alicia did not understand some of the language in it, so she asked Dr. Williams for an explanation.

Critical Thinking

97. How might Dr. Williams explain "The lesion does not appear to invade the underlying and associated . . ."?

98. The dysplastic changes extend to the surgical margin, which is the outline out to which the removal of the cancer will take place. What determines the surgical margin?

Pharmacological Terms

Aside from surgery and radiation, cancer treatment includes three other **modalities** (methods)—**chemotherapy,** use of drugs to treat cancer, **biological therapy,** use of agents that enhance the body's own immune response in fighting tumor growth, and **gene therapy,** the use of cells from a laboratory to change the course of a disease (much of this is still experimental). Both chemotherapy and biological therapy have side effects, such as hair loss, nausea, and so on. Gene therapy is just in its beginning stages and long-term results are not known yet. The other four cancer treatments may be used together or separately during the course of a protocol. There are many researchers working on new cancer therapies, such as the inhibition of *angiogenesis*, the process in the body of supplying blood to tumors.

Radiation and chemotherapy must be specifically directed so as not to harm healthy cells while destroying unhealthy ones. Biological therapy targets cells that are receptive to the substances being injected.

For more information on gene therapy, go to the Human Genome Project Web site (http://www.ornl.gov/sci/techresources/Human_Genome/medicine/genetherapy.shtml).

MORE ABOUT . . .

Angiogenesis Inhibitor Therapy

Angiogenesis is the formation of new blood vessels controlled by chemicals produced in the body. Because tumors cannot grow or spread without the formation of new blood vessels and a blood supply, scientists are trying to find ways to stop angiogenesis. Angiogenesis is not a frequent process in adults, but it does occur in women each month as new vessels form in the lining of the uterus during the menstrual cycle. In addition, angiogenesis is necessary for the regeneration of tissue during wound healing. Unfortunately new blood vessel generation can provide cancer cells with oxygen and nutrients, allowing these cells to grow and spread to other parts of the body.

The objective of angiogenesis inhibitor therapy in cancer treatment is to arrest and/or block the chemicals responsible for beginning the new blood vessel formation process. Some drugs block vascular endothelial cell production directly or by obstructing the endothelial cells' ability to break down the extracellular matrix, allowing cancer cells to migrate.Researchers have answered many questions about angiogenesis, but many questions still remain. Studies continue trying to determine if inhibiting angiogenesis can be a long-term solution to slowing down or preventing the growth and spread of cancer in humans. Currently, new drugs being tested are in clinical trials and a few drugs have been approved by the U.S. Food and Drug Administration (FDA) for use on certain types of cancers.

VOCABULARY REVIEW

In the previous section, you learned terms relating to pharmacology. Before going on to the exercises, review the terms below and refer to the previous section if you have any questions. Pronunciations are provided for certain terms. Sometimes information about where the word came from is included after the term. The etymologies (word histories) are for your information only. You do not need to memorize them.

Term	Meaning
biological therapy	Treatment of cancer with agents from the body that increase immune response.
chemotherapy [KĒM-ō-thār-ă-pē, KĒ-mō-thār-ă-pē] chemo-, chemical + therapy	Treatment of cancer using drugs.
gene therapy	Method of treatment using genetically changed cells to cure or lessen the symptoms of disease.
modality [mō-DĂL-ĭ-tē]	Method of treatment.

CASE STUDY

Finding Another Cancer

Alicia went for a six-month gynecological checkup. Her pap smear was normal. She encouraged her sister, Margo, to see Dr. Williams. Margo is 15 years younger than Alicia. Margo goes to the gynecologist only when she has a problem. She has never had a mammogram. Dr. Williams shows Margo how to do breast self-examination and tells her that he feels a small lump on the side of her breast. This was confirmed with a mammogram and a biopsy. After a lumpectomy, Margo was told that the cancer had spread to one lymph node, which was also removed. Chemotherapy is recommended, along with biological therapy in the form of a weekly injection.

Critical Thinking

99. Why did the surgeon recommend chemotherapy?

100. How might the biological therapy help Margo?

TERMINOLOGY IN ACTION

A male patient has a blood test. It indicates there is an unusually high PSA level. His doctor recommends a biopsy to see if he has cancer. What type of cancer does the doctor suspect might be present. A female patient has a normal Pap smear. If it had been abnormal, what type of cancer would be suspected? Name the most virulent type of skin cancer. What type of cancer is most often caused by smoking?

USING THE INTERNET

Go to the American Cancer Society's Web site (www.cancer.org) and write a paragraph about cancer prevention. Also, list three types of treatment for cancer discussed at that site.

CHAPTER REVIEW

The material that follows is to help you review this chapter.

Complete the Sentence

Circle the term that best describes the *italicized* description of the correct answer.

101. The patient was treated with *a bombarding of tumors with rays that damage the DNA of cells* and had positive result after the treatment was completed. (chemotherapy, protocol, radiation)

102. The physician remarked that the lesion appeared *to be formed in tight clusters* and was found to be abnormal. (necrotic, nodular, verrucous)

103. A biopsy revealed that the tumor was *hard and densely packed* just as the pathologist suspected. (scirrhous, papillary, pleomorphic)

104. Dr. Jacobs noted that the dysplastic lesion appeared *intensely colored* and this concern warranted further evaluation. (hyperlplastic, hypoplastic, hyperchromatic)

105. One of the purposes of the TNM system of categorizing tumors is to determine *the degree of tumor spread* within the body. (carcinoma in situ, stage, grade)

Root Out the Meaning

Separate the following terms into word parts and define each word as well as each word part.

106. carcinogenic _____

107. carcinolytic _____

108. carcinoma _____

109. carcinophobia _____

110. mutagen _____

111. oncogenesis _____

112. oncogenic _____

113. oncogenous _____

114. oncofetal _____

115. oncology _____

116. oncolysis _____

117. oncosis _____

118. radioactive _____

119. radiodiagnosis _____

120. radiograph _____

121. radiographer _____

122. radiographic _____

123. radiogram _____

124. radiography _____

125. radiology _____

126. radiologist _____

127. radiometer _____

128. radiopaque _____

129. radiopathology _____

130. radioresistant _____

131. radiopharmaceutical _____

132. radiosensitive _____

133. radiotoxiemia _____

134. genoblast _____

135. glioblastoma _____

136. glioma _____

137. fibrosarcoma _____

138. medulloblastoma _____

139. melanoma _____

140. nephrosarcoma _____

141. neuroblastoma _____

142. osteosarcoma _____

143. retinoblastoma _____

144. rhabdomyosarcoma _____

145. sarcoma _____

Complete the Sentence

Circle the term that best describes the *italicized* description of the correct answer.

146. Timothy Clemons' physician indicated that the skin cancer on his forehead would be removed by *fulguration.* (destruction by burning tissue, destruction by freezing tissue, destruction by high-frequency current)

147. Karen Smartley has to make a decision about how her breast tumor will be removed before she has surgery. Her physician is recommending the *surgical removal of a localized tumor.* (resectioning, excisional biopsy, lumpectomy)

148. The tumor was found to be *growing uncontrollably* through out the body. (encapsulating, metastasizing, mutating)

149. The medical term for *abnormal tissue growth* is _____. (anaplasia, apoptosis, dysplasia)

Check Your Spelling

For each of the following terms, place a C if the spelling is correct. If it is not, write the correct spelling in the space provided.

150. chondocarcoma _____

151. milanocytoma _____

152. astrocytoma _____

153. rabbdomyosarcoma _____

154. neuroblastoma _____

155. inflamatory _____

DEFINITIONS

Define the following terms, combining forms and suffixes. Review the chapter before starting. Make sure you know how to pronounce each term as you define it.

TERM

156. alveolar [ăl-VĒ-ō-lăr]

157. anaplasia [ăn-ă-PLĀ-zhē-ă]

158. anaplastic [ăn-ă-PLĂS-tŏk]

159. apoptosis [ă-pŏp-Tō-sĭs]

160. benign [bĕ-NĪN]

161. biological therapy

162. blast(o)

163. -blast

164. brush biopsy

165. carcin(o)

166. carcinoma in situ [kăr-sĭ-NŌ-mă ĭn SĪ-tū]

167. chemotherapy [KĔM-ō-thār-ă-pē, KĒ-mō-thār-ă-pē]

168. cryosurgery [krī-ō-SĔR-jĕr-ē]

169. cystic [SĬS-tĭk]

170. cytoplasm [SĪ-tō-plăzm]

171. dedifferentiated [dē-DĬF-ĕr-ĕn-shē-Ā-tĕd]

172. differentiated [dĭf-ĕr-ĔN-shē-ā-tĕd]

173. diffuse [dĭ-FYŪS]

174. dysplasia [dĭs-PLĀ-zhē-ă]

175. dysplastic [dĭs-PLĂS-tĭk]

176. electrocauterization [ē-LĔK-trō-CĂW-tĕr-ĭ-ZĀ-shŭn]

177. encapsulated [ĕn-KĂP-sū-lā-tĕd]

178. epidermoid [ĕp-ĭ-DĔR-mŏyd]

179. excisional biopsy [ĕk-SĬZH-shŭn-l BĪ-ŏp-sē]

180. exenteration [ĕks-ĕn-tĕr-Ā-shŭn]

181. exfoliative [ĕks-FŌ-lē-ā-tĭv] biopsy

182. follicular [fŏl-LĬK-yū-lăr]

183. fulguration [fŭl-gū-RĀ-shŭn]

184. fungating [FŬNG-āt-ĭng]

185. gene therapy

186. grade

187. heteroplasia [HĔT-ĕr-ō-PLĀ-zē-ă]

188. hyperchromatic [HĪ-pĕr-krō-MĂT-ĭk]

189. hyperplastic [hī-pĕr-PLĂS-tĭk]

190. hypoplastic [HĪ-pō-PLĂS-tĭk]

191. incisional [ĭn-SĬZH-ŭn-l] biopsy

192. inflammatory [ĭn-FLĂM-ă-tōr-ē]

193. invasive [ĭn-VĀ-sĭv]

194. lumpectomy [lŭm-PĔK-tō-mē]

195. malignant [mă-LĬG-nănt]

196. medullary [MĔD-ū-lăr-ē]

197. metastasis [mě-TĂS-tă-sĭs]

198. mitosis [mī-TŌ-sĭs]

199. modality [mō-DĂL-ĭ-tē]

200. muta

201. mutagen(o)

202. mutation [myū-TĀ-shŭn]

203. necrotic [ně-KRŎT-ĭk]

204. needle biopsy

205. neoplasm [NĒ-ō-plăzm]

206. nodular [NŌD-yū-lăr]

207. -oma (plural -omata)

208. onc(o)

209. oncogene [ŎNG-kō-jēn]

210. papillary [PĂP-ĭ-lăr-ē]

211. -plasia

212. -plasm

213. -plastic

214. pleomorphic [plē-ō-MŌR-fĭk]

215. polypoid [PŎL-ĭ-pŏyd]

216. protocol [PRŌ-tō-kŏl]

217. radi(o)

218. radiation [RĀ-dē-Ā-shŭn]

219. resectioning [rē-SĔK-shŭn-ĭng]

220. sarcoma [săr-KŌ-mă]

221. scirrhous [SKĬR-ŭs]

222. solid tumor

223. stage

224. teratoma [tĕr-ă-TŌ-mă]

225. TNM system

226. tumor [TŪ-mŏr]

227. tylectomy [tī-LĔK-tō-mē]

228. ulcerating [ŬL-sĕr-ā-tĭng]

229. undifferentiated [ŬN-dĭf-ĕr-ĔN-shē-ā-tĕd]

230. verrucous [vě-RŪ-kōs]

Abbreviations

Write the full meaning of each abbreviation.

231. ALL

232. AML

233. bx

234. CA

235. CEA

236. chemo

237. CLL

238. CML

239. DES

240. DNA

241. DRE

242. ER

243. METS, mets

244. NHL

245. PSA

246. rad

247. RNA

248. RT

249. TNM

250. T_X

251. XRT

Answers to Chapter Exercises

1. Yes. Early detection is important; and skin changes can occur fairly rapidly.
2. breast and uterine, cervical, or ovarian
3. dedifferentiated
4. benign
5. invasive
6. malignant
7. deoxyribonucleic acid (DNA)
8. oncogene
9. teratoma
10. sarcoma
11. metastasis
12. carcinogen
13. metastasis
14. C
15. carcinoma
16. C
17. deoxyribonucleic
18. cytoplasm
19. b
20. g
21. h
22. a
23. c
24. d
25. e
26. f
27. prostate
28. Early detection improves the chances of survival.
29. radiotherapy
30. osteoma
31. erythroblast
32. cystoadenocarcinoma
33. meningioma
34. lymphoma
35. gland
36. immature nerve cell
37. muscle tissue
38. retina (eye)
39. lymph cells
40. blast
41. onco
42. muta
43. radi
44. carcino
45. andr(o), masculine + blast(o), immature cell (testicular) + oma, tumor
46. carcin(o), cancer + -genesis, production of

47. mut(a), genetic change + -genesis, production of
48. onc(o), tumor + -gene, element that controls inherited traits
49. radi(o)- x-rays + -therapy, treatment
50. radi(o), x-ray + -necr(o), death + -osis abnormal condition
51. hyper-, above normal + nephr(o), kidney + -oma, tumor
52. lei(o), smooth + my(o), muscle + sarc(o), connective tissue + -oma, tumor
53. aden(o), gland + carcin(o), cancer + -oma, tumor
54. onc(o), tumor + -logist, one who practices
55. onc(o), tumor + -cyte, cell
56. aden(o), gland + -oma, tumor
57. astr(o), star shaped + cyt(o), cell + -oma, tumor
58. chondr(o), cartilage + sarc(o), connective tissue + -oma
59. lip(o), fatty + sarc(o), connective tissue + -oma
60. lymph(o), lymph + -oma, tumor
61. yes, dysplasia
62. no, carcinoma in situ
63. breast
64. prostate
65. prostate
66. uterus and cervix
67. cystic
68. hyperchromatic
69. protocol
70. necrotic
71. verrucous
72. to find further cancer early
73. no, because metastasized cancer needs aggressive treatment
74. carcinoma in situ, carcinoma
75. adenocarcinoma
76. nephrosarcoma
77. basal cell carcinoma or melanoma
78. medulloblastoma, glioma, astrocytoma
79. leukemia
80. lymphoma, Burkitt's lymphoma, Hodgkin's disease, non-Hodgkin's lymphoma
81. osteosarcoma
82. liposarcoma

83. glioblastoma
84. astrocytoma
85. Self-examination, regular check-ups, colonoscopy, mammogram, and avoidance of carcinogens should be in each student's paragraph.
86. breast, skin
87. alveolar
88. C
89. dysplastic
90. medullary
91. C
92. d
93. e
94. b
95. c
96. a
97. This means the cancer has not spread.
98. how far the cancer extends out to healthy tissue
99. Margo's cancer had metastasized. There was no guarantee that all the cancer was removed.
100. Increased immune responses might attack cancer cells.
101. radiation
102. nodular
103. scirrhous
104. hyperchromatic
105. stage
106. carcin(o), cancer + -gen, producing + -ic, pertaining to
107. carcin(o), cancer + -lytic, destroying
108. carcin(o), cancer + -oma, tumor
109. carcin(o), cancer + -phobia, fear of
110. mut(a), genetic change + -gen, producing
111. onc(o), tumor + -genesis, production of
112. onc(o), tumor + -gen, producing + -ic, pertaining to
113. onc(o), tumor + -gen, producing + -ous, pertaining to
114. onc(o), tumor + -fetal, pertaining to fetal tissue
115. onc(o), tumor + -logy, study of
116. onc(o), tumor + -lysis, destruction of

117. onc(o), tumor + -osis, condition, state, process
118. radi(o), x-ray + -active, emitting alpha, gamma, or beta
119. radi(o), x-ray + -diagnosis, determination of condition
120. radi(o), x-ray + -graph, recording instrument
121. radi(o), x-ray + -grapher, a technologist trained to take
122. radi(o), x-ray + graph, instrument + -ic pertaining to
123. radi(o), x-ray + -gram, a recording
124. radi(o), x-ray + -graphy, process of recording
125. radi(o), x-ray + -logy, study of
126. radi(o), x-ray + -logist, one who practices
127. radi(o), x-ray + -meter, instrument used to measure
128. radi(o), x-ray + -opaque, inability to be penetrated
129. radi(o), x-ray + path(o), disease + -logy,

130. radi(o), x-ray + -resistant, less affected by
131. radi(o), x-ray + -pharmaceutical, drug
132. radi(o), x-ray + -sensitive, receptive to
133. radi(o), x-ray + -toxi(o), poisoning + -emia, blood
134. gen(o), producing + -blast, immature cell (ovum)
135. gli(o), neuroglia + blast(o), immature cell + -oma, tumor
136. gli(o), neuroglia + -oma, tumor
137. fibr(o), fibrous + sarc(o), connective tissue + -oma
138. medull(o), medulla + blast(o), immature cell + -oma, tumor
139. melan(o), black + -oma, tumor
140. nephr(o), kidney + sarc(o), connective tissue + -oma
141. neur(o), nerve + blast(o), immature cell + -oma
142. oste(o), bone + sarc(o), connective tissue + -oma

143. retin(o), retina + blast(o), immature cell + -oma
144. rhabd(o), rod shaped + my(o), muscle + sarc(o), connective tissue + -oma
145. sarc(o), connective tissue + -oma
146. destruction by high-frequency current
147. lumpectomy
148. metastasizing
149. dysplasia
150. chondrosarcoma
151. melanocytoma
152. C
153. rhabdomyosarcoma
154. C
155. inflammatory
156–251. Answers are available in the vocabulary reviews in this chapter.

Diagnostic Imaging, Radiation Oncology, and Surgery

After studying this chapter, you will be able to:

19.1 List the types of diagnostic imaging

19.2 Explain the uses of radiation therapy

19.3 List the types of surgery and some important surgical tools

19.4 Define the combining forms and suffixes used in building words that relate to diagnostic imaging and surgery

19.5 Identify the meaning of related abbreviations

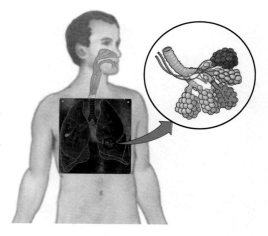

Radiology or **roentgenology** is the medical specialty that analyzes the results of imaging tests. The medical specialty that uses radioactive substances to view or to treat diseases is known as **nuclear medicine.** Either a radiologist or a nuclear medicine physician is a specialist in radiology. Generally, physicians do not administer the tests or treatment. Radiologic technologists are certified and registered by the American Registry of Radiologic Technologists (ARRT) in the following specialties:

- Radiographers who produce diagnostic images via conventional, CT, MRI, or ultrasound technologies.
- Nuclear medicine technologists who image nuclear scans to provide a diagnosis.
- Radiation therapists who administer ionizing radiation to patients to cure or relieve symptoms associated with cancer.

Each radiologic technologist works under the direction of a board-certified specialist in radiology. **Radiography** is the production of diagnostic images. **Cineradiography** allows a radiologist to view a sequence of images showing how tissues or organs work in an individual.

Diagnostic Imaging

Historically, if a doctor tried to diagnose an internal ailment, surgery was the only way to actually see the tissue and organs of a person. With the advent of imaging, it is now possible to view the interior of the human body without invasive procedures. **Imaging** is the production of visual output using x-rays, sound waves, or magnetic fields. **Diagnostic imaging**

> The Web site (www.radiologyinfo.org) provides an explanation of the types of radiation therapy.

is the use of imaging to diagnose problems in the interior of a part of the body without surgery. The three major types of imaging are:

1. *X-ray technology* was the earliest form of imaging. It now ranges from black and white images produced by electromagnetic radiation to computer-enhanced images on a computerized axial tomography (CAT) scan. X-ray technology is widely used in dentistry and for numerous diagnostic situations such as bone fractures, tumor locations, and many other conditions.
2. *Ultrasonography* uses sound waves to produce a visual image of an area of the body's interior. Ultrasonography is routinely used to view the womb of a pregnant women.
3. *Magnetic resonance imaging* (MRI) uses a magnet to obtain images of an area of the body.

Radiology

In the early twentieth century, **x-rays** were discovered and the first images of the inside of a living person were made. X-rays are high-energy electromagnetic **radiation,** energy from the interior of a substance carried by a stream of electrically charged particles. There are three types of radioactive particles:

- **Gamma rays** have the most penetrating ability of the three types.
- **Alpha rays** have the least penetrating ability.
- **Beta rays** fall somewhere in the middle in penetrating ability.

The use of x-rays increased dramatically until it was discovered that extensive exposure to radiation could cause health problems (cancer, birth defects, and so on). Later, lower doses of x-rays that are considered safe dramatically altered the way disease is diagnosed. Now, x-rays are commonly used to detect pathology throughout the body and to treat certain diseases.

X-rays show images in black, white, and gray (Figure 19-1). They are useful for showing abnormalities such as broken bones, internal anomalies, or dental abnormalities, as well as for use in treating certain diseases.

X-rays reveal internal images by exposure of a picture on a photographic plate. The x-rays are directed toward the patient and when they travel through the patient, they come to the plate placed directly behind. Patients are positioned so that the best image may be obtained. Substances of the body may be **radiolucent,** allowing x-rays to pass through quickly (air is radiolucent), or **radiopaque,** blocking or absorbing x-rays (bone is radiopaque). In between radiolucent and radiopaque, there are many degrees of absorbability or resistance to the passage of x-rays. For example, fat is fairly absorbent; blood, lymph, and water are more so. Radiolucent substances appear black on x-ray images and radiopaque substances appear white. Substances in between radiolucent and radiopaque appear in various shades of gray.

X-rays can be dangerous, particularly to people who administer them in a clinical setting. X-rays cannot be seen, heard, touched, or smelled. They cannot travel through lead, a very dense substance, so that the use of lead vests or aprons is very common for radiologic technologists and for radiation therapists. Also, lead vests are often used to cover parts of the patient's body not being x-rayed. X-rays **ionize,** change neutral particles to positively charged **ions,** and, in doing so, destroy cancer cells and slow the growth of tumors. Control of x-rays has become more sophisticated; however, damage to surrounding tissue almost invariably occurs during *radiation therapy,* the

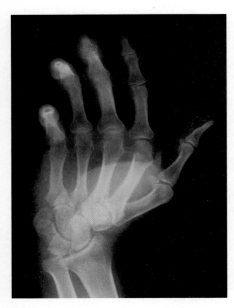

FIGURE 19-1 X-ray of an arthritic hand.

For an x-ray of human bones, go to www.accessexcellence.org/RC/VL/xrays.

use of x-rays to destroy cancer cells. Long-term, unprotected exposure to x-rays can cause cancer.

The use of computers has enhanced radiologic techniques. Not only is the detail of x-rays increased, but computer-guided x-rays can photograph at various angles and can photograph certain body parts (such as the heart) while they are working. Common procedures in cardiology which use computer imaging, such as cardiac catheterization, are discussed in Chapter 6. **Tomography,** the production of three-dimensional images, provides much anatomical and diagnostic information. **CT (computed tomography)** or **CAT (computerized axial tomography) scans** show a series of images conveyed to the computer as detailed pictures of slices of an organ or body part.

PET (positron emission tomography) scans are imaging tests that show the distribution of substances in tissue. They are often used to diagnose brain disorders. This is accomplished by bombarding the area being x-rayed with x-rays at many different angles. The computer interprets the normal density of various parts of the body and the density of a solution ingested. The result is a clear image of minute sections able to show abnormalities in detail.

Fluoroscopy is another imaging technique using x-rays. Instead of a photographic plate, the image is projected onto a fluorescent screen that shows visual images as light rays that are emitted when the x-rays pass through a patient. Fluoroscopy allows for observation of a body part in motion.

X-ray equipment varies depending on the intended use. For example, dental x-rays are taken with a machine that points the radiation to an area of the mouth. Chest x-rays are generally taken on a large plate that covers the front of the chest. CAT scans and PET scans also aim x-rays at particular body areas. The equipment for these scans is attached to a computer on which the image is shown.

The clarity of x-rays can be enhanced if a *contrast medium*, a dense substance that shows up as white on the x-ray film, is used for a particular area of the body. **Barium** and **iodine** substances are ingested to provide a dense substance in a particular area. A *barium swallow* is used for examination of the hypopharynx and the esophagus. A *barium enema* is the insertion of barium into the rectum and colon for a lower GI series.

Iodine is used in many imaging tests to highlight the interior of a cavity, tube, or vessel:

- *Angiography* is imaging of the blood vessels and chambers of the heart after an iodine substance is inserted through a catheter to the heart.
- *Digital subtraction angiography (DSA)* is a two-step imaging process described in Chapter 6.
- *Magnetic resonance angiography* is the imaging of the flow of blood through vessels.
- *Arteriography* is the imaging of arteries usually in the brain (usually to detect blockages).
- *Arthrography* is the imaging of joints after injection of an iodine substance.
- *Cholangiography* is an examination of the gallbladder and bile ducts.
- *Cholecystography* is an image taken after an iodine substance is swallowed and it reaches the gallbladder and bile ducts.
- *Hysterosalpingography* is imaging of the fallopian tubes after injection of a contrast medium containing iodine.
- *Lymphangiography* is imaging of the lymphatic vessels.

A commercial Web site (www.petscaninfocenter.com) gives detailed information about PET scans.

- *Myelography* is imaging of the spinal cord to examine disks and check for anomalies.
- *Pyelography* is the imaging of the renal pelvis and urinary tract.
- *Venography* is the imaging of any vein after injection of a contrast medium.

Ultrasonography

Ultrasonography or *sonography* is the use of sound waves to produce images showing the interior of the body. An **ultrasound** image or a **sonogram** results when high-frequency sound waves are reflected off the body part being observed. The waves are received by a detector that converts them to electrical impulses, which can then be seen on a video monitor. The images produced have become clearer as the technology has advanced. Ultrasonography is a noninvasive method of observation. The equipment used for ultrasonography usually consists of a wand, which is attached to a monitor on which the image is seen, that is moved back and forth over the area being observed. It is used most frequently in monitoring fetal development during pregnancy (Figure 19-2). It is also commonly used for diagnosis, as in *echocardiography*, a test used in cardiovascular diagnosis, and ultra-sonography can be helpful in diagnosing disorders of many other organs (kidney, breast, uterus, gallbladder). A special type of ultrasound unit called a doppler is used on blood vessels.

Ultrasonography is also being commercialized in shopping malls where, for a fee, pregnant women can get a video image done by an ultrasound machine. Some women are having multiple ultrasounds to record the growth of their fetuses. Since no long-term studies have been done of frequent ultrasounds, and since many of the operators of this equipment in a shopping mall setting are unqualified to read ultrasounds, this practice is discouraged by medical professionals.

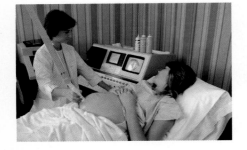

FIGURE 19-2 A pregnant woman having an ultrasound.

To learn more about ultrasounds, go to http://ultrasound.medical-information.org.

Magnetic Resonance Imaging (MRI)

Magnetic resonance imaging (MRI) creates images by tracking the magnetic properties within the nuclei of various cells. As the cells move, some atoms respond to magnetic fields and emit radio waves that produce an image. MRIs are commonly used to diagnose various tumors, defects in the cardiovascular system, and brain anomalies. MRIs do not use x-rays and, therefore, are considered safe and effective. Most MRIs do not require a contrast medium, but one may be used to enhance a scan in certain cases such as in viewing blood vessels. MRI equipment generally consists of a tube into which the patient is placed. While the patient is lying absolutely still, the magnet in the equipment obtains the scan.

Nuclear Medicine

Nuclear medicine uses radioactivity to test and treat disease. Radioactive chemicals, combined with blood or urine specimens *in vitro* (in a test tube), can reveal the presence of various hormones and drugs. Such information is used to monitor the use of medications with potentially harmful side effects. One test in particular, a **radioimmunoassay (RIA)**, is a common "drug" test, often given to participants in sports events, applicants for a job, or others who require regular drug testing. A radioimmunoassay is also used to determine the amount of a medication left in the body after a certain period of time. This information is useful in determining the correct dosage of certain medications. Lead-lined vials and syringes are used to protect workers from exposure.

Other studies in nuclear medicine are done *in vivo* (in the body). The basic goal of an in vivo test is to trace **radionuclides** (radioactive substances) ingested by the patient as they travel through the body. **Tracer studies** trace a specific **radiopharmaceutical** (combination of a chemical and a radionuclide designed to travel to a specific organ) while it makes its way through the organ. In this way, the function of an organ is imaged for observation and treatment. Similarly, a *scanner* (machine capable of creating **scans** or images) tracks the movement of radiopharmaceuticals within an organ to show how the organ functions. Common scans are:

- A *blood and heart scan*, a tracing of blood flow through the heart for diagnosing heart disease.
- A *bone scan* for bone cancer.

- A *brain scan*, for detecting anomalies in the brain that would allow a radiopharmaceutical to pass the BBB (blood-brain barrier).
- A *gallium scan*, using a specific radionuclide (gallium-67) to locate tumors and cysts.
- A *thyroid scan*, scanning the thyroid gland for thyroid cancer and function.

An **uptake test** in nuclear medicine is used to determine how quickly a radiopharmaceutical is absorbed by a particular organ or body part, as in a radioactive iodine uptake of the thyroid gland. A *perfusion study* in nuclear medicine tracks the passage of radiopharmaceuticals throughout the capillaries of the lungs, revealing any clots. A perfusion study may be used in combination with a ventilation study, which tracks an inhaled gas as it fills the air sacs of the lungs.

Radiation Oncology

Radiation oncology or *radiation therapy* is the specialty of those who treat benign and cancerous tumors. The goal of radiation therapy is to cure the patient or relieve the symptoms while sparing as much healthy tissue as possible. Radiation therapy is also used to relieve pain, thereby making the patient's remaining time more comfortable.

X-rays and radionuclides are potentially dangerous in high doses. They can cause damage and death to cells at which they are aimed. Cells that are treated with high-dose radiation are **irradiated.** Irradiation of cells is used in treating diseases with abnormal tissue growth, such as cancer. Radiation is given in doses necessary to penetrate and destroy the malignant cells. The radiation is measured in **rads** (radiation *absorbed dose*), which in turn is measured in **grays (gy)**, each gray equaling 100 rads. Tissue to be irradiated is either **radiosensitive** (as are most lymphomas), needing fewer grays to kill cells, or **radioresistant** (as are most sarcomas), needing more grays to kill cells.

Radiation is transmitted to cells using various techniques and machines depending on the location of the cancerous cells needing treatment. A *linear accelerator* is an *external beam machine* used to emit radioactive particles in a straight line directed at a malignancy. A *betatron* is a circular machine for delivery of radioactive material. A **stereotactic frame** is a device placed around the patient to direct a radiation beam to a specific spot in the brain.

In addition to equipment, radiotherapy may be delivered directly in **brachytherapy,** the implanting of radioactive elements directly into a tumor (**interstitial therapy**) or into an adjacent cavity (**intracavitary therapy**). Another type of radiotherapy is the introduction of radioactive materials that have a specific use (as radioactive iodine in thyroid therapy) when placed in the bloodstream. In the case of the thyroid, it is the only body organ to use iodine, so the treatment affects only the thyroid even though the material travels through the bloodstream.

Radiation therapy may be beneficial and even lifesaving, but it does have potential side effects. Some temporary effects are listed below:

- *alopecia*, loss of hair
- *nausea*, *vomiting*, or *diarrhea*
- *radiation anemia*, suppression of red blood cell production after treatment with radioactive material

- *inflammations* of the skin, mucous membranes, or epithelial tissue due to breakdown of tissue exposed to the radiation
- **malaise,** general ill feeling

Radiologists always need to have the clearest possible images for analysis. Correct positioning of the patient to provide the best views is the technologist's job. An image may be taken anterior-posterior (A/P), from front to back. It may be taken with the patient prone, supine, or in any body position. (Chapter 3 discusses directional terms and body planes.)

VOCABULARY REVIEW

In the previous section, you learned terms relating to diagnostic imaging. Before going on to the exercises, review the terms below and refer to the previous section if you have any questions. Pronunciations are provided for certain terms. Sometimes information about where the word came from is included after the term. The etymologies (word histories) are for your information only. You do not need to memorize them.

Term	Meaning
alpha [ĂL-fă] **rays**	Type of radioactive particle that has a low ability to penetrate the body.
barium [BĂ-rē-ŭm] Greek *barys*, heavy	Contrast medium that shows up as white on an x-ray.
beta [BĀ-tă] **rays**	Type of radioactive particle that has a medium ability to penetrate the body.
brachytherapy [brăk-ē-THĀR-ă-pē] brachy-, short + therapy	Implanting of radioactive elements directly into a tumor or tissue.
CAT (computerized axial tomography) scan	Scan that shows images as detailed slices of a body part or organ.
cineradiography [SĬN-ĕ-rā-dē-ŎG-ră-fē] cine-, movement + radiography	Radiography of tissues or organs in motion.
CT (computed tomography) scan	CAT scan.
diagnostic imaging	Use of imaging techniques in diagnosing illness.
fluoroscopy [flūr-ŎS-kō-pē] fluoro-, light + -scopy, observing	X-ray in which the image is projected onto a fluorescent screen.
gamma [GĂ-mă] **rays**	Commonly used radioactive particles with high penetrating ability.
gray (gy)	Unit of measure equal to 100 rads.
imaging [ĬM-ă-jĭng]	Production of a visual output using x-rays, sound waves, or magnetic fields.
interstitial [ĭn-tĕr-STĬSH-ăl] **therapy**	Substance is placed within the tissue or tumor.
intracavitary [ĬN-tră-CĂV-ĭ-tār-ē] **therapy** intra-, within + cavit(y)	Brachytherapy in which the radioactive substance is placed in a cavity near a cancerous lesion.

Term	Meaning
iodine [Ī-ō-dīn]	Substance used in radiopharmaceuticals for contrast medium and radiation therapy.
ion [Ī-ŏn]	Positively charged particle used to ionize tissue.
ionize [Ī-ŏn-īz]	To destroy cells by changing neutral particles to ions using x-rays.
irradiated [ĭ-RĀ-dē-āt-ĕd]	Treated with radiation.
magnetic resonance imaging (MRI)	Imaging produced by tracking the magnetic properties in the nuclei of various cells.
malaise [mă-LĀZ]	General feeling of illness.
nuclear medicine	Medical specialty for treating diseases with radioactive substances.
PET (positron emission tomography) scan	A series of images that shows the distribution of substances through tissue.
rad [răd] **(radiation absorbed dose)**	Unit of radioactive substance that can be absorbed in a particular period of time.
radiation [RĀ-dē-Ā-shŭn] From Latin *radius*, beam	Energy carried by a stream of particles from a substance.
radiography [RĀ-dē-ŎG-ră-fē] radio-, radiation + -graphy	Production of diagnostic images.
radioimmunoassay (RIA) [RĀ-dē-ō-ĬM-ū-nō-ĂS-sā] radio- + immuno-, immunity + assay	In vitro test to determine the amount of drugs or medication left in the body.
radiology [RĀ-dē-ŎL-ō-jē] radio- + -logy, study of	Medical specialty in diagnostic imaging and radiation treatment.
radiolucent [RĀ-dē-ō-LŪ-sĕnt] radio- + Latin *lucens*, shining	Able to be easily penetrated by x-rays.
radionuclide [RĀ-dē-ō-NŪ-klĭd] radio- + nucl(ear)	Radioactive substance.
radiopaque [RĀ-dē-ō-PĀK] radi-, radiation + -opaque	Not able to be easily penetrated by x-rays.
radiopharmaceutical [RĀ-dē-ō-făr-mă-SŪ-tĭ-kăl] radio- + pharmaceutical	Chemical substance containing radioactive material.
radioresistant [RĀ-dē-ō-rē-ZĬS-tĕnt] radio- + resistant	Not greatly affected by radiation.
radiosensitive [RĀ-dē-ō-SĔN-sĭ-tĭv] radio- + sensitive	Easily affected by radiation.
roentgenology [RĔNT-gĕn-ŎL-ō-jē] roentgeno-, roentgen + -logy	Radiology.
scan	Image obtained from the interior of the body.

Term	Meaning
sonogram [SŎN-ō-grăm] sono-, sound + -gram, a recording	Ultrasound image.
stereotactic [STĔR-ē-ō-TĂK-tĭk] **frame** stereo-, three-dimensional + Greek *taxis*, frame	Headgear worn by patients needing pinpoint accuracy in the treatment of brain anomalies.
tomography [tō-MŎG-ră-fē] Greek *tomos*, cutting + -graphy	Type of imaging that produces three-dimensional images.
tracer study	Image that traces the passage of a radio-pharmaceutical through an organ or tissue.
ultrasonography [ŬL-tră-sō-NŎG-ră-fē] ultra-, beyond + sono- + -graphy	Use of sound waves to produce images of the interior of a body.
ultrasound [ŬL-tră-sŏwnd] ultra- + sound	Image resulting from ultrasonography; produced by sound waves.
uptake [ŬP-tāk]	Speed of absorption of a radiopharmaceutical by a particular organ or body part.
x-ray [ĔKS-rā]	High-energy particles of radiation from the interior of a substance.

CASE STUDY

Diagnosing a Disease

Nina Thorman made an appointment with her internist to discuss some weakness on her left side. After testing her reflexes and discussing her symptoms, her doctor referred her to a neurologist. Two weeks later while talking to the neurologist, Nina discovered that a series of tests might be necessary because some diseases (particularly neurological ones) are diagnosed by a process of elimination. (For example, multiple sclerosis does not show up in blood or urine tests, but does have several indicators that allow a neurologist to arrive at a diagnosis.) Nina was given an MRI to determine if a brain tumor or other brain anomaly was affecting her on one side. The MRI showed some plaque on her brain. After a series of other tests, including a spinal tap to obtain CSF (cerebral spinal fluid) for analysis, the neurologist told Nina that she has multiple sclerosis. They discussed plans for management of the disease.

Critical Thinking

1. Why did the internist refer Nina to a neurologist for testing, rather than ordering an MRI himself?
2. Why was an MRI ordered as opposed to an x-ray?

DIAGNOSTIC IMAGING TERMS EXERCISES

Match the correct definition on the right with the term on the left.

3. ____ ultrasound
4. ____ radiography
5. ____ PET scan
6. ____ CAT scan

a. blood-brain barrier
b. drug test
c. in a test tube
d. imaging of a joint

7. ____ cineradiography

8. ____ arthrography

9. ____ radioimmunoassay

10. ____ in vitro

11. ____ BBB

12. ____ betatron

13. ____ alopecia

e. loss of hair

f. imaging showing slices of tissue

g. imaging showing movement of substances

h. device for delivering radiation

i. imaging of tissues or organs in motion

j. image using sound waves

k. the production of diagnostic images

Matching

Write the letter of the meaning of each of the diagnostic imaging terms in the space provided.

14. ____ sonogram

15. ____ tomography

16. ____ tracer study

17. ____ radiology

18. ____ magnetic resonance imaging (MRI)

19. ____ diagnostic imaging

20. ____ fluoroscopy

21. ____ CT scan

22. ____ stereotactic frame

23. ____ roentgenology

a. image that traces the passage of a radiopharmaceutical through an organ or tissue.

b. use of imaging techniques in diagnosing illness.

c. medical specialty in diagnostic imaging and radiation treatment.

d. CAT scan

e. ultrasound image.

f. radiology

g. imaging produced by tracking the magnetic properties in the nuclei of various cells

h. headgear worn by patients needing pinpoint accuracy in the treatment of brain anomalies.

i. x-ray in which the image is projected onto a fluorescent screen.

j. type of imaging that produces three-dimensional images.

Surgical Terms

Types of Surgery

Surgery is the removal of tissue, manipulation of tissue, or insertion of a device or transplanted body part or tissue. There are many types of surgery:

- **Preventative,** designed to prevent further disease (as in removal of a cancerous lesion likely to spread).
- **Manipulative** or **closed,** changed without incision (as in the alignment of a fracture).
- **Diagnostic,** helping to finalize a diagnosis (as in the removal of sample tissue for microscopic diagnosis or biopsy).
- **Minimally invasive,** with the smallest possible incision (as in surgeries that use laparoscopes).
- **Reconstructive** or **cosmetic,** designed to improve on or return a part of the body to its original functioning and/or appearance.

- **Cryogenic,** involving the use of freezing to destroy tissue.
- **Cauterizing,** involving the use of heat to destroy tissue.

Surgery and **operations,** the removal, transplant, or manipulation of tissue performed in surgery, can be described according to location on the body, obstruction being removed, machine or techniques being used, or where it is performed. Abdominal surgery is performed on the abdomen; craniofacial surgery is performed on the cranium and facial bones; hip surgery usually means repair or replacement of a hip; transplant surgery is the removal of and insertion of a body part or tissue; and dental surgery is performed on the mouth and gums. Cataract surgery is the removal of a lens of the eye, and **Mohs' surgery** is the removal of a carcinoma after mapping with a chemical to establish the narrowest possible margin of affected tissue. *Endoscopic* and *laparoscopic* surgeries are performed with the use of a camera attached to a lighted probe. *Inpatient* surgery takes place in the hospital with the patient admitted for one or more nights. *Ambulatory* or *outpatient* surgery takes place in a hospital, clinic, or office without admission to a hospital.

The American Society for Aesthetic Plastic Surgery's Web site (www.surgery.org) provides detailed information about plastic surgery.

Surgical Implements

In the centuries before anesthesia and x-rays, surgery was basically performed using a knife and a lot of guesswork (Figure 19-3). Later, **aseptic** (germ-free) environments and instruments contributed to a gradually increasing surgical survival rate. Surgical implements include cutting and dissecting instruments, clamping devices, retracting, dilating, and probing instruments, injecting and suturing implements, and equipment to protect the surgical staff.

Cutting and dissecting instruments include various types of **scalpels** (knives), **surgical scissors,** and **curette** (also *curet*), sharp-edged instruments for scraping tissue. Surgical **clamps** or **forceps** are used to grasp and hold or remove something during surgery. Forceps may be placed around something (such as a baby's temple) to aid in pulling the baby out through the birth canal. Clamps are used to grab and hold tissue in place or to apply pressure to a blood vessel to control bleeding. **Retractors** are used to hold a surgical wound open, **dilators** are used to enlarge an opening, and **probes** are used to explore body cavities or to clear blockages. Hollow needles are used in surgery to inject or extract material. **Suture needles** and **needle holders** allow the surgeon to bind the surgical wound after surgery by sewing suturing material through the wound. **Staples** are another suturing implement. New glues and other materials can be used to suture without needles or staples.

Individuals participating in the surgical procedure must wear personal surgical protective clothing that includes scrub gowns or outfits (pants and top), protective headgear, face shields, protective glasses, and masks (Figure 19-4). Those people who will be performing or assisting in the surgery must also wear sterile gowns and latex or vinyl gloves. All must follow hospital and government rules (set by OSHA, Occupational Safety and Health Administration) and guidelines for **standard precautions** (set by the CDC, Centers for Disease Control and Prevention) with regard to blood and body fluids to prevent the spread of disease. Standard precautions are slightly more detailed than the previous universal precautions set by the government.

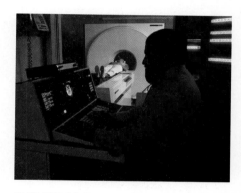

FIGURE 19-3 A technician operating an MRI scanner.

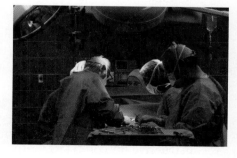

FIGURE 19-4 Surgery being performed in an aseptic environment.

VOCABULARY REVIEW

In the previous section, you learned terms relating to surgery. Before going on to the exercises, review the terms below and refer to the previous section if you have any questions. Pronunciations are provided for certain terms. Sometimes information about where the word came from is included after the term. These etymologies (word histories) are for your information only. You do not need to memorize them.

Term	Meaning
aseptic [ā-SĔP-tĭk] a-, without + sepsis, presence of pathogens	Germ-free.
cauterizing [KĂW-tĕr-īz-ĭng] From Greek *kauterion*, branding iron	Destroying tissue by burning.
clamps [klămps]	Implement used to grasp a body part during surgery.
closed	Performed without an incision.
cosmetic	Designed to improve the appearance of an exterior body part.
cryogenic [krī-ō-JĔN-ĭk] cryo-, cold + -genic, producing	Destroying tissue by freezing.
curette [kyū-RĔT]	Sharp instrument for scraping tissue.
diagnostic [dī-ăg-NŎS-tĭk]	Helping to finalize a diagnosis.
dilator [DĪ-lā-tōr]	Implement used to enlarge an opening.
forceps [FŌR-sĕps] Latin, tongs	Surgical implement used to grasp and remove something.
manipulative [mă-NĬP-yū-lā-tĭv]	Done without an incision, as in the reduction of a fracture.
minimally invasive	Done with the smallest incision possible, such as the clearing of arterial blockages with tiny probes that use lasers.
Mohs' [mōhz] **surgery** After Frederic Mohs (1910–2002), U.S. surgeon	Removal of a carcinoma after mapping with a chemical to establish the narrowest possible margin of affected tissue.
needle holder	Surgical forceps used to hold and pass a suturing needle through tissue.
operation	Any surgical procedure, such as the removal, transplant, or manipulation of tissue.
preventative [prē-VĔN-tă-tĭv]	Designed to stop or prevent disease.
probe	Sharp device for exploring body cavities or clearing blockages.
reconstructive [rē-cŏn-STRŬC-tĭv]	Designed to restore a body part to its original state or appearance.

Term	Meaning
retractor [rē-TRĂK-tōr]	An instrument used to hold back edges of tissue and organs to expose other tissues or body parts; especially used in surgery.
scalpel [SKĂL-pl] Latin *scalpellum*, small knife	Knife used in surgery or dissection.
standard precautions	Guidelines issued by the Centers for Disease Control for preventing the spread of disease.
staples	Metal devices used to suture surgical incisions.
surgery [SĔR-jĕr-ē]	Removal, transplant, or manipulation of tissue.
surgical scissors	Scissors used for cutting and dissecting tissue during surgery.
suture [SŪ-chūr] needles	Needles used in closing surgical wounds by sewing.

CASE STUDY

Outpatient Surgery

James Wilson, an 80-year-old, scheduled his yearly appointment with his ophthalmologist. James has had cataracts but they were not yet ready to be removed. However, at this visit, the ophthalmologist suggested that removal of the right cataract and insertion of an intraocular lens would be a fast and comfortable solution to Mr. Wilson's ever-diminishing sight. The medical assistant scheduled Mr. Wilson for surgery at the Eye and Ear Center, a local outpatient clinic. The day of the surgery, Mr. Wilson was greeted by a patient care technician who escorted him into the surgical area. There he was given a surgical gown and covers for his shoes and head. The doctor, anesthesiologist, and nurse all were in the operating room scrubbed and ready for surgery. Later that day, after several hours of rest and observation, Mr. Wilson's son picked him up to take him home.

Critical Thinking

24. Is Mr. Wilson's surgery an example of preventative, diagnostic, or cosmetic surgery?
25. Cataract operations are simple and localized in one eye. Why is it necessary for the doctors and assistants to be surgically aseptic?

SURGICAL TERMS EXERCISES

Know the Equipment

Write the name of the instrument that is being defined in each statement below.

forceps   clamps   probe   surgical scissors   curette   dilator   needle holder   retractor   staples   surgical needles

26. Sharp instrument for scraping tissue: _____
27. Needles used in closing surgical wounds by sewing: _____
28. Device for exploring body cavities or clearing blockages: _____
29. Surgical forceps used to pass a suturing needle through tissue: _____

30. Instrument used to hold back edges of tissue and body organs to expose other

    tissues or body parts: _____

31. Instrument used to grasp a body part especially during surgery: _____

32. Implement used to enlarge an opening: _____

33. Surgical implement used to grasp and remove: _____

34. Metal devices used to suture surgical openings: _____

35. Scissors used for cutting and dissecting tissue during surgery: _____

Combining Forms and Abbreviations

The lists below include combining forms, suffixes, and abbreviations that relate specifically to diagnostic imaging and surgery. Pronunciations are provided for the examples.

COMBINING FORM	MEANING	EXAMPLE
cine	movement	*cineradiography* [SĬN-ĕ-rā-dē-ŎG-ră-fē], radiography of an organ in motion
electr(o)	electric; electricity	*electrocardiogram* [ē-lĕk-trō-KĂR-dē-ō-grăm], graphic record of heart's electrical currents
fluor(o)	light; luminous	*fluoroscopy* [flūr-ŎS-kō-pē], deep tissue examination by x-ray
micr(o)	small; microscopic	*microsurgery* [mī-krō-SĔR-jĕr-ē], surgery performed using magnification by a microscope
radi(o)	radiation	*radiopaque* [RĀ-dē-ō-PĀK], impenetratable to radiation
son(o)	sound	*sonogram* [SŎN-ō-grăm], ultrasound image
ultra	beyond	*ultrasound* [ŬL-tră-sŏwnd], imaging using sound frequencies beyond a certain frequency

SUFFIX	MEANING	EXAMPLE
-centesis	puncture	*amniocentesis* [ăm-nē-ō-sĕn-TĒ-sĭs], retrieval of amniotic fluid through a needle inserted into the amnion
-clasis	breaking	*osteoclasis* [ŎS-tē-ō-KLĂ-sĭs], intentional breaking of a bone
-clast	breaking	*osteoclast* [ŎS-tē-ō-klăst], instrument for breaking a bone
-ectomy	removal of	*appendectomy* [ăp-pĕn-DĔK-tō-mē], removal of the appendix
-gram	a recording	*sonogram* [SŎN-ō-grăm], ultrasound image

SUFFIX	MEANING	EXAMPLE
-graph	recording instrument	*electroencephalograph* [ē-LĔK-trō-ĕn-SĔF-ă-lō-grăf], system for recording the brain's electrical activity
-graphy	process of recording	*ultrasonography* [ŬL-tră-sō-NŎG-ră-fē], imaging by the use of sound waves
-opsy	a viewing	*biopsy* [BĪ-ŏp-sē], removal of tissue from a living patient for examination
-ostomy	opening	*colostomy* [kō-LŎS-tō-mē], surgical opening in the colon
-pexy	fixation done surgically	*nephropexy* [NĔF-rō-pĕk-sē], surgical fixation of a floating kidney
-plasty	surgical repair	*rhinoplasty* [RĪ-nō-plăs-tē], plastic surgery of the nose
-rrhaphy	surgical suturing	*herniorrhaphy* [hĕr-nē-ŌR-ă-fē], surgical repair of a hernia
-scope	instrument for observing	*microscope* [MĪ-krō-skōp], instrument for viewing small objects
-scopy	a viewing	*microscopy* [mĭ-KRŎS-kō-pē], use of microscopes
-stomy	opening	*nephrostomy* [nĕ-FRŎS-tō-mē], surgical opening between the kidney and the exterior of the body
-tome	cutting segment	*osteotome* [ŎS-tē-ō-tōm], instrument for cutting bone
-tomy	cutting operation	*laparotomy* [LĂP-ă-RŎT-ō-mē], incision in the abdomen

ABBREVIATION	MEANING	ABBREVIATION	MEANING
Ba	barium	DSA	digital subtraction angiography
BaE	barium enema	ERCP	endoscopic retrograde cholangiopancreatography
CAT	computerized axial tomography	Fx	fracture
C-spine	cervical spine (film)	gy	unit of radiation equal to 100 rads
CT	computed tomography	IVC	intravenous cholangiography
CXR	chest x-ray	IVP	intravenous pyelogram
IVU	intravenous urography	rad	radiation absorbed dose
MRA	magnetic resonance angiography	RAI	radioactive iodine
MRI	magnetic resonance imaging	RIA	radioimmunoassay

ABBREVIATION	MEANING	ABBREVIATION	MEANING
MUGA	multigated acquisition scan	SPECT	single photon emission computed tomography
NMR	nuclear magnetic resonance (imaging)	U/S	ultrasound
PET	positron emission tomography	V/Q	ventilation perfusion scan
r	roentgen	XRT	radiation therapy
Ra	radium		

CASE STUDY

Receiving Treatment

Molly Pearl is 80 years old and is having frequent bouts of dizziness, has fallen five times, and is losing some feeling in her limbs. Her gerontologist has referred her to a clinic for neurological disorders where she is given a number of tests including an MRI and a CAT scan. The results of the tests show abnormalities that contribute to her symptoms.

Critical Thinking

36. Why do some imaging tests require the use of a contrast medium?
37. In what part of Molly Pearl's body did the MRI likely show abnormalities?

COMBINING FORMS AND ABBREVIATIONS EXERCISES

Build Your Medical Vocabulary

Complete the terms below by adding a suffix from the list in this section.

38. Kidney removal: nephr_____
39. Recording of the heart: cardio_____
40. Imaging of an artery: arterio_____
41. Suture of a vein: phlebo_____
42. Surgical fixing of the bladder: cysto_____
43. Instrument for viewing the uterus: hystero_____
44. Creation of an opening into the bladder: cysto_____
45. Cutting of a nerve: neuro_____

Root Out the Meaning

Separate the following terms into word parts and define each word part.

46. cineangiocardiography _____
47. cineradiography _____
48. electrodiagnosis _____
49. electroencephalography _____
50. electrolysis _____
51. electrophoresis _____
52. electrophysiology _____
53. electrosurgery _____
54. fluoroscopy _____
55. microscope _____

56. radiotherapy _____

57. radiopharmaceutical _____

58. sonogram _____

59. microsurgery _____

60. radiology _____

61. amniocentesis _____

62. colocentesis _____

63. thoracocentesis _____

64. arthroclasia _____

65. osteoclasis _____

66. vasectomy _____

67. cholecystogram _____

68. electromyogram _____

69. mammogram _____

70. venogram _____

71. angiography _____

72. colonography _____

73. hysteroplasty _____

74. dermatoplasty _____

75. keratoplasty _____

USING THE INTERNET

The governmental Agency for Health Care Policy and Research (www.ahcpr.gov/consumer/surgery/surgery.htm) maintains a Web site containing information about surgery. Go to the site and find at least five questions to ask your doctor before you have surgery.

CHAPTER REVIEW

The material that follows is to help you review this chapter.

Root Out the Meaning

Separate the following terms into word parts and define each word part.

76. electrocauterization _____

77. electrochemotherapy _____

78. electrodesiccation _____

79. fluorometry _____

80. fluoroscope _____

81. fluoroscopic _____

82. microscopy _____

83. radiography _____

84. sonography _____

85. sonographer _____

86. ultrasonography _____

87. ultrasound _____

88. arthrocentesis _____

89. pericardiocentesis _____

90. pleurocentesis _____

91. clastic _____

92. adenoidectomy _____

93. endarterectomy _____

94. laryngectomy _____

95. lobectomy _____

96. mastectomy _____

97. pneumonectomy _____

98. prostatectomy _____

99. onychectomy _____

100. mammography _____

101. nephrosonography _____

102. colostomy _____

103. ileostomy _____

104. craniostomy _____

105. cystolithotomy _____

106. episiotomy _____

107. laryngotracheotomy _____

108. phlebotomy _____

109. tenotomy _____

110. tracheotomy _____

111. bronchoplasty _____

112. dermatoautoplasty _____

113. neuroplasty _____

114. rhinoplasty _____

115. tenomyoplasty _____

116. angiorrhaphy _____

117. colpoperineorrhaphy _____

118. neurorrhaphy _____

119. hysteropexy _____

120. nephropexy _____

121. pleuropexy _____

122. endoscope _____

123. laparoscope _____

124. arthroscopy _____

125. colonoscopy _____

126. sigmoidoscopy _____

127. adenotome _____

128. dermatome _____

129. mammotome _____

Complete the Sentence

Circle the term that best describes the *italicized* description of the correct answer

130. The roentogram required the use of *radioactive particles with high penetrating ability* in order to properly produce the visual needed to diagnose the condition. (alpha rays, beta rays, gamma rays)

131. The radiologist performed the *implantation of radioactive elements directly into the tumor* to reduce the size and hopefully eliminate the tumor altogether. (interstitial therapy, brachytherapy, intercavitary therapy)

132. A routine x-ray was not appropriate for the diagnosis of injured tissue because the tissue is *easily penetrated by x-rays*. (radiopaque, radiosensitive, radiolucent)

133. The small intestine was illuminated by the *contrast medium that showed up as white on the x-ray*. (barium, iodine, radionuclide)

134. _____ are *guidelines issued by the Centers of Disease Control for preventing the spread of disease*. (aseptic procedures, standard precautions, or preventive procedures)

135. The patient hoped surgery *designed to restore a body part to its original state of appearance* would be successful. (cosmetic, manipulative, reconstructive)

True or False

Indicate in the blank whether the statement is true (T) or false (F).

136. ____ Mohs' surgery is the removal of a carcinoma after mapping with a chemical to establish the narrowest possible margin of affected tissue. T F

137. ____ The destruction of tissue by burning is called cryocautery. T F

138. ____ Ultrasonography and sonography refer to the same process. T F

139. ____ Arthrography is the imaging of joints after injection of an iodine substance. T F

140. ____ A gallium scan, using a specific radionuclide (gallium-76) is used to locate tumors and cysts. T F

141. ____ An example of a manipulated or closed surgery would be correcting a simple dislocated joint. T F

Check Your Spelling

For each of the following terms, place a C if the spelling is correct. If it is not, write the correct spelling in the space provided.

142. kriogenic _____

143. suture _____

144. currette _____

145. interstitial _____

DEFINITIONS

Define the following terms, combining forms, and suffixes. Review the chapter before starting. Make sure you know how to pronounce each term as you define it.

TERM

146. alpha [ĂL-fă] rays

147. aseptic [ā-SĔP-tĭk]

148. barium [BĂ-rē-ŭm]

149. beta [BĀ-tă] rays

150. brachytherapy [brăk-ē-THĀR-ă-pē]

151. CAT (computerized axial tomography) scan

152. cauterizing [KĂW-tĕr-īz-ĭng]

153. -centesis

154. cine

155. cineradiography [SĬN-ĕ-rā-dē-ŎG-ră-fē]

156. clamps [klămps]

157. -clasis

158. -clast

159. closed

160. cosmetic

161. cryogenic [krī-ō-JĔN-ĭk]

162. CT (computed tomography) scan

163. curette [kyū-RĔT]

164. diagnostic [dī-ăg-NŎS-tĭk]

165. diagnostic imaging

166. dilator [DĪ-lā-tor]

167. -ectomy

168. electr(o)

169. fluor(o)

170. fluoroscopy [flūr-ŎS-kō-pē]

171. forceps [FŌR-sĕps]

172. gamma [GĂ-mă] rays

173. -gram

174. -graph

175. -graphy

176. gray (gy)
177. imaging [ĬM-ă-jĭng]
178. interstitial [ĭn-tĕr-STĬSH-ăl] therapy
179. intracavitary [ĬN-tră-CĂV-ĭ-tār-ē] therapy
180. iodine [Ī-ō-dĭn]
181. ion [Ī-ŏn]
182. ionize [Ī-ŏn-īz]
183. irradiated [ĭ-RĀ-dē-āt-ĕd]
184. magnetic resonance imaging (MRI)
185. malaise [mă-LĀZ]
186. manipulative [mă-NĬP-yū-lā-tĭv]
187. micr(o)
188. minimally invasive
189. Mohs' [mōhz] surgery
190. needle holder
191. nuclear medicine
192. operation
193. -opsy
194. -ostomy
195. PET (positron emission tomography) scan

196. -pexy
197. -plasty
198. preventative [prē-VĔN-tă-tĭve]
199. probe
200. rad [răd] (radiation absorbed dose)
201. radiation [RĀ-dē-Ā-shŭn]
202. radi(o)
203. radiography [RĀ-dē-ŎG-ră-fē]
204. radioimmunoassay (RIA) [RĀ-dē-ō-ĬM-ū-nō-ĂS-sā]
205. radiology [RĀ-dē-ŎL-ō-jē]
206. radiolucent [RĀ-dē-ō-LŪ-sĕnt]
207. radionuclide [RĀ-dē-ō-NŪ-klīd]
208. radiopaque [RĀ-dē-ō-PĀK]
209. radiopharmaceutical [RĀ-dē-ō-făr-mă-SŪ-tĭ-kăl]
210. radioresistant [RĀ-dē-ō-rē-ZĬS-tĕnt]
211. radiosensitive [RĀ-dē-ō-SĔN-sĭ-tĭv]
212. reconstructive [rē-cŏn-STRŬC-tĭv]
213. retractor [rē-TRĂK-tōr]
214. roentgenology [RĔNT-gĕn-ŎL-ō-jē]

215. -rrhaphy
216. scalpel [SKĂL-pl]
217. scan
218. -scope
219. -scopy
220. son(o)
221. sonogram [SŎN-ō-grăm]
222. standard precautions
223. staples
224. stereotactic [STĒR-ē-ō-TĂK-tĭk] frame
225. -stomy
226. surgery [SĔR-jĕr-ē]
227. surgical scissors
228. suture [SŪ-chūr] needles
229. -tome
230. tomography [tō-MŎG-ră-fē]
231. -tomy
232. tracer study
233. ultra
234. ultrasonography [ŬL-tră-sō-NŎG-ră-fē]
235. ultrasound [ŬL-tră-sŏwnd]
236. uptake [ŬP-tāk]
237. x-ray [ĔKS-rā]

Abbreviations

Write the full meaning of each abbreviation.

238. BA
239. BaE
240. CAT
241. C-spine
242. CT
243. CXR
244. DSA
245. ERCP
246. Fx

247. gy
248. IVC
249. IVP
250. IVU
251. MRA
252. MRI
253. MUGA
254. NMR
255. PET

256. r
257. Ra
258. rad
259. RAI
260. RIA
261. SPECT
262. U/S
263. V/Q
264. XRT

Answers to Chapter Exercises

1. Neurologists specialize in diagnosing central nervous system disorders, partially through imaging.
2. to check for brain anomalies not viewable on an x-ray
3. j
4. k
5. g
6. f
7. i
8. d
9. b
10. c
11. a
12. h
13. e
14. e
15. j
16. a
17. c
18. g
19. b
20. i
21. d
22. h
23. f
24. diagnostic
25. Any surgery requires aseptic conditions.
26. curette
27. surgical needles
28. probe
29. needle holder
30. retractor
31. clamps
32. dilator
33. forceps
34. staples
35. surgical scissors
36. to highlight certain areas of the body or to follow motion within the body
37. brain
38. nephrectomy
39. cardiogram
30. arteriography
41. phleborrhaphy
42. cystopexy
43. hysteroscope
44. cystostomy
45. neurotomy
46. cine, movement + angi(o), vessels + cardi(o), heart + -graphy, process of recording

47. cine, movement + radi(o), radiation + -graphy, process of recording
48. electr(o), electricity + -diagnosis, determining the nature of the medical problem
49. electr(o), electricity + encephal(o), brain + -graphy, process of recording
50. electr(o), electricity + -lysis, destruction
51. electr(o), electricity + -phoresis, carrying, transmission
52. electr(o), electricity + -physiology, functions, activities
53. electr(o), electricity + -surgery, treatment by operation or manipulation
54. fluor(o), light, luminous + -scopy, use of an instrument for observing
55. micr(o), small + -scope, instrument for observing
56. radi(o), radiation + -therapy, treatment
57. radi(o), radiation + -pharmaceutical, drug
58. son(o), sound + -gram, a recording
59. micr(o), small + -surgery, treatment by operation or manipulation
60. radi(o), radiation + -logy, study
61. amni(o), amnion + -centesis, puncture
62. col(o), colon + -centesis, puncture
63. thorac(o), chest + -centesis, puncture
64. arthr(o), joint + -clasia, breaking
65. oste(o), bone + -clasis, breaking
66. vas(o), vas deferens + -ectomy, removal of
67. cholecyst(o), gallbladder + -gram, a recording
68. electr(o), electricity, electrical + my(o), muscle + -gram, a recording
69. mamm(o), breast + -gram, a recording
70. ven(o), vein + -gram, a recording
71. angi(o), vessel + -graphy, process of recording

72. colon(o), colon + -graphy, process of recording
73. hyster(o), uterus + -plasty, surgical repair
74. dermat(o), skin + -plasty, surgical repair
75. kerat(o), cornea + -plasty, surgical repair
76. electr(o), electricity + -cauterization, destroying tissue
77. electr(o), electricity + chem(o), chemical + -therapy, treatment
78. electr(o), electricity + -desiccation, drying, destroying, or sealing tissue
79. fluor(o), light, luminous + -metry, measurement
80. fluor(o), light, luminous + -scope, instrument for observing
81. fluor(o), light, luminous + -scopic, pertaining to an instrument for observing
82. micr(o), small + -scopy, use of an instrument for observing
83. radi(o), radiation + -graphy, process of recording
84. son(o), sound + -graphy, process of recording
85. son(o), sound + -grapher, technician trained in
86. ultra, beyond + son(o), sound + -graphy, process of recording
87. ultra, beyond + -sound, noise
88. arthr(o), joint + -centesis, puncture
89. peri-, around + cardi(o), heart + -centesis, puncture
90. pleur(o), pleura + -centesis, puncture
91. clast(o), breaking + -ic, pertaining to
92. adenoid(o), adenoids + -ectomy, removal of
93. end(o), within + arter(o), artery + -ectomy, removal of
94. laryng(o), larynx + -ectomy, removal of
95. lob(o), lobe + -ectomy, removal of
96. mast(o), breast + -ectomy, removal of
97. pneumon(o), lung + -ectomy, removal of

98. prostat(o), prostate gland + -ectomy, removal of
99. onych(o), nail + -ectomy, removal of
100. mamm(o), breast + -graphy, process of recording
101. nephr(o), kidney + son(o), sound + -graphy, process of recording
102. col(o), colon + -stomy, opening
103. ile(o), ileum + -stomy, opening
104. crani(o), cranium + -stomy, opening
105. cyst(o), bladder + lith(o), stone + -tomy, cutting operation
106. episi(o), vulva + -tomy, cutting operation
107. laryng(o), larynx + trache(o), trachea + -tomy, cutting operation
108. phleb(o), vein + -tomy, cutting operation
109. ten(o), tendin + -tomy, cutting operation
110. trache(o), trachea + -tomy, cutting operation
111. bronch(o), bronchus + -plasty, surgical repair

112. dermat(o), skin + aut(o), self + -plasty, surgical repair
113. neur(o), nerve + -plasty, surgical repair
114. rhin(o), nose + -plasty, surgical repair
115. ten(o), tendin + my(o), muscle + -plasty, surgical repair
116. angi(o), vessel + -rrhaphy, surgical suturing
117. colp(o), vagina + perine(o), perineum + -rrhaphy, surgical suturing
118. neur(o), nerve + -rrhaphy, surgical suturing
119. hyster(o), uterus + -pexy, surgical fixation
120. nephr(o), kidney + -pexy, surgical fixation
121. pleur(o), pleura + -pexy, surgical fixation
122. end(o), within + -scope, instrument for observing
123. lapar(o), abdominal wall + -scope, instrument for observing
124. arthr(o), joint + -scopy, use of an instrument for observing
125. colon(o), colon + -scopy, use of an instrument for observing

126. sigmoid(o), sigmoid colon + -scopy, use of an instrument for observing
127. aden(o), glandular tissue + -tome, cutting instrument
128. derm(a), skin tissue + tome, cutting instrument
129. mamm(o), breast tissue + -tome, cutting instrument
130. gamma rays
131. brachytherapy
132. radiolucent
133. barium
134. standard precautions
135. reconstructive
136. T
137. F
138. T
139. T
140. F
141. T
142. cryogenic
143. C
144. curette
145. C
146–254. Answers are available in the vocabulary reviews in this chapter.

CHAPTER 20

Terms in Psychiatry

▶ PSYCHIATRY
▶ PSYCHOLOGY

After studying this chapter, you will be able to:

20.1 Describe common mental disorders

20.2 Define combining forms and suffixes used in building words that relate to mental disorders

20.3 Identify the meaning of related abbreviations

20.4 Name the common tests, procedures, and treatments used in treating mental disorders

20.5 Recognize common pharmacological agents used in treating psychiatric ailments

Psychiatric Disorders Terms

Psychiatric or mental disorders (disorders of the mind) can have many causes. Heredity often plays a role. Environmental stresses may also contribute to mental illness, or medication taken for other ailments may be the underlying cause of symptoms. With the advent of sophisticated diagnostic imaging, some mental disorders that result from damage to the brain can be assessed by imaging or by physical testing (as of neurological responses). Most mental disorders, however, must be assessed by a specialist trained in understanding how a group of symptoms equals a mental disorder and how to treat that disorder. Many mental disorders are also diseases of the nervous system, such as Alzheimer's disease, and are covered in Chapter 8. Treatment usually involves either medication or psychotherapy (talk therapy) or a combination of both. It may also involve surgery or electroshock therapy (EST).

Psychiatry (Figure 20-1) is the medical specialty that diagnoses and treats mental disorders, usually ones that require medication. A *psychiatrist* is a medical doctor specializing in psychiatry. Psychiatrists sometimes provide talk therapy, often in combination with medication. Nonmedical practitioners who treat mental disorders using psychotherapy alone are called *psychologists, psychotherapists* (Figure 20-2), **therapists,** or **social workers.** These people may have a master's degree or a doctorate. They usually have had extensive training in **psychology,** the profession that studies human behavior and nonmedical treatments of mental disorders. Such training gives them the ability to practice **psychotherapy,** treatment of mental disorders with verbal and nonverbal communication as opposed to treatment with medication alone. Psychotherapy is also known as *talk therapy*.

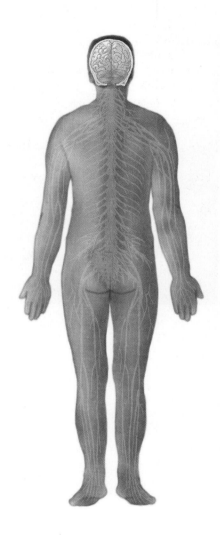

The American Psychiatric Association (www.psych.org) is the premier organization for psychiatrists.

615

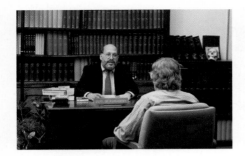

FIGURE 20-1 A psychiatrist talking to a patient.

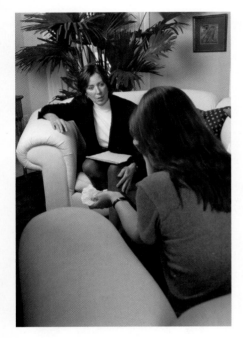

FIGURE 20-2 A psychotherapist talking to a patient.

MORE ABOUT . . .

Phobias

Many people have very specific phobias. Descriptive terms for those phobias are formed by adding the suffix *-phobia* to a combining form that indicates the item about which the patient is phobic. For example, extreme fear of bees (api-) is apiphobia; extreme fear of darkness (nycto-) is nyctophobia; fear of heights (acro-) is acrophobia; and fear of the number thirteen (triskaideka-) is triskaidekaphobia.

Although phobias are symptoms of many mental disorders, having a phobia does not necessarily indicate disease. Rather, it may be as a result of a traumatic experience or the influence of someone else's phobia.

Dementia Symptoms

Mental disorders often include many types of emotional and behavioral symptoms. They may arise from an existing physical ailment, or they may lead to a physical ailment. Symptoms of emotional illnesses may include:

- **aggressiveness,** attacking forcefulness
- **agitation,** abnormal restlessness
- **ambivalence,** feeling of conflicting emotions about the same person or issue, as love–hate, pleasure–pain, and tenderness–cruelty
- **anxiety,** abnormal worry
- **catalepsy,** trancelike state with holding of one pose for a long time
- *defensiveness,* psychological process that enables an individual to deny, displace, or repress something that causes anxiety
- **deliriousness,** mental confusion, often with hallucinations that last for a brief period, as during a high fever
- **delusional,** having false beliefs resulting from disordered thinking
- **dementia,** disorder, particularly in older adulthood, with multiple cognitive defects, loss of intellectual functioning resulting in memory loss, and loss of decision-making abilities
- **depression,** condition with feelings of despair, loneliness, and low self-esteem
- **paranoia,** abnormal distrust of others
- **phobia,** obsessive fear of something
- **psychosis,** extreme disordered thinking

These terms all relate to some sort of mental or personality disorder. Some of the symptoms, such as depression and anxiety, are also the name of a disorder.

Mental Disorders

The American Psychiatric Association publishes the *Diagnostic and Statistical Manual of Mental Disorders*, currently in its fourth edition (1994). A full revision is being worked on and is expected to be ready in 2010. Known informally as DSM-IV, it lists the criteria on which mental disorders are diagnosed and categorized. The major mental disorders are as follows:

- *Anxiety disorder* and *panic disorder*—Anxiety disorder is a condition with chronic unrealistic fear over a period of time, usually affecting concentration and sleep, and causing fatigue. Panic disorder is a condition with recurring *panic attacks*, short periods of intense and immobilizing fear. While having an attack, patients may feel they are suffering from shortness of breath and/or chest pain. Such attacks can mimic the symptoms of a heart attack, adding to the extreme fright experienced by the patient.

- *Alcohol/substance abuse*—Alcohol or substance abuse is a condition in which the patient uses alcohol or drugs recurrently and its use has affected the patient's ability to function at school or work and at home. Such patients are **addicts,** people who have difficulty avoiding alcohol or drugs.

- **Obsessive-compulsive disorder (OCD)**—Obsessive-compulsive disorder (OCD) is a condition with persistent thoughts and ideas that lead to tendencies to perform acts that are recurrent, time-consuming, repetitive, and ritualistic. This disorder usually involves a patient who is a perfectionist and inflexible. If severe, this can interfere with the patient's ability to function normally in daily life.

- **Dissociative disorders**—Dissociative disorders include a gradual or sudden loss of the ability to integrate memory, identity, and other mental abilities with the environment. Patients may have more than one identity or may become depersonalized to an extreme degree.

- **Post-traumatic stress disorder (PTSD)**—PTSD is a condition of extreme traumatic stress that may occur and last for years after a traumatic incident or a period of time in an extremely stressful environment. Prisoners of war, victims of torture, combat veterans, child abuse victims, and crime victims are just some of the people who are vulnerable to PTSD. PTSD does not necessarily show up immediately. It may take years before it develops.

- *Eating disorders*—Eating disorders include conditions with grossly disturbed eating habits. In **anorexia nervosa,** patients refuse to eat enough to maintain a normal body weight, usually accompanied by a distorted body image and an obsessive need to lose weight even, in some cases, to the point of starvation and death. No matter how thin the individual is, they perceive themselves as physically fat. **Bulimia nervosa** is a condition in which the patient binges (eats uncontrollably) and then purges (forces regurgitation). **Pica** is a condition in which the patient (usually a young child) eats nonnutritive substances, such as paint, clay, or sand, for a long period of time.

- **Mental retardation** (or developmental disability)—Usually a condition of birth, such as Down syndrome, mental retardation includes far below average intellectual functioning to the point of inability to care for oneself thoroughly and inability to function within a certain range of academic skills.

> The National Association for Retarded Children is known as the ARC (www.thearc.org). It is an advocacy group and provider of information on intellectual and developmental disabilities.

- *Mood disorders*—Mood disorders include conditions in which the patient has abnormal moods or mood swings. Depression, when it is diagnosed as clinical depression, is a disabling disorder with a loss of interest and pleasure in almost all activities. A clinically depressed person can become suicidal, in danger of killing him- or herself. **Manic** patients have moods that become dangerously elevated to the point of inability to work, sleep, concentrate, and maintain normal relationships. **Bipolar** or **manic-depressive** or **mixed-episode disorders** include drastic swings between manic and depressive moods.

  Bipolar disorder can usually be controlled with medication and those with this disorder can often lead productive lives. Those with the disorder who do not respond to or do not take their medication account for a large number of people with mental illness. Many people with untreated bipolar disorder are prevalent in the community and homeless shelters. Government funding has been decreasing in this area. As a result, allied health workers are seeing many of these patients in ambulatory care areas.

- *Personality disorders*—Personality disorders are conditions in which a destructive pattern of behavior is part of a maladjusted person's everyday life. Included in personality disorders are obsessive-compulsive behavior, the characteristics of which are perfectionism and inflexibility; paranoia, extreme, unfounded mistrust of others; *dependency*, abnormal submissiveness, particularly in adulthood; *narcissism*, unusual preoccupation with oneself; *histrionic*, emotional, immature, and given to irrational outbursts; schizoid, emotionally cold and aloof; and **sociopathy** or *antisocial* behavior, having an unusually callous disregard for others and without moral standards.

- **Schizophrenia**—Schizophrenia has many degrees of severity. Most schizophrenics experience some hallucinations such as imagined inner voices directing their lives. New medications have made it possible for many schizophrenics to function in society. The most prominent symptom of schizophrenia is psychosis that interferes with the activities of daily living. A childhood mental disorder with morbid self-absorption, **autism,** is sometimes thought to have some of the same symptoms as schizophrenia.

- **Somatoform disorders**—Somatoform disorders include physical symptoms having a psychological basis. **Hypochondria** is the preoccupation with imagined illnesses in the patient's body. Somatoform disorders also include intense preoccupation with imagined physical defects in one's body.

Some mental difficulties do not rise to the level of a mental disorder and usually do not require medication for an extended period of time. For example, depression may be situational, as in the death of a loved one. In that case, it would not be classified as clinical depression. Patients with anxiety disorder have levels of anxiety that interfere with their overall functioning. Many people have anxieties that do not prevent them from functioning. Such people are said to have **neuroses,** behavioral conditions that the person has learned to cope with and that do not overwhelmingly affect daily functioning.

There are some mental disorders that affect functioning at a certain level but may go untreated for long periods of time since they do not include very obviously abnormal behaviors. *Attention-deficit disorder (ADD)* and *adult ADD* usually result in distracted behavior, such as an inability to focus at a high level. These disorders can range from mild to severe and are often very treatable with medication.

The National Alliance for Research on Schizophrenia and Depression (www.narsad.org) has information on advances in treatment and causes.

VOCABULARY REVIEW

In the previous section, you learned terms relating to psychiatric disorders. Before going on to the exercises, review the following terms and refer to the previous section if you have any questions. Pronunciations are provided for certain terms. Sometimes information about where the word came from is included after the term. The etymologies (word histories) are for your information only. You do not need to memorize them.

Term	Definition
addict [ĂD-ĭkt]	One who is dependent on a substance (usually illegal, as narcotics) on a recurring basis.
aggressiveness [ă-GRĔS-ĭv-nĕs]	Abnormal forcefulness toward others.
agitation [ă-jĭ-TĀ-shŭn]	Abnormal restlessness.
ambivalence [ăm-BĬV-ă-lĕns]	Feeling of conflicting emotions about a person or issue.
anorexia nervosa [ăn-ō-RĔK-sē-ă nĕr-VŌ-să]	Eating disorder in which the patient refuses to eat enough to sustain a minimum weight.
anxiety [āng-ZĪ-ĕ-tē]	Abnormal worry.
autism [ĂW-tĭzm]	Mental disorder usually beginning in early childhood with morbid self-absorption and difficulty in perceiving reality.
bipolar [bī-PŌ-lăr] **disorder**	Condition with drastic mood swings over a period of time.
bulimia nervosa [bū-LĒM-ē-ă, byū-LĒM-ē-ā, bū-LĬM-ē-ă, byū-LĬM-ē-ă nĕr-VŌ-să]	Eating disorder with extreme overeating followed by purging.
catalepsy [KĂT-ă-lĕp-sē]	Trancelike state with holding of one pose for a long period of time.
deliriousness [dē-LĒR-ē-ŭs-nĕs]	Mental confusion, often with hallucinations, usually having a physical cause such as a high fever.
delusional [dē-LŪ-zhŭn-ăl]	Having false beliefs resulting from disordered thinking.
dementia [dē-MĔN-shē-ă]	Disorder, particularly in older adulthood, with multiple cognitive defects.
depression [dē-PRĔSH-ŭn]	Disabling condition with a loss of interest and pleasure in almost all activities.
dissociative [dĭ-SŌ-sē-ă-tĭv] **disorder**	Condition with a gradual or sudden loss of the ability to integrate memory, identity, and other mental abilities with the environment.
hypochondria [hī-pō-KŎN-drē-ă]	Condition of preoccupation with imagined illnesses in the patient's body.
manic [MĂN-ĭk]	Having a dangerously elevated mood.
manic-depressive [MĂN-ĭk dē-PRĔ-sĭv] **disorder**	See *bipolar disorder*.
mental retardation	Condition with below average intellectual functioning.
mixed-episode disorder	See *bipolar disorder*.
neurosis (*pl.*, neuroses) [nū-RŌ-sĭs (nū-RŌ-sēz)]	Behavior condition that usually involves anxiety that a patient can cope with and that does not rise to the level of psychosis.

Term	Definition
obsessive-compulsive disorder (OCD)	Condition with obsessive-compulsive feelings.
paranoia [păr-ă-NŎY-ă]	Extreme unfounded mistrust of others.
phobia [FŌ-bē-ă]	Irrational or obsessive fear of something.
pica [PĪ-kă]	Eating disorder in which the patient compulsively eats nonnutritive substances, such as clay and paint.
post-traumatic stress disorder (PTSD)	Condition of extreme traumatic stress that can occur and last for years after a traumatic time or incident.
psychiatry [sī-KĪ-ă-trē]	Medical specialty concerned with the diagnosis and treatment of mental disorders.
psychology [sī-KŎL-ō-jē]	Profession that studies human behavior and treats mental disorders.
psychosis [sī-KŌ-sĭs]	Extreme disordered thinking.
psychotherapy [sī-kō-THĀR-ă-pē]	Treatment of mental disorders with verbal and nonverbal communication.
schizophrenia [skĭz-ō-FRĒ-nē-ă]	Condition with recurring psychosis, with hallucinations.
social worker	Nonmedical professional who is trained as an advocate for people (such as the elderly or children) and may also be trained in the treatment of mental disorders.
sociopathy [SŌ-sē-ō-păth-ē]	Extreme callous disregard for others.
somatoform [SŌ-mă-tō-fŏrm, sō-MĂT-ō-fŏrm] disorders	Mental disorders including physical symptoms that have a psychological base.
therapist [THĀR-ă-pĭst]	Nonmedical professional trained in the treatment of mental disorders through talk therapy.

CASE STUDY

Working with Addiction

Alfred Willett has returned to the Drug Treatment Center (DTC) at a local hospital. Alfred, 50 years old, has been an inpatient for alcoholism at the DTC two times in the past. He had been sober for four years, but recently he started using both alcohol and cocaine.

Since returning to his addictions, Alfred's health has declined. The DTC has Alfred see the in-house physician for a check-up and one of the staff psychologists for an evaluation. His health history reveals that he is diabetic and has a smoker's cough. The current checkup finds a slight loss of hearing, but nothing else that is significant since his last inpatient admission four years ago.

Before Alfred can take advantage of the group and individual therapies available at DTC, he must first stay in the detoxification unit where he will be helped to rid his system of alcohol and cocaine. Often this withdrawal period is painful. A total withdrawal from alcohol can cause DT (*delirium tremens*).

Critical Thinking

1. What is the medical term for Alfred's behavior?
2. Why would both a physical and psychological evaluation be necessary?

Match the definition on the right with the term on the left.

3. _____ defensiveness

4. _____ paranoia

5. _____ phobia

6. _____ agitation

7. _____ ambivalence

8. _____ catalepsy

9. _____ delusional

10. _____ aggressiveness

11. _____ anxiety

12. _____ delirious

a. obsessive fear of something

b. abnormal restlessness

c. abnormal forcefulness

d. abnormal worry

e. psychological process that enables one to deny, displace, or repress something

f. abnormal distrust of others

g. feeling of conflicting emotions about a person or issue

h. mental confusion often with hallucinations

i. trancelike state with holding of one pose for a long time

j. having false beliefs resulting from disordered thinking

Spell It Correctly

For each of the following words, write C if the spelling is correct. If it is not, write the correct spelling.

13. psychiotrist _____

14. paranoia _____

15. ankxiety _____

16. boulimia _____

17. schitzophrenia _____

18. hypochondria _____

19. catolepsy _____

20. dementia _____

Combining Forms and Abbreviations

The lists below include combining forms, suffixes, and abbreviations that relate specifically to psychiatry. Pronunciations are provided for the examples.

COMBINING FORM	MEANING	EXAMPLE
hypn(o)	sleep	*hypnosis* [hĭp-NŌ-sĭs], artificially induced trancelike state
neur(o), neuri	nerve, nervous system	*neurosis* [nū-RŌ-sĭs], psychological condition with abnormal anxiety
psych(o), psyche	mind, mental	*psychosocial* [sī-kō-SŌ-shŭl], pertaining to both the psychological and social aspects
schiz(o)	split, schizophrenia	*schizophasia* [skĭz-ō-FĀ-zhē-ă], disordered speech of some schizophrenics

SUFFIX	MEANING	EXAMPLE
-mania	abnormal impulse toward	*hypermania* [HĪ-pĕr-MĀ-nē-ă], extreme impulsivity toward someone or something
-philia	craving for, affinity for	*necrophilia* [nĕk-rō-FĬL-ē-ă], abnormal affinity for the dead

SUFFIX	MEANING	EXAMPLE
-phobia	abnormal fear of	*claustrophobia* [klăw-strō-FŌ-bē-ǎ], abnormal fear of confined spaces
-phoria	feeling	*euphoria* [yū-FŌR-ē-ǎ], feeling of well-being

ABBREVIATION	MEANING	ABBREVIATION	MEANING
AA	Alcoholics Anonymous	IQ	intelligence quotient
AAMR	American Association on Mental Retardation	MHA	Mental Health Association
ADD	Attention Deficit Disorder	NAMH	National Association of Mental Health
APA	American Psychiatric Association	NARC	National Association for Retarded Children
DSM	Diagnostic and Statistical Manual of Mental Disorders	NIMH	National Institute of Mental Health
DT	delirium tremens	OCD	obsessive-compulsive disorder
ECT	electroconvulsive therapy	PTSD	post-traumatic stress disorder
EQ	emotional "intelligence" quotient	TDM	therapeutic drug monitoring
EST	electroshock therapy		

CASE STUDY

Moving on in Treatment

DTC's patients come from all age and social groups. Once Alfred is released from the detoxification unit, he starts at Level 1, the level with the least personal freedom and with the most intensive scrutiny. All of Alfred's visitors and any packages he receives are examined for drugs. Alfred is given daily urine tests. He is encouraged to participate in a self-help organization such as AA, which holds meetings once a week at DTC.

Critical Thinking

21. Many people drink alcohol in moderation. Do you think Alfred can learn to be a moderate drinker?
22. How is drug monitoring being applied in Alfred's case?

COMBINING FORMS AND ABBREVIATIONS EXERCISES

Build Your Medical Vocabulary

Add one of the following suffixes to complete the term: -mania, -philia, -phobia.

23. Unnatural attraction to dead people: necro _____

24. Disorder with intense desire to steal: klepto _____

25. Unnatural fear of public places: agora _____

26. Unnatural attraction to children: pedo _____

Write the abbreviation(s) that best fits the description for each item below.

27. Self-help organization: _____

28. Test of intelligence: _____

29. Type of therapy: _____

30. Type of mental disorder: _____

31. Official diagnostic manual: _____

Psychiatric Treatment Terms

Usually before treatment starts, either a clear diagnosis is made or the patient is put through a series of psychological tests designed to reveal intellectual ability and social functioning, along with an analysis of personality traits. Tests such as the *Stanford-Binet IQ Test* (testing intellectual ability) and the *Thematic Apperception Test* (testing personality traits) are widely used. The *Rorschach Test* asks patients to interpret an ink blot thereby revealing certain personality traits. The *Minnesota Multiphasic Personality Inventory* is a test of personality traits used at many stages of diagnosis and treatment.

Treatment of mental disorders is often based on a combination of psychopharmacology, the science that deals with medications to treat mental disorders, and psychotherapy. Psychotherapists have developed a number of techniques for changing patterns of thought and behavior. For children, **play therapy,** having a child reveal feelings through play, can provide a guide to treatment. Some therapists use **biofeedback,** a method of measuring physical responses (blood pressure or brain waves, for example) to emotional issues, and then use these responses to retrain the client to better recognize and deal with these stressors. Others use **hypnosis,** a state of semiconsciousness in which the patient may be able to reveal hidden thoughts and may be open to suggestions from the person performing the hypnosis. **Psychoanalysis** attempts to have the patient bring unconscious emotions to the surface to deal with them. **Behavior therapy** is the changing of a destructive pattern of behavior by substitution of a beneficial pattern of behavior. **Group therapy** involves a small group of people led by a trained psychotherapist who guides discussions among the participants in an attempt to get them to be open and to change personality problems in long discussions with others.

Various treatment centers around the country treat drug and alcohol addiction as well as eating disorders and many other mental disorders. Most use medications, behavior therapy or **behavior modification,** and individual talk as well as group therapy.

Electroshock therapy (EST) or **electroconvulsive therapy (ECT)** is the use of electric current to a specific area of the brain that changes the brain's electrical activity or "scrambles" the communication from that area to the thought processes. This is only used for very severe cases that have failed to respond to medication and/or therapy. This treatment has made some drastic changes over the years. In the past, patients receiving this treatment were literally strapped to a table and electrodes were placed on their head. Patients would often have grand mal seizures as the current flowed through the brain. A piece of rubber was

MORE ABOUT...

EQ

In recent years, a number of experiments have been done to prove that emotional "intelligence" (EQ) may be more valuable than the traditional intelligence quotient (IQ). One such experiment followed a class of an Ivy League college for ten years. At first, the class was given a personality test that revealed what the researchers thought would be the most important factors for success in life. Over the ten years, it was found that the people with the highest IQ and the lowest EQ were the most unsuccessful, while the people with the lowest IQ and the highest EQ did very well in their lives and in their interpersonal relationships. The statistical results indicate that the bottom third of the class led the most successful lives in terms of careers and personal relationships.

usually placed in the mouth to prevent them from biting their tongue. Today, EST patients receive a general anesthetic. They also have milder or fewer seizures since the current is now controlled by more sophisticated equipment.

VOCABULARY REVIEW

In the previous section, you learned terms relating to psychiatric treatment. Before going on to the exercises, review the terms below and refer to the previous section if you have any questions. Pronunciations are provided for certain terms. Sometimes information about where the word came from is included after the term. The etymologies (word histories) are for your information only. You do not need to memorize them.

Term	Definition
behavior modification	Substitution of a beneficial behavior pattern for a destructive behavior pattern.
behavior therapy	Therapy that includes the use of behavior modification.
biofeedback [bī-ō-FĒD-băk]	Method of measuring physical responses to emotional issues.
electroconvulsive [ē-LĔK-trō-kŏn-VŬL-sĭv] **therapy (ECT)**	See *electroshock therapy.*
electroshock [ē-LĔK-trō-shŏk] **therapy (EST)** electro-, electrical + shock	Passing of electric current through a specific area of the brain to change or "scramble" communication from that area to the thought processes.
group therapy	Talk therapy under the leadership of a psychotherapist in which the members of the group discuss their feelings and try to help each other improve.
hypnosis [hĭp-NŌ-sĭs] Greek *hypnos*, sleep + -osis, condition	State of semiconsciousness.
play therapy	Revealing of feelings through play with a trained therapist.
psychoanalysis [sī-kō-ă-NĂL-ĭ-sĭs] psycho-, psychological + analysis	Therapy that attempts to have patients bring unconscious emotions to the surface to deal with them.

CASE STUDY

Dealing with Life Changes

Alfred's psychological evaluation reveals that he started abusing alcohol and drugs again about three months after his wife left him. He is the superintendent of a large apartment building and relations with the tenants have worsened. The psychologist observes that Alfred is having trouble dealing with the recent changes in his life. She also feels that counseling to help him deal with these changes would benefit him. At the moment, she suspects that he is depressed, but she does not speak to the staff psychiatrist about prescribing medication until he has been reevaluated after detoxification.

Critical Thinking

32. Why might it be easier to determine if Alfred suffers from depression after the process of detoxification?

33. Why is counseling used in combination with medications?

PSYCHIATRIC TREATMENT TERMS EXERCISES

Explain the type of therapy and when and/or with whom it would be useful.

34. play therapy _____

35. biofeedback _____

36. hypnosis _____

37. behavior therapy _____

38. group therapy _____

39. electroshock therapy _____

Pharmacological Terms

Psychopharmacology is the science that deals with medications that affect the emotions. *Pharmacokinetics* is the study of the action of drugs on the body. Many beneficial drugs have been developed that stop or slow the progress of neurotic and psychotic behavior. **Antianxiety agents** generally calm anyone with moderate anxiety. **Antipsychotic agents** relieve the agitation and, sometimes, the disordered thinking of psychotics. **Antidepressants** control the effects of clinical depression on a patient. **Ataractics** and **tranquilizers** relieve anxiety. Many of these psychopharmaceuticals have possible harmful side effects, such as impaired liver or kidney function. For that reason, many patients on such drugs need to have **therapeutic drug monitoring (TDM),** the regular measurement of blood for levels and effectiveness of prescribed medicines. Drug monitoring is also used to detect illegal substances in the blood or urine of addicts in treatment. Table 20-1 lists common psychopharmaceuticals used in treatment.

Illegal drugs can have a negative effect on emotions. *Mind-altering substances, psychedelics,* or *hallucinogens* are illegal substances that produce disturbed thoughts and illusions in a normal person. Most illegal substances are mind-altering to a greater or lesser degree. Because illegal drugs are not monitored, many addicts die each year after an **overdose,** a toxic dose of a substance. People also use legal drugs in illegal doses to get "high," having a feeling of temporary euphoria. The well-publicized "war on drugs" is an attempt to limit access to such drugs while dissuading addicts from using drugs. A relatively recent development in the illegal use of drugs is

TABLE 20-1 Some Agents Used in Psychopharmacology

Drug Class	Purpose	Generic	Trade Name
antianxiety agent, ataractic, tranquilizer, sedative	to relieve anxiety	alprazolam diazepam lorazepam temazepam	Xanax Valium Ativan Restoril
antidepressant	to relieve clinical depression	fluoxetine sertraline paroxetidine	Prozac Zoloft Paxil
antipsychotic	to relieve agitation and some psychoses	aripiprazole clozapine risperidone olanzapine ziprasidene haloperidol	Abilify Clozaril Risperdal Zyprexa Geodon Haldol

the explosion of sales of prescription drugs over the Internet. Many drugs can be obtained without legal prescriptions. This had led to addictions and overdoses.

VOCABULARY REVIEW

In the previous section, you learned terms about pharmacology. Before going on to the exercises, review the terms below and refer to the previous section if you have any questions. Pronunciations are provided for certain terms. Sometimes information about where the word came from is included after the term. The etymologies (word histories) are for your information only. You do not need to memorize them.

Term	Definition
antianxiety agent	Tranquilizer.
antidepressant [ĂN-tē-dē-PRĔS-ănt]	Agent that controls the effects of clinical depression.
antipsychotic [ĂN-tē-sī-KŎT-ĭk] **agent**	Agent that relieves agitation and some psychoses.
ataractic [ă-tă-RĂK-tĭk]	Tranquilizer.
overdose [Ō-vĕr-dōs]	Toxic dose of a substance.
psychopharmacology [sī-kō-FĂR-mă-KŎL-ō-jē]	Science that deals with medications that affect the emotions.
therapeutic drug monitoring (TDM)	Taking of regular blood or urine tests to track drug use and effectiveness of medication.
tranquilizer [TRĂNG-kwĭ-lī-zĕr]	Medication used to relieve anxiety.

CASE STUDY

Talking to a Therapist

After three weeks, Alfred seems quite depressed. He is having trouble relating to the other patients. Alfred's psychologist prescribes therapy sessions three times a week, but does not ask the psychiatrist for antidepressant medications at this time. The psychologist encourages Alfred to express his feelings about his children and his ex-wife, while also encouraging him to understand why his marriage broke up.

Critical Thinking

40. Medication for mental disorders is often regarded as a quick fix. What does it NOT accomplish?

41. The circumstances in Alfred's life could certainly depress someone, but Alfred is not being diagnosed with the mental disorder depression. Why did the psychologist prescribe psychotherapy?

PHARMACOLOGICAL TERMS EXERCISES

Fill in the blanks.

42. An ataractic is a type of _____.

43. A medication used to relieve agitation and some psychoses is a(n) _____.

44. A mind-altering substance is a(n) _____.

45. The science that studies the actions of drugs on the body is _____.

USING THE INTERNET

Go to the American Psychological Association's Web site (www.apa.org). Find information about three mental disorders and describe each in a paragraph.

CHAPTER REVIEW

The material that follows is to help you review this chapter.

DEFINITIONS

Define the following terms, combining forms, and suffixes. Review the chapter before starting. Make sure you know how to pronounce each term as you define it.

TERM

46. addict [ĂD-ĭkt]
47. aggressiveness [ă-GRĔS-ĭv-nĕs]
48. agitation [ă-jĭ-TĀ-shŭn]
49. ambivalence [ăm-BĬV-ă-lĕns]
50. anorexia nervosa [ăn-ō-RĔK-sē-ă nĕr-VŌ-să]
51. antianxiety agent
52. antidepressant [ĂN-tē-dē-PRĔS-ănt]
53. antipsychotic [ĂN-tē-sī-KŎT-ĭk] agent
54. anxiety [ăng-ZĪ-ĕ-tē]
55. ataractic [ă-tă-RĂK-tĭk]
56. autism [ĂW-tĭzm]
57. behavior modification
58. behavior therapy
59. biofeedback [bī-ō-FĒD-băk]
60. bipolar [bī-PŌ-lăr] disorder
61. bulimia nervosa [bū-LĒM-ē-ă, byū-LĒM-ē-ă, bū-LĬM-ē-ă, byū-LĬM-ē-ă nĕr-VŌ-să]
62. catalepsy [KĂT-ă-lĕp-sē]
63. deliriousness [dē-LĒR-ē-ŭs-nĕs]
64. delusional [dĕ-LŪ-zhŭn-ăl]
65. dementia [dē-MĔN-shē-ă]
66. depression [dē-PRĔSH-ŭn]

67. dissociative [dĭ-SŌ-sē-ă-tĭv] disorder
68. electroconvulsive [ē-LĔK-trō-kŏn-VŬL-sĭv] therapy (ECT)
69. electroshock [ē-LĔK-trō-shŏk] therapy (EST)
70. group therapy
71. hypn(o)
72. hypnosis [hĭp-NŌ-sĭs]
73. hypochondria [hī-pō-KŎN-drē-ă]
74. -mania
75. manic [MĂN-ĭk]
76. manic-depressive [MĂN-ĭk dē-PRĔ-sĭv] disorder
77. mental retardation
78. mixed-episode disorder
79. neur(o), neuri
80. neurosis (pl., neuroses) [nū-RŌ-sĭs, nū-RŌ-sēz]
81. obsessive-compulsive disorder (OCD)
82. overdose [Ō-vĕr-dōs]
83. paranoia [păr-ă-NŎY-ă]
84. -philia
85. phobia [FŌ-bē-ă]
86. -phobia
87. -phoria

88. pica [PĪ-kă]
89. play therapy
90. post-traumatic stress disorder (PTSD)
91. psych(o), psyche
92. psychiatry [sī-KĪ-ă-trē]
93. psychoanalysis [sī-kō-ă-NĂL-ĭ-sĭs]
94. psychology [sī-KŎL-ō-jē]
95. psychopharmacology [sī-kō-FĂR-mă-KŎL-ō-jē]
96. psychosis [sī-KŌ-sĭs]
97. psychotherapy [sī-kō-THĀR-ă-pē]
98. schiz(o)
99. schizophrenia [skĭz-ō-FRĒ-nē-ă]
100. social worker
101. sociopathy [SŌ-sē-ō-păth-ē]
102. somatoform [SŌ-mă-tō-fŏrm, sō-MĂT-ō-fŏrm] disorders
103. therapeutic drug monitoring (TDM)
104. therapist [THĀR-ă-pĭst]
105. tranquilizer [TRĂNG-kwĭ-lĭ-zĕr]

Abbreviations

Write the full meaning of each abbreviation.

ABBREVIATION		
106. AA	112. ECT	118. NARC
107. AAMR	113. EQ	119. NIMH
108. ADD	114. EST	120. OCD
109. APA	115. IQ	121. PTSD
110. DSM	116. MHA	122. TDM
111. DT	117. NAMH	

Answers to Chapter Exercises

1. alcohol/substance abuse, addiction
2. to see if a physical problem or another mental disorder is causing some of Alfred's problems
3. e
4. f
5. a
6. b
7. g
8. i
9. j
10. c
11. d
12. h
13. psychiatrist
14. C
15. anxiety
16. bulimia
17. schizophrenia
18. C
19. catalepsy
20. C
21. No, addiction is a mental disorder; addicts do not usually have enough control.

22. daily urine tests and checking all packages and visitors
23. necrophilia
24. kleptomania
25. agoraphobia
26. pedophilia
27. AA
28. IQ
29. ECT or EST
30. PTSD, ADD, or OCD
31. DSM
32. Drugs and alcohol can produce symptoms of other mental disorders.
33. Alfred needs to talk about his problems. Talk therapy can help a patient deal realistically with the actual stressors in his or her life.
34. observing and talking through play—children
35. measuring physical responses to psychological situations—for individuals who can be retrained to deal with stressors
36. state of semiconsciousness in which the patient may be able

to reveal hidden thoughts and may be open to suggestions from the person performing the hypnosis
37. retraining of behavior—for anyone with destructive patterns of behavior that cause severe problems
38. talking out problems to a group of people with similar difficulties—for anyone needing psychological and social support
39. use of electric current to affect the brain—for anyone whose serious mental disorder has not responded to all other types of treatment
40. dealing with issues underlying the mental disorder
41. Alfred's depression was due to situations in his life, not to the mental disorder.
42. tranquilizer
43. antipsychotic
44. psychedelic or hallucinogen
45. pharmacokinetics
46–122. Answers are available in the vocabulary reviews in this chapter.

Terms in Dental Practice

After studying this chapter, you will be able to:

21.1   Name the parts of the body treated in dentistry
21.2   Describe the function of each body part treated in dentistry
22.2   Define combining forms used in building words that relate to dental practice
22.3   Identify the meaning of related abbreviations
22.4   Name the common diagnostic, pathological, and treatment terms related to dental practice
22.5   Recognize common pharmacological agents used in dental practice

Terms in Dental Care

Dental practice (also known as *dentistry* or *odontology*) is the profession that studies, diagnoses, and treats the teeth and gums and any other parts of the oral cavity and facial structure that interact with teeth and gums. Dental practice includes prevention, diagnosis, and treatment, including both reconstructive and cosmetic surgery. **Dentists** are trained practitioners generally assisted by *dental hygienists,* licensed health care professionals who have completed extensive educational and clinical preparation in preventive oral health care, by *dental assistants* who take x-rays, assist the dentist in providing treatment, and perform general office tasks, and by dental laboratory *technicians* who work in the dental lab creating fixed or removable prosthetic devices such as crowns or bridges. Figure 21-1 shows a patient being treated by a dentist and a dental hygienist assisting the dentist.

The oral cavity is part of the digestive system. Teeth and gums help masticate or chew food in the beginning of the digestive process. They are also important to speech and general appearance. The **gums** or **gingivae** surround the bony **sockets** that hold the teeth in place. The gingivae are dense fibrous tissue that attach to and surround the necks of the teeth and adjacent alveolar bone of the jaw inside the oral cavity.

Infants are born with no visible teeth but they usually have 20 primary teeth that have formed inside the gums. **Primary teeth** or **deciduous teeth** begin to erupt through the gum tissue at regular intervals at about six months. The twenty primary teeth, ten in the upper jaw and ten in the lower jaw, are usually all in place by age three. **Pedodontists** are dentists who specialize in treating children. Early good dental hygiene can also affect the development of the hard palate and facial structure. Then, at about age six, the **secondary**

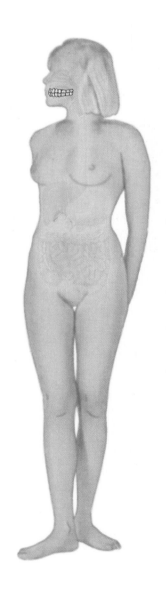

The American Dental Hygienist's Association (www.adha.org) gives good tips on prevention of tooth decay.

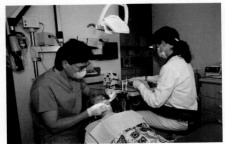

FIGURE 21-1 Dental hygienist assisting the dentist.

or **permanent teeth** begin to develop and push the primary teeth out of their sockets at regular intervals. Ultimately, by as late as the mid-twenties, most people have gone through the teething process, and all thirty-two permanent teeth have developed. Permanent teeth are not replaced by the body if they are lost (Figure 21-2).

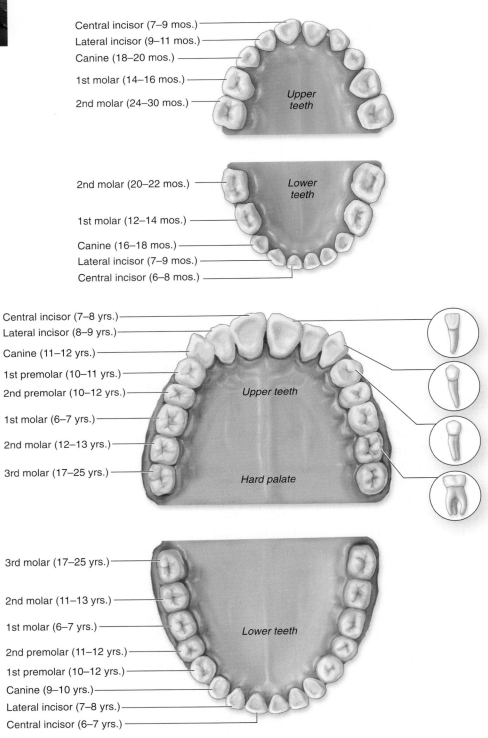

Central incisor (7–9 mos.)
Lateral incisor (9–11 mos.)
Canine (18–20 mos.)
1st molar (14–16 mos.)
2nd molar (24–30 mos.)

Upper teeth

2nd molar (20–22 mos.)
1st molar (12–14 mos.)
Canine (16–18 mos.)
Lateral incisor (7–9 mos.)
Central incisor (6–8 mos.)

Lower teeth

Central incisor (7–8 yrs.)
Lateral incisor (8–9 yrs.)
Canine (11–12 yrs.)
1st premolar (10–11 yrs.)
2nd premolar (10–12 yrs.)
1st molar (6–7 yrs.)
2nd molar (12–13 yrs.)
3rd molar (17–25 yrs.)

Upper teeth

Hard palate

3rd molar (17–25 yrs.)
2nd molar (11–13 yrs.)
1st molar (6–7 yrs.)
2nd premolar (11–12 yrs.)
1st premolar (10–12 yrs.)
Canine (9–10 yrs.)
Lateral incisor (7–8 yrs.)
Central incisor (6–7 yrs.)

Lower teeth

FIGURE 21-2 Primary and Secondary Teeth.

Each tooth has a **crown,** the part projecting above the jawline, and a **root,** the part below the jawline. The crown consists of an outer layer of glossy, hard, white **enamel,** and an inner layer of hard bony substance called **dentin** surrounding the central portion of the tooth, the **pulp cavity.** The pulp cavity contains connective tissue, blood vessels, and nerves called the **pulp,** the life source of the tooth. The pulp extends down into the root of the tooth. **Root canals** are tubular structures that carry the blood vessels and nerves from the bottom of the jaw up into the pulp cavity. The root of the tooth is held in place by **cementum,** a bony material surrounding the root, and a *periodontal ligament*, fibrous material that connects the cementum to the jawbone.

The average human has three types of primary teeth and four types of secondary teeth. Primary teeth include incisors, cuspids, and molars. The *first molar* sits next to the cuspid, and the *second molar* sits at the back of a child's jaw. These molars are sometimes called *premolars*. **Incisors** are the cutting teeth on either side of the center line of the jaw. The **central incisors** are the teeth on either side of the center line—two on top and two on bottom. Next, are the **lateral incisors** or second incisors. The **cuspid,** a tooth with a sharp-pointed projection called a **cusp** sits next to the lateral incisor. Cuspids are also known as **canines** or **eyeteeth.** There are three **molars.** The **first molar** sits next to the cuspid, and the **second molar** sits at the back of a child's jaw. These molars are sometimes called **premolars.**

The types of secondary teeth include incisors, cuspids, and molars, as well as **bicuspids.** The secondary teeth also have central and lateral incisors, followed by one cuspid tooth. Next to each cuspid tooth is a **first bicuspid,** followed by a **second bicuspid.** Bicuspids are so named because they each have two cusps.

Permanent teeth include a first, second, and **third molar** on each side of the jaw, both top and bottom. The third molar is popularly known as a *wisdom tooth*, because it usually appears after a person is fully grown.

In dental care, the outer surfaces of teeth are referred to in special terms. The *labial* surfaces are the parts of the teeth nearest the inner lip that meet when the mouth is closed. The *buccal* surface is on the side of teeth nearest the cheek. The lingual surface is the inside surface of teeth nearest the tongue. The *mesial* surface is the short side of the tooth nearest the midline of the jawline, and the distal surface is the short side of the tooth farthest from the midline of the jawline. Figure 21-3 shows the names used for the surfaces of teeth.

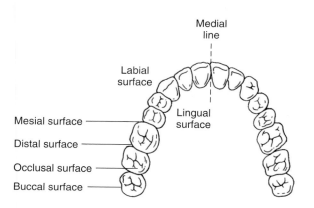

FIGURE 21-3 Dental work on tooth surfaces is usually labeled by the name of the tooth surface.

VOCABULARY REVIEW

In the previous section, you learned terms related to dental care. Before going on to the exercises, review the terms below and refer to the previous section if you have any questions. Pronunciations are provided for certain terms. Sometimes information about where the word came from is included after the term. The etymologies (word histories) are for your information only. You do not need to memorize them.

Term	Definition
bicuspid [bī-KŬS-pĭd] bi-, two + Latin *cuspis*, point	Fourth and fifth tooth from the median of the jawline with two cusps.
canine [KĀ-nīn]	Cuspid.
cementum [sĕ-MĔN-tŭm] Latin *caementum*, quarry stone	Bony material surrounding the root of the tooth.
central incisor	Tooth on either side of the center jawline.
crown [krŏwn]	Part of the tooth projecting above the jawline.
cusp [kŭsp] Latin *cuspis*, tooth	Sharp-pointed tooth projection.
cuspid [KŬS-pĭd]	Third tooth from the midline of the jawline with a cusp.
deciduous teeth [dĕ-SĬD-yū-ŭs] Latin *deciduus*, falling off	Primary teeth.
dentin [DĔN-tĭn] Latin *dens*, tooth	Inner bony layer of the crown of a tooth.
dentist [DĔN-tĭst]	Practitioner trained in dentistry.
enamel [ē-NĂM-ĕl]	Glossy, hard, white outer covering of teeth.
eyetooth [Ī-tūth]	Cuspid.
first bicuspid	Fourth tooth from the midline of the jawline.
first molar	Sixth tooth from the midline of the jawline.
gingivae [JĬN-jĭ-vī]	Gum tissue.
gums [gŭmz]	Dense fibrous tissue that attaches to and surrounds the necks of the teeth and adjacent alveolar bone of the jaw inside the oral cavity.
incisor [ĭn-SĪ-zĕr]	First and second tooth next to the midline of the jawline.
lateral incisor	Second tooth from the midline of the jawline.
molar [MŌ-lăr]	Any of the three teeth at the back of the mouth furthest from the midline of the jawline.
pedodontist [pē-dō-DŎN-tĭst] ped-, child + odont-, tooth	Dentist specializing in the treatment of children's teeth.
permanent teeth	Second set of teeth that erupt at regular intervals starting at around age six.

Term	Definition
premolar [prē-MŌ-lăr] pre-, before + molar	Molar in primary teeth.
primary teeth	First set of teeth that erupt at regular intervals between six months and age three.
pulp [pŭlp]	Connective tissue, blood vessels, and nerves that fill the pulp cavity. The life source of the tooth.
pulp cavity	Center portion of a tooth.
root [rūt]	Portion of the tooth that lies below the jawline.
root canal	Tubular structure holding blood vessels and nerves between the pulp cavity and the jawline.
second bicuspid	Fifth tooth from the midline of the jawline.
second molar	Second to last tooth at the back of the mouth.
secondary teeth	Permanent teeth.
socket	Bony space in the jawline out of which teeth erupt above the jawline.
third molar	Molar furthest from the midline of the jawline.

CASE STUDY

Getting a Checkup

Leila Secor made an appointment for a dental cleaning and checkup. Leila, a 42-year-old mother of two, had lost several teeth after the birth of her youngest child 8 years ago. During pregnancy, the mother's calcium is used first for fetal development. Her own teeth and gums may weaken as a result. Leila now goes to the dentist regularly, and her teeth and gums have improved. Her dentist, Dr. Jack, examined her teeth and gums and pronounced everything in order. The hygienist then cleaned Leila's teeth carefully, and instructed her on a few areas Leila might want to floss more thoroughly.

Critical Thinking

1. Are gums important to teeth?
2. Why is diet particularly important for pregnant women's dental health?

TERMS IN DENTAL CARE EXERCISES

Check Your Knowledge

Circle T for true or F for false.

3. Wisdom teeth are only secondary teeth. T F
4. The pulp of a tooth is the gum. T F
5. Primary teeth erupt through the gums all at once. T F
6. The outer layer of a tooth is the enamel. T F
7. The buccal surface is the side nearest the lip. T F

Combining Forms and Abbreviations

The lists below include combining forms and abbreviations that relate specifically to dentistry. Pronunciations are provided for the examples.

COMBINING FORM	MEANING	EXAMPLE
dent(o), denti	tooth	*dentilabial* [DĔN-tǐ-LĀ-bē-ă], relating to both teeth and lips
gingiv(o)	gum	*gingivitis* [jǐn-jǐ-VĪ-tǐs], inflammation of the gums
odont(o)	tooth	*odontorrhagia* [ō-dǒn-tō-RĀ-jē-ă], profuse bleeding after an extraction

ABBREVIATION	MEANING	ABBREVIATION	MEANING
CDA	certified dental assistant	dmf	decayed, missing, or filled (primary teeth)
DDS	doctor of dental surgery	DMF	decayed, missing, or filled (permanent teeth)
def	decayed, extracted, or filled (primary teeth)	RDH	registered dental hygienist
DEF	decayed, extracted, or filled (permanent teeth)	TMJ	temporomandibular joint

CASE STUDY

Replacing Fillings

Leila's dentist updated her chart by putting in the date and type of service. He noticed that six teeth were marked DMF, but she has not needed further extractions or fillings in over eight years. Leila has two fillings that are over 20 years old. Her dentist made a note on the chart to take x-rays on the next visit to check the condition of those two fillings.

Critical Thinking

8. Why is it important to date a particular type of dental service?
9. Does Leila have two old fillings in her primary teeth?

COMBINING FORMS AND ABBREVIATIONS EXERCISES

Find a Match

Match the definition on the right with the correct term on the left.

10. ____ dentiform

11. ____ odontopathy

a. tooth disease

b. tooth-shaped

12. ____ dentalgia

13. ____ gingivectomy

14. ____ odontology

c. dentistry

d. toothache

e. surgical resectioning of the gums

Diagnostic, Pathological, and Treatment Terms

Most dental work begins with prevention of tooth decay, **cavities,** or **caries,** gradual decay and disintegration of teeth, and **gingivitis** or gum disease. Preventive measures include:

- *Brushing* teeth and gums twice daily to remove **plaque,** the sticky, colorless layer of bacteria that forms on the crowns and root surfaces of teeth causing tooth decay and periodontal (gum) disease
- *Flossing,* using a thin dental tape or string to clean between the teeth and under the gum line helps to remove plaque and food particles.
- Using *antimicrobial mouth rinses and toothpastes* reduces the bacterial count and inhibits bacterial activity in dental plaque.
- Using *fluoride mouth rinse and fluoride toothpaste* provides extra protection against tooth decay.
- Applying *sealants,* a plastic resin is applied to the depressions and grooves (pits and fissures) on chewing surfaces of molars and bicuspids. The sealant acts as a barrier, protecting enamel from plaque and acids.

Tooth decay in infants or toddlers can be caused by going to sleep with bottles in their mouth. As soon as a baby's first teeth appear—usually by age six months or so—the child is susceptible to decay. This condition is often referred to as baby bottle tooth decay or early childhood caries. In some unfortunate cases, infants and toddlers may experienced severe tooth decay that requires dental restorations or extractions.

Once tooth decay (caries) has begun, the earlier it is caught the better the outcome. Dental x-rays reveal the beginnings of decay at and below the surface of teeth (Figure 21-4). They can also reveal any problems with the normal growth of permanent teeth, such as an *impacted wisdom tooth,* a third molar so tightly wedged into the jawbone that it is unable to erupt or break through the surface of the gums thoroughly. Tooth decay can cause toothaches or **odontalgia,** which can be quite painful. Early tooth decay that has not invaded the central portion of the tooth usually receives a **filling,** a dental restoration. Filling includes **drilling,** cutting away some of the tooth structure, removing the decayed area, and placing into the space medication and restoration material. There are several dental filling options:

- Dental **amalgam** is a mixture of metal alloys. It is durable, easy to use, highly resistant to wear, and relatively inexpensive in comparison to other materials.
- *Composite* fillings are a mixture of glass or quartz filler in a resin medium that produces a tooth-colored filling.
- *Glass ionomers* are translucent, tooth-colored materials made of a mixture of acrylic acids and fine glass powders that are used to fill cavities, particularly those on the root surfaces of teeth.

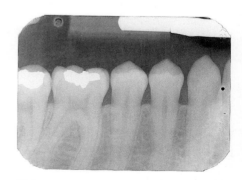

FIGURE 21-4 Dental x-rays can show decay as well as existing fillings.

- *All-porcelain (ceramic)* dental materials include porcelain, ceramic or glasslike fillings crowns or veneers. A *veneer* is a very thin shell of porcelain that can replace or cover part of the enamel of the tooth. These restorations are particularly desirable because their color and translucency mimic natural tooth enamel.
- *Porcelain-fused-to-metal* provides strength to a crown or bridge. These restorations are very strong and durable.
- *Gold alloys* contain gold, copper, and other metals that result in a strong, effective filling, crown, or bridge.

A mixture of metals or other substances that are designed to prevent further tooth erosion. If decay is deeper within the tooth, affecting the nerve tissue, an **abscess,** infection and swelling of the soft tissue of the jaw, may result.

In some cases, the tooth must be removed partially or totally. If nerve tissue must be removed, root canal work is performed. *Root canal work* is the removal of pulp tissue and affected nerves in the root canals. Medication is applied and the affected canals are sealed off. **Endodontists** are dentists who specialize in root canal work.

When teeth are damaged by severe trauma or decayed to the extent that they cannot be restored, replacement or artificial teeth are used. **Dentures** are dental prostheses that can be permanently held in place or can be removable. Dentures are either **partial,** replacing one or more but not all teeth, or **full,** replacing a whole set of teeth (Figure 21-5). Partials are attached to other teeth with clasps and are removable for cleaning. A **bridge,** sometimes called a fixed partial denture, is a restoration which replaces or spans the space where one or more teeth have been lost. There are two types of bridges, fixed and removable. Fixed bridges are bonded into place and can only be removed by the dentist. Removable bridges can be taken out for cleaning. Dentists use a process of impressions, molding, shaping, and color-matching substances that are then made into dentures or bridges in a dental laboratory before being placed into the patient's mouth. Missing teeth may also be replaced with dental **implants,** artificial teeth that have extensions set into bone. Implants are expensive and, while some people will have an entire mouth filled with implants, they are more commonly used for just a few teeth. *Prosthodontics* is the branch of dentistry that deals with the construction of artificial devices for replacing missing teeth or other structures in the mouth and jaw. The *prosthodontist* specializes in the practice of prosthodontics.

Gum disease (periodontal disease) is classified according to the severity of the disease. The two major stages are *gingivitis* and *periodontitis*. Gingivitis is a milder and reversible form of periodontal disease that only affects the gums. Gingivitis may lead to more serious, destructive forms of periodontal disease called periodontitis. Gingivitis and periodontitis, inflammation and infection of the tissue that supports the teeth, can result from too much plaque, other medical conditions, or general poor dental hygiene and health. **Periodontists** are specialists who treat gum disease, often by surgically removing diseased tissue and calcified plaque in a process called scaling. Signs and symptoms of periodontal disease include:

- Gums that bleed easily
- Red, swollen, tender gums
- Gums that have pulled away from the teeth

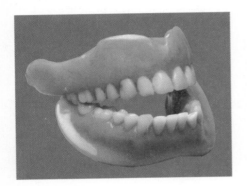

FIGURE 21-5 A full set of dentures.

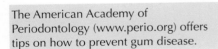

The American Academy of Periodontology (www.perio.org) offers tips on how to prevent gum disease.

- Persistent bad breath or bad taste
- Permanent teeth that are loose or separating
- Any change in the way your teeth fit together when you bite
- Any change in the fit of partial dentures

It is possible to have periodontal disease and have no warning signs. That is one reason why regular dental checkups and periodontal examinations are very important. Good oral hygiene is essential to help keep periodontal disease from becoming more serious or recurring necessary to reduce the inflammation before gums can be thoroughly treated.

Orthodontists are dentists who specialize in **orthodontics,** the correction and prevention of irregularities in the alignment and appearance of teeth. They can correct **malocclusions,** abnormal closure of the top teeth in relation to the bottom teeth, such as an overbite. Malocclusions may be corrected with surgical removal of any teeth that are crowding other teeth or with **braces,** appliances that put pressure on the teeth to move them slowly into place. There is much debate between orthodontists and child developmental experts regarding thumb-sucking. The child development experts argue the benefits of the child being able to take control of his/her emotions and well-being. The orthodontists are quick to point out the damage that is done to the developing hard palate and tooth alignment.

Some dentists also treat **temporomandibular joint (TMJ) dysfunction,** pain in the jawline due to dislocation or joint problems that prevent this complex system of muscles, ligaments, discs, and bones from working together properly. Treatments for this pain may include stress reducing exercises, muscle relaxants, or wearing a mouth protector to prevent teeth grinding *(bruxism)*.

Other dentists perform cosmetic dentistry by replacing and manipulating broken, discolored, or disfigured teeth. Still others treat discolored teeth with bleaching products to whiten them. Most dental stains are caused by age, tobacco, coffee or tea, antibiotics, such as tetracycline, or excess fluoride. Cosmetic treatment may include:

The American Association of Orthodontists (www.braces.org) has a public information Web site.

- *Bleaching:* Chairside bleaching involves several sessions. A bleaching agent is applied to the teeth, and a special light may be used to enhance the action of the agent. At-home bleaching may involve the use mouth trays and a peroxide containing gel.
- *Bonding:* Composite resin is molded onto the teeth to change their color and to reshape them.
- **Porcelain veneers:** Shell-like facings can be bonded onto stained teeth.
- **Whitening toothpastes:** While some whitening toothpastes effectively keep the teeth cleaner and, therefore, looking whiter, some are more abrasive than others.

VOCABULARY REVIEW

In the previous section, you learned terms relating to dental diagnosis, pathology, and treatment. Before going on to the exercises, review the following terms and refer to the previous section if you have any questions. Pronunciations are provided for certain terms. Sometimes information about where the word came from is included after the term. The etymologies (word histories) are for your information only. You do not need to memorize them.

Term	Definition
abscess [ĂB-sĕs]	Infection and swelling of the soft tissue of the jaw.
amalgam [ă-MĂL-găm]	Mixture of metals or other alloys used as fillings.
braces [BRĀ-sĕz]	Appliances that straighten teeth slowly.
bridge [brĭdj]	Fixed or removable dental restoration replacing missing teeth.
caries [KĀR-ēz]	Tooth decay.
cavity [KĂV-ĭ-tē]	Tooth decay.
dentures [DĔN-chūrs]	Artificial replacement teeth.
drilling	Cutting of tooth structure and removal of the decayed area of a tooth with a small dental drill.
endodontist [ĕn-dō-DŎN-tĭst]	Dentist who specializes in root canal work.
filling	An amalgam or other restorative material placed into a drilled space to prevent further tooth decay.
fluoride [FLŪR-īd]	Substance given as a topical application or mouthwash to prevent tooth decay.
full	Complete (set of dentures).
gingivitis [jĭn-jĭ-VĪ-tĭs]	Inflammation of the gums.
implant	Artificial replacement tooth that has an extension set into bone.
malocclusions [măl-ō-KLŪ-zhŭns]	Abnormal closures of the top teeth in relation to the bottom teeth.
odontalgia [ō-dŏn-TĂL-jē-ă]	Tooth pain.
orthodontics [ōr-thō-DŎN-tĭks]	Dental specialty concerned with the correction and prevention of irregularities in the placement and appearance of teeth.
partial	One or more artificial replacement teeth.
periodontist [PĔR-ē-ō-DŎN-tĭst]	Dentist who specializes in the treatment of gum disease.
plaque [plăk]	Microorganisms that grow on the crowns and along the roots of teeth, causing decay of teeth and breakdown of gums.
temporomandibular [TĔM-pŏ-rō-măn-DĬB-yū-lăr] joint (TMJ) dysfunction	Pain in the jawline due to dislocation of the joint.

CASE STUDY

Feeling Pain

Leila was pleased with the results of her dental visit. She asked the receptionist to remind her when her next six-month appointment was needed. The reminder postcards keep Leila on track. Two months after her visit, Leila felt a slight pain in one of her teeth. She thought she felt some food stuck between her teeth, so she flossed and the pain went away. A few days later, on a Saturday, Leila felt queasy and noticed a dull ache in the same tooth that had hurt a couple of days ago. Leila called the dentist's office and got an appointment for Monday morning. By Monday morning, the dull ache had become a painful toothache. The dentist took x-rays and saw that an abscess had formed at the root apex (end) of a tooth containing one of the old fillings.

He explained to Leila that her tooth could be extracted totally (requiring a partial denture, bridge, or a dental implant) or could be partially removed and an artificial crown put in its place. Leila chose to have the crown, thereby saving as much of her natural tooth as possible. In either case, because the abscess is an infection, a root canal would have to be performed. If the crown were just cosmetic, no root canal work would be needed.

Critical Thinking

15. What type of specialist is Leila likely to have to see before the crown is put in place?
16. Will Leila have to remove the crown daily for cleaning?

DIAGNOSTIC, PROCEDURAL, AND LABORATORY TERMS EXERCISES

Review the Information

Fill in the blanks.

17. Two types of dental prostheses are _____ and _____.
18. Amalgam is a material used to _____ teeth.
19. Abnormal closure of the top teeth in relation to the bottom teeth is called a _____.
20. Microorganisms that cause decay form _____ around the teeth and gums.
21. A specialist in the treatment of gum disease is a _____.
22. A fixed dental appliance that replaces one or more teeth is a(n) _____.
23. The dental specialist concerned with correcting the alignment of teeth is a(n) _____.
24. DEF is the abbreviation for _____.
25. Another term for tooth decay is _____.

Pharmacological Terms

Dentists provide local anesthetics during certain treatments, such as drilling. The most commonly used are **Novocaine,** which is injected near the site being treated, and **nitrous oxide,** a gas inhaled by the patient. Nitrous oxide is also known as *laughing gas* because it produces laughing in some patients. If a dentist needs to prescribe antibiotics or painkillers after a procedure, there are limitations to the number and strengths they can prescribe.

VOCABULARY REVIEW

In the previous section, you learned terms relating to pharmacology. Before going on, review the terms below and refer to the previous section if you have any questions.

Term	Definition
nitrous oxide [NĪ-trŭs ŎK-sīd]	An anesthetic gas inhaled by the patient.
Novocaine [NŌ-vă-kān]	An anesthetic injected near the site being treated.

USING THE INTERNET

Go to the American Dental Association's Web site (www.ada.org). Find an article about preventive dentistry. Write a brief paragraph summarizing the information you have read.

CHAPTER REVIEW

The material that follows is to help you review this chapter.

Understanding Dental Terms

Write the letter of the answer in the space provided. Not all answers will be used.

26. _____ number of primary teeth
27. _____ number of secondary teeth
28. _____ buccal
29. _____ near the tongue
30. _____ labial

a. lingual
b. near the cheek
c. near the lip
d. mesial
e. 32
f. 20

Fill in the Blank

Write the word that best completes the sentence.

31. You would visit a(n) _____ for braces.
32. A(n) _____ treats gum disease.
33. Root canals are performed by _____.
34. _____ specialize in dental treatment for children.
35. Gingivitis would be treated by a(n) _____.
36. A dental specialist in the replacement of missing teeth is a(n) _____.
37. The dental _____ is a licensed member of the dental health team who may perform extensive preventive treatment for patients.

Spell It Correctly

Write the correct spelling in the blank to the right of any misspelled words. If the word is already correctly spelled, write C.

38. temparomandibuler _____
39. dicidous _____
40. bycusped _____
41. moler _____
42. inciser _____
43. partial _____
44. flourid _____
45. vener _____
46. gingevas _____

47. amalgum _____
48. bridge _____
49. inplant _____
50. seelant _____
51. composit _____
52. permanent _____
53. hygeinest _____
54. prosthadontist _____
55. Novicain _____

DEFINITIONS

Define the following terms and combining forms. Review the chapter before starting. Make sure you know how to pronounce each term as you define it.

TERM

56. abscess [ĂB-sĕs]
57. amalgam [ă-MĂL-găm]
58. bicuspid [bī-KŬS-pĭd]
59. braces [BRĀ-sĕz]
60. bridge [brĭdj]
61. canine [KĀ-nīn]
62. caries [KĀR-ēz]
63. cavity [KĂV-ĭ-tē]
64. cementum [sĕ-MĔN-tŭm]
65. central incisor
66. crown [krŏwn]
67. cusp [kŭsp]
68. cuspid [KŬS-pĭd]
69. deciduous [dē-SĬD-yū-ŭs] teeth
70. dent(o), denti
71. dentin [DĔN-tĭn]
72. dentist [DĔN-tĭst]
73. dentures [DĔN-chūrs]
74. drilling
75. enamel [ē-NĂM-ĕl]
76. endodontist [ĕn-dō-DŎN-tĭst]

77. eyetooth [Ī-tūth]
78. filling
79. first bicuspid
80. first molar
81. fluoride [FLŪR-ĭd]
82. full
83. gingiv(o)
84. gingivae [JĬN-jĭ-vī]
85. gingivitis [jĭn-jĭ-VĪ-tĭs]
86. gums [gŭmz]
87. implant
88. incisor [ĭn-SĪ-zĕr]
89. lateral incisor
90. malocclusions [măl-ō-KLŪ-zhŭnz]
91. molar [MŌ-lăr]
92. nitrous oxide [NĪ-trŭs ŎK-sīd]
93. Novocaine [NŌ-vă-kān]
94. odont(o)
95. odontalgia [ō-dŏn-TĂL-jē-ă]
96. orthodontics [ōr-thō-DŎN-tĭks]

97. partial
98. pedodontist [pē-dō-DŎN-tĭst]
99. periodontist [PĔR-ē-ō-DŎN-tĭst]
100. permanent teeth
101. plaque [plăk]
102. premolar [prē-MŌ-lăr]
103. primary teeth
104. pulp [pŭlp]
105. pulp cavity
106. root [rūt]
107. root canal
108. second bicuspid
109. second molar
110. secondary teeth
111. socket
112. temporomandibular [TĔM-pō-rō-măn-DĬB-yū-lăr] joint (TMJ) dysfunction
113. third molar

Abbreviations

Write the full meaning of each abbreviation.

ABBREVIATION

114. DDS
115. def
116. DEF

117. dmf
118. DMF
119. RDH

120. TMJ

Answers to Chapter Exercises

1. Yes, they hold the teeth in place.
2. Teeth need calcium to remain healthy, and the embryo needs calcium to grow inside the womb. A pregnant woman usually requires a diet rich in calcium as well as other nutrients.
3. T
4. F
5. F
6. T
7. F
8. to know how old fillings are and to know when cleanings are needed
9. No, her primary teeth fell out long ago.
10. b
11. a
12. d
13. e
14. c
15. an endodontist
16. No, a crown is permanent.
17. dentures, implants
18. fill
19. malocclusion
20. plaque
21. periodontist
22. bridge
23. orthodontist
24. decayed, extracted, or filled
25. caries
26. f
27. e
28. b
29. a
30. c
31. othodontist
32. periodontist
33. endodontists
34. pedodontists
35. periodontist
36. prosthodontist
37. hygienist
38. temporomandibular
39. deciduous
40. bicuspid
41. molar
42. incisor
43. C
44. fluoride
45. veneer
46. gingivae
47. amalgam
48. C
49. implant
50. sealant
51. composite
52. C
53. hygienist
54. prosthodontist
55. Novocaine
56–120. Answers are available in the vocabulary reviews in this chapter.

CHAPTER 22
Terms in Pharmacology

▶ PHARMACOLOGY

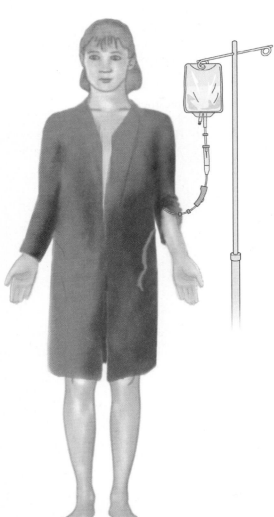

After studying this chapter, you will be able to:

22.2   Describe the source and types of drugs

22.3   List various generic and trade names for common drugs

22.4   Identify the various ways drugs are administered

22.5   Describe some of the ways in which drugs affect the body

22.6   Identify the meaning of related abbreviations

Drug Sources, Types, Function, and Administration

Drugs are biological or chemical agents. They are *therapeutic* when they are used to cure, alleviate, diagnose, treat, or prevent illness. They are *addictive* or habit-forming when they are used in unregulated and excessive quantities to stimulate or depress someone's moods. Therapeutic drugs are also called **medicines** or **medications.**

Drugs come from plants, animals, or through chemical synthesis in a laboratory. **Vitamins,** organic substances found in food, are also a form of drugs. The federal *Food and Drug Administration (FDA)* regulates the testing, manufacture, content, and distribution of all drugs that are not part of or derived from food. The FDA has an approval process that is intended to exclude drugs that may cause more harm than they can cure. It evaluates data submitted by pharmaceutical companies to determine the safety or harmful effects of a drug, and to ensure the drug provides effective treatment. In recent years, there have been questions about the efficacy of the FDA's approval and monitoring processes. Congress is studying new ways to ensure the independence of the FDA. The standards for approval are set by an independent committee in publications collected and published as the *United States Pharmacopeia (U.S.P.)*. When the letters U.S.P. follow a drug name on the package, it means that the drug has met the stringent standards set by the committee.

Aside from the Pharmacopeia, doctors generally use one of two references in gathering drug information. The first, the *Hospital Formulary*, lists drugs that are approved for patient care in that particular facility. The use of formularies grew out of the need to control health care costs under managed care systems. The second, the *Physician's Desk Reference (PDR)*, is a widely used reference for physicians. The PDR lists drugs by their drug class, and includes information such as indication for use, known side effects, appropriate dosages, and routes of administration.

Pharmacology is the science that studies, develops, and tests drugs. Some of the scientists who work in pharmacology specialize in the various subdivisions of the field. For example, *medicinal chemistry* is the study of new drugs, their structure, and how they work. **Pharmacodynamics** is the study of how drugs affect the body. **Toxicology** is the study of harmful effects of drugs on the body and of **antidotes,** substances able to cancel out unwanted effects. **Pharmacokinetics** is the study of how drugs are **absorbed, metabolized** (chemically changed so it can be used in the body), and **excreted** over time. Since the mapping of the human genome and ability to use stem cells, new drug therapies are being developed all the time. Many foresee a day when genetically developed drugs and therapies will be the preferred method for preventing and curing disease.

Some drugs are available **over-the-counter (OTC),** sold without a doctor's **prescription,** which is an order for medication with the dosages, directions, route, and timing of administration included. Prescription drugs are dispensed by a **pharmacist** or **druggist** in a pharmacy or drug store. Figure 22-1 shows a pharmacist who is filling a prescription. Drugs are also available from mail-order companies and from companies on the Internet. Drugs usually come with instructions about how and how often to take the medication and a listing of the potential side effects. Sometimes other drugs or even foods are **contraindicated** (advised against) to be taken along with the medication being given.

Drugs can have several different names. First is a chemical name that describes the chemical formula of the drug. Second is a **generic** name that is the official name of the drug and is often a shortened or simpler version of the chemical name for legal purposes. Third is a **trade, brand,** or **proprietary**

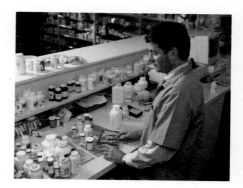

FIGURE 22-1 Pharmacist filling a prescription.

The publishers of the PDR run a Web site (www.gettingwell.com) where it is possible to search for information about specific drugs.

MORE ABOUT . . .

Pain Management and Controlled Substances

In the past, many in the medical community regarded chronic pain as only a symptom. Often, practitioners told patients much of it was in their heads. In recent years, chronic pain has come to be regarded as a long-term condition in need of management both for the quality of life such management offers and for the attempt to prevent the pain from becoming debilitating. Many pain medications have been developed and are effective along with therapies, such as acupuncture, biofeedback, physical therapy, massage therapy, and others. Unfortunately, the most effective medications are also the drugs most likely to be abused or to become addictive. The federal government regards narcotics and other medications, such as Vicodin, Oxycontin, sedatives, and various strong muscle relaxants, as controlled substances. This means that patients can only receive a limited number of pills in a specified time period. Also, physicians who prescribe and pharmacists who fulfill an inordinate number of prescriptions of controlled substances often come under scrutiny. For more information on pain management, visit the WebMD section on this issue (www.webmd.com/pain-management/default.htm).

name that is given and copyrighted by the manufacturer for a specific drug. Each drug has only one chemical name and only one generic name, but it may have many trade names. For example, acetylsalicylic acid is the chemical name for *aspirin*, the generic name packaged under various trade names, such as Bayer aspirin. Table 22-1 lists some generic and trade names of drugs according to their function (what class of drug it is). Many insurance companies will only pay for generic drugs or the least expensive alternatives. Pharmacies generally check a patient's insurance before filling any prescription. Federal laws also may limit the number of pills of certain restricted drugs that may be filled at any one time. Restricted drugs, called *controlled substances*, are usually narcotics or other addictive drugs that may be easily abused.

Dosages of drugs vary depending on the age, size, severity of symptoms, and other medications in use. Some drugs are tapered; that is, they are given at a higher dose initially and then the dose is gradually reduced as the symptoms subside. Many drugs are synthesized to perform like substances in the body. For example, manufactured **hormones** (chemical substances in the body that form in one organ and have an effect on another organ or part) are widely used in hormone replacement therapy. Many drugs are derived from plant material. Many drugs have been in use for centuries, such as aloe vera for infections. Today there are many people who prefer to use plant-based remedies instead of certain drugs. For example, St. John's Wort (a plant derivative) is widely used for cases of mild depression. The use of alternative drug therapies should always be checked with a physician. Herbal remedies can have side effects and can be contraindicated in certain cases, such as drug interaction with other prescription drugs.

Drugs are classified by their use in the body. For example, **antibiotics** or **anti-infectives** stop or slow the growth of harmful microorganisms, such as bacteria, fungi, or parasites. However, when antibiotics are overused, microbes become resistant to the antibiotic and infections can become harder to treat. Some physicians are trying to limit the prescribing of antibiotics only to those people who really need them. Subclassifications of antibiotics include the more specific purposes of the drug, as an **antifungal** is an antibiotic that kills fungi. Table 22-1 lists the major drug classes, their functions, and generic and trade name examples for each class.

Drugs come in many forms—pills, liquids, semiliquids, suppositories, foams, lotions, creams, powders, transdermal patches, sprays, or gases—depending on how the drug is to be administered to the patient. Pills or tablets (usually stored in a small bottle called a **vial**) may be available as the standard solid small tablet or they may be in the form of capsules, a tablet with a gelatin covering encasing a powder or a liquid. They may also be coated (**enteric-coated** capsules dissolve slowly in the intestine so as not to irritate the stomach) or delayed- or timed-release (as with a transdermal patch), which spreads the dosage of the medicine gradually over a period of hours. Pills may also be in the form of lozenges, tablets meant to be dissolved slowly in the mouth, not swallowed. Tablets and some liquids can also be placed **sublingually,** under the tongue, or **buccally,** inside the cheek, where they are left to dissolve. **Oral administration** is the most common method for giving pills and some liquids.

Liquid and semiliquid drugs may come in various forms, such as syrups, heavy solutions of sugar, flavoring, and water added to the medication,

TABLE 22-1 Pharmacological Agents, Their Functions, and Examples

Drug Class	Purpose	Generic	Trade Name
analgesic	relieves pain without causing loss of consciousness	acetaminophen	Tylenol
anesthetic	produces a lack of feeling either locally or generally throughout the body	lidocaine procaine	Novacaine Xylocaine
antacid	neutralizes stomach acid	calcium carbonate and magnesia alumina, magnesia, simethicone	Rolaids Mylanta
antianemic	replaces iron	ferrous sulfate erythropoietin	Feosol, Slow Fe Procrit
antianginal	dilates coronary arteries to increase blood flow and reduce angina	nitroglycerine	Nitrocot
antianxiety	relieves anxiety	alprazolam lorazepam	Xanax Ativan
antiarrhythmic	controls cardiac arrhythmias	quinidine amiodarone	Cardioquin, Quinaglute Cordarone
antibiotic, anti-infective, antibacterial	destroys or inhibits the growth of harmful microorganisms	ciprofloxacin levofloxacin amoxicillin penicillin	Cipro Levaquin Amoxil, Wymox various
anticholinergic	blocks certain nerve impulses and muscular reactions, as in the movements of Parkinson's disease, or in cases of nausea	atropine homatropine propantheline	Atropair Homapin Pro-Banthine
anticoagulant	prevents blood clotting	warfarin sodium heparin dipyrimadole	Coumadin various Persantine
anticonvulsant	inhibits convulsions	phenytoin clonazepam carbamazepine	Dilantin Klonipin Tegetrol
antidepressant	prevents or relieves symptoms of depression	fluoxentine sertraline paroxetine	Prozac Zoloft Paxil
antidiabetic	lowers blood sugar or increases insulin sensitivity	insulin glyburide rosiglitazone	Humulin, Novolin Diabeta, Micronase Avandia
antidiarrheal	prevents or slows diarrhea	bismuth subsalicylate loperamide	Pepto-Bismol Imodium
antiemetic	prevents or relieves nausea and vomiting	dimenhydrenate meclizine	Dramamine Bonine, Antivert

(continued)

TABLE 22-1 Pharmacological Agents, Their Functions, and Examples (cont.)

Drug Class	Purpose	Generic	Trade Name
antifungal	destroys or inhibits fungal growth	tolnaftate ketoconazole	Tinactin, Desenex Nizoral
antihistamine	slows allergic reactions by counteracting histamines	loratidine diphenhydramine fexofenadine	Claritin Benadryl Allegra
antihypertensive	controls high blood pressure	clonidine prazosin guanethidine metoprolol	Catapres Minipress Ismelin Lopressor
anti-inflammatory, **nonsteroidal anti-inflammatory drug (NSAID)**	counteracts inflammations	ibuprofen naprosyn valdecoxib	Advil, Motrin Aleve Bextra
antineoplastic	destroys malignant cells	cyclophosphamide vincristine doxorubicin	Cytoxan Oncovin Adriamycin
antiparkinson	controls symptoms of Parkinson's disease	levodopa benztropine biperiden	Sinemet Cogentin Akineton
antipsychotic	controls symptoms of schizophrenia and some psychoses	aripiprazole risperidone olanzapine	Abilify Risperdal Zyprexa
antipyretic	reduces fever	acetylsalicylic acid (aspirin)	Bayer, Excedrin, various
antitubercular	decreases growth of microorganisms that cause tuberculosis	isoniazid ethambutol rifampin	Laniazid Myambutol Rifadin
antitussive, expectorant	prevents or relieves coughing	guaifenesin dextromethorphan	Humibid, Robitussin Vicks Formula 44
antiulcer	relieves and heals ulcers	cimetidine omeprazole ranitidine	Tagamet Prilosec Zantac
antiviral	controls the growth of viral microorganisms	didanosine zidovudine amantadine	Videx AZT, Retrovir Symmetrel
barbiturate	controls epileptic seizures	pentobarbital secobarbital	Nembutal Seconal
bronchodilator	dilates bronchial passages	albuterol ephredrine	Ventolin Bronkaid, Primatene
decongestant	reduces nasal congestion and/or swelling	pseudoephedrine	Drixoral, Sudafed
diuretic	increases excretion of urine	furosemide bumetanide	Lasix Bumex
hemostatic	controls or stops bleeding	aminocaproic acid recombinant factor VIIa	Amicar NovoSeven

TABLE 22-1 Pharmacological Agents, Their Functions, and Examples (cont.)

Drug Class	Purpose	Generic	Trade Name
hypnotic, sedative	produces sleep or a hypnotic state	diazepam zolpidem methaqualone	Valium Ambien Quaalude
hypoglycemic	lowers blood glucose levels	glucagon	Glucagon Diagnostic Kit
laxative	loosens stool and promotes normal bowel elimination	psyllium bisacodyl docusate	Metamucil Dulcolax, Theralax Therevac
vasodilator	decreases blood pressure by relaxing blood vessels	hydralazine enalapril benazepril	Apresoline Vasotec Lotensin

and emulsions, suspensions of oil or fat in water along with the medication. Liquids can be swallowed, sprayed (as on a wound or in an inhalant form), or injected. They may also be released directly into the body from an implantable drug pump controlled by the patient. This method is usually used to administer pain control medication to chronically ill patients. Patients with diabetes can use a pump to release amounts of insulin as needed rather than in a specific dose. Specific types of liquid and semiliquid medications are:

- *elixir*, oral liquid dissolved in alcohol
- *tincture*, topical liquid dissolved in alcohol
- *solution*, drug dissolved in liquid
- *suspension*, drug particles suspended in liquid, must shake before administration
- *emulsion*, drug particles suspended with oil or fat in water
- *lozenge*, drug in a candy-like base, dissolves slowly and coats the oral pharynx
- *syrup*, oral liquid drug in a thick solution, coats the oral pharynx

Drugs that are meant to go throughout the body are *systemic* (able to travel throughout the bloodstream to affect any part of the body); for example, aspirin tablets are taken internally for various pains. **Suppositories,** drugs mixed with a semisolid melting substance, are inserted into the

MORE ABOUT . . .

Drugs

When doctors prescribe drugs, the pharmacist usually provides instructions regarding side effects and what to avoid (incompatible or contraindicated with certain other drugs, alcohol, and so on). Those instructions do not usually discuss what types of food can interact with drugs. The National Consumers League and the Food and Drug Administration have published a brochure listing potentially harmful drug-food combinations. For example, grapefruit juice taken along with certain heart drugs can be fatal. Cheeses and sausages contain the substance tyramine, which can cause extremely high blood pressure when taken along with certain antidepressants.

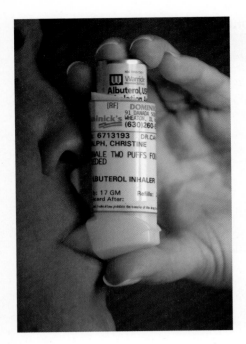

FIGURE 22-2 Patient using an inhaler.

vagina, rectum, or urethra are either topical or systemic drugs. Foams are generally inserted into the vagina. Lotions and creams are applied **topically** to the surface of the skin. Topical drugs are meant to work where they are placed. Powders may be inserted into a gelatin capsule or mixed with a liquid. Liquids or gases can be administered in **inhalation** form in which tiny droplets are inhaled through an inhaler (Figure 22-2), nebulizer, or spray. Inhalants are usually given in metered doses (for example, 2 puffs q4h). Sprays can be applied topically to the skin, into the nose (*intranasal*), or into the mouth.

Injection of a drug is called **parenteral administration.** Parenteral administration may be done by health care professionals or someone trained to administer it. Parenteral administration is medication that does not go through the gastrointestinal system. Most drugs given by parenteral administration are meant for systemic use. The closer to the bloodstream, the faster the drug will work. Some parenteral administration is topical; for example, **intradermal** or **intracutaneous** administration is the injection of a needle or **syringe** just beneath the outer layer of skin to check for local reactions. **Subcutaneous** administration is injection of the substance into the fatty layer of tissue below the outer portion of the skin. **Intramuscular** administration is the injection of drugs deep into the muscles. Intravenous administration is the injection of drugs through an **intravenous (IV)** tube. Generally the liquid drugs are titrated, put into solution in a specific volume. An IV **infusion** is the slow intravenous administration of a drug so that fluid is added to the bloodstream at a slow and steady rate. IV tubes can also be put into a pump system controlled by the patient. Figure 22-3 shows the methods of parenteral administration. There are other types of parenteral injection that can only be performed by a physician. These types of injection are: **intracardiac** (directly into heart muscle), **intra-arterial** (directly into an artery), **intraspinal** or **intrathecal** (directly into spinal spaces as in a case of severe pain or cancer), and **intraosseus** (directly into bone). For steroids and **anesthetics,** injections are done *intra-articularly,* or directly into a joint.

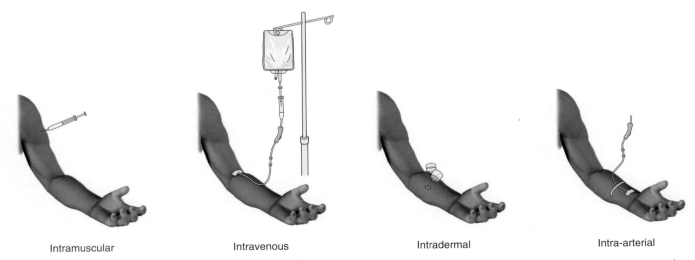

| Intramuscular | Intravenous | Intradermal | Intra-arterial |

FIGURE 22-3 Parenteral administration is the general term for administration by injection. These are only some types of parenteral administration.

VOCABULARY REVIEW

In the previous section, you learned terms relating to pharmacology. Before going on to the exercises, review the terms below and refer to the previous section if you have any questions. Pronunciations are provided for certain terms. Sometimes information about where the word came from is included after the term. These etymologies (word histories) are for your information only. You do not need to memorize them.

Term	Definition
absorb [ăb-SŎRB]	To take into.
analgesic [ăn-ăl-JĒ-zĭk] From Greek *analgesia*, insensibility	Drug that lessens or blocks pain.
anesthetic [ăn-ĕs-THĔT-ĭk]	Drug that causes temporary loss of ability to perceive sensations at a conscious level.
antacid [ănt-ĂS-ĭd] ant-, against + acid	Drug that lessens or neutralizes acidity.
antibacterial [ĂN-tē-băk-TĒR-ē-ăl] anti-, against + bacterial	Drug that stops or slows bacterial growth.
antibiotic [ĂN-tē-bī-ŎT-ĭk] anti- + Greek *biosis*, life	Drug that stops or slows the growth of harmful microorganisms.
antidiabetic [ĂN-tē-dī-ă-BĔT-ĭk] anti- + diabetic	Drug that lowers blood sugar or increases insulin sensitivity.
antidote [ĂN-tē-dōt] Greek *antidotos*, given against	Substance able to cancel out unwanted effects of another substance.
antifungal [ĂN-tē-FŬNG-găl] anti- + fungal	Drug that stops or slows the growth of fungus.
antihistamine [ĂN-tē-HĬS-tă-mēn] anti- + histamine	Drug that reduces the action of histamines; used in allergy treatments.
anti-infective [ĂN-tē-ĭn-FĔK-tĭv]	See *antibiotic*.
antitubercular [ĂN-tē-tū-BĔR-kyū-lăr] anti- + tubercular	Drug that stops the spread of tuberculosis.
antiviral [ĂN-tē-VĪ-răl] anti- + viral	Drug that stops or slows the spread of a virus.
brand name	See *trade name*.
buccally [BŪK-ăl-lē] Latin *bucca*, cheek	Inside the cheek.
contraindicated [kŏn-tră-ĭn-dĭ-KĀ-tĕd] contra- + indicated	Inadvisable to use; said especially of a drug that might cause complications when used in combination with other drugs or when used on a patient with a particular set of symptoms.
drug [drŭg]	Biological or chemical agents that can aid or alter body functions.

Term	Definition
druggist [DRŬG-ĭst]	See *pharmacist*.
enteric-coated [ĕn-TĒR-ĭk]	Having a coating (as on a capsule) that prevents stomach irritation.
excrete [ĕks-KRĒT]	To separate out and expel.
generic [jĕ-NĂR-ĭk]	Shortened version of a chemical name; official drug name.
hormone [HŌR-mōn]	Chemical substance in the body that forms in one organ and moves to another organ or part on which the substance has an effect; manufactured version of that chemical substance.
infusion [ĭn-FYŪ-zhŭn]	Administration of a fluid through an intravenous tube at a slow and steady rate.
inhalation [ĭn-hă-LĀ-shŭn]	Taking in of drugs in a fine spray of droplets.
intra-arterial [ĬN-tră-ăr-TĒ-rē-ăl]	Injected directly into an artery.
intracardiac [ĬN-tră-KĂR-dē-ăk] intra-, within + cardiac	Injected directly into heart muscle.
intracutaneous [ĬN-tră-kyū-TĀ-nē-ŭs] intra- + (sub)cutaneous	Injected just beneath the outer layer of skin.
intradermal [ĬN-tră-DĔR-măl] intra- + dermal	See *intracutaneous*.
intramuscular [ĬN-tră-MŬS-kyū-lăr] intra- + muscular	Injected deep into muscle tissue.
intraosseus [ĬN-tră-ŎS-ē-ŭs] intra- + Latin *os*, bone	Injected directly into bone.
intraspinal [ĬN-tră-SPĪ-năl] intra- + spinal	Injected directly into spinal spaces.
intrathecal [ĬN-tră-THĒ-kăl] intra- + Greek *theke*, box	See *intraspinal*.
intravenous [ĬN-tră-VĒ-nŭs] **(IV)** intra- + venous	Administered through a tube into a vein.
medication, medicine [mĕd-ĭ-KĀ-shŭn, MĔD-ĭ-sĭn]	Drug that serves a therapeutic purpose.
metabolize [mĕ-TĂB-ō-līz]	To change chemically or physically so as to make useful.
nonsteroidal anti-inflammatory drug (NSAID)	Anti-inflammatory drug that does not include steroids.
oral administration	Swallowing of pills or liquids via the mouth.
over-the-counter (OTC)	Available for sale without a doctor's prescription.
parenteral [pă-RĔN-tēr-ăl] **administration**	Administration of a drug by injection.
pharmacist [FĂR-mă-sĭst]	Person licensed to dispense medications.

Term	Definition
pharmacodynamics [FĂR-mă-kō-dī-NĂM-ĭks] pharmaco-, drugs + dynamics	Study of how drugs affect the body.
pharmacokinetics [FĂR-mă-kō-kĭ-NĔT-ĭks] pharmaco- + kinetics	Study of how the body absorbs, metabolizes, and excretes drugs.
pharmacology [făr-mă-KŎL-ō-jē] pharmaco- + -logy, study	Science that studies, develops, and tests new drugs.
prescription [prē-SKRĬP-shŭn]	Order given by a doctor for medication dosage, route, and timing of administration.
proprietary [prō-PRĬ-ĕ-tār-ē] **name**	See *trade name*.
subcutaneous [sŭb-kyū-TĀ-nē-ŭs] sub-, under + Latin *cutis*, skin	Injected into the fatty layer of tissue beneath the outer layer of skin.
sublingually [sŭb-LĬNG-gwă-lē] sub- + Latin *lingua*, tongue	Under the tongue.
suppository [sŭ-PŎZ-ĭ-tōr-ē] Latin *suppositorium*, placed underneath	Drug mixed with a semisolid melting substance meant for administration by insertion into the vagina, rectum, or urethra.
syringe [sĭ-RĬNJ] Greek *syrinx*, tube	Instrument used for injection or withdrawal of fluids.
topically [TŎP-ĭ-căl-lē]	On the surface of the skin.
toxicology [tŏk-sĭ-KŎL-ō-jē] toxico-, poison + -logy	Study of harmful effects of drugs.
trade name	Name copyrighted by the manufacturer for a particular version of a drug.
vial [VĪ-ăl] Greek *phiale*, drinking cup	A small receptacle for holding liquid or pill medications.
vitamin [VĪT-ă-mĭn] Latin *vita*, life + amine	Organic substance found in food.

DRUG SOURCES, TYPES, FUNCTION, AND ADMINISTRATION EXERCISES

Follow the Route

Name the route of drug administration or type of drug from its description.

1. Drug is administered via a semisolid into the rectum: _____

2. Drug is administered via vapor or gas into the nose or mouth: _____

3. Drug is administered under the tongue: _____

4. Drug is applied locally on skin or mucous membrane: _____

5. Drug is injected through a syringe under the skin, into a vein, into a muscle, or into a body cavity: _____

6. Drug is given by mouth and absorbed through the stomach or intestinal wall: _____

Find the Class

Give the class (not the name) of a drug that does the following. For example: stops diarrhea = antidiarrheal.

7. prevents/stops angina: _____

8. increases excretion of urine: _____

9. reduces blood pressure: _____

10. corrects abnormal heart rhythms: _____

11. relieves symptoms of depression: _____

12. prevents blood clotting: _____

13. promotes vomiting: _____

14. relieves pain: _____

15. neutralizes stomach acid: _____

CASE STUDY

Getting an Evaluation

Many elderly people go to different doctors for different ailments without being monitored by one regular physician. Some people take so many medications that it affects their health adversely. Helen Metrone is an 86-year-old woman with high blood pressure, a tendency to retain water, skin allergies, and minor heart disease. Her preferred provider organization (PPO) allows her to see different doctors. Helen likes to go to various doctors. She almost always gets new prescriptions because of her symptoms. Often, she neglects to tell each doctor what medications she is already taking. When asked to list her medications, Helen will put one or two that she can remember. Also, Helen sometimes forgets which pills she has already taken in one day. This has led to several instances of fainting, disorientation, and dizziness. Helen's family is very concerned. They are looking into an assisted living arrangement where a nurse would give Helen her medication. They have also made an appointment with a gerontologist to review Helen's medications, outlook, and general health.

Critical Thinking

16. Why is it important for patients to inform their physician of all medications they are taking?

17. Why is it important for Helen to understand the instructions that come with her medication?

Combining Forms and Abbreviations

The lists below include combining forms and abbreviations that relate specifically to pharmacology. Pronunciations are provided for the examples. Many of these abbreviations are no longer used in the hospital because of the confusion they create. The Joint Commission for Hospital Accreditation has actually prohibited the use of some of them. But they are still used in many physician practices so it is a good idea to be familiar with them. See Appendix B for a further discussion of abbreviations.

COMBINING FORM	MEANING	EXAMPLE
chem(o)	chemical	*chemotherapy* [KĒ-mō-thār-ă-pē], treatment of a disease with chemical substances
pyret(o)	fever	*pyretogenous* [pī-rĕ-TŎJ-ĕ-nŭs], causing fever
tox(o), toxi, toxico	poison	*toxicogenic* [TŎK-sĭ-kō-JĔN-ĭk], caused by a poison

ABBREVIATION	MEANING	ABBREVIATION	MEANING
aa, $\overline{aa}$	of each	a.u., AU	each ear (Latin *auris uterque*)
a.c.	before meals (Latin *ante cibum*), usually one-half hour preceding a meal	BID, b.i.d.	twice a day (Latin *bis in die*)
ad	up to	c, $\overline{c}$	with
a.d., AD	right ear (Latin *auris dexter*)	cap., caps.	capsule
ad lib	freely (Latin *ad libitum*), as often as desired	cc., cc	cubic centimeter
AM, a.m., A	morning (Latin *ante meridiem*)	comp.	compound
a.s., AS	left ear (Latin *auris sinister*)	cx	contraindicated
DAW	dispense as written	ml	milliliter
dil.	dilute	n., noct.	night (Latin *nocte*)
disc, DC, dc	discontinue	non rep.	do not repeat
disp.	dispense	NPO	nothing by mouth
div.	divide	NPO p MN	nothing by mouth after midnight
DW	distilled water	N.S., NS	normal saline
D₅W	dextrose 5% in water	NSAID	nonsteroidal anti-inflammatory drug
dx, Dx	diagnosis	N&V	nausea and vomiting
elix.	elixir	o.d., OD	right eye (Latin *oculus dexter*)
e.m.p.	as directed (Latin *ex modo praescripto*)	oint., ung.	ointment, unguent
ex aq.	in water	o.l.	left eye
ext.	extract	o.s.	left eye (Latin *oculus sinister*)
FDA	Food and Drug Administration	OTC	over the counter
fld. ext.	fluid extract	o.u.	each eye
FUO	fever of unknown origin	oz.	ounce
g, gm	gram	p	post, after
gr	grain, gram	p.c.	after meals (Latin *post cibum*), one-half hour after a meal
gtt	drop	PDR	*Physician's Desk Reference*
H	hypodermic	PM, p.m., P	afternoon (Latin *post meridiem*)
h.	every hour (Latin *hora*)	p.o.	by mouth (Latin *per os*)
h.s.	at bedtime (Latin *hora somni*, hour of sleep)	PRN, p.r.n.	repeat as needed (Latin *pro re nata*)
IM	intramuscular	pulv., pwdr	powder
inj	injection	qam	every morning

ABBREVIATION	MEANING	ABBREVIATION	MEANING
IV	intravenous	q.d.	every day (Latin *quaque dies*)
mcg	microgram	q.h.	every hour
mEq	milliequivalent	q.i.d.	four times a day
mg	milligram	QNS	quantity not sufficient
q.o.d.	every other day	susp.	suspension
q.s.	sufficient quantity	sym, Sym, Sx	symptom
R	rectal	syr.	syrup
Rx	prescription	tab.	tablet
s, s̄	without	tbsp.	tablespoonful
Sig.	patient directions such as route and timing of medication (Latin *signa*, inscription)	t.i.d.	three times a day
SL	sublingual	tinct., tr.	tincture
sol., soln.	solution	TPN	total parenteral nutrition
s.o.s.	if there is need	TPR	temperature, pulse, respirations
sp.	spirit	tsp.	teaspoonful
ss, s̄s̄	one-half	U, u	unit
stat	immediately	u.d.	as directed
subc, subq, s.c.	subcutaneously	ung.	ointment
supp., suppos	suppository	U.S.P.	*United States Pharmacopeia*

CASE STUDY

Visiting a Specialist

Helen finally did go to a gerontologist—this time with her niece. Her niece brought along a list of all her medications. The doctor advised coming off several of the medications over the next few weeks. The gerontologist also asked Helen to see her in three weeks for a medication evaluation. She asked Helen to bring in the prescription vials, but her niece also had her regular nurse provide the following list of her medications.

> Lopressor 10 mg. b.i.d.
> Synthroid 50 mcg q.d.
> Motrin as needed
> Lasix 10 mg. b.i.d.

NDC 0075-1505-43

Nasacort®
(triamcinolone acetonide) U.S. Pat. No. 49999999999

Black's Pharmacy   #3333 ph. 879-000-0000
36 Main St.
Norfolk, VA 34444

Rx: **666777**   Dr. Esteves, Marion D.
       St: B3456789

Use 2 sprays in each nostril once daily.

Nasacort Nasal inhaler RHO

You may refill this script 10 times before 4/26/XXXX.

Critical Thinking

18. How many times a day does Helen take Synthroid?
19. How many milligrams of Lopressor does Helen take daily?

COMBINING FORMS AND ABBREVIATIONS EXERCISES

Check Your Knowledge

Give abbreviations for the following.

20. three times a day _____

21. before meals _____

22. intramuscular _____

23. two times a day _____

24. intravenous _____

25. nothing by mouth _____

26. after meals _____

27. every hour _____

28. every morning _____

29. at bedtime _____

30. four times a day _____

31. when requested _____

32. every day _____

33. drops _____

Find the Root

Add the combining form to complete the word.

34. Resistance to the effects of chemicals: _____ resistance

35. Treatment of fever: _____ therapy

36. Study of poisons: _____ logy

USING THE INTERNET

Go to the FDA's Web site (www.fda.gov/opacom/hpnews.html) and find information about the approval of at least one drug. Explain what the medication is for. In addition, describe at least one new procedure aimed at monitoring drug safety once the drug is on the market.

CHAPTER REVIEW

The material that follows is to help you review this chapter.

True or False

Circle T for true or F for false.

37. All medications require a prescription. T F
38. IM medications go into an IV. T F
39. Trade name and brand name are the same. T F
40. The most common method of drug administration is oral. T F
41. A tablet used sublingually is inserted under the tongue. T F
42. A parenteral administration is the injection of a medication. T F
43. A capsule is a small solid tablet. T F
44. A suppository can only be used rectally. T F
45. You should never swallow a suppository. T F

Understanding Pharmacological Terms

Write the letter of the correct definition in the space provided.

46. ____ analgesic
47. ____ antidiarrheal
48. ____ antipyretic
49. ____ antidepressant
50. ____ antacid
51. ____ antiarrhythmic
52. ____ antianemic
53. ____ antianginal
54. ____ antianxiety
55. ____ antitussive

a. relieves heart pain
b. normalizes heart rhythm
c. reduces fever
d. relieves nervousness and feelings of dread
e. works on a mood disorder
f. relieves pain
g. relieves indigestion
h. relieves bouts of loose bowels
i. prevents or relieves coughing
j. replaces iron

Understanding Pharmacological Terms

Write the letter of the correct definition in the space provided.

56. ____ diuretic
57. ____ hypoglycemic
58. ____ laxative
59. ____ bucally
60. ____ generic
61. ____ brand name
62. ____ intramuscular

a. injected into the fatty layer of the skin
b. on the skin surface
c. under the tongue
d. offical drug name
e. increase excretion of urine
f. lowers blood glucose
g. loosens stool and promotes bowel elimination

63. ____ intradermal

64. ____ topically

65. ____ subcutaneous

66. ____ sublingually

h. trade name

i. inside the cheek

j. into the muscle

k. beneath outer layer of skin (between layers)

Know the Abbreviations

For the following prescriptions, describe the timing and amount of the dosage.

67. Zyrtec 10 mg q d

68. Amoxicillin 500 mg bid for 10 days

69. Cymbalta 60 mg at hs

70. Relpax 40 mg prn for migraine

DEFINITIONS

Define the following terms and abbreviations. Make sure you know the proper pronunciations of terms. The blue words in curly brackets are references to the Spanish glossary available online at www.mhhe.com/medterm3e.

TERM

71. absorb [ăb-SŎRB]

72. analgesic [ăn-ăl-JĒ-zĭk] {analgésico}

73. anesthetic [ăn-ĕs-THĔT-ĭk] {anestésico}

74. antacid [ănt-ĂS-ĭd] {antiácido}

75. antibacterial [ĂN-tē-băk-TĒR-ē-ăl] {antibacteriano}

76. antibiotic [ĂN-tē-bī-ŎT-ĭk] {antibiótico}

77. antidiabetic [ĂN-tē-dī-ă-BĔT-ĭk] {antidiabético}

78. antidote [ĂN-tē-dōt] {antidote}

79. antifungal [ĂN-tē-FŬNG-găl] {antifúngico}

80. antihistamine [ĂN-tē-HĬS-tă-mēn] {antihistamina}

81. anti-infective [ĂN-tē-ĭn-FĔK-tĭv]

82. antitubercular [ĂN-tē-tū-BĔR-kyū-lăr]

83. antiviral [ĂN-tē-VĪ-răl]

84. brand name

85. buccally [BŬK-ăl-lē]

86. chem(o)

87. contraindicated [kŏn-tră-ĭn-dĭ-KĀ-tĕd]

88. drug [drŭg] {droga}

89. druggist [DRŬG-ĭst] {boticario}

90. enteric-coated [ĕn-TĒR-ĭk]

91. excrete [ĕks-KRĒT]

92. generic [jĕ-NĀR-ĭk] {genérico}

93. hormone [HŎR-mōn] {hormona}

94. infusion [ĭn-FYŪ-zhŭn]

95. inhalation [ĭn-hă-LĀ-shŭn]

96. intra-arterial [ĬN-tră-ăr-TĒ-rē-ăl]

97. intracardiac [ĬN-tră-KĂR-dē-ăk]

98. intracutaneous [ĬN-tră-kyū-TĀ-nē-ŭs]

99. intradermal [ĬN-tră-DĔR-măl]

100. intramuscular [ĬN-tră-MŬS-kyū-lăr]

101. intraosseus [ĬN-tră-ŎS-ē-ŭs]

102. intraspinal [ĬN-tră-SPĪ-năl]

103. intrathecal [ĬN-tră-THĒ-kăl]

104. intravenous [ĬN-tră-VĒ-nŭs] (IV) {intravenoso (IV)}

105. medication, medicine [mĕd-ĭ-KĀ-shŭn, MĔD-ĭ-sĭn] {medicación, medicina}

106. metabolize [mĕ-TĂB-ō-līz]

107. nonsteroidal anti-inflammatory drug (NSAID) {agentes de antiiflamatorios no esteroideos, AINE}

108. oral administration

109. over-the-counter (OTC)

110. parenteral [pă-RĔN-tēr-ăl] administration

111. pharmacist [FĂR-mă-sĭst]

112. pharmacodynamics
[FĂR-mă-kō-dī-NĂM-ĭks]

113. pharmacokinetics
[FĂR-mă-kō-kĭ-NĔT-ĭks]

114. pharmacology
[făr-mă-KŎL-ō-jē]
{farmacología}

115. prescription
[prē-SKRĬP-shŭn]
{prescripción}

116. proprietary
[prō-PRĪ-ĕ-tār-ē] name

117. pyret(o)

118. subcutaneous
[sŭb-kyū-TĀ-nē-ŭs]

119. sublingually
[sŭb-LĬNG-gwă-lē]

120. suppository
[sŭ-PŎZ-ĭ-tōr-ē]
{supositorio}

121. syringe [sĭ-RĬNJ] {jeringa}

122. topically [TŎP-ĭ-căl-lē]

123. tox(o), toxi, toxico

124. toxicology [tŏk-sĭ-KŎL-ō-jē]
{toxicología}

125. trade name

126. vial [VĪ-ăl] {vial}

127. vitamin [VĪT-ă-mĭn]
{vitamina}

Abbreviations

Write the full meaning of each abbreviation

ABBREVIATION

128. aa, a̅a̅
129. a.c.
130. ad
131. a.d., AD
132. ad lib
133. AM, a.m., A
134. a.s., AS
135. a.u., AU
136. BID, b.i.d.
137. c, c̅
138. cap., caps.
139. cc., cc
140. comp.
141. cx
142. DAW
143. dil.
144. disc, DC, dc
145. disp.
146. div.
147. DW
148. D$_5$W
149. dx, Dx
150. elix.

151. e.m.p.
152. ex aq.
153. ext.
154. FDA
155. fld. ext.
156. FUO
157. g, gm
158. gr
159. gtt
160. H
161. h.
162. h.s.
163. IM
164. inj
165. IV
166. mcg
167. mEq
168. mg
169. ml
170. n., noct.
171. non rep.
172. NPO
173. NPO p MN

174. N.S., NS
175. NSAID
176. N&V
177. o.d., OD
178. oint., ung.
179. o.l.
180. o.s.
181. OTC
182. o.u.
183. oz.
184. p
185. p.c.
186. PDR
187. PM, p.m., P
188. p.o.
189. PRN, p.r.n.
190. pulv., pwdr
191. qam
192. q.d.
193. q.h.
194. q.i.d.
195. QNS
196. q.o.d.

197. q.s.

198. R

199. RX

200. s, s̄

201. Sig.

202. SL

203. Sol., soln.

204. s.o.s.

205. sp.

206. ss, s̄s̄

207. stat

208. subc, subq, s.c.

209. supp., suppos

210. susp.

211. sym, Sym, Sx

212. syr.

213. tab.

214. tbsp.

215. t.i.d.

216. tinct., tr.

217. TPN

218. TPR

219. tsp.

220. U, u

221. u.d.

223. ung.

224. U.S.P.

Answers to Chapter Exercises

1. suppository
2. inhalation
3. sublingually
4. topically
5. parenteral
6. oral administration
7. antianginal
8. diuretic
9. antihypertensive, vasodilator
10. antiarrhythmic
11. antidepressant
12. anticoagulant
13. antiemetic
14. analgesic
15. antacid
16. Medications can cause interactions or side effects.
17. Instructions, such as "take with food," can help avoid side effects.
18. once
19. 20 mg.
20. t.i.d.
21. a. c.
22. IM
23. b.i.d.
24. IV

25. NPO
26. p.c.
27. q.h. or h.
28. qam
29. h.s.
30. q.i.d.
31. ad lib
32. q.d.
33. gtt
34. chemoresistance
35. pyretotherapy
36. toxicology
37. False
38. False
39. True
40. True
41. True
42. True
43. False
44. False (vaginal or rectal depending on type)
45. True
46. f
47. h
48. c
49. e

50. g
51. b
52. j
53. a
54. d
55. i
56. e
57. f
58. g
59. i
60. d
61. h
62. j
63. k
64. b
65. a
66. c
67. Zyrtec 10 mg every day
68. Amoxicillin 500 mg twice a day for 10 days
69. Cymbalta 60 mg at bedtime
70. Relpax 40 mg as needed
71–224. Answers are available in the vocabulary reviews in this chapter.

Terms in Complementary and Alternative Medicine

After studying this chapter, you will be able to:

23.1   Define complementary and alternative medicine
23.2   Describe some of the historical aspects of complementary and alternative medicine
23.3   List the five major classifications of complementary and alternative medicines

What Is Complementary and Alternative Medicine?

Most medical practices in the United States are run under *conventional medicine* standards. These standards include most of the practices learned in medical schools and endorsed by national organizations, such as the American Medical Association (AMA). However, other types of medical practice are used to treat, heal, and prevent illness and promote well-being in large areas of the world, as well as by many practitioners in the United States. When such practices are used in combination or alongside conventional medicine, they are called **complementary medicine.** When they are used instead of conventional medicine, they are called **alternative medicine.** Some forms of complementary or alternative medicine are considered *holistic medicine*, treatment of the whole person, including physical, nutritional, environmental, social, and emotional needs.

History of Alternative Medicine

Since the times of the earliest humans, people have healed themselves physically or spiritually using whatever was available to them in their environment. In most cases, minor injuries and infections were treated with mechanical techniques or plants (which are the source of many current traditional medicines). Gradually, knowledge of treatment and healing was passed down through generations. Some people became experts in certain treatments; for example, some women became midwives, assisting other women in childbirth. Spiritual healers also had a place in the treatment of both physical and mental illnesses. The lifespan of the average human was fairly short since many people had no protection from disease or from the natural elements.

Around the world, various cultures developed fairly sophisticated understandings of human health. For over 2,000 years, Chinese practitioners

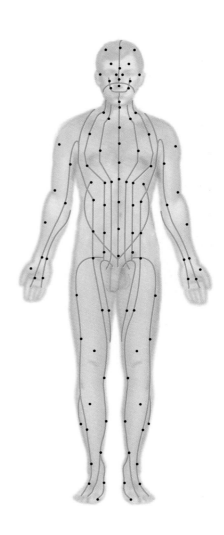

The National Institute of Health runs a National Center for Complementary and Alternative Medicine (NCCAM) and offers updated information on its Web site (www.nccam.nih.gov).

have helped people with *acupuncture* and various medicinal herbs. In India, *ayurvedic medicine* is practiced widely. It is based on a holistic view of the human body and mind. Many other cultures have long traditions of physical and spiritual healing.

Hippocrates is generally regarded as the founder of conventional medical practice. He lived in ancient Greece and instituted the Hippocratic Oath (discussed in Chapter 1). Since then, conventional medicine has developed— and is continuing to develop—cures based on examination, diagnosis, and treatment with medicines, various mechanical techniques, and/or surgery. Conventional medicine took a great leap forward in the mid-1800s when Joseph Lister, a British surgeon, began to understand and promote antiseptic surgery. Once antisepsis was understood thoroughly, many more lives were saved. From the early days of conventional medicine, it was most available to those with the money to go to professionals. In modern times, some countries consider health care a universal right, and others have made health care much more widely available than it has been in the past.

For centuries, many individuals did not have easy access to conventional medicine. Therefore, they turned to whatever folk medicine was available to them. Some of the practices in folk medicine were effective and some were not. Over time, some practitioners of conventional medicine as well as practitioners of alternative medicine have tried to incorporate those practices from folk medicine and from other cultures that seemed to be effective.

Because of heightened interest in alternative medicine, the government's National Institutes of Health has set up the National Center for Complementary and Alternative Medicine (NCCAM) to provide information, support research, and set standards. It is estimated that as much as 40 percent of the U.S. population uses some form of alternative or complementary medicine.

Types of Complementary and Alternative Medicine

NCCAM classifies **CAM** (complementary and alternative medicine) practices into five major types:

1. **Alternative medical systems,** which are complete systems of theory and practice.
2. **Mind-body interventions,** which use the mind's capacity to affect bodily function and symptoms.
3. **Biologically based therapies,** which use substances found in nature, such as herbs, foods, and vitamins.
4. **Manipulative** and **body-based therapies,** which are based on manipulation and/or movement of one or more parts of the body. This is sometimes called *natural healing*.
5. **Energy therapies,** which involve the use of energy fields.

Alternative Medical Systems

There are four major alternative medicine systems:

1. **Homeopathic medicine** is a system that believes that "like cures like." Patients are treated with small, highly diluted quantities of medicinal substances that would actually cause those symptoms at higher doses.

It is theorized that the body reacts by healing itself in response to the smaller doses.

2. **Naturopathic medicine** theorizes that there is healing power within the body that can maintain and restore health. Naturopathic practitioners work to support this healing power through the use of nutritional counseling, supplements, exercise, and a combination of treatments from other alternative medicine practices.

3. **Traditional Chinese medicine** (TCM) is based on a concept of balanced *qi* (pronounced "chee"), or vital energy. It is believed that this energy regulates a person's spiritual, emotional, mental, and physical balance through two opposing forces—yin (negative energy) and yang (positive energy). Disease is thought to result from yin and yang becoming imbalanced. Among the components of TCM are **acupuncture** (Figure 23-1), herbal and nutritional therapy, exercises, meditation, and massage. *Qi Gong* is one type of TCM that combines movement, meditation, and breathing.

4. **Ayurveda** emphasizes body, mind, and spirit in combination to prevent and treat disease. It has been practiced in India for 5,000 years and includes nutritional and herbal remedies and physical movement as well as meditation.

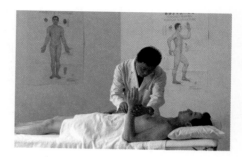

The Web site of the National Center for Homeopathy (www.homeopathic.org) provides information on this type of therapy.

FIGURE 23-1 Acupuncturist treating a client.

Mind-Body Interventions

Mind-body intervention techniques use the power of the mind to affect changes in body function and symptoms. Some mind-body interventions have moved from being part of complementary medicine and have become part of conventional medicine. Examples of this are behavioral therapy, which is widely used in certain mental illnesses and patient support groups and is now considered routine as part of the treatment of chronic illness.

Other techniques of mind-body intervention remain in the complementary and alternative medicine sphere. Meditation has been used on the Indian subcontinent for centuries. In studies, it has been shown that meditation can affect blood pressure and body temperature as well as other body functions. Prayer is regarded as an effective healing technique in some cases. Various therapies that use music, dance, and other creative outlets are used to change the course of some illnesses. In general, the power of the mind has been shown to play a role in the course of a disease.

Biologically Based Therapies

Biologically based therapies use food, herbs, vitamins, and minerals to relieve symptoms, maintain health, and, in some cases, cure diseases. Traditional Chinese medicine as well as medicines of other cultures have long used herbs to cure ailments and relieve symptoms. Many practitioners in the United States now use some of this ancient knowledge as well as more recent theories about vitamins, minerals, and dietary practices to provide guidance for preventing or healing disease. In addition, individuals are taking herbs and vitamins, often without specific guidance. The use of a particular substance for healing commonly spreads by word of mouth. For example, some people find relief from depression using the herb St. John's Wort. Others use various minerals and vitamin combinations to relieve joint pain. Still others find that some plant extracts raise energy levels. There are problems with herbal medications in that they are not controlled by the FDA. Also many individuals forget to mention they are taking herbals to their physicians, either because they do not think they are important or because they forget they are taking them. Sometimes they do not tell the doctor because they think the doctor will not approve. This can lead to complications and drug interactions. It is very important to convey this information to your physician to prevent interactions or overtreating for your condition.

Manipulation and Body-Based Methods

The two major types of manipulation or body-based methods are **chiropractic** and **therapeutic massage.** Chiropractic focuses primarily on the relationship between alignment of the body (particularly of the spine) and overall health. Chiropractors attempt to align the spine by moving the body in various ways, especially by turning the neck so as to position it properly (Figure 23-2).

Chiropractic uses many treatments and modalities in addition to manipulation by force. Some of the other chiropractic modalities or treatments include light force adjustments, activators, special tables for traction, and drop tables that allow the chiropractor to use less force to accomplish the same adjustment. Some chiropractors use a computerized tool called a precision adjuster that first measures the alignment and the problem areas then delivers a specific force to adjust the spin in the direction needed. They may also use the application of hot and cold, electrical stimulation and magnets to relax the muscles allowing the body to go back into alignment easier and stay in alignment longer.

Therapeutic massage (Figure 23-3) stimulates the skin, muscles, and connective tissue by manipulation. It promotes healing and a feeling of well-being. There are many different types of therapeutic massage techniques and modalities. Massage therapy has been around for a long time. There are many styles and types of massages and massage strokes, including Swedish massage, relaxation massage, deep tissue massage, therapeutic massage, pregnancy massage, reflexology, aromatherapy, infant massage, geriatric massage, sports massage and many, many others. All massage starts with touch. The style, depth, speed, and type of stroke is what makes the major difference. A relaxation massage is mostly long, gentle, gliding strokes called *effleurage*. A deep tissue or therapeutic massage will use effleurage strokes but will also include *petrissage* (kneading

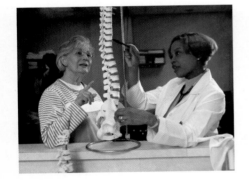

FIGURE 23-2 A chiropractor explaining treatment to a patient.

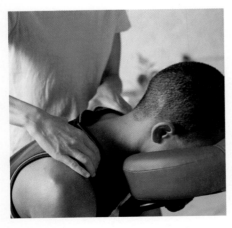

FIGURE 23-3 A massage therapist giving a back massage.

strokes or compression), *friction,* and *tapotement* (percussion or tapping of the body). It is important for clients to find a massage therapist that has a touch and technique that they like. It is also a good idea for clients to check the therapist's credentials and training. A deep tissue massage does not have to hurt to go deep. Some therapists add scented essential oils to help the client relax depending on the goal of the massage. For example lavender is relaxing and can help a client relax.

Massage therapy can help with a lot of physical problems. It is also contraindicated in some conditions. For example, in an acute injury, the injured area should not be massaged for 48 hours. Pregnant women should not get a massage in the first trimester. If either the therapist or client is not sure if a particular massage is contraindicated, a medical doctor should be consulted. It is also important that the therapist know of any medical conditions so as not to harm the client unintentionally. A massage therapist may ask for a note from the physician before giving a client a massage.

Energy Therapies

Energy therapies are divided into two types. The first, **biofield therapy,** attempts to affect the energy fields that are assumed to surround the human body. One example of a biofield therapy is **therapeutic touch,** the laying on of hands. It is based on the belief that passing the healer's hands through the energy fields surrounding the body will help heal imbalances. Another example is **reiki,** a Japanese form of therapy in which energy is passed from the healer to the patient, who is thought to be healed in this process. There are many other types of energy therapies, such as *quantum touch* and *healing touch,* which are used successfully to help some people.

The second type of energy therapy is **bioelectromagnetic-based therapy.** This involves the use of electromagnetic fields, such as pulsed fields, magnetic fields, or AC- or DC-current fields.

> The American Chiropractic Association (www.amerchiro.org) is the largest organization promoting chiropractic care.

Alternative Medicine Coding

Coding systems have been developed for use in CAM and nursing. An ABC coding system for CAM can be found at Alternative Link's Web site (www.alternativelink.com). It is estimated that there are 3 million alternative healthcare practitioners in the United States. The market for their services is continuing to increase. Currently, many insurance companies will pay for chiropractic care but not for many of the other CAM therapies. However, as the popularity of many of these methods increases, the willingness of health insurance companies to pay for alternative services will also increase. As it increases, coding for CAM will become standardized.

VOCABULARY REVIEW

In the previous section, you learned terms relating to complementary and alternative medicine. Before going on to the exercises, review the following terms and refer to the previous section if you have any questions. Pronunciations are provided for certain terms. Sometimes information about where the word came from is included after the term. These etymologies (word histories) are for your information only. You do not need to memorize them.

Term	Definition
acupuncture [ă-kyū-PŬNK-chūr]	Originally Chinese therapy that uses fine needles.
alternative medical system	Complete system of medical treatment outside the realm of conventional medicine.
alternative medicine	Medical therapies outside the realm of conventional medicine.
ayurveda [ī-yūr-VĀ-dă, ī-yūr-VĒ-dă]	Holistic alternative medicine system originally from India.
bioelectromagnetic-based therapy	Type of energy therapy that uses electromagnetic fields.
biofield therapy	Type of energy therapy that attempts to affect energy fields.
biologically based therapy	The use of foods, herbs, vitamins, and minerals to heal or prevent disease.
body-based therapy	See *manipulative therapy*.
CAM	Complementary and alternative medicine.
chiropractic [kī-rō-PRĂK-tĭk]	Therapy based on alignment of the body (particularly the spine).
complementary medicine	A nonconventional medical practice used in combination with conventional medicine.
energy therapy	Therapy that uses energy fields.
homeopathic [hō-mē-ō-PĂTH-ĭk] medicine	Medical system that uses diluted doses of substances to stimulate immunity.
manipulative therapy	Therapy that uses manipulation of the body to treat patients.
mind-body intervention	Therapy that uses the power of the mind to affect the body.
naturopathic [nă-chūr-ō-PĂTH-ĭk] medicine	Therapy that uses the body's own healing powers to maintain and restore health.
reiki [RĀ-kē]	Therapy that uses touch from a healer.
therapeutic massage	Stimulates the skin, muscles, and tissue to promote healing.
therapeutic touch	The laying on of hands to promote healing.
traditional Chinese medicine	Various practices that promote balance between yin and yang to promote and maintain health.

Working in a CAM office

Julie started a new job as an office assistant to Dr. Mira Sanchez, a chiropractor with a small practice. Dr. Sanchez shares an office with Jim Wilson, a trained massage therapist, and Fouad Sharma, a nutritional counselor who often recommends herbal preparations. Julie will serve as receptionist and office clerk for all three practitioners. An important part of Julie's job is to take medical histories of new patients as well as to explain to patients about insurance reimbursement if any is available.

Critical Thinking

1. Should the medical histories include a list of medications?
2. Julie knows a lot about vitamins and herbs. Should she discuss any of these with patients?

COMPLEMENTARY AND ALTERNATIVE MEDICINE EXERCISES

Fill in the Blank

Complete the sentences below.

3. Originally a system of Indian medicine, _____ is now a type of alternative medical system.

4. In traditional Chinese medicine, balance between _____ and _____ is considered essential.

5. Spinal manipulation is routinely performed by _____.

6. Therapeutic touch uses _____ fields while therapeutic _____ uses manipulation.

7. Any type of alternative therapy used in conjunction with conventional medicine is called _____ medicine.

8. Stimulating immunity by using diluted doses takes place in _____ medicine.

9. A Japanese energy therapy is called _____.

10. St. John's Wort is used to relieve _____.

USING THE INTERNET

Go to NCCAM's Web site (www.nccam.nih.gov) and find information about one type of complementary or alternative medicine. Explain how the therapy is expected to heal or prevent disease.

CHAPTER REVIEW

The material that follows is to help you review this chapter.

DEFINITIONS

Define the following terms. Review the chapter before starting. Make sure you know how to pronounce each term as you define it.

Answers to Chapter Exercises

1. Yes, because herbal preparations and vitamins can interact with medications.
2. No, Julie does not have the necessary training to recommend any supplements.
3. ayurveda
4. yin, yang
5. chiropractors
6. energy, massage
7. complementary
8. homeopathic
9. reiki
10. depression
11–30. Answers are available in the vocabulary reviews in this chapter.

APPENDIX

Combining Forms, Prefixes, and Suffixes

Listed below are the word parts that appear throughout this textbook. The page numbers given in the index next to each word part indicate those pages on which the parts are defined and an example is also given there of how they are used in a medical term. When a combining form ends in a vowel, the vowel is surrounded with parentheses only in those cases where the term may also appear used in words without the vowel. For example: abdomin(o) represents the combining form used both in *abdominoskeletal* and in *abdominal*.

a-, without,
ab-, abs-, away from,
abdomin(o), abdomen,
acanth(o), spiny; thorny,
acetabul(o), cup-shaped hip socket,
acromi(o), end point of the scapula,
actin(o), light,
-ad, toward,
ad-, toward, to,
aden(o), gland,
adenoid(o), adenoid, gland,
adip(o), fat,
adren(o), adrenal glands,
aer(o), air; gas,
agglutin(o), agglutinin,
alge, algesi, algio, algo, pain,
-algia, pain,
alveol(o), air sac, alveolus,
ambi-, both, around,
amni(o), amnion,
amyl(o), starch,
an-, without,
an(o), anus,
ana-, up, toward,
andr(o), masculine,
angi(o), vessel,
ankyl(o), bent, crooked,
ante-, before,
anti-, against,
aort(o), aorta,
apo-, derived, separate,
append(o), appendic(o), appendix,
arteri(o), artery,
arteriol(o), arteriole,
arthr(o), joint, articulation,
-asthenia, weakness,
ather(o), plaque; fatty substance,
atri(o), atrium,
audi(o), audit(o), hearing,

aur(i), aur(o), auricul(o), ear, hearing,
aut(o)-, self,

bacill(i), bacilli; bacteria,
bacteri(o), bacteria,
balan(o), glans penis,
bar(o), weight; pressure,
bas(o), basi(o), base,
bi-, twice, double,
bil(o), bili, bile,
bio, life,
-blast, immature, forming,
blast(o), immature cells,
blephar(o), eyelid,
brachi(o), arm,
brachy-, short,
brady-, slow,
bronch(o), bronchi, bronchus,
bronchiol(o), bronchiole,
bucc(o), cheek,
burs(o), bursa,

cac(o), bad; ill,
calc(o), calci(o), calcium,
calcane(o), heel bone,
cali(o), calic(o), calix,
capn(o), carbon dioxide,
carcin(o), cancer,
cardi(o), heart; esophageal opening of the stomach,
carp(o), wrist bones,
cata-, down,
cec(o), cecum,
-cele, hernia,
celi(o), abdomen,
-centesis, puncture,
cephal(o), head,
cerebell(o), cerebellum,
cerebr(o), cerebrum,

cerumin(o), wax,
cervic(o), neck; cervix,
cheil(o), chil(o), lip,
chem(o), chemical,
chir(o), hand,
chlor(o), chlorine, green,
chol(e), cholo, bile,
cholangi(o), bile vessel,
cholecyst(o), gallbladder,
choledoch(o), common bile duct,
chondri(o), chondr(o), cartilage,
chore(o), dance,
chrom, chromat, chromo, color,
chrono, time,
chyl(o), chyle, a digestive juice,
chym(o), chyme, semifluid present during digestion,
-cidal, destroying, killing,
-cide, destroying, killing,
cine(o), movement,
circum-, around,
-clasis, breaking,
-clast, breaking,
co-, col-, com-, con-, cor-, together,
cochle(o), cochlea,
col(o), colon(o), colon,
colp(o), vagina,
condyl(o), knob, knuckle,
coni(o), dust,
conjunctiv(o), conjunctiva,
contra-, against,
cor(o), core(o), pupil,
corne(o), cornea,
cortic(o), cortex,
costi, costo, rib,
crani(o), cranium,
crin(o), secrete,
-crine, secreting,
-crit, separate,

cry(o), cold,
crypt(o), hidden; obscure,
cyan(o), blue,
cycl(o), circle; cycle; ciliary body,
cyst(o), cysti, bladder, cyst, cystic duct,
cyt(o), cell,
-cyte, cell,
-cytosis, condition of cells,

dacry(o), tears,
dactyl(o), fingers, toes,
de-, away from,
dent(i) , dento, tooth,
derm(o), derma, dermat(o), skin,
-derma, skin,
-desis, binding,
dextr(o), right, toward the right,
di-, dif-, dir-, dis-, not, separated,
dia-, through,
dips(o), thirst,
dors(o), dorsi, back,
duoden(o), duodenum ,
dynamo, force; energy,
-dynia, pain,
dys-, abnormal; difficult,

echo, reflected sound,
ect(o)-, outside,
-ectasia, expansion; dilation,
-ectasis, expanding; dilating,
-ectomy, removal of,
-edema, swelling,
electr(o), electricity; electric,
-ema, condition,
-emesis, vomiting,
-emia, blood,
-emic, relating to blood,
encephal(o), brain,
end(o)-, within,
enter(o), intestines,
eosin(o), red; rosy,
epi-, over,
epididym(o), epididymis,
epiglott(o), epiglottis,
episi(o), vulva,
ergo, work,
erythr(o), red, redness,
esophag(o), esophagus,
-esthesia, sensation,
esthesio, sensation, perception,
ethmo, ethmoid bone,
etio, cause,
eu-, well, good, normal,
ex-, out of, away from,
exo-, external, on the outside,
extra-, without, outside of,

fasci(o), fascia,
femor(o), femur,
fibr(o), fiber,
fluor(o), light; luminous; fluorine,

-form, in the shape of,
fungi, fungus,

galact(o), milk,
gangli(o), ganglion,
gastr(o), stomach,
-gen, producing, coming to be,
gen(o), producing; being born,
-genesis, production of,
-genic, producing,
gero, geront(o), old age,
gingiv(o), gum,
gli(o), neuroglia,
-globin, protein,
-globulin, protein,
glomerul(o), glomerulus,
gloss(o), tongue,
gluc(o), glucose,
glyc(o), sugars,
glycogen(o), glycogen,
gnath(o), jaw,
gonad(o), sex glands,
gonio, angle,
-gram, a recording,
granulo, granular,
-graph, recording instrument,
-graphy, process of recording,
gyn(o), gyne, gyneco, women,

hem(a), hemat(o), hemo, blood,
hemangi(o), blood vessel,
hemi-, half,
hepat(o), hepatic(o), liver,
hidr(o), sweat,
histi(o), histo, tissue,
home(o), homo, same; constant,
humer(o), humerus,
hydr(o), hydrogen, water,
hyper-, above normal; overly,
hypn(o), sleep,
hypo-, below normal,
hyster(o), uterus, hysteria,

-iasis, pathological condition or
    state,
iatr(o), physician; treatment,
-ic, pertaining to,
ichthy(o), dry; scaly; fish,
-ics, treatment, practice, body of
    knowledge,
idio, distinct; unknown,
ile(o), ileum,
ili(o), ilium,
immun(o), safe; immune,
infra-, positioned beneath,
inguin(o), groin,
inter-, between,
intra-, within,
ir(o), irid(o), iris,
ischi(o), ischium,
-ism, condition, disease, doctrine,

iso-, equal, same,
-itis (pl. -itides), inflammation,

jejun(o), jejunum,

kal(i), potassium,
karyo, nucleus,
kerat(o), cornea,
ket(o); keton(o), ketone; acetone,
kin(o), kine, movement,
kinesi(o), kineso, motion,
-kinesia, movement,
-kinesis, movement,
kyph(o), humpback,

labi(o), lip,
lacrim(o), tears,
lact(o), lacti, milk,
lamin(o), lamina,
lapar(o), abdominal wall,
laryng(o), larynx,
latero, lateral, to one side,
leiomy(o), smooth muscle,
-lepsy, condition of having seizures,
-leptic, having seizures,
lepto, light, frail, thin,
leuk(o), white,
lingu(o), tongue,
lip(o), fat,
lith(o), stone,
lob(o), lobe of the lung,
log(o), speech, words, thought,
-logist, one who practices,
-logy, study, practice,
lumb(o), lumbar,
lymph(o), lymph,
lymphaden(o), lymph nodes,
lymphangi(o), lymphatic vessels,
lys(o), dissolution,
-lysis, destruction of,
-lytic, destroying,

macr(o), large; long,
mal-, bad; inadequate,
-malacia, softening,
mamm(o), breast,
-mania, obsession,
mast(o), breast,
mastoid(o), mastoid process,
maxill(o), maxilla,
meato, meatus,
medi(o), middle; medial plane,
mediastin(o), mediastinum,
medull(o), medulla,
meg(a), megal(o), large; million,
-megaly, enlargement,
melan(o), black; dark,
mening(o), meninges,
men(o), menstruation,
mes(o), middle; median,
meta-, after,

metacarp(o), metacarpal,
-meter, measuring device,
metr(o), uterus,
-metry, measurement,
micr(o), small; microscopic;
　one-millionth; tiny,
mio, smaller; less,
mon(o)-, single,
morph(o), structure; shape,
muc(o), mucus,
multi-, many,
muta, genetic change,
mutagen(o), genetic change,
my(o), muscle,
myc(o), fungus,
myel(o), spinal cord; bone marrow,
myring(o), eardrum, middle ear,

narco, sleep; numbness,
nas(o), nose,
necr(o), death; dying,
nephr(o), kidney,
neur(i), neuro, nerve,
noct(i), night,
normo, normal,
nucle(o), nucleus,
nyct(o), night,

ocul(o), eye,
odont(o), tooth,
-oid, like, resembling,
olig(o)-, few; little; scanty,
-oma (pl. -omata), tumor, neoplasm,
oncho, onc(o), tumor,
onych(o), nail,
oo, egg,
oophor(o), ovary,
ophthalm(o), eye,
-opia, vision,
-opsia, vision,
-opsy, view of,
opt(o), optic(o), eye; sight,
or(o), mouth,
orch(o), orchi(o), orchido, testis,
orth(o), straight; normal,
-osis (pl. -oses), condition, state, process,
osseo, ossi, bone,
ossicul(o), ossicle,
ost(e), osteo, bone,
-ostomy, opening,
ot(o), ear,
ov(i), ovo, egg; ova,
ovari(o), ovary,
ox(o), oxi, oxygen,
-oxia, oxygen,
oxy, sharp; acute; oxygen,
pachy, thick,
pan-, pant(o)-, all, entire,
pancreat(o), pancreas,
par(a)-, beside; abnormal; involving
　two parts,

-para, bearing,
parathyroid(o), parathyroid,
-paresis, slight paralysis,
-parous, producing; bearing,
patell(o), knee,
path(o), disease,
-pathy, disease,
ped(o), pedi, foot; child,
pelvi(o), pelvo, pelvic bone; hip,
-penia, deficiency,
-pepsia, digestion,
per-, through, intensely,
peri-, around, about, near,
pericardi(o), pericardium,
perine(o), perineum,
peritone(o), peritoneum,
-pexy, fixation, usually done surgically,
phac(o), phak(o), lens,
-phage, -phagia, -phagy, eating,
　devouring,
phag(o), eating; devouring; swallowing,
phalang(o), finger or toe bone,
pharmaco, drugs; medicine,
pharyng(o), pharynx,
-phasia, speaking,
-pheresis, removal,
-phil, attraction; affinity for,
-philia, attraction; affinity for,
phleb(o), vein,
-phobia, fear,
phon(o), sound; voice; speech,
-phonia, sound,
-phoresis, carrying,
-phoria, feeling; carrying,
phot(o), light,
phren(o), phreni, phrenico, mind;
　diaphragm,
-phrenia, of the mind,
-phthisis, wasting away,
-phylaxis, protection,
physi, physio, physical; natural,
-physis, growing,
physo, air; gas; growing,
phyt(o), plant,
pil(o), hair,
-plakia, plaque,
-plasia, formation,
-plasm, formation,
plasma, plasmo, plasmat(o), plasma,
-plastic, forming,
-plasty, surgical repair,
-plegia, paralysis,
-plegic, one who is paralyzed,
pleur(o), pleura, rib; side; pleura,
pluri-, several, more,
-pnea, breath,
pneum(a), pneumat(o), pneumo,
　pneumon(o), lungs; air; breathing,
pod(o), foot,
-poiesis, formation,
-poietic, forming,

-poietin, one that forms,
poikilo, varied; irregular,
poly-, many,
-porosis, lessening in density,
post-, after, following,
pre-, before,
pro-, before, forward,
proct(o), anus,
prostat(o), prostate gland,
pseud(o), false,
psych(o), psyche, mind,
-ptosis, falling down; drooping,
pub(o), pubis,
pulmon(o), lung,
pupill(o), pupil,
pyel(o), renal pelvis,
pylor(o), pylorus,
pyo, pus,
pyret(o), fever,
pyro, fever; fire; heat,

quadra-, quadri-, four,

rachi(o), spine,
radi(o), radiation; x-ray; radius,
re-, again, backward,
rect(o), rectum,
ren(i), reno, kidney,
retin(o), retina,
retro-, behind, backward,
rhabd(o), rod-shaped,
rhabdomy(o), striated muscle,
rhin(o), nose,
-rrhage, discharging heavily,
-rrhagia, heavy discharge,
-rrhaphy, surgical suturing,
-rrhea, a flowing, a flux,
-rrhexis, rupture,

sacr(o), sacrum,
salping(o), tube,
sarco, fleshy tissue; muscle,
scapul(o), scapula,
-schisis, splitting,
schisto, split,
schiz(o), split; division,
scler(o), sclera, hardness; hardening, white
　of the eye,
scoli(o), crooked; bent,
-scope, instrument for observing,
-scopy, use of an instrument for
　observing,
scot(o), darkness,
seb(o), fat,
semi-, half,
sial(o), salivary glands; saliva,
sialaden(o), salivary gland,
sidero, iron,
sigmoid(o), sigmoid colon,
sito, food; grain,
somat(o), body,

somn(o), somni, sleep,
-somnia, sleep,
son(o), sound,
-spasm, contraction,
spasmo, spasm,
sperm(a), spermato, spermo, semen;
   spermatozoa,
spher(o), round; spherical,
sphygm(o), pulse,
spin(o), spine,
spir(o), breath; breathe,
splanchn(o), splanchni, viscera,
splen(o), spleen,
spondyl(o), vertebra,
squamo, scale; squamous,
-stalsis, contraction,
staphyl(o), grapelike clusters,
-stasis, stopping; constant,
-stat, agent to maintain a state,
-static, maintaining a state,
steat(o), fat,
steno, narrowness,
-stenosis, narrowing,
stere(o), three-dimensional,
stern(o), sternum,
steth(o), chest,
stom(a), stomat(o), mouth,
-stomy, opening,
strepto, twisted chains; streptococci,
styl(o), peg-shaped,
sub-, less than, under, inferior,
super-, more than, above, superior,
supra-, above, over,
syl-, sym-, syn-, sys-, together,

synov(o), synovial membrane,
syring(o), tube,

tachy-, fast,
tars(o), tarsus,
tel(o), tele(o), distant; end; complete,
ten(o), tendin(o), tendo, tenon(o), tendon,
terato, monster (as a malformed fetus),
test(o), testis,
thalam(o), thalamus,
therm(o), heat,
thorac(o), thoracico, thorax, chest,
thromb(o), blood clot,
thym(o), thymus gland,
thyr(o), thyroid gland,
tibi(o), tibia,
-tome, cutting instrument, segment,
-tomy, cutting operation,
tono, tension; pressure,
tonsill(o), tonsils,
top(o), place; topical,
tox(i), toxico, toxo, poison; toxin,
trache(o), trachea,
trachel(o), neck
trans-, across, through,
trich(o), trichi, hair,
trigon(o), trigone,
-trophic, nutritional,
tropho, food; nutrition,
-trophy, nutrition,
-tropia, turning,
-tropic, turning toward,
-tropy, condition of turning toward,
tympan(o), eardrum, middle ear,

uln(o), ulna,
ultra-, beyond, excessive,
un-, not,
uni-, one,
ur(o), urin(o), urine,
ureter(o), ureter,
urethr(o), urethra,
-uria, urine,
uter(o), uterus,
uve(o), uvea,

vag(o), vagus nerve,
vagin(o), vagina,
varico, varicosity,
vas(o), blood vessel, duct,
vasculo, blood vessel,
veni, ven(o), vein,
ventricul(o), ventricle,
-version, turning,
vertebr(o), vertebra,
vesic(o), bladder,
vivi, life,
vulv(o), vulva,

xanth(o), yellow,
xeno, stranger,
xer(o), dry,
xiph(o), sword; xiphoid,

zo(o), life,
zym(o), fermentation; enzyme,

APPENDIX

B Abbreviations—Ones to Use and Ones to Avoid

Recently, medical abbreviations have been linked to some of the worst medical errors, particularly those involving wrong doses of medication. As a result, the Joint Commission on Accreditation of Hospital Organizations (JCAHO) has come up with a list of nine prohibited abbreviations plus several as recommended for elimination in medical communication. For the prohibited abbreviations, it is suggested that the full words be substituted. Table A-1 shows the prohibited abbreviations, what they can be confused with, and what should be substituted. Table A-2 shows suggested replacements for abbreviations that have the potential to cause medical errors. JCAHO has also suggested that each healthcare organization come up with their own list of frequently used and potentially misunderstood abbreviations.

TABLE A-1 Prohibited Abbreviations

Abbreviation	Potential Problem	Solution
1. U (for unit)	Mistaken as zero, four or cc.	Write or speak "unit"
2. IU (for international unit)	Mistaken as IV (intravenous) or 10 (ten).	Write or speak "international unit"
3. Q.D. (once daily) 4. Q.O.D. (every other day)	Mistaken for each other. The period after the Q can be mistaken for an "I" and the "O" can be mistaken for "I".	Write or speak "daily" and "every other day"
5. Trailing zero (X.0 mg) [*Note: Prohibited only for medication-related notations*]; 6. Lack of leading zero (.X mg)	Decimal point is missed and dosage is either too large or too small.	Never write a zero by itself after a decimal point (X mg), and always use a zero before a decimal point (0.X mg)
7. MS 8. MSO$_4$ 9. MgSO$_4$	Can mean morphine sulfate or magnesium sulfate. Potentially confused for one another.	Write or speak "morphine sulfate" or "magnesium sulfate"

TABLE A-2 Suggested Additional Abbreviations to Avoid.

Abbreviation	Potential Problem	Solution
µg (for microgram)	Mistaken for mg (milligrams) resulting in one thousand-fold dosing overdose.	Write "mcg" or speak microgram
H.S. (for half-strength or Latin abbreviation for bedtime)	Mistaken for either half-strength or hour of sleep (at bedtime). q.H.S. mistaken for every hour. All can result in a dosing error.	Write out or speak "half-strength" or "at bedtime"
T.I.W. (for three times a week)	Mistaken for three times a day or twice weekly resulting in an overdose.	Write or speak "3 times weekly" or "three times weekly"
S.C. or S.Q. (for subcutaneous)	Mistaken as SL for sublingual, or "5 every".	Write or speak "Sub-Q","subQ, or "subcutaneously"
D/C (for discharge)	Interpreted as discontinue whatever medications follow (typically discharge meds).	Write "discharge"
c.c. (for cubic centimeter)	Mistaken for U (units) when poorly written.	Write or speak "ml" for milliliters
A.S., A.D., A.U. (Latin abbreviation for left, right, or both ears)	Mistaken for OS, OD, and OU, etc.).	Write or speak "left ear," "right ear" or "both ears"

Listed below are the medical abbreviations that you should learn while studying medical terminology.

ABBREVIATION	MEANING	ABBREVIATION	MEANING
−	minus/concave	AGN	acute glomerulonephritis
+	plus/convex	AH	abdominal hysterectomy
aa, āā	of each	AIDS	acquired immunodeficiency syndrome
AA	Alcoholics Anonymous	AIH	artificial insemination homologous
AB	abortion	A-K	above the knee
ABG	arterial blood gases	ALL	acute lymphocytic leukemia
a.c.	before meals (Latin *ante cibum*), usually one-half hour preceding	ALS	amyotrophic lateral sclerosis
acc.	accommodation	ALT, AT	alanine transaminase
AcG	accelerator globulin	AM, a.m., A	morning (Latin *ante meridiem*)
Ach	acetylcholine	AMI	acute myocardial infarction
ACTH	adrenocorticotropic hormone	AML	acute myelogenous leukemia
ad	up to	AP	anteroposterior
a. d., AD	right ear (Latin *auris dexter*)	A&P	auscultation and percussion
ADD	attention deficit disorder	APTT	activated partial thromboplastin time
ad lib	freely (Latin *ad libitum*), as often as desired	ARD	acute respiratory disease
ADH	antidiuretic hormone	ARDS	adult respiratory distress syndrome
AF	atrial fibrillation	ARF	acute respiratory failure, acute renal failure
AFB	acid-fast bacillus (causes tuberculosis)	ARMD	age-related macular degeneration
AFP	alpha-fetoprotein	a. s., AS	left ear (Latin *auris sinister*)
A/G	albumin/globulin	AS	aortic stenosis

ABBREVIATION	MEANING	ABBREVIATION	MEANING
ASCVD	arteriosclerotic cardiovascular disease	CCU	coronary care unit
ASD	atrial septal defect	CDA	certified dental assistant
ASHD	arteriosclerotic heart disease	CEA	carcinogenic embryonic antigen
ASIS	anterior superior iliac spine	CHD	coronary heart disease
AST	aspartic acid transaminase	chemo	chemotherapy
ATN	acute tubular necrosis	CHF	congestive heart failure
a. u., AU	each ear (Latin *auris uterque*)	CIS	carcinoma in situ
AV	atrioventricular	Cl	chlorine
AZT	Azidothymidine	CLL	chronic lymphocytic leukemia
B	bilateral	CML	chronic myelogenous leukemia
B-K	below the knee	CMV	cytomegalovirus
Ba	barium	CNS	central nervous system
BaE	barium enema	CO	cardiac output
baso	basophil	COLD	chronic obstructive lung disease
BBB	blood-brain barrier	comp.	compound
BCP	biochemistry panel	COPD	chronic obstructive pulmonary disease
BE	barium enema	CP	cerebral palsy
BID, b.i.d.	twice a day (Latin *bis in die*)	CPK	creatine phosphokinase
BMT	bone marrow transplant	CPR	cardiopulmonary resuscitation
BNO	bladder neck obstruction	CRF	chronic renal failure
BP	blood pressure	CRH	corticotropin-releasing hormone
BPH	benign prostatic hypertrophy	CS, C-section	caesarean section
bpm	beats per minute	CSF	cerebrospinal fluid
BS	breath sounds	C-spine	cervical spine (film)
BUN	blood urea nitrogen	CT	computed tomography
bx	biopsy	CT or CAT scan	computerized (axial) tomography
c, c̄	with	CTA	clear to auscultation
C-section	caesarean section	CTS	carpal tunnel syndrome
C-spine	cervical spine (film)	CVA	cerebrovascular accident
C_1	first cervical vertebra	CVD	cerebrovascular disease
ca	calcium	cx	contraindicated
CA	carcinoma	Cx	cervix
CABG	coronary artery bypass graft	CXR	chest x-ray
CAD	coronary artery disease	cysto	cystoscopy
cap., caps.	capsule	D	diopter
CAPD	continuous ambulatory peritoneal dialysis	D_1	first dorsal vertebra
CAT	computerized axial tomography	D & C	dilation and curettage
cath	catheter	DDS	doctor of dental surgery
CBC	complete blood count	DIC	disseminated intravascular coagulation
cc., cc	cubic centimeter	d.t.d.	give of such doses

Abbreviation	Meaning	Abbreviation	Meaning
D_5W	dextrose 5% in water	ECT	electroconvulsive therapy
DAW	dispense as written	EDC	expected date of confinement (delivery)
dB	decibel	EEG	electroencephalogram
DDS	doctor of dental surgery	EENT	eye, ear, nose, and throat
def	decayed, extracted, or filled (primary teeth)	EGD	esophagogastroduodenoscopy
DEF	decayed, extracted, or filled (permanent teeth)	EIA, ELISA	Enzyme-linked immunosorbent assay
DES	diethylstilbestrol	elix.	elixir
diff	differential blood count	EMB	endometrial biopsy
dil.	dilute	EMG	electromyogram
disc, D. C., dc	discontinue	e.m.p.	as directed
disp.	dispense	ENT	ear, nose, and throat
div.	divide	eos	eosinophils
DJD	degenerative joint disease	EQ	emotional "intelligence" quotient
DLE	discoid lupus erythematosus	ER	estrogen receptor
DM	diabetes mellitus	ERCP	endoscopic retrograde cholangiopancreatography
dmf	decayed, missing, or filled (primary teeth)	ERT	estrogen replacement therapy
DMF	decayed, missing, or filled (permanent teeth)	ESR	erythrocyte sedimentation rate
DNA	deoxyribonucleic acid	ESRD	end-stage renal disease
DOE	dyspnea on exertion	EST	electroshock therapy
DPT	diphtheria, pertussis, tetanus (combined vaccination)	ESWL	extracorporeal shock wave lithotripsy
DRE	digital rectal exam	ET tube	endotracheal intubation tube
DSA	digital subtraction angiography	ETT	exercise tolerance test
DSM	*Diagnostic and Statistical Manual of Mental Disorders*	ex aq.	in water
DT	delirium tremens	ext.	extract
DTR	deep tendon reflex	FDA	Food and Drug Administration
DUB	dysfunctional uterine bleeding	FEF	forced expiratory flow
DVA	distance visual acuity	FEV	forced expiratory volume
DVT	deep venous thrombosis	FHT	fetal heart tones
DW	distilled water	fld. ext.	fluid extract
dx, Dx	diagnosis	FSH	follicle-stimulating hormone
EBV	Epstein-Barr virus	FUO	fever of unknown origin
ECC	endocervical curettage	FVC	forced vital capacity
ECCE	extracapsular cataract extraction	fx, Fx	fracture
ECG, EKG	electrocardiogram	g, gm	gram
ECHO	echocardiogram	G	gravida (pregnancy)

ABBREVIATION	MEANING	ABBREVIATION	MEANING
G-CSF	granulocyte colony-stimulating factor	IgM	immunoglobulin M
GERD	gastroesophageal reflux disease	IM	intramuscular
GH	growth hormone	IMV	intermittent mandatory ventilation
GI	gastrointestinal	inj	injection
GM-CSF	granulocyte macrophage colony-stimulating factor	IOL	intraocular lens
GOT	glutamic oxaloacetic transaminase	IPPB	intermittent positive pressure breathing
gr	grain, gram	IOP	intraocular pressure
gtt	drop	IQ	intelligence quotient
GTT	glucose tolerance test	IRDS	infant respiratory distress syndrome
Gy	unit of radiation equal to 100 rads	IRV	inspiratory reserve volume
gyn	gynecology	IUD	intrauterine device
H	hypodermic	IV	intravenous
h.	every hour (Latin *hora*)	IVC	intravenous cholangiography
h.s.	hour of sleep (Latin *hora somni*)	IVP	intravenous pyelogram
HBOT	hyperbaric oxygen therapy	IVU	intravenous urography
HCG	human chorionic gonadotropin	K+	potassium
HCT, Hct	hematocrit	KUB	kidney, ureter, bladder
HD	hemodialysis	L	left
HDL	high-density lipoprotein	L_1	first lumbar vertebra
HGB, Hgb, HB	hemoglobin	LDH	lactate dehydrogenase
HIV	human immunodeficiency virus	LDL	low-density lipoprotein
HR	heart rate	LH	luteinizing hormone
HRT	hormone replacement therapy	LLL	left lower lobe [of the lungs]
HSG	hysterosalpingography	LMP	last menstrual period
HSO	hysterosalpingoophorectomy	LP	lumbar puncture
HSV	herpes simplex virus	LUL	left upper lobe [of the lungs]
IBD	inflammatory bowel disease	LV	left ventricle
IBS	irritable bowel syndrome	LVH	left ventricular hypertrophy
ICCE	intracapsular cataract cryoextraction	M.	mix
ICD	International Classification of Diseases	MBC	maximal breathing capacity
ICP	intracranial pressure	mcg	microgram
IDDM	insulin-dependent diabetes mellitus	MCH	mean corpuscular hemoglobin
IgA	immunoglobulin A	MCHC	mean corpuscular hemoglobin concentration
IgD	immunoglobulin D	MCP	metacarpophalangeal
IgE	immunoglobulin E	MCV	mean corpuscular volume
IgG	immunoglobulin G	MDI	metered dose inhaler

ABBREVIATION	MEANING	ABBREVIATION	MEANING
mEq	milliequivalent	oint., ung.	ointment, unguent
METS, mets	metastases	o.l., OL	left eye
mg	milligram	OM	otitis media
MI	mitral insufficiency; myocardial infarction	o.s., OS	left eye
ml	milliliter	OT	oxytocin
mono	monocyte	OTC	over the counter
MR	mitral regurgitation	o.u., OU	each eye
MRA	magnetic resonance angiography	oz.	ounce
MRSA	A form of staphylococcus aureus that is resistant to a common group of antibiotics that include methicillin, penicillin, and amoxicillin	p	post, after
MRI	magnetic resonance imaging	P	para (live births)
MS	multiple sclerosis	P	phosphorus
MS	mitral stenosis	p.c.	after meals (Latin *post cibum*), one-half hour after a meal
MSH	melanocyte-stimulating hormone	PA	posteroanterior
MUGA	multiple-gated acquisition scan	PAC	premature atrial contraction
multip	multiparous	Pap smear	Papanicolaou smear
MVP	mitral valve prolapse	PCP	Pneumocystis carinii pneumonia
n., noct.	night (Latin, *nocte*)	PCV	packed cell volume
NG	nasogastric	PDR	*Physician's Desk Reference*
N.S., NS	normal saline	PE tube	polyethylene ventilating tube (placed in the eardrum)
N&V	nausea and vomiting	PED	penile erectile dysfunction
Na+	sodium	PEEP	positive end expiratory pressure
NHL	non-Hodgkin's lymphoma	PERRL, PERRLA	pupils equal, round, reactive to light (and accommodation)
NIDDM	noninsulin-dependent diabetes mellitus	PET	positron emission tomography
NMR	nuclear magnetic resonance (imaging)	PFT	pulmonary function tests
non rep.	do not repeat	PG	prostaglandins
NPO	nothing by mouth	pH	power of hydrogen concentration
NPO p MN	nothing by mouth after midnight	PID	pelvic inflammatory disease
NSAID	nonsteroidal anti-inflammatory drug	PIP	proximal interphalangeal joint
NVA	near visual acuity	PKU	phenylketonuria
OA	osteoarthritis	PLT	platelet count
OB	obstetrics	PM, p.m., P	afternoon (Latin *post meridiem*)
OCD	obsessive-compulsive disorder	PMN, poly	polymorphonuclear neutrophil
OCP	oral contraceptive pill	PMP	previous menstrual period
o.d., OD	right eye	PMS	premenstrual syndrome

ABBREVIATION	MEANING	ABBREVIATION	MEANING
PNS	peripheral nervous system	RNA	ribonucleic acid
PND	paroxysmal nocturnal dyspnea; postnasal drip	ROM	range of motion
p.o.	by mouth (Latin *per os*)	RT	radiation therapy
PRN, p.r.n.	repeat as needed (Latin *pro re nata*)	RUL	right upper lobe [of the lungs]
PSA	prostate-specific antigen	RP	retrograde pyelogram
PSIS	posterior superior iliac spine	Rx	prescription
PT	prothrombin time	s,$\bar{s}$	without
PTCA	percutaneous transluminal coronary angioplasty	SA	sinoatrial
PTH	parathyroid hormone, parathormone	SAH	subarachnoid hemorrhage
PTSD	post-traumatic stress disorder	SARS	severe acute respiratory syndrome
PTT	partial thromboplastin time	seg	segmented mature white blood cells
pulv., pwdr.	powder	SG	specific gravity
PUVA	psoralen—ultraviolet A light therapy	SGOT	serum glutamic oxaloacetic transaminase
PVC	premature ventricular contraction	SGPT	serum gluamic pyruvic transaminase
PPD	purified protein derivative	SIDS	sudden infant death syndrome
primip	primiparous	Sig.	patient directions such as route and timing of medication (Latin signa, inscription)
PRL	prolactin	SL	sublingual
qam	every morning	SLE	systemic lupus erythematosus
q.d.	every day (Latin *quaque dies*)	SNOMED	Systematized Nomenclature of Medicine
q.h.	every hour	SOB	shortness of breath
q.i.d.	four times a day	sol., soln.	solution
q.o.d.	every other day	SOM	serous otitis media
QNS	quantity not sufficient	s.o.s.	if there is need
q. s.	sufficient quantity	sp.	spirit
r	roentgen	SPECT	single photon emission computed tomography
R	rectal	SPP	suprapubic prostatectomy
R	right	SR; sed. rate	sedimentation rate
RA	rheumatoid arthritis	ss, $\bar{ss}$	one-half
Ra	radium	stat	immediately
rad	radiation absorbed dose	STH	somatotropin hormone
RAI	radioactive iodine	subc, subq, s.c.	subcutaneously
RBC	red blood cell count	supp., suppos.	suppository
RD	respiratory disease	susp.	suspension
RDH	registered dental hygienist	SV	stroke volume
RDS	respiratory distress syndrome	sym, Sym, Sx	symptoms
RIA	radioimmunoassay	syr.	syrup
RLL	right lower lobe [of the lungs]	T_1	first thoracic verterbra

ABBREVIATION	MEANING	ABBREVIATION	MEANING
TC	total cholesterol	TURP	transurethral resection of the prostate
t.i.d.	three times a day	Tx	treatment
tab.	tablet	UA	urinalysis
T&A	tonsillectomy and adenoidectomy	UC	uterine contractions
TAH-BSO	total abdominal hysterectomy with bilateral salpingo-oophorectomy	u.d.	as directed
tal.	such	UGI(s)	uppergastrointestinal (series)
tal. dos.	such doses	ung.	ointment
TAT	Thematic Apperception Test	URI	upper respiratory infection
TB	tuberculosis	U/S	ultrasound
tbsp.	tablespoonful	U.S.P.	*United States Pharmacopeia*
TC	total cholesterol	UTI	urinary tract infection
TDM	therapeutic drug monitoring	U, u	unit
TIA	transient ischemic attack	VC	vital capacity
tinct., tr.	tincture	VCU, VCUG	voiding cystourethrogram
TLC	total lung capacity	VF	visual field
TMJ	temporomandibular joint	VLDL	very low-density lipoprotein
TNM	tumor, nodes, metastasis	V/Q, V/Q scan	ventilation/perfusion scan
tPA, TPA	tissue plasminogen activator	VRE	A form of enterococcus that is resistant to most antibiotics
TPN	total parenteral nutrition	VSD	ventricular septal defect
TPR	temperature, pulse, and respiration	VT	ventricular tachycardia
TSH	thyroid-stimulating hormone	WAIS	Wechsler Adult Intelligence Scale
tsp.	teaspoonful	WBC	white blood cell count
TSS	toxic shock syndrome	XRT	x-ray or radiation therapy
TUIP	transurethral incision of the prostate	ZDV	ZDV
TUNA	transurethral needle ablation		

APPENDIX

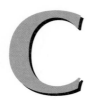

Glossary of Key Terms

The following glossary includes the key terms found throughout this text. The Spanish terms in blue for selected key terms are references to the Spanish Glossary available online at www.mhhe.com/medterm3e.

A

abdominal [ăb-DŎM-ĭ-năl] **cavity** Body space between the abdominal walls, above the pelvis, and below the diaphragm.

abdominocentesis [ăb-DŎM-ĭ-nō-sĕn-TĒ-sĭs] Incision into the abdomen to remove fluid or relieve pressure.

abortifacient [ă-bōr-tĭ-FĀ-shĕnt] {abortifaciente} Medication to prevent implantation of an ovum.

abortion [ă-BŌR-shŭn] {aborto} Premature ending of a pregnancy.

abruptio placentae [ăb-RŬP-shē-ō plă-SĔN-tē] Breaking away of the placenta from the uterine wall.

abscess [ĂB-sĕs] {absceso} Localized collection of pus and other exudate, usually accompanied by swelling and redness; infection and swelling of the soft tissue of the jaw.

absence seizure Mild epileptic seizure consisting of brief disorientation with the environment.

absorb [ăb-SŎRB] To take into.

absorption [ăb-SŎRP-shŭn] {absorción} Passing of nutrients into the bloodstream.

acetabulum [ăs-ĕ-TĂB-yū-lŭm] {acetábulo} Cup-shaped depression in the hip bone into which the top of the femur fits.

acetone [ĂS-ĕ-tōn] {acetona} Type of ketone normally found in urine in small quantities; found in larger quantities in diabetic urine.

acetylcholine [ăs-ē-tĭl-KŌ-lēn] {acetilcolina} Chemical that stimulates cells.

achalasia [ăk-ă-LĀ-zhē-ă] {acalasia} Inability of a muscle, particularly the cardiac sphincter, to relax.

achlorhydria [ā-klōr-HĪ-drē-ă] Lack of hydrochloric acid in the stomach.

acidosis [ăs-ĭ-DŌ-sĭs] {acidosis} Abnormal release of ketones in the body.

acne [ĂK-nē] {acné} Inflammatory eruption of the skin, occurring in or near sebaceous glands on the face, neck, shoulder, or upper back.

acne vulgaris [vŭl-GĀR-ĭs] {acne vulgar} See acne.

acquired active immunity Resistance to a disease acquired naturally or developed by previous exposure or vaccination.

acquired immunodeficiency [ĬM-yū-nō-dē-FĬSH-ĕn-sē] **disease (AIDS)** Most widespread immunosuppressive disease; caused by the HIV virus.

acquired passive immunity Inoculation against disease or poison, using antitoxins or antibodies from or in another person or another species.

acromegaly [ăk-rō-MĔG-ă-lē] {acromegalia} Abnormally enlarged features resulting from a pituitary tumor and hypersecretion of growth hormone.

acromion [ă-KRŌ-mē-ŏn] {acromion} Part of the scapula that connects to the clavicle.

actinic keratosis [ăk-TĬN-ĭk KĔR-ă-tō-sĭs] Overgrowth of horny skin that forms from over-exposure to sunlight; sunburn.

acupuncture [ă-kyū-PŬNK-chūr] Originally Chinese therapy that uses fine needles.

Adam's apple {manzana de Adán} Thyroid cartilage, supportive structure of the larynx; larger in males than in females; protrusion in the neck caused by a fold of thyroid cartilage.

addict [ĂD-ĭkt] One who is dependent on a substance (usually illegal, as narcotics) on a recurring basis.

Addison's [ĂD-ĭ-sŏnz] **disease** Underactivity of the adrenal glands.

adenectomy [ă-dĕ-NĔK-tō-mē] Removal of a gland.

adenohypophysis [ĂD-ĕ-nō-hī-PŎF-ĭ-sĭs] Anterior lobe of the pituitary gland.

adenoidectomy [ĂD-ĕ-nŏy-DĔK-tō-mē] {adenoidectomía} Removal of the adenoids.

adenoiditis [ĂD-ĕ-nŏy-DĪ-tĭs] {adenoiditis} Inflammation of the adenoids.

adenoids [ĂD-ĕ-nŏydz] {adenoids} Collection of lymphoid tissue in the nasopharynx; pharyngeal tonsils.

adipose [ĂD-ĭ-pōs] {adipose} Fatty; relating to fat.

adrenal cortex [ă-DRĒ-năl KŎR-tĕks] Outer portion of the adrenal gland; helps control metabolism, inflammations, sodium and potassium retention, and effects of stress.

adrenal gland {adrenal} One of two glands, each of which is situated on top of each kidney.

adrenal medulla [mĕ-DŪL-lă] Inner portion of adrenal glands; releases large quantities of hormones during stress.

adrenalectomy [ă-drē-năl-ĔK-tō-mē] {adrenalectomía} Removal of an adrenal gland.

adrenaline [ă-DRĔ-nă-lĭn] {adrenalina} Epinephrine; secreted by adrenal medulla.

adrenocorticotropic [ă-DRĒ-nō-KŌR-tĭ-kŏ-TRŌ-pĭk] **hormone (ACTH)** Hormone secreted by anterior pituitary; involved in the control of the adrenal cortex.

aerotitis media [ăr-ō-TĪ-tĭs MĒ-dē-ă] Inflammation of the middle ear caused by air pressure changes, as in air travel.

afferent [ĂF-ĕr-ĕnt] **(sensory) neuron** Neuron that carries information from the sensory receptors to the central nervous system.

afterbirth [ĂF-tĕr-bĭrth] {secundina} Placenta and membranes that are expelled from the uterus after birth.

agglutination [ă-glū-tĭ-NĀ-shŭn] {aglutinación} Clumping of cells and particles in blood.

agglutinogen [ă-glū-TĬN-ō-jĕn] {aglutinógeno} Substances that cause agglutination.

aggressiveness [ă-GRĔS-ĭv-nĕs] Abnormal forcefulness toward others.

agitation [ă-jĭ-TĀ-shŭn] Abnormal restlessness.

agnosia [ăg-NŌ-zē-ă] {agnosia} Inability to receive and understand outside stimuli.

agranulocyte [ā-GRĂN-yū-lō-sīt] {agranulocito} Leukocyte with nongranular cytoplasm.

AIDS [ādz] *See* acquired immunodeficiency syndrome.

albinism [ĂL-bĭ-nĭzm] {albinismo} Rare, congenital condition causing either partial or total lack of pigmentation.

albumin [ăl-BYŪ-mĭn] {albúmina} 1. Simple protein; when leaked into urine, may indicate a kidney problem. 2. Simple protein found in plasma.

albuminuria [ăl-byū-mĭ-NŪ-rē-ă] {albuminuria} Presence of albumin in urine, usually indicative of disease.

aldosterone [ăl-DŎS-tĕr-ōn] {aldosterona} Hormone secreted by adrenal cortex; mineralocorticoid.

alimentary [ăl-ĭ-MĔN-tĕr-ē] **canal** Muscular tube from the mouth to the anus; digestive tract; gastrointestinal tract.

allergen [ĂL-ĕr-jĕn] {alergeno} Substance to which exposure causes an allergic response.

allergy [ĂL-ĕr-jē] {alergia} Production of IgE antibodies against an allergen.

allograft [ĂL-ō-grăft] {aloinjerto} *See* homograft.

alopecia [ăl-ō-PĒ-shē-ă] {alopecia} Lack of hair in spots; baldness.

alopecia areata [ăl-ō-PĒ-shē-ă ă-rē-Ā-tă] Loss of hair in patches.

alpha [ĂL-fă] **cells** Specialized cells that produce glucagon in the pancreas.

alpha rays Type of radioactive particles that have a low ability to penetrate the body.

alpha-hydroxy [ĂL-fă-hī-DRŎK-sē] **acid** Agent added to cosmetics to improve the skin's appearance.

alternative medical system Complete system of medical treatment outside the realm of conventional medicine.

alternative medicine Medical therapies outside the realm of conventional medicine.

alveolar [ăl-VĒ-ō-lăr] Forming small sacs.

alveolus (*pl.*, **alveoli**) [ăl-VĒ-ō-lŭs (ăl-VĒ-ō-lī)] {alvéolo} Air sac at the end of each bronchiole.

Alzheimer's [ĂLTS-hī-mĕrz] **disease** A type of degenerative brain disease causing thought disorders, gradual loss of muscle control, and, eventually, death.

amalgam [ă-MĂL-găm] Mixture of metals or other substances used in fillings.

ambivalence [ăm-BĬV-a-lens] Feeling of conflicting emotions about a person or issue.

amenorrhea [ā-mĕn-ŏ-RĒ-ă] {amenorrea} Lack of menstruation.

amino [ă-MĒ-nō] **acid** {aminoácido} Chemical compound that results from digestion of complex proteins.

amnesia [ăm-NĒ-zē-ă] {amnesia} Loss of memory.

amniocentesis [ĂM-nē-ō-sĕn-TĒ-sĭs] {amniocentesis} Removal of a sample of amniotic fluid through a needle injected in the amniotic sac.

amnion [ĂM-nē-ŏn] {amnios} Innermost membrane of the sac surrounding the fetus during gestation.

amniotic [ăm-nē-ŎT-ĭk] {amniótico} **fluid** Fluid surrounding the fetus and held by the amnion.

amphiarthrosis (*pl.*, **amphiarthroses**) [AM-fi-ar-THRO-sis (AM-fi-ar-THRO-ses)] {anfiartrosis} Cartilaginous joint having some movement at the union of two bones.

amputation [ĂM-pyū-TĀ-shŭn] {amputación} Cutting off of a limb or part of a limb.

amylase [ĂM-ĭl-ās] {amilasa} Enzyme that is part of pancreatic juice and saliva and that begins the digestion of carbohydrates.

amyotrophic lateral sclerosis [ā-mī-ō-TRŌ-fĭk LĂT-ĕr-ăl sklĕ-RŌ-sĭs] **(ALS)** Degenerative disease of the motor neurons leading to loss of muscular control and death.

anacusis [ăn-ă-KŪ-sĭs] {anacusia} Loss of hearing.

anal [Ā-năl] **canal** Part of the digestive tract extending from the rectum to the anus.

anal fistula [Ā-năl FĬS-tyū-lă] Small opening in the anal canal through which waste matter can leak.

anal fistulectomy [Ā-năl fĭs-tyū-LĔK-tō-mē] Removal of an anal fistula.

analgesic [ăn-ăl-JĒ-zĭk] {analgésico} Agent that relieves or eliminates pain.

anaphylaxis [ĂN-ă-fĭ-LĂK-sĭs] {anafilaxia o anafilaxis} Life-threatening allergic reaction.

anaplasia [ăn-ă-PLĀ-zē-ă] Loss of cell differentiation.

anaplastic [ăn-ă-PLĂS-tĭk] Reverting to a more immature form.

anastomosis [ă-NĂS-tō-MŌ-sĭs] {anastomosis} Surgical connection of two blood vessels to allow blood flow between them; surgical union of two hollow structures.

androgen [ĂN-drō-jĕn] {andrógeno} Any male hormone, such as testosterone.

anemia [ă-NĒ-mē-ă] {anemia} Condition in which red blood cells do not transport enough oxygen to the tissues.

anesthetic [ăn-ĕs-THĚT-ĭk] {anestésico} 1. Agent that relieves pain by blocking nerve sensations. 2. Agent that causes loss of feeling or sensation. 3. Drug that causes temporary loss of ability to perceive sensations at a conscious level.

aneurysm [ĂN-yū-rĭzm] {aneurisma} Abnormal widening of an artery wall that bursts and releases blood; ballooning of the artery wall caused by weakness in the wall.

angina [ĂN-jī-nă, ăn-JĪ-nă] {angina} Angina pectoris.

angina pectoris [PĚK-tōr-ĭs, pĕk-TŌR-ĭs] {angina de pecho} Chest pain, usually caused by a lowered oxygen or blood supply to the heart.

angiocardiography [ăn-jē-ō-kăr-dē-ŎG-ră-fē] Viewing of the heart and its major blood vessels by x-ray after injection of a contrast medium.

angiography [ăn-jē-ŎG-ră-fē] Viewing of the heart's major blood vessels by x-ray after injection of a contrast medium.

angioplasty [ĂN-jē-ō-plăs-tē] {angioplastia} Opening of a blocked blood vessel, as by balloon dilation.

angioscopy [ăn-jē-ŎS-kō-pē] {angioscopia} Viewing of the interior of a blood vessel using a fiberoptic catheter inserted or threaded into the vessel.

angiotensin [ăn-jē-ō-TĚN-sĭn] **converting enzyme (ACE) inhibitor** Medication used for heart failure and other cardiovascular problems; acts by dilating arteries to lower blood pressure and makes the heart pump easier.

anisocytosis [ăn-Ī-sō-sī-TŌ-sĭs] {anisocitosis} Condition with abnormal variation in the size of red blood cells.

ankle [ĂNG-kl] {tobillo} Hinged area between the lower leg bones and the bones of the foot.

ankyloglossia [ĂNG-kĭ-lō-GLŎS-ē-ă] {anquiloglosia} Condition of the tongue being partially or completely attached to the bottom of the mouth.

ankylosis [ĂNG-kĭ-LŌ-sĭs] {anquilosis} Stiffening of a joint, especially as a result of disease.

anorchism [ăn-ŌR-kĭzm], **anorchia** [-kē-ă] {anorquia} Congenital absence of one or both testicles.

anorexia nervosa [ăn-ō-RĔK-sē-ă nĕr-VŌ-să] Eating disorder in which the patient refuses to eat enough to sustain a minimum weight; eating disorder with extreme weight loss.

anovulation [ăn-ŏv-yū-LĀ-shŭn] Lack of ovulation.

antacid [ănt-ĂS-ĭd] {antiácido} Drug that lessens or neutralizes acidity.

anteflexion [ăn-tē-FLĚK-shŭn] Bending forward, as of the uterus.

anterior [ăn-TĒR-ē-ōr] At or toward the front (of the body).

anthracosis [ăn-thră-KŌ-sĭs] {antracosis} Lung disease caused by long-term inhalation of coal dust; black lung disease.

antianginal [ăn-tē-ĂN-jĭ-năl] Agent used to relieve or prevent attacks of angina.

antianxiety agent Tranquilizer.

antiarrhythmic [ăn-tē-ā-RĬTH-mĭk] Agent used to help normalize cardiac rhythm.

antibacterial [ĂN-tē-băk-TĒR-ē-ăl] {antibacteriano} Agent that kills or slows the growth of bacteria.

antibiotic [ĂN-tē-bī-ŎT-ĭk] {antibiótico} Agent or drug that kills or slows the growth of harmful microorganisms.

antibody [ĂN-tē-bŏd-ē] {anticuerpo} Specialized protein that fights disease; also called immunoglobulin.

anticlotting *See* anticoagulant.

anticoagulant [ĂN-tē-kō-ĂG-yū-lĕnt] Agent that prevents the formation of dangerous blood clots.

anticonvulsant [ĂN-tē-kŏn-VŬL-sănt] Agent that lessens or prevents convulsions.

antidepressant [ĂN-tē-dē-PRĔS-ĕnt] Agent that controls the effects of clinical depression.

antidiabetic [ĂN-tē-dī-ă-BĔT-ĭk] {antidiabético} Drug that lowers blood sugar or increases insulin sensitivity.

antidiarrheal [ăn-tē-dī-ă-RĒ-ăl] Agent that controls loose, watery stools.

antidiuretic [ĂN-tē-dī-yū-RĔT-ĭk] **hormone (ADH)** Posterior pituitary hormone that increases water reabsorption.

antidote [ĂN-tē-dōt] {antidoto} Substance able to cancel out unwanted effects of another substance.

antiemetic [ĂN-tē-ĕ-MĔT-ĭk] Agent that prevents vomiting.

antifungal [ĂN-tē-FŬNG-ăl] {antifúngico} Agent or drug that kills or slows the growth of fungi.

antigen [ĂN-tĭ-jĕn] {antígeno} Any substance that can provoke an immune response.

antiglobulin [ĂN-tē-GLŎB-yū-lĭn] **test** Test for antibodies on red blood cells.

antihistamine [ĂN-tē-HĬS-tă-mēn] {antihistamina} 1. Agent that controls allergic reactions by blocking the effectiveness of histamines in the body. 2. Drug that reduces the action of histamines; used in allergy treatments.

antihyperglycemic [ĂN-tē-HĪ-pĕr-glī-SĒ-mĭk] Agent that lowers blood glucose.

antihypertensive Agent that helps control high blood pressure.

antihypoglycemic [ĂN-tē-HĪ-pō-glī-SĒ-mĭk] Agent that raises blood glucose.

anti-infective [ĂN-tē-ĭn-FĔK-tĭv] *See* antibiotic.

anti-inflammatory (corticosteroids) Agent that reduces inflammation.

anti-inflammatory Agent that relieves the symptoms of inflammations.

antipruritic [ĂN-tē-prū-RĬT-ĭk] Agent that controls itching.

antipsychotic [ĂN-tē-sī-KŎT-ĭk] **agent** Agent that relieves agitation and some psychoses.

antiseptic Agent that kills or slows the growth of microorganisms.

antispasmodic [ăn-tē-spăz-MŎD-ĭk] Pharmacological agent that relieves spasms; also decreases frequency of urination; agent that controls intestinal tract spasms.

antitoxin [ăn-tē-TŎK-sĭn] {antitoxina} Antibodies directed against a particular disease or poison.

antitubercular [ăn-tē-tū-BĔR-kyū-lăr] Drug that stops the spread of tuberculosis.

antitussives [ăn-tē-TŬS-sĭvs] Agents that control coughing.

antiviral [ăn-tē-VĪ-răl] Drug that stops or slows the spread of a virus.

anuresis [ăn-yū-RĒ-sĭs] Abnormal retention of urine.

anuria [ăn-YŪ-rē-ă] {anuria} Lack of urine formation.

anus [Ā-nŭs] {ano} Place at which feces exit the body.

anxiety [ănks-ZĪ-ĕ-tē] Abnormal worry.

aorta [ā-OR-tă] {aorta} Largest artery of the body; artery through which blood exits the heart.

aortic regurgitation [rē-GŬR-jĭ-TĀ-shŭn] **or reflux** [RĒ-flŭks] Backward flow or leakage of blood through a faulty aortic valve.

aortic stenosis [stĕ-NŌ-sĭs] Narrowing of the aorta.

aortic valve Valve between the aorta and the left ventricle.

aortography [ā-ōr-TŎG-ră-fē] Viewing of the aorta by x-ray after injection of a contrast medium.

apex [Ā-pĕks] {apex} Topmost section of the lung.

Apgar [ĂP-găr] **score** A rating of a newborn's Activity, Pulse, Grimace, Appearance, Respiration.

aphagia [ă-FĀ-jē-ă] {afagia} Inability to swallow.

aphakia [ă-FĀ-kē-ă] {afaquia} Absence of a lens.

aphasia [ă-FĀ-zē-ă] {afasia} Loss of speech.

apnea [ĂP-nē-ă] {apnea} Cessation of breathing.

apocrine [ĂP-ō-krĭn] **glands** Glands that appear during and after puberty and secrete sweat, as from the armpits.

apoptosis [ā-pŏp-TŌ-sĭs] Normal death of cells.

appendage [ă-PĔN-dĭj] {apéndice} Any body part (inside or outside) either subordinate to a larger part or having no specific central function.

appendectomy [ăp-pĕn-DĔK-tō-mē] Removal of the appendix.

appendicitis [ă-pĕn-dĭ-SĪ-tĭs] Inflammation of the appendix.

appendix [ă-PĔN-dĭks] {apéndice} Wormlike appendage to the cecum.

apraxia [ă-PRĂK-sē-ă] {apraxia} Inability to properly use familiar objects.

arachnoid [ă-RĂK-nŏyd] {aracnoideo} Middle layer of meninges.

areola [ă-RĒ-ō-lă] {aréola} Darkish area surrounding the nipple on a breast.

arrhythmia [ă-RĬTH-mē-ă] {arritmia} Irregularity in the rhythm of the heartbeat.

arterial [ăr-TĒR-ē-ăl] **blood gases** Laboratory test that measures the levels of oxygen and carbon dioxide in arterial blood.

arteriography [ăr-tēr-ē-ŎG-ră-fē] Viewing of a specific artery by x-ray after injection of a contrast medium.

arteriole [ăr-TĒ-rē-ōl] {arteriola} A tiny artery connecting to a capillary.

arteriosclerosis [ăr-TĒR-ē-ō-sklĕr-Ō-sĭs] {arteriosclerosis} Hardening of the arteries.

arteriotomy [ăr-tēr-ē-ŎT-ō-mē] Surgical incision into an artery, especially to remove a clot.

arteritis [ăr-tēr-Ī-tĭs] {arteritis} Inflammation of an artery or arteries.

artery [ĂR-tēr-ē] {arteria} A thick-walled blood vessel that, in systemic circulation, carries oxygenated blood away from the heart.

arthralgia [ăr-THRĂL-jē-ă] {artralgia} Severe joint pain.

arthritis [ăr-THRĪ-tĭs] {artritis} Any of various conditions involving joint inflammation.

arthrocentesis [ĂR-thrō-sĕn-TĔ-sĭs] {artrocentesis} Removal of fluid from a joint with use of a puncture needle.

arthrodesis [ăr-thrō-DĒ-sĭs] Surgical fusion of a joint to stiffen it.

arthrography [ăr-THRŎG-ră-fē] Radiography of a joint.

arthroplasty [ĂR-thrō-plăs-tē] Surgical replacement or repair of a joint.

arthroscopy [ăr-THRŎS-kō-pē] Examination with an instrument that explores the interior of a joint.

articular [ăr-TĬK-yū-lăr] **cartilage** Cartilage at a joint.

articulation [ăr-tĭk-yū-LĀ-shŭn] {articulación} Point at which two bones join together to allow movement.

asbestosis [ăs-bĕs-TŌ-sĭs] {asbestosis} Lung disorder caused by long-term inhalation of asbestos (as in construction work).

ascites [ă-SĪ-tēs] {ascitis} Fluid buildup in the abdominal and peritoneal cavities.

aseptic [ā-SĔP-tĭk] Germ-free.

aspermia [ā-SPĔR-mē-ă] {aspermia} Inability to produce sperm.

aspiration [ăs-pĭ-RĀ-shŭn] {aspiración} Biopsy in which fluid is withdrawn through a needle by suction.

asthenopia [ăs-thĕ-NŌ-pē-ă] {astenopía} Weakness of the ocular or ciliary muscles that causes the eyes to tire easily.

asthma [ĂZ-mă] {asma} Chronic condition with obstruction or narrowing of the bronchial airways.

astigmatism [ā-STĬG-mă-tĭzm] {astigmatismo} Distortion of sight because of lack of focus of light rays at one point on the retina.

astringent [ăs-TRĬN-jĕnt] Agent that removes excess oils and impurities from the surface of skin.

astrocyte, astroglia [ĂS-trō-sīt, ăs-TRŎG-lē-ă] {astrocito, astroglia} A type of neuroglia that maintains nutrient and chemical levels in neurons.

astrocytoma [ĂS-trō-sī-TŌ-mă] {astrocitoma} Type of glioma formed from astrocytes.

asystole [ā-SĬS-tō-lē] {asistolia} Cardiac arrest.

ataractic [ă-tă-RĂK-tĭk] Tranquilizer.

ataxia [ā-TĂK-sē-ă] {ataxia} Condition with uncoordinated voluntary muscular movement, usually resulting from disorders of the cerebellum or spinal cord.

atelectasis [ăt-ĕ-LĔK-tă-sĭs] {atelectasia} Collapse of a lung or part of a lung.

atherectomy [ăth-ĕ-RĔK-tō-mē] Surgical removal of an atheroma.

atheroma [ăth-ĕr-Ō-mă] {ateroma} A fatty deposit (plaque) in the wall of an artery.

atherosclerosis [ĂTH-ĕr-ō-sklĕr-ō-sĭs] {aterosclerosis} Hardening of the arteries caused by the buildup of atheromas.

atlas [ĂT-lăs] {atlas} First cervical vertebra.

atresia [ă-TRĒ-zhē-ă] {atresia} Abnormal narrowing, as of the ureters or urethra.

atrial fibrillation [fĭ-brĭ-LĀ-shŭn] An irregular, usually rapid, heartbeat caused by overstimulation of the AV node.

atrioventricular [Ā-trē-ō-věn-TRĬK-yū-lăr] **bundle** Bundle of fibers in the interventricular septum that transfer charges in the heart's conduction system; also called bundle of His.

atrioventricular block Heart block; partial or complete blockage of the electrical impulses from the atrioventricular node to the ventricles.

atrioventricular (AV) node Specialized part of the interatrial septum that sends a charge to the bundle of His.

atrioventricular valve One of two valves that control blood flow between the atria and ventricles.

atrium (*pl.*, **atria**) [Ā-trē-ŭm (Ā-trē-ă)] {atrium} Either of the two upper chambers of the heart.

atrophy [ĂT-rō-fē] {atrofia} Wasting away of tissue, organs, and cells, usually as a result of disease or loss of blood supply.

audiogram [ĂW-dē-ō-grăm] {audiograma} Graph that plots the acoustic frequencies being tested.

audiologist [ăw-dē-ŎL-ō-jĭst] {audiólogo} Specialist in evaluating hearing function.

audiometry [ăw-dē-ŎM-ě-trē] {audiometría} Measurement of acoustic frequencies using an audiometer.

auditory ossicles [ĂW-dĭ-tōr-ē ŎS-ĭ-klz] Three specially shaped bones in the middle ear that anchor the eardrum to the tympanic cavity and that transmit vibrations to the inner ear.

aura [ĂW-ră] {aura} Group of symptoms that precede a seizure.

auricle [ĂW-rĭ-kl] {auricular} Funnel-like structure leading from the external ear to the external auditory meatus; also called pinna.

auscultation [ăws-kŭl-TĀ-shŭn] {auscultación} Process of listening to body sounds via a stethoscope.

autism [ĂW-tĭzm] Mental disorder usually beginning in early childhood with morbid self-absorption and difficulty in perceiving reality.

autograft [ĂW-tō-grăft] {autoinjerto} Skin graft using skin from one's own body.

autoimmune [ăw-tō-ĭ-MYŪN] **disease** Any of a number of diseases, such as rheumatoid arthritis, lupus, and scleroderma, caused by an autoimmune response.

autoimmune response Overactivity in the immune system against oneself causing destruction of one's own healthy cells.

autonomic [ăw-tō-NŎM-ĭk] **nervous system** Part of the peripheral nervous system that carries impulses from the central nervous system to glands, smooth muscles, cardiac muscle, and various membranes.

axis [ĂK-sĭs] {axis} Second cervical vertebra.

axon [ĂK-sŏn] {axon} Part of a nerve cell that conducts nerve impulses away from the cell body.

ayurveda [ī-yūr-VĒ-dă] Holistic alternative medicine system originally from India.

azoospermia [ā-zō-ō-SPĚR-mē-ă] {azoospermia} Semen without living sperm.

azotemia [ăz-ō-TĒ-mē-ă] {azoemia} *See* uremia.

B

Babinski's [bă-BĬN-skēs] **reflex** Reflex on the plantar surface of the foot.

bacilli (*sing.*, **bacillus**) [bă-SĬL-Ī (bă-SĬL-ŭs)] {bacillo} A type of bacteria.

bacterial endocarditis Bacterial inflammation of the inner lining of the heart.

bacterial meningitis [měn-ĭn-JĪ-tĭs] Meningitis caused by a bacteria; pyrogenic meningitis.

balanitis [băl-ă-NĪ-tĭs] {balanitis} Inflammation of the glans penis.

balloon catheter dilation Insertion of a balloon catheter into a blood vessel to open the passage so blood can flow freely.

balloon valvuloplasty [VĂL-vyū-lō-PLĂS-tē] Procedure that uses a balloon catheter to open narrowed orifices in cardiac valves.

barium [BĂ-rē-ŭm] Contrast medium that shows up as white on an x-ray.

Bartholin's [BĂR-thō-lěnz] **gland** One of two glands on either side of the vagina that secrete fluid into the vagina.

basal cell carcinoma [BĀ-săl sěl kăr-sĭn-Ō-mă] Slow-growing cancer of the basal cells of the epidermis, usually a result of sun damage.

basal ganglia [BĀ-săl GĂNG-glē-ă] Large masses of gray matter within the cerebrum.

base [bās] {base} Bottom section of the lung.

basophil [BĀ-sō-fĭl] {basófilo} Leukocyte containing heparin and histamine.

basophilia [bā-sō-FĬL-ē-ă] {basofilia} Condition with an increased number of basophils in the blood.

behavior modification Substitution of a beneficial behavior pattern for a destructive behavior pattern.

behavior therapy Therapy that includes the use of behavior modification.

Bell's palsy [PĂWL-zē] Paralysis of one side of the face; usually temporary.

benign [bě-NĬN] Encapsulated; not malignant.

beta [BĀ-tă] **blocker** Agent that lowers blood pressure by reducing contraction strength of the heart muscle; slows heartbeat.

beta [BĀ-tă] **cells** Specialized cells that produce insulin in the pancreas.

beta rays Type of radioactive particles that have a medium ability to penetrate the body.

bicuspid [bī-KŬS-pĭd] Fourth and fifth tooth from the median of the jawline with two cusps.

bicuspid [bī-KŬS-pĭd] **valve** Atrioventricular valve on the left side of the heart.

bile [bīl] {bilis} Yellowish-brown to greenish fluid secreted by the liver and stored in the gallbladder; aids in fat digestion.

bilirubin [bĭl-ĭ-RŪ-bĭn] {bilirubina} Substance produced in the liver; elevated levels may indicate liver disease or hepatitis when found in urine; pigment contained in bile.

Billroth's [BĬLL-rŏths] **I** Excision of the pylorus.

Billroth's II Resection of the pylorus with the stomach.

biochemistry panel Common group of automated tests run on one blood sample.

bioelectromagnetic-based therapy Type of energy therapy using electromagnetic fields.

biofeedback [bī-ō-FĒD-băk] Method of measuring physical responses to emotional issues.

biofield therapy Type of energy therapy that attempts to affect energy fields.

biological therapy Treatment of cancer with agents from the body that increase immune response.

biologically-based therapy The use of foods, herbs, vitamins, and minerals to heal or prevent disease.

biopsy [BĪ-ŏp-sē] {biopsia} Excision of tissue for microscopic examination.

bipolar [bī-PŌ-lăr] **disorder** Condition with drastic mood swings over a period of time.

birth control pills or implants Medication that controls the flow of hormones to block ovulation.

birthmark Lesion (especially a hemangioma) visible at or soon after birth; nevus.

B lymphocytes [LĬM-fō-sīts], **B cells** Lymphocyte that manufactures antibodies.

black lung *See* anthracosis.

blackhead {punto negro} *See* comedo.

bladder [BLĂD-ĕr] {vejiga} Organ where urine collects before being excreted from the body.

bladder cancer Malignancy of the bladder.

blepharitis [blĕf-ă-RĪ-tĭs] {blefaritis} Inflammation of the eyelid.

blepharochalasis [blĕf-ă-rō-KĂL-ă-sĭs] Loss of elasticity of the eyelid.

blepharoplasty [BLĔF-ă-rō-plăst-ē] Surgical repair of the eyelid.

blepharoptosis [blĕf-ă-RŎP-tō-sĭs] Drooping of the eyelid.

blepharospasm [BLĔF-ă-rō-spăzm] Involuntary eyelid movement; excessive blinking.

blindness {ceguera} Loss or absence of vision.

blood [blŭd] {sangre} Essential fluid made up of plasma and other elements that circulates throughout the body (arteries, veins, capillaries, and heart); delivers nutrients to and removes waste from the body's cells.

blood chemistry Test of plasma for presence of a particular substance such as glucose.

blood culture Test of a blood specimen in a culture medium to observe for particular microorganisms.

blood indices [IN-di-sez] Measurement of the characteristics of red blood cells.

blood pressure Measure of the force of blood surging against the walls of the arteries.

blood sugar, blood glucose Test for glucose in blood.

blood [blŭd] **system** Body system that includes blood and all its component parts.

blood types or groups Classification of blood according to its antigen and antibody qualities.

blood vessel Any of the tubular passageways in the cardiovascular system through which blood travels.

body {cuerpo} Middle portion of the uterus; middle section of the stomach.

body-based therapy *See* manipulative therapy.

bone {hueso} Hard connective tissue that forms the skeleton of the body.

bone grafting Transplantation of bone from one site to another.

bone head Upper, rounded end of a bone.

bone marrow biopsy Extraction of bone marrow, by means of a needle, for observation.

bone marrow transplant Injection of donor bone marrow into a patient whose diseased cells have been killed through radiation and chemotherapy.

bone phagocyte [FĂG-ō-sīt] Bone cell that ingests dead bone and bone debris.

bone scan Radiographic or nuclear medicine image of a bone.

bony necrosis [BŌN-ē nĕ-KRŌ-sĭs] Death of portions of bone.

bowel [bŏw-l] {intestino} Intestine.

Bowman's capsule Capsule surrounding a glomerulus and serving as a collection site for urine.

braces [BRĀ-sĕz] Appliances that straighten teeth slowly.

brachytherapy [brāk-ē-THĀR-ă-pē] Implanting of radioactive elements directly into a tumor or tissue.

bradycardia [brād-ē-KĂR-dē-ă] {bradicardia} Heart rate of fewer than 60 beats per minute.

bradypnea [brād-ĭp-NĒ-ă] {bradipnea} Abnormally slow breathing.

brain [brān] {cerebro} Body organ responsible for controlling the body's functions and interactions with outside stimuli.

brain contusion [kŏn-TŪ-shŭn] Bruising of the surface of the brain without penetration.

brainstem {tronco encefálico} One of the four major divisions of the brain; division that controls certain heart, lung, and visual functions.

brand name *See* trade name.

breech [brēch] Birth canal position with feet or buttocks first.

bridge [brĭdj] Partial that is attached to other teeth.

Bright's disease Inflammation of the glomeruli that can result in kidney failure.

bronchial alveolar lavage [BRŎNG-kē-ăl ăl-VĒ-ō-lăr lă-VĂZH] Retrieval of fluid for examination through a bronchoscope.

bronchial brushing Retrieval of material for biopsy by insertion of a brush through a bronchoscope.

bronchiole [BRŎNG-kē-ōl] {bronquiolo} Fine subdivision of the bronchi made of smooth muscle and elastic fibers.

bronchitis [brŏng-KĪ-tĭs] {bronquitis} Inflammation of the bronchi.

bronchodilators [brŏng-kō-dī-LĀ-tōrz] Agents that dilate the walls of the bronchi.

bronchography [brŏng-KŎG-ră-fē] {broncografía} Radiological picture of the trachea and bronchi.

bronchoplasty [BRŎNG-kō-plăs-tē] Surgical repair of a bronchus.

bronchoscope [BRŎNG-kō-skōp] {broncoscopio} Device used to examine airways.

bronchospasm [BRŎNG-kō-spăzm] {broncoespasmo} Sudden contraction in the bronchi that causes coughing.

bronchus (*pl.,* **bronchi**) [BRŎNG-kŭs (BRŎNG-kī)] {bronquio} One of the two airways from the trachea to the lungs.

bruit [brū-Ē] {ruido} Sound or murmur, especially an abnormal heart sound heard on auscultation, especially of the carotid artery.

brush biopsy The passing of a catheter with bristles into the ureter to gather cells for examination.

buccally [BŪK-ăl-lē] Inside the cheek.

bulbourethral [BŬL-bō-yū-RĒ-thrăl] **gland** *See* Cowper's gland.

bulimia [bū-LĒM-ē-ă] Eating disorder with bingeing and purging.

bulimia nervosa [BŪ-lēm-ē-ă, BŪ-lĭm-ē-ă nĕr-VŌ-să] Eating disorder with extreme overeating followed by purging.

bulla (*pl.*, **bullae**) [BŬL-ă (BŬL-ī)] {bulla} Bubble-like blister on the surface of the skin.

bundle of His [hĭz, hĭs] *See* atrioventricular bundle.

bunion [BŬN-yŭn] {bunio} An inflamed bursa at the foot joint, between the big toe and the first metatarsal bone.

bunionectomy [bŭn-yŭn-ĔK-tō-mē] {bunionectomía} Removal of a bunion.

burn {quemadura} Damage to the skin caused by exposure to heat, chemicals, electricity, radiation, or other skin irritants; bubble-like blister on the surface of the skin caused by exposure to heat, chemicals, electricity, radiation, or other skin irritants.

bursa (*pl.*, **bursae**) [BŬR-să (BŬR-sē)] {bursa} Sac lined with a synovial membrane that fills the spaces between tendons and joints.

bursectomy [bŭr-SĔK-tō-mē] {bursectomía} Removal of a bursa.

bursitis [bŭr-SĪ-tĭs] {bursitis} Inflammation of a bursa.

bypass A structure (usually a vein graft) that creates a new passage for blood to flow from one artery to another artery or part of an artery; used to create a detour around blockages in arteries.

C

calcaneus [kăl-KĀ-nē-ŭs] {calcáneo} Heel bone.

calcar [KĂL-kăr] {calcar} Spur.

calcitonin [kăl-sĭ-TŌ-nĭn] {calcitonia} Hormone secreted by the thyroid gland and other endocrine glands; helps control blood calcium levels.

calcium [KĂL-sē-ŭm] {calcio} Mineral important in the formation of bone.

calcium channel blocker Medication that lessens the ability of calcium ions to enter heart and blood vessel muscle cells; used to lower blood pressure and normalize some arrhythmias.

calices, calyces (*sing.*, **calix, calyx**) [KĂL-ĭ-sēz (KĀ-lĭks)] {calices, *sing.*, cáliz} Cup-shaped structures in the renal pelvis for the collection of urine.

callus [KĂL-ŭs] {callo} Mass of hard skin that forms as a cover over broken skin on certain areas of the body, especially the feet and hands.

CAM Complementary and alternative medicine.

cancellous [KĂN-sĕ-lŭs] **bone** {canceloso} Spongy bone with a latticelike structure.

candidiasis [kăn-dĭ-DĪ-ă-sĭs] {candidiasis} Yeastlike fungus on the skin, caused by Candida; characterized by pruritus, white exudate, peeling, and easy bleeding; examples are thrush and diaper rash.

canine [KĀ-nīn] Cuspid.

capillary [KĂP-ĭ-lăr-ē] {capilar} A tiny blood vessel that forms the exchange point between the arterial and venous vessels.

carbon dioxide (CO₂) {dióxido de carbono} Waste material transported in the venous blood.

carbuncle [KĂR-bŭng-kl] {carbunco} Infected area of the skin producing pus and usually accompanied by fever.

carcinoma in situ [kăr-sĭ-NŌ-mă ĭn SĪ-tū] Localized malignancy that has not spread; contained at a site without spreading.

cardiac arrest Sudden stopping of the heart; also called asystole.

cardiac catheterization [kăth-ĕ-tĕr-ĭ-ZĀ-shŭn] Process of passing a thin catheter through an artery or vein to the heart to take blood samples, inject a contrast medium, or measure various pressures.

cardiac cycle Repeated contraction and relaxation of the heart as it circulates blood within itself and pumps it out to the rest of the body or the lungs.

cardiac enzyme tests/studies Blood tests for determining levels of enzymes during a myocardial infarction; serum enzyme tests.

cardiac MRI Viewing of the heart by magnetic resonance imaging.

cardiac [KĂR-dē-ăk] **muscle** Striated involuntary muscle of the heart.

cardiac scan Process of viewing the heart muscle at work by scanning the heart of a patient into whom a radioactive substance has been injected.

cardiac tamponade [tăm-pō-NĂD] Compression of the heart caused by fluid accumulation in the pericardial sac.

cardiomyopathy [KĂR-dē-ō-mī-ŎP-ă-thē] {cardiomiopatía} Disease of the heart muscle.

cardiopulmonary [KĂR-dē-ō-PŬL-mō-nĕr-ē] **bypass** Procedure used during surgery to divert blood flow to and from the heart through a heart-lung machine and back into circulation.

cardiotonic [KĂR-dē-ō-TŎN-ĭk] Medication for congestive heart failure; increases the force of contractions of the myocardium.

cardiovascular [KĂR-dē-ō-VĂS-kyū-lăr] Relating to or affecting the heart and blood vessels.

cardiovascular [KĂR-dē-ō-VĂS-kyū-lăr] **system** Body system that includes the heart and blood vessels; circulatory system.

caries [KĂR-ēz] Tooth decay.

carotid [kă-RŎT-ĭd] **artery** Artery that transports oxygenated blood to the head and neck.

carpal [KĂR-păl] **tunnel syndrome** Pain and paresthesia in the hand due to repetitive motion injury of the median nerve.

carpus, carpal [KĂR-pŭs, KĂR-păl] **bone** Wrist; wrist bone.

cartilage [KĂR-tĭ-lăj] {cartílago} Flexible connective tissue found in joints, fetal skeleton, and the lining of various parts of the body.

cartilaginous [kăr-tĭ-LĂJ-ĭ-nŭs] **disk** Thick, circular mass of cartilage between the vertebrae of the spinal column.

casting {colado} Forming of a cast in a mold; placing of fiberglass or plaster over a body part to prevent its movement.

castration [kăs-TRĀ-shŭn] {castración} Removal of the testicles.

casts Materials formed in urine when protein accumulates; may indicate renal disease.

CAT (computerized axial tomography) scan Scan that shows images as detailed slices of a body part or organ.

catalepsy [KĂT-ă-lĕp-sē] Trancelike state with holding of one pose for a long period of time.

cataract [KĂT-ă-răkt] {catarata} Cloudiness of the lens of the eye.

catecholamines [kăt-ĕ-KŌL-ă-mēnz] {catecolaminas} Hormones, such as epinephrine, released in response to stress.

cathartic [kă-THĂR-tĭk] Agent that induces vomiting; also a strong laxative for emptying the bowels.

cauterization [kăw-tĕr-ĭ-ZĀ-shŭn] {cauterización} Removal or destruction of tissue using chemicals or devices, such as laser-guided equipment.

cauterize [KĂW-tĕr-īz] {cauterizar} To apply heat to an area to cause coagulation and stop bleeding.

cauterizing [KĂW-tĕr-īz-ĭng] Destroying tissue by burning.

cavity [KĂV-ĭ-tē] Tooth decay.

cecum [SĒ-kŭm] {ciego} Pouch at the top of the large intestine connected to the bottom of the ileum.

cell [sĕl] Smallest unit of a living structure.

cell body Part of a nerve cell that has branches or fibers that reach out to send or receive impulses.

cell-mediated immunity Resistance to disease mediated by T cells.

cellulitis [sĕl-yū-LĪ-tĭs] {celulitis} Severe inflammation of the dermis and subcutaneous portions of the skin, usually caused by an infection that enters the skin through an opening, such as a wound; characterized by local heat, redness, pain, and swelling.

cementum [sē-MĔN-tŭm] Bony material surrounding the root of the tooth.

central incisor Tooth on either side of the center jawline.

central nervous system The brain and spinal cord.

cerebellitis [sĕr-ĕ-bĕl-Ī-tĭs] {cerebelitis} Inflammation of the cerebellum.

cerebellum [sĕr-ĕ-BĔL-ŭm] One of the four major divisions of the brain; division that coordinates musculoskeletal movement.

cerebral angiogram X-ray of the brain's blood vessels after a dye is injected.

cerebral cortex [SĔR-ĕ-brăl KŌR-tĕks] Outer portion of the cerebrum.

cerebral infarction [SĔR-ĕ-brăl ĭn-FĂRK-shŭn] *See* cerebrovascular accident.

cerebral palsy [SĔR-ĕ-brăl PĂWL-zē] Congenital disease caused by damage to the cerebrum during gestation or birth and resulting in lack of motor coordination.

cerebrospinal [SĔR-ē-brō-spī-năl] **fluid (CSF)** Watery fluid that flows throughout the brain and around the spinal cord.

cerebrovascular [SĔR-ē-brō-VĂS-kyū-lăr] **accident (CVA)** Neurological incident caused by disruption in the normal blood supply to the brain; stroke.

cerebrum [SĔR-ĕ-brŭm, sĕ-RĒ-brŭm] {cerebrum} One of the four major divisions of the brain; division involved with emotions, memory, conscious thought, moral behavior, sensory interpretations, and certain bodily movement.

cerumenous [sĕ-RŪ-mĭn-ŭs] **glands** Glands that secrete a waxy substance on the surface of the ear.

cervical [SĔR-vĭ-kl] **vertebrae** Seven vertebrae of the spinal column located in the neck.

cervicitis [sĕr-vĭ-SĪ-tĭs] Inflammation of the cervix.

cervix [SĔR-vĭks] {cervix} Protective part of uterus, located at the bottom and protruding through the vaginal wall; contains glands that secrete fluid into the vagina.

cesarean [sĕ-ZĀ-rē-ăn] **section** Surgical removal of the fetus through the abdomen.

chalazion [kă-LĀ-zē-ŏn] {chalazión} Nodular inflammation that usually forms on the eyelid.

chancroids [SHĂNG-krŏyds] Bacterial infection that can be sexually transmitted; results in sores on the penis, urethra, or anus.

cheeks {carrillos} Walls of the oral cavity.

cheilitis [kī-LĪ-tĭs] {queilitis} Inflammation of the lips.

cheiloplasty [KĪ-lō-plăs-tē] Repair of the lips.

chemistry profile *See* blood chemistry.

chemotherapy [KĒ-mō-THĂR-ă-pē] Treatment of cancer that uses drugs or chemicals to destroy malignant cells.

cherry angioma [ăn-jē-Ō-mă] A dome-shaped vascular angioma lesion that usually occurs in the elderly.

Cheyne-Stokes respiration [chān stōks rĕs-pĭ-RĀ-shŭn] Irregular breathing pattern with a period of apnea followed by deep, labored breathing that becomes shallow, then apneic.

chiropractic [kī-rō-PRĂK-tĭk] Therapy based on alignment of the body (particularly the spine).

chiropractor [kī-rō-PRĂK-tōr] {quiropráctico} Health care professional who works to align the spinal column so as to treat certain ailments.

chlamydia [klă-MĬD-ē-ă] {clamidia} Sexually transmitted bacterial infection affecting various parts of the male or female reproductive systems; the bacterial agent itself.

chloasma [klō-ĂZ-mă] {cloasma} Group of fairly large, pigmented facial patches, often associated with pregnancy.

cholangiography [kō-lăn-jē-ŎG-ră-fē] X-ray of the bile ducts.

cholangitis [kō-lăn-JĪ-tĭs] {colangitis} Inflammation of the bile ducts.

cholecystectomy [KŌ-lē-sĭs-TĔK-tō-mē] Removal of the gallbladder.

cholecystitis [KŌ-lē-sĭs-TĪ-tĭs] {colecistitis} Inflammation of the gallbladder.

cholecystography [kō-lē-sĭs-TŎG-ră-fē] {colecistografía} X-ray of the gallbladder.

choledocholithotomy [kō-LĔD-ō-kō-lĭ-THŎT-ō-mē] Removal of stones from the common bile duct.

cholelithiasis [KŌ-lē-lĭ-THĪ-ă-sĭs] Gallstones in the gallbladder.

cholelithotomy [KŌ-lē-lĭ-THŎT-ō-mē] Removal of gallstones.

cholelithotripsy [kō-lē-LĬTH-ō-trĭp-sē] Breaking up or crushing of stones in the body, especially gallstones.

cholesteatoma [kō-lĕs-tē-ă-TŌ-mă] Fatty cyst within the middle ear.

cholesterol [kō-LĔS-tĕr-ōl] {colesterol} Fatty substance present in animal fats; cholesterol circulates in the bloodstream, sometimes causing arterial plaque to form.

chondromalacia [KŎN-drō-mă-LĀ-shē-ă] {condromalacia} Softening of cartilage.

chorion [KŌ-rē-ŏn] {corion} Outermost membrane of the sac surrounding the fetus during gestation.

choroid [KŌ-rŏyd] {coroides} Thin posterior membrane in the middle layer of the eye.

chronic bronchitis Recurring or long-lasting bouts of bronchitis.

chronic obstructive pulmonary disease Disease of the bronchial tubes or lungs with chronic obstruction.

chyme [kīm] {quimo} Semisolid mass of partially digested food and gastric juices that passes from the stomach to the small intestine.

cicatrix [SĬK-ă-trĭks] {cicatriz} Growth of fibrous tissue inside a wound that forms a scar; also, general term for scar.

cilia [SĬL-ē-ă] Hairlike extensions of a cell's surface that usually provide some protection by sweeping foreign particles away.

ciliary [SĬL-ē-ăr-ē] **body** Thick anterior membrane in the middle layer of the eye.

cineradiography [SĬN-ē-ră-dē-ŎG-ră-fē] Radiography of tissues or organs in motion.

circumcision [sĕr-kŭm-SĬZH-ŭn] {circuncisión} Removal of the foreskin.

cirrhosis [sĭr-RŌ-sĭs] {cirrosis} Liver disease, often caused by alcoholism.

clamps [klămps] Implement used to grasp a body part during surgery.

claudication [klăw-dĭ-KĀ-shŭn] {claudicación} Limping caused by inadequate blood supply during activity; usually subsides during rest.

clavicle [KLĂV-ĭ-kl] {clavicula} Curved bone of the shoulder that joins to the scapula; collar bone.

climacteric [klī-MĂK-tēr-ĭk] {climaterio} Period of hormonal changes just prior to menopause.

clitoris [KLĬT-ō-rĭs] {clítoris} Primary organ of female sexual stimulation, located at the top of the labia minora.

closed Performed without an incision.

closed fracture Fracture with no open skin wound.

coagulant [kō-ĂG-yū-lĕnt] Clotting agent.

coagulation [kō-ăg-yū-LĀ-shŭn] {coagulación} Changing of a liquid, especially blood, into a semi-solid.

coarctation [kō-ărk-TĀ-shŭn] **of the aorta** Abnormal narrowing of the aorta.

cobalt [KŌ-băwlt] Radioactive substance used in radiation therapy.

coccyx [KŎK-sĭks] {cóccix} Small bone consisting of four fused vertebrae at the end of the spinal column; tailbone.

cochlea [KŎK-lē-ă] {caracol} Snail-shaped structure in the inner ear that contains the organ of Corti.

coitus [KŌ-ĭ-tŭs] {coito} Sexual intercourse.

cold sore Eruption around the mouth or lips; herpes simplex virus Type 1.

colectomy [kō-LĔK-tō-mē] {colectomía} Removal of the colon.

colic [KŎL-ĭk] {cólico} Gastrointestinal distress, especially of infants.

colitis [kō-LĪ-tĭs] {colitis} Inflammation of the colon.

collagen [KŎL-lă-jĕn] {colágeno} Major protein substance that is tough and flexible and that forms connective tissue in the body.

Colles' [kōlz] **fracture** Fracture of the lower end of the radius.

colon [KŌ-lŏn] {colon} Major portion of the large intestine.

colonoscopy [kō-lŏn-ŎS-kō-pē] {colonoscopia} Examination of the colon using an endoscope.

colostomy [kō-LŎS-tō-mē] {colostomía} Creation of an opening from the colon into the abdominal wall.

colposcopy [kŏl-PŎS-kō-pē] Examination of the vagina with a colposcope.

coma [KŌ-mă] {coma} Abnormally deep sleep with little or no response to stimuli.

comedo (*pl.*, **comedos, comedones**) [KŎM-ē-dō, kō-MĒ-dō (KŎM-ē-dōz, kō-mē-DŌ-nĕz)] Open hair follicle filled with bacteria and sebum; common in acne; blackhead.

comminuted [KŎM-ĭ-nū-tĕd] **fracture** Fracture with shattered bones.

compact bone Hard bone with a tightly woven structure.

complementary medicine A nonconventional medical practice used in combination with conventional medicine.

complete blood count (CBC) Most common blood test for a number of factors.

complex fracture Fracture with part of the bone displaced.

complicated fracture Fracture involving extensive soft tissue injury.

compound fracture Fracture with an open skin wound; open fracture.

compression fracture Fracture of one or more vertebrae caused by compressing of the space between the vertebrae.

computerized (axial) tomography (CT or CAT) scan Radiographic imaging that produces cross-sectional images.

concussion [kŏn-KŪSH-ŭn] {concusión} Brain injury due to trauma.

condom [KŎN-dŏm] {condón} Contraceptive device consisting of a rubber or vinyl sheath placed over the penis or as a lining that covers the vaginal canal that blocks contact between the sperm and the female sex organs.

condom catheter [KĂTH-ĕ-tĕr] Disposable catheter for urinary sample collection or incontinence.

conduction system Part of the heart containing specialized tissue that sends charges through heart fibers, causing the heart to contract and relax at regular intervals.

conductivity [kŏn-dŭk-TĬV-ĭ-tē] {conductividad} Ability to transmit a signal.

condyle [KŎN-dīl] Rounded surface at the end of a bone.

condyloma [kŏn-dĭ-LŌ-mă] {condiloma} Growth on the external genitalia.

cones [kōnz] {conos} Specialized receptor cells in the retina that perceive color and bright light.

congenital [kŏn-JĔN-ĭ-tăl] **heart disease** Heart disease (usually a type of malformation) that exists at birth.

congestive [kŏn-JĔS-tĭv] **heart failure** Inability of the heart to pump enough blood out during the cardiac cycle; collection of fluid in the lungs results.

conization [kō-nĭ-ZĀ-shŭn] {conización} Removal of a cone-shaped section of the cervix for examination.

conjunctiva (*pl.*, **conjunctivae**) [kŏn-JŬNK-tĭ-vă (kŏn-JŬNK-tĭ-vē)] {conjuntiva} Mucous membrane lining the eyelid.

conjunctivitis [kŏn-jŭnk-tĭ-VĪ-tĭs] {conjuntivitis} Inflammation of the conjunctiva of the eyelid.

connective [kŏn-NĔK-tĭv] **tissue** Fibrous substance that forms the body's supportive framework.

constipation [kŏn-stĭ-PĀ-shŭn] {constipación} Difficult or infrequent defecation.

constriction [kŏn-STRĬK-shŭn] {constricción} Compression or narrowing caused by contraction, as of a vessel.

contact lenses Corrective lenses worn on the surface of the eye.

contraception [kŏn-tră-SĔP-shŭn] {anticoncepción} Method of controlling conception by blocking access or interrupting reproductive cycles; birth control.

contracture [kŏn-TRĂK-chŭr] Extreme resistance to the stretching of a muscle.

contraindicated [kŏn-tră-ĭn-dĭ-KĀ-tĕd] Inadvisable to use; said especially of a drug that might cause complications when used in combination with other drugs or when used on a patient with a particular set of symptoms.

convolutions [kŏn-vō-LŪ-shŭnz] {circunvolución} Folds in the cerebral cortex; gyri.

copulation [kŏp-yū-LĀ-shŭn] {copulación} Sexual intercourse.

cordotomy [kŏr-DŎT-ō-mē] {cordotomía} Removing part of the spinal cord.

corium [KŌ-rē-ŭm] {corium} *See* dermis.

corn {callo} Growth of hard skin, usually on the toes.

cornea [KŌR-nē-ă] {cornea} Transparent anterior section of the eyeball that bends light in a process called refraction.

coronal [KŌR-ō-năl] **plane** Imaginary line that divides the body into anterior and posterior positions.

coronary angioplasty *See* angioplasty.

coronary [KŌR-ō-năr-ē] **artery** Blood vessel that supplies oxygen-rich blood to the heart.

coronary artery disease Condition that reduces the flow of blood and nutrients through the arteries of the heart.

coronary bypass surgery *See* bypass.

corpus callosum [KŌR-pŭs kă-LŌ-sŭm] Bridge of nerve fibers that connects the two hemispheres of the cerebrum.

corpus luteum [KŌR-pŭs LU-te-um] Structure formed after the graafian follicle fills with a yellow substance that secretes estrogen and progesterone.

cortex [KŌR-tĕks] {corteza} Outer portion of the kidney.

corticosteroid [KŌR-tĭ-kō-STĔR-ŏyd] {corticosteroide} Agent with anti-inflammatory properties.

corticosteroids [KŌR-tĭ-kō-STĔR-ŏydz] Steroids produced by the adrenal cortex.

cortisol [KŌR-tĭ-sōl] {cortisol} Hydrocortisone.

cosmetic Designed to improve the appearance of an exterior body part.

Cowper's [KŎW-pĕrs] **gland** One of two glands below the prostate that secrete a fluid to lubricate the inside of the urethra.

crackles [KRĂK-ls] Popping sounds heard in lung collapse or other conditions; rales.

cranial [KRĀ-nē-ăl] **cavity** Space in the head that contains the brain.

cranial [KRĀ-nē-ăl] **nerves** Any of 12 pairs of nerves that carry impulses to and from the brain.

craniectomy [krā-nē-ĔK-tō-mē] {cranietomía} Removal of a part of the skull.

craniotomy [krā-nē-ŎT-ō-mē] {craneotomía} Incision into the skull.

cranium [KRĀ-nē-ŭm] {cráneo} Bony structure that the brain sits in.

creatine [KRĒ-ă-tēn] {creatina} Substance found in urine; elevated levels may indicate muscular dystrophy.

creatinine [krē-ĂT-ĭ-nēn] {creatinina} A component of creatine.

crepitation, crepitus [krĕp-ĭ-TĀ-shŭn, KRĔP-ĭ-tŭs] Noise made by rubbing together of bones.

crest {cresta} Bony ridge.

Crohn's [krōnz] **disease** Type of irritable bowel disease with no ulcers.

cross-sectional plane Imaginary line that intersects the body horizontally.

croup [krūp] {crup} Acute respiratory syndrome in children or infants accompanied by seal-like coughing.

crown [krŏwn] Part of the tooth projecting above the jawline.

crust {costar} Hard layer, especially one formed by dried pus, as in a scab.

cryogenic [krī-ō-JĔN-ĭk] Destroying tissue by freezing.

cryoretinopexy [krī-ō-rĕ-tĭn-nō-PĔKS-ē] Fixing of a torn retina using extreme cold.

cryosurgery [krī-ō-SĔR-jĕr-ē] {criocirugía} 1. Surgery that removes tissue by freezing it with liquid nitrogen. 2. Destruction by freezing.

cryptorchism [krĭp-TŌR-kĭzm] Birth defect with the failure of one or both of the testicles to descend into the scrotal sac.

CT (computed tomography) scan CAT scan.

culdocentesis [KŬL-dō-sĕn-tē-sĭs] Taking of a fluid sample from the base of the pelvic cavity to see if an ectopic pregnancy has ruptured.

culdoscopy [kŭl-DŎS-kō-pē] Examination of the pelvic cavity using an endoscope.

curettage [kyū-rĕ-TĂHZH] Removal of tissue from an area, such as a wound, by scraping.

curette [kyū-RĔT] Sharp instrument for scraping tissue.

Cushing's [KŬSH-ǐngs] **syndrome** Group of symptoms caused by overactivity of the adrenal glands.

cusp [kŭsp] Sharp-pointed tooth projection.

cuspid [KŬS-pǐd] Third tooth from the median of the jawline with a cusp.

cuticle [KYŪ-tǐ-kl] {cutícula} Thin band of epidermis that surrounds the edge of nails, except at the top.

cyanosis [sī-ă-NŌ-sǐs] {cianosis} Bluish or purplish coloration, as of the skin, caused by inadequate oxygenation of the blood.

cyst [sǐst] {quiste} Abnormal sac containing fluid.

cystectomy [sǐs-TĔK-tō-mē] {cistectomía} Surgical removal of the bladder.

cystic [SĬS-tǐk] Filled with fluid.

cystic fibrosis [SĬS-tǐk fī-BRŌ-sǐs] Disease that causes chronic airway obstruction and also affects the bronchial tubes.

cystitis [sǐs-TĪ-tǐs] {cistitis} Inflammation of the bladder.

cystocele [SĬS-tō-sēl] {cistocele} Hernia of the bladder.

cystolith [SĬS-tō-lǐth] {cistolito} Bladder stone.

cystopexy [SĬS-tō-pĕk-sē] Surgical fixing of the bladder to the abdominal wall.

cystoplasty [SĬS-tō-plăs-tē] Surgical repair of the bladder.

cystorrhaphy [sǐs-TŌR-ă-fē] {cistorrafia} Suturing of a damaged bladder.

cystoscope [SĬS-tō-skōp] {cistoscopio} Tubular instrument for examining the interior of the bladder.

cystoscopy [sǐs-TŎS-kō-pē] The insertion of a cystoscope to examine the bladder with light.

cytoplasm [SĪ-tō-plăzm] Outer portion of a cell surrounding the nucleus.

cytotoxic [sī-tō-TŎK-sǐk] **cell** T cell that helps in destruction of infected cells throughout the body.

D

dacryoadenitis [DĂK-rē-ō-ăd-ĕ-NĪ-tǐs] Inflammation of the lacrimal glands.

dacryocystectomy [dăk-rē-ō-sǐs-TĔK-tō-mē] Removal of a lacrimal sac.

dacryocystitis [DĂK-rē-ō-sǐs-TĪ-tǐs] Inflammation of a tear duct.

deafness Loss or absence of hearing.

debridement [dā-brēd-MŎN] Removal of dead tissue from a wound.

decibel [DĔS-ǐ-bĕl] {decibel} Measure of the intensity of sound.

deciduous [dĕ-SĬD-yū-ŭs] **teeth** Primary teeth.

decongestants [dē-kŏn-JĔST-ănts] Agents that relieve mucus congestion of the upper respiratory tract.

decubitus (*pl.*, **decubiti**) [dĕ-KYŪ-bǐ-tŭs (dĕ-KYŪ-bǐ-tī)] {decubiti} **ulcer** Chronic ulcer on skin over bony parts that are under constant pressure; pressure sore.

dedifferentiated [dē-DĬF-ĕr-ĕn-shē-Ā-tĕd] Lacking in normal orderly cell arrangement.

deep Away from the surface (of the body).

deep vein thrombosis [thrŏm-BŌ-sǐs] Formation of a thrombus (clot) in a deep vein, such as a femoral vein.

defecation [dĕ-fĕ-KĀ-shŭn] {defecación} Release of feces from the anus.

degenerative arthritis Arthritis with erosion of the cartilage.

deglutition [dē-glū-TĬSH-ŭn] {deglución} Swallowing.

deliriousness [dē-LĬR-ē-ŭs-nĕs] Mental confusion, often with hallucinations, usually having a physical cause such as a high fever.

delusional [dē-LŪ-zhŭn-ăl] Having false beliefs resulting from disordered thinking.

dementia [dē-MĔN-shē-ă] {demencia} 1. Deterioration in mental capacity, usually in the elderly. 2. Disorder, particularly in older adulthood, with multiple cognitive defects.

demyelination [dē-MĪ-ĕ-lǐ-NĀ-shŭn] {desmielinación} Destruction of myelin sheath, particularly in MS.

dendrite [DĔN-drīt] {dendrita} A thin branching extension of a nerve cell that conducts nerve impulses toward the cell body.

densitometer [dĕn-sǐ-TŎM-ĕ-tĕr] Device that measures bone density using light and x-rays.

dentin [DĔN-tǐn] Inner bony layer of the crown of a tooth.

dentist [DĔN-tǐst] Practitioner trained in dentistry.

dentures [DĔN-tyŭrs] Artificial replacement teeth.

depigmentation [dē-pǐg-mĕn-TĀ-shŭn] Loss of color of the skin.

depolarization [dē-pō-lă-rǐ-ZĀ-shŭn] {despolarización} Contracting state of the myocardial tissue in the heart's conduction system.

depression [dē-PRĔSH-ŭn] Disabling condition with a loss of interest and pleasure in almost all activities.

dermabrasion [dĕr-mă-BRĀ-zhŭn] {dermabrasión} Removal of wrinkles, scars, tattoos, and other marks by scraping with brushes or emery papers.

dermatitis [dĕr-mă-TĪ-tǐs] {dermatitis} Inflammation of the skin.

dermatochalasis [DĔR-mă-tō-kă-LĀ-sǐs] {dermatocalasia} Loss of elasticity of the eyelid.

dermatology [dĕr-mă-TŎL-ō-jē] {dermatologia} Medical specialty that deals with diseases of the skin.

dermis [DĔR-mǐs] {dermis} Layer of skin beneath the epidermis containing blood vessels, nerves, and some glands.

diabetes [dī-ă-BĒ-tēz] {diabetes} *See* Type I diabetes, Type II diabetes.

diabetes insipidus [ǐn-SĬP-ǐ-dŭs] Condition caused by hyposecretion of antidiuretic hormone.

diabetes mellitus [MĔL-ǐ-tŭs, mĕ-LĪ-tŭs] *See* Type I diabetes, Type II diabetes.

diabetic nephropathy [dī-ă-BĔT-ǐk nĕ-FRŎP-ă-thē] Kidney disease due to diabetes.

diabetic neuropathy [nū-RŎP-ă-thē] Loss of sensation in the extremities due to diabetes.

diabetic retinopathy [rĕt-ǐ-NŎP-ă-thē] Gradual loss of vision due to diabetes.

diagnostic [dī-ăg-NŎS-tǐk] Helping to finalize a diagnosis.

diagnostic imaging Use of imaging techniques in diagnosing illness.

dialysis [dī-ĂL-ǐ-sǐs] {diálisis} Method of filtration used when kidneys fail.

diaphoresis [DĪ-ă-fō-RĒ-sĭs] {diaforesis} Excretion of fluid by the sweat glands; sweating.

diaphragm [DĪ-ă-frăm] {diafragma} Muscle that divides the abdominal and thoracic cavities; membranous muscle between the abdominal and thoracic cavities that contracts and relaxes during the respiratory cycle; contraceptive device that covers the cervix and blocks sperm from entering; used in conjunction with spermicide.

diaphysis [dī-ĂF-ĭ-sĭs] {diáfisis} Long middle section of a long bone; shaft.

diarrhea [dī-ă-RĒ-ă] {diarrea} Loose, watery stool.

diarthroses (*sing.*, **diarthrosis**) [dī-ăr-THRŌ-sēz (dī-ăr-THRŌ-sĭs)] Freely movable joints.

diastole [dī-ĂS-tō-lē] {diástole} Relaxation phase of a heartbeat.

diencephalon [dī-ĕn-SĔF-ă-lŏn] {diencéfalo} One of the four major structures of the brain; it is the deep portion of the brain and contains the thalamus.

differentiated [dĭf-ĕr-ĔN-shē-ā-tĕd] Growing in an orderly fashion.

diffuse [dĭ-FYŪS] Spreading evenly.

digestion [dī-JĔS-chŭn] {digestión} Conversion of food into nutrients for the body and into waste products for release from the body.

digestive [dī-JĔS-tĭv] **system** Body system that includes all organs of digestion and waste excretion, from the mouth to the anus.

digital subtraction angiography Use of two angiograms done with different dyes to provide a comparison between the results.

dilator [DĪ-lā-tōr] Implement used to enlarge an opening.

diopter [dī-ŎP-tĕr] Unit of refracting power of a lens.

diphtheria [dĭf-THĒR-ē-ă] {difteria} Acute infection of the throat and upper respiratory tract caused by bacteria.

diplopia [dĭ-PLŌ-pē-ă] {diplopía} Double vision.

discoid lupus erythematosus (DLE) [DĬS-kŏyd LŪ-pŭs ĕr-ĭ-THĔM-ă-tō-sŭs] Mild form of lupus.

disk [dĭsk] {disco} *See* cartilaginous disk.

diskography [dĭs-KŎG-ră-fē] {discografía} Radiographic image of an intervertebral disk by injection of a contrast medium into the center of the disk.

dislocation {dislocación} Movement of a joint out of its normal position as a result of an injury or sudden, strenuous movement.

dissociative [dĭ-sō-sē-Ă-tĭv] **disorder** Condition with a gradual or sudden loss of the ability to integrate memory, identity, and other mental abilities with the environment.

distal [DĬS-tăl] Away from the point of attachment to the trunk.

diuretic [dī-yū-RĔT-ĭk] Pharmacological agent that increases urination; medication that promotes the excretion of urine.

diverticula [dī-vĕr-TĬK-yū-lă] Small pouches in the intestinal walls.

diverticulectomy [dī-vĕr-tĭk-ū-LĔK-tō-mē] Removal of diverticula.

diverticulitis [DĪ-vĕr-tĭk-yū-LĪ-tĭs] {diverticulitis} Inflammation of the diverticula.

diverticulosis [DĪ-vĕr-tĭk-yū-LŌ-sĭs] {diverticulosis} Condition in which diverticula trap food or bacteria.

dopamine [DŌ-pă-mēn] {dopamina} Substance in the brain or manufactured substance that helps relieve symptoms of Parkinson's disease.

Doppler [DŎP-lĕr] **ultrasound** Ultrasound test of blood flow in certain blood vessels.

dorsal [DŌR-săl] At or toward the back of the body.

dorsal [DŌR-săl] **cavity** Main cavity on the back side of the body containing the cranial and spinal cavities.

dorsal vertebrae Thoracic vertebrae.

drilling Cutting of a decayed area out of a tooth with a small dental drill.

drug [drŭg] {droga} Biological or chemical agents that can aid or alter body functions.

druggist [DRŬG-ĭst] {boticario} *See* pharmacist.

ductless gland Endocrine gland.

ductus arteriosus [DŬK-tŭs ăr-tēr-ē-Ō-sŭs] Structure in the fetal circulatory system through which blood flows to bypass the fetus's nonfunctioning lungs.

ductus venosus [vĕn-Ō-sŭs] Structure in the fetal circulatory system through which blood flows to bypass the fetal liver.

duodenal [DŪ-ō-DĒ-năl] **ulcer** Ulcer in the duodenum.

duodenum [dū-ō-DĒ-nŭm] {duodeno} Top part of the small intestine where chyme mixes with bile, pancreatic juices, and intestinal juice to continue the digestive process.

dura mater [DŪ-ră MĂ-tĕr] Outermost layer of meninges.

duritis [dū-RĪ-tĭs] Inflammation of the dura mater.

dwarfism [DWŎRF-ĭzm] {enanismo} Abnormally stunted growth caused by hyposecretion of growth hormone, congenital lack of a thyroid gland, or a genetic defect.

dyscrasia [dĭs-KRĀ-zē-ă] {discrasia} Any disease with abnormal particles in the blood.

dysentery [DĬS-ĕn-tĕr-ē] {disentería} Irritation of the intestinal tract with loose stools.

dysmenorrhea [dĭs-mĕn-ōr-Ē-ă] {dismenorrea} Painful menstruation.

dyspareunia [dĭs-pă-RŪ-nē-ă] {dispareunia} Painful sexual intercourse due to any of various conditions, such as cysts, infection, or dryness, in the vagina.

dyspepsia [dĭs-PĔP-sē-ă] {dispepsia} Indigestion.

dysphagia [dĭs-FĀ-jē-ă] {disfagia} Difficulty in swallowing.

dysphasia [dĭs-FĀ-zē-ă] {disfasia} Speech difficulty.

dysphonia [dĭs-FŌ-nē-ă] {disfonía} Hoarseness usually caused by laryngitis.

dysplasia [dĭs-PLĀ-zē-ă] Abnormal tissue growth.

dysplastic [dĭs-PLĂS-tĭk] Abnormal in cell appearance.

dyspnea [dĭsp-NĒ-ă] {disnea} Difficult breathing.

dysrhythmia [dĭs-RĬTH-mē-ă] {disritmia} Abnormal heart rhythm.

dystonia [dĭs-TŌ-nē-ă] {distonia} Abnormal tone in tissues.

dysuria [dĭs-YŪ-rē-ă] {disuria} Painful urination.

E

ear [ēr] {oreja, oído} Organ of hearing.

eardrum [ĒR-drŭm] {tambor de oído} Oval, semitransparent membrane that moves in response to sound waves and produces vibrations.

ecchymosis (*pl.*, **ecchymoses**) [ĕk-ĭ-MŌ-sĭs (ĕk-ĭ-MŌ-sēz)] {equimosis} Purplish skin patch (bruise) caused by broken blood vessels beneath the surface.

eccrine [ĔK-rĭn] **glands** {glándulas ecrinas} Sweat glands that occur all over the body, except where the apocrine glands occur.

echocardiography [ĕk-ō-kăr-dē-ŎG-ră-fē] {ecocardiografía} Use of sound waves to produce images showing the structure and motion of the heart.

eczema [ĔK-zĕ-mă] {eccema} Severe inflammatory condition of the skin, usually of unknown cause.

edema [ĕ-DĒ-mă] {edema} Retention of water in cells, tissues, and cavities, sometimes due to kidney disease.

efferent [ĔF-ĕr-ĕnt] **(motor) neuron** Neuron that carries information to the muscles and glands from the central nervous system.

ejaculation [ē-jăk-yū-LĀ-shŭn] {eyaculación} Expulsion of semen outside the body.

ejection fraction Percentage of the volume of the contents of the left ventricle ejected with each contraction.

elbow [ĔL-bō] {codo} Joint between the upper arm and the forearm.

electrocardiography [ē-lĕk-trō-kăr-dē-ŎG-ră-fē] Use of the electrocardiograph in diagnosis.

electrocauterization [ē-LĔK-trō-CĂW-tĕr-ĭ-ZĀ-shŭn] Destruction by burning tissue.

electroconvulsive [ē-LĔK-trō-kŏn-VŬL-sĭv] **therapy (ECT)** *See* electroshock therapy.

electrodesiccation [ē-LĔK-trō-dĕ-sĭ-KĀ-shŭn] Drying with electrical current.

electroencephalogram (EEG) [ē-LĔK-trō-ĕn-SĔF-ă-lō-grăm] {electroencefalógrafo} Record of the electrical impulses of the brain.

electrolyte [ē-LĔK-trō-līt] {electrólito} Any substance that conducts electricity and is decomposed by it.

electromyogram [ē-lĕk-trō-MĪ-ō-grăm] {electromiógrafo} A graphic image of muscular action using electrical currents.

electrophoresis [ē-lĕk-trō-FŌR-ē-sĭs] {electroforesis} Process of separating particles in a solution by passing electricity through the liquid.

electroshock [ē-LĔK-trō-shŏk] **therapy (EST)** Passing of electric current through a specific area of the brain to change or "scramble" communication from that area to the thought processes.

elimination [ē-lĭm-ĭ-NĀ-shŭn] The conversion of waste material from a liquid to a semisolid and removal of that material via defecation.

embolectomy [ĕm-bō-LĔK-tō-mē] {embolectomía} Surgical removal of an embolus.

embolic [ĕm-BŎL-ĭk] **stroke** Sudden stroke caused by an embolus.

embolus [ĔM-bō-lŭs] {émbolo} Mass of foreign material blocking a vessel; clot from somewhere in the body that blocks a small blood vessel in the brain.

embryo [ĔM-brē-ō] Fertilized ovum until about 10 weeks of gestation.

emesis [ĕ-MĒ-sĭs] {emesis} *See* regurgitation.

emollient [ē-MŎL-ē-ĕnt] Agent that smooths or softens skin.

emphysema [ĕm-fă-SĒ-mă] {enfisema} Chronic condition of hyperinflation of the air sacs; often caused by prolonged smoking.

empyema [ĕm-pī-Ē-mă] {empiema} Pus in the pleural cavity.

emulsification [ē-MŬL-sĭ-fĭ-KĀ-shŭn] Breaking down of fats.

enamel [ē-NĂM-ĕl] Glossy, white outer covering of teeth.

encapsulated [ĕn-KĂP-sū-lā-tĕd] Held within a capsule; benign.

encephalitis [ĕn-sĕf-ă-LĪ-tĭs] {encefalitis} Inflammation of the brain.

encephalogram [ĕn-SĔF-ă-lō-grăm] {encefalograma} Record of the radiographic study of the ventricles of the brain.

endarterectomy [ĕnd-ăr-tĕr-ĔK-tō-mē] Surgical removal of the diseased portion of the lining of an artery.

endocarditis [ĔN-dō-kăr-DĪ-tĭs] {endocarditis} Inflammation of the endocardium, especially an inflammation caused by a bacterial (for example, staphylococci) or fungal agent.

endocardium [ĕn-dō-KĂR-dē-ŭm] {endocardio} Membranous lining of the chambers and valves of the heart; the innermost layer of heart tissue.

endocrine [ĔN-dō-krĭn] **gland** {glándula endocrina} Gland that secretes substances into the bloodstream instead of into ducts.

endocrine [ĔN-dō-krĭn] **system** Body system that includes glands which secrete hormones to regulate certain body functions.

endodontist [ĕn-dō-DŎN-tĭst] Dentist who specializes in root canal work.

endolymph [ĔN-dō-lĭmf] {endolinfa} Fluid inside the membranous labyrinth.

endometriosis [ĔN-dō-mē-trē-Ō-sĭs] {endometriosis} Abnormal condition in which uterine wall tissue is found in the pelvis or on the abdominal wall.

endometrium [ĔN-dō-MĒ-trē-ŭm] {endometrio} Inner mucous layer of the uterus.

endoscope [ĔN-dō-skōp] {endoscopio} Tube used to view a body cavity.

endosteum [ĕn-DŎS-tē-ŭm] {endostio} Lining of the medullary cavity.

endothelium [ĕn-dō-THĒ-lē-ŭm] {endotelio} Lining of the arteries that secretes substances into the blood.

endotracheal intubation [ĕn-dō-TRĀ-kē-ăl ĭn-tū-BĀ-shŭn] **(ET)** Insertion of a tube through the nose or mouth, pharynx, and larynx and into the trachea to establish an airway.

endovascular [ĕn-dō-VĂS-kyū-lăr] **surgery** Any of various procedures performed during cardiac catheterization, such as angioscopy and atherectomy.

end-stage renal disease (ESRD) The last stages of kidney failure.

energy therapy Therapy using energy fields.

enteric-coated [ĕn-TĒR-ĭk] Having a coating (as on a capsule) that prevents stomach irritation.

enteritis [ĕn-tĕr-Ī-tĭs] {enteritis} Inflammation of the small intestine.

enucleation [ē-nū-klē-Ā-shŭn] {enucleación} Removal of an eyeball.

enuresis [ĕn-yū-RĒ-sĭs] {enuresis} Urinary incontinence.

enzyme [ĔN-zīm] {enzima} Protein that causes chemical changes in substances in the digestive tract.

enzyme-linked immunosorbent assay (EIA, ELISA) Test used to screen blood for the presence of antibodies to different viruses or bacteria.

eosinophil [ē-ō-SĬN-ō-fĭl] {eosinófilo} Type of granulocyte.

eosinophilia [Ē-ō-sĭn-ō-FĬL-ē-ă] {eosinofilia} Condition with an abnormal number of eosinophils in the blood.

epicardium [ĕp-ĭ-KĂR-dē-ŭm] {epicardio} Outermost layer of heart tissue.

epidermis [ĕp-ĭ-DĔRM-ŭs] {epidermis} Outer portion of the skin containing several strata.

epidermoid [ĕp-ĭ-DĔR-mŏyd] Resembling epithelial cells.

epididymectomy [ĔP-ĭ-dĭd-ĭ-MĔK-tō-mē] Removal of an epididymis.

epididymis [ĕp-ĭ-DĬD-ĭ-mĭs] {epidídimo} Group of ducts at the top of the testis where sperm are stored.

epididymitis [ĕp-ĭ-dĭd-ĭ-MĪ-tĭs] {epididimitis} Inflammation of the epididymis.

epidural [ĕp-ĭ-DŪR-ăl] **space** Area between the pia mater and the bones of the spinal cord.

epigastric [ĕp-ĭ-GĂS-trĭk] **region** Area of the body immediately above the stomach.

epiglottis [ĕp-ĭ-GLŎ-tĭs] {epiglotis} Cartilaginous flap that covers the larynx during swallowing to prevent food from entering the airway; movable flap of tissue that covers the trachea.

epiglottitis [ĕp-ĭ-glŏt-Ī-tĭs] {epiglotitis} Inflammation of the epiglottis.

epilepsy [ĔP-ĭ-LĔP-sē] Chronic recurrent seizure activity.

epinephrine [ĔP-ĭ-NĔF-rĭn] {epinefrina} Hormone released by the adrenal medulla in response to stress; adrenaline.

epiphora [ĕ-PĬF-ō-ră] {epífora} Excessive tearing.

epiphyseal [ĕp-ĭ-FĬZ-ē-ăl] **plate** Cartilaginous tissue that is replaced during growth years, but eventually calcifies and disappears when growth stops.

epiphysitis [ĕ-pĭf-ĭ-SĪ-tĭs] {epifisitis} Inflammation of the epiphysis.

epispadias [ĕp-ĭ-SPĀ-dē-ăs] {epispadias} Birth defect with abnormal opening of the urethra on the top side of the penis.

epistaxis [ĔP-ĭ-STĂK-sĭs] Bleeding from the nose, usually caused by trauma or a sudden rupture of the blood vessels of the nose.

epithalamus [ĔP-ĭ-THĂL-ă-mŭs] {epitálamo} One of the parts of the diencephalon; serves as a sensory relay station.

epithelial [ĕp-ĭ-THĒ-lē-ăl] **tissue** Tissue that covers or lines the body or its parts.

equilibrium [ē-kwĭ-LĬB-rē-ŭm] {equilibrio} Sense of balance.

erosion {erosion} Wearing away of the surface of the skin, especially when caused by friction.

eructation [ē-rŭk-TĀ-shŭn] {eructación} Belching.

erythroblastosis fetalis [ĕ-RĬTH-rō-blăs-TŌ-sĭs fē-TĂL-ĭs] Incompatibility disorder between a mother with Rh negative and a fetus with Rh positive.

erythrocyte [ĕ-RĬTH-rō-sīt] {eritrocito} Mature red blood cell.

erythrocyte sedimentation rate (ESR) Test for rate at which red blood cells fall through plasma.

erythropenia [ĕ-rĭth-rō-PĒ-nē-ă] {eritropenia} Disorder with abnormally low number of red blood cells.

erythropoietin [ĕ-rĭth-rō-PŎY-ĕ-tĭn] {eritropoyetina} Hormone released by the kidneys to stimulate red blood cell production.

esophagitis [ĕ-sŏf-ă-JĪ-tĭs] {esofagitis} Inflammation of the esophagus.

esophagoplasty [ĕ-SŎF-ă-gō-plăs-tē] {esofagoplastia} Repair of the esophagus.

esophagoscopy [ĕ-sŏf-ă-GŎS-kō-pē] {esofagoscopia} Examination of the esophagus with an esophagoscope.

esophagus [ĕ-SŎF-ă-gŭs] {esófago} Part of the alimentary canal from the pharynx to the stomach.

esotropia [ĕs-ō-TRŌ-pē-ă] {esotropía} Deviation of one eye inward.

essential hypertension High blood pressure without any known cause.

estrogen [ĔS-trō-jĕn] {estrógeno} One of the primary female hormones produced by the ovaries.

ethmoid [ĔTH-mŏyd] **bone** Irregular bone of the face attached to the sphenoid bone.

ethmoid sinuses Sinuses on both sides of the nasal cavities between each eye and the sphenoid sinus.

eupnea [yūp-NĒ-ă, YŪP-nē-ă] {eupnea} Normal breathing.

eustachian [yū-STĀ-shŭn, yū-STĀ-kē-ăn] **tube** Tube that connects the middle ear to the pharynx.

euthanasia [yū-thă-NĀ-zē-ă] Assisting in the suicide of or putting a person with an incurable or painful disease to death.

evoked potentials [ē-VŎKT pō-TĔN-shăls] Record of the electrical wave patterns observed in an EEG.

exanthematous [ĕks-zăn-THĔM-ă-tŭs] **viral disease** Viral disease that causes a rash on the skin.

excisional biopsy [ĕk-SĬZH-shŭn-l BĪ-ŏp-sē] Removal of tumor and surrounding tissue for examination.

excitability [ĕk-SĪ-tă-BĬL-ĭ-tē] {excitabilidad} Ability to respond to stimuli.

excoriation [ĕks-KŌ-rē-Ā-shŭn] {excoriación} Injury to the surface of the skin caused by a scratch, abrasion, or burn, usually accompanied by some oozing.

excrete [ĕks-KRĔT] To separate out and expel.

exenteration [ĕks-ĕn-tĕr-Ā-shŭn] Removal of an organ, tumor, and surrounding tissue.

exfoliative biopsy The scraping of skin cells from the skin surface for examination.

exhalation [ĕks-hă-LĀ-shŭn] {exahalación} Breathing out.

exocrine [ĔK-sō-krĭn] **gland** {exocrine} 1. Any gland that releases substances through ducts to a specific location. 2. Gland that secretes through ducts toward the outside of the body.

exophthalmos, exophthalmus [ĕk-sŏf-THĂL-mōs] {exoftalmía} Abnormal protrusion of the eyeballs; abnormal protrusion of the eyes typical of Graves' disease.

exostosis [ĕks-ōs-TŌ-sĭs] {exostosis} Abnormal bone growth capped with cartilage.

exotropia [ĕk-sō-TRŌ-pē-ă] Deviation of one eye outward.

expectorants [ĕk-SPĔK-tō-rănts] Agents that promote the coughing and expelling of mucus.

expiration [ĕks-pĭ-RĀ-shŭn] {espiración} Exhalation.

external fixation device Device applied externally to hold a limb in place.

external nares [NĂR-ēz] *See* nostrils.

external respiration Exchange of air between the body and the outside environment.

extracorporeal shock wave lithotripsy (ESWL) Breaking of kidney stones by using shock waves from outside the body.

exudate [ĔKS-yū-dāt] {exudado} Any fluid excreted out of tissue, especially fluid excreted out of an injury to the skin.

eye [ī] {ojo} Organ of sight.

eyebrow [Ī-brŏw] {ceja} Clump of hair, usually about a half an inch above the eye, that helps to keep foreign particles from entering the eye.

eyelashes [Ī-lăsh-ĕz] {pestaña} Group of hairs protruding from the end of the eyelid; helps to keep foreign particles from entering the eye.

eyelid [Ī-lĭd] {párpado} Moveable covering over the eye.

eyestrain {vista fatigada} Asthenopia.

eyetooth [Ī-tūth] Cuspid.

F

fainting *See* syncope.

fallopian [fă-LŌ-pē-ăn] **tube** One of the two tubes that lead from the ovaries to the uterus; uterine tube.

farsightedness {hiperopía} Hyperopia.

fascia (*pl.*, **fasciae**) [FĂSH-ē-ă (FĂSH-ē-ē)] {fascia} Sheet of fibrous tissue that encloses muscles.

fasting blood sugar Test for glucose in blood following a fast of 12 hours.

fatty acid Acid derived from fat during the digestive process.

feces [FĒ-sēz] {heces} Semisolid waste that moves through the large intestine to the anus, where it is released from the body.

femoral [FĔM-ō-răl, FĒ-mō-răl] **artery** An artery that supplies blood to the thigh.

femur [FĒ-mūr] {fémur} Long bone of the thigh.

fertilization [FĔR-tĭl-ĭ-ZĀ-shŭn] Union of an egg cell(s) with sperm.

fetus [FĒ-tŭs] Developing product of conception from 8 weeks to birth.

fever blister Eruption around the mouth or lips; herpes simplex virus Type 1.

fibrillation [fĭ-brĭ-LĀ-shŭn] {fibrilación} Random, chaotic, irregular heart rhythm.

fibrin [FĪ-brĭn] **clot** Clot-forming threads formed at the site of an injury during coagulation where platelets clump together with various other substances.

fibrinogen [fĭ-BRĬN-ō-jĕn] {fibrinógeno} Protein in plasma that aids in clotting.

fibroid [FĪ-brŏyd] {fibroide} Benign tumor commonly found in the uterus.

fibula [FĬB-yū-lă] {peroné} Smallest long bone of the lower leg.

filling An amalgam placed into a drilled space to prevent further tooth decay.

filtration [fĭl-TRĀ-shŭn] {filtración} Process of separating solids from a liquid by passing it through a porous substance.

fimbriae [FĬM-brē-ē] {fimbrias} Hairlike ends of the uterine tubes that sweep the ovum into the uterus.

first bicuspid Fourth tooth from the median of the jawline.

first molar Sixth tooth from the median of the jawline.

first-degree burn Least severe burn, causes injury to the surface of the skin without blistering.

fissure [FĬSH-ūr] {fisura} 1. Deep slit in the skin. 2. Deep furrow or slit (as in bone). 3. One of many indentations of the cerebrum; sulcus.

fistula [FĬS-tyū-lă] {fistula} Abnormal opening in tissue.

flaccid [FLĂK-sĭd] {fláccido} Without tone; relaxed.

flagellum [flă-JĔL-ŭm] {flagelo}Tail at the end of a sperm that helps it move.

flat bones Thin, flattened bones that cover certain areas, as of the skull.

flatulence [FLĂT-yū-lĕns] {flatulencia} Gas in the stomach or intestines.

flatus [FLĂ-tŭs] {flato} Gas in the lower intestinal tract that can be released through the anus.

fluoride [FLŪR-ĭd] Substance given as a mouth wash to prevent tooth decay.

fluoroscopy [flŭr-ŎS-kō-pē] X-ray in which the image is projected onto a fluorescent screen.

flutter {aleteo} Regular but very rapid heartbeat.

Foley catheter Indwelling catheter held in place by a balloon that inflates inside the bladder.

follicle-stimulating hormone (FSH) Hormone necessary for maturation of oocytes and ovulation; hormone released by the anterior pituitary to aid in production of ova and sperm.

follicular [fŏl-LĬK-yū-lăr] Containing glandular sacs.

Fontan's [FŎN-tănz] **operation** Surgical procedure that creates a bypass from the right atrium to the main pulmonary artery; Fontan's procedure.

fontanelle [FŎN-tă-nĕl] {fontanela} Soft, membranous section on top of an infant's skull.

foramen [fō-RĂ-mĕn] {agujero} Opening or perforation through a bone.

foramen magnum [MĂG-nŭm] Opening in the occipital bone through which the spinal cord passes.

foramen ovale [ō-VĂ-lĕ] Opening in the septum of the fetal heart that closes at birth.

forceps [FŌR-sĕps] Surgical implement used to grasp and remove something.

foreskin [FŌR-skĭn] {prepucio} Fold of skin at the top of the labia minora; flap of skin covering the glans penis; removed by circumcision in many cultures.

fossa (*pl.*, **fossae**) [FŎS-ă (FŎS-ē)] {fosa} Depression, as in a bone.

fovea centralis [FŌ-vē-ă sĕn-TRĂL-ĭs] Depression in the center of the macula lutea; perceives sharpest images.

fracture [FRĂK-chūr] {fractura} A break, especially in a bone.

frenulum [FRĔN-yū-lŭm] {frenillo} Mucous membrane that attaches the tongue to the floor of the mouth.

frontal [FRŬN-tăl] **bone** Large bone of the skull that forms the top of the head and forehead.

frontal lobe One of the four parts of each hemisphere of the cerebrum.

frontal [FRŬN-tăl] **plane** Imaginary line that divides the body into anterior and posterior positions.

frontal sinuses Sinuses above the eyes.

fulguration [fŭl-gŭ-RĀ-shŭn] {fulguración} Destruction of tissue using electric sparks or by high-frequency current.

full [fŭl] Complete (set of dentures).

fundus [FŬN-dŭs] {fondo} Top portion of the uterus; upper portion of the stomach.

fungating [FŬNG-āt-ĭng] Growing in a mushroomlike pattern.

furuncle [FYŬ-rŭng-kl] {furúnculo} Localized skin infection, usually in a hair follicle and containing pus; boil.

G

gait [gāt] {marcha} Manner of walking.

gallbladder [GĂWL-blăd-ĕr] {vesícula biliar} Organ on lower surface of liver; stores bile.

gallop {galope} Triple sound of a heartbeat, usually indicative of serious heart disease.

gallstones {cálculo biliar} Calculi in the gallbladder.

gamete [GĂM-ēt] {gameto} Sex cell; *see* ovum.

gamma globulin [GĂ-mă GLŎB-yū-lĭn] 1. Globulin that arises in lymphatic tissue and functions as part of the immune system. 2. Antibodies given to prevent or lessen certain diseases.

gamma rays Commonly used radioactive particles with high penetrating ability.

gangliitis [găng-glē-Ī-tĭs] {ganglitis} Inflammation of a ganglion.

ganglion (*pl.*, **ganglia, ganglions**) [GĂNG-glē-ŏn (-ă, -ŏns)] {ganglion} Any group of nerve cell bodies forming a mass or a cyst in the peripheral nervous system; usually forms in the wrist.

gangrene [GĂNG-grēn] {gangrena} Death of an area of skin, usually caused by loss of blood supply to the area.

gastrectomy [găs-TRĔK-tō-mē] {gastrectomia} Removal of part or all of the stomach.

gastric bypass *See* gastric resection.

gastric resection or gastric bypass Removal of part of the stomach and repair of the remaining part.

gastritis [găs-TRĪ-tĭs] {gastritis} Inflammation of the stomach.

gastroenteritis [GĂS-trō-ĕn-tĕr-Ī-tĭs] {gastroenteritis} Inflammation of the stomach and small intestine.

gastroscopy [găs-TRŎS-kō-pē] {gastrocopia} Examination of the stomach using an endoscope.

gene therapy Method of treatment using genetically changed cells to cure or lessen the symptoms of disease.

generic [jĕ-NĂR-ĭk] {genérico} Shortened version of a chemical name.

genetics [jĕ-NĔT-ĭks] Science of biological inheritance.

genital herpes *See* herpes simplex virus Type 2.

geriatric [JĔR-ē-Ă-trĭk] Of or relating to old age.

gerontology [JĔR-ŏn-TŎL-ō-jē] Medical specialty that diagnoses and treats disorders of old age.

gestation [jĕs-TĀ-shŭn] {gestación} Period of fetal development from fertilization until delivery; usually about 40 weeks.

gigantism [JĪ-găn-tĭzm] {gigantismo} Abnormally fast and large growth caused by hypersecretion of growth hormone.

gingivae [JĬN-jĭ-vē] Gums.

gingivitis [jĭn-jĭ-VĪ-tĭs] Inflammation of the gums.

gland {glándula} Any organized mass of tissue secreting or excreting substances.

glans penis [glănz PĒ-nĭs] Sensitive area at the tip of the penis.

glaucoma [glăw-KŌ-mă] {glaucoma} Any of various diseases caused by abnormally high eye pressure.

glioblastoma multiforme [GLĪ-ō-blăs-TŌ-mă MŬL-tĭ-fŏrm] Most malignant type of glioma.

glioma [glī-Ō-mă] {glioma} Tumor that arises from neuroglia.

globin [GLŌ-bĭn] {globina} Protein molecule; in the blood, a part of hemoglobin.

globulin [GLŎB-yū-lĭn] {globulina} Any of a family of proteins in blood plasma.

glomerulonephritis [glō-MĂR-yū-lō-nĕf-RĪ-tĭs] Inflammation of the glomeruli of the kidneys.

glomerulus (*pl.*, **glomuleri**) [glō-MĂR-yū-lĭs (glō-MĂR-yū-lī)] {glomérulo} Group of capillaries in a nephron.

glossectomy [glŏ-SĔK-tō-mē] Removal of the tongue.

glossitis [glŏ-SĪ-tĭs] {glositis} Inflammation of the tongue.

glossorrhaphy [glŏ-SŎR-ă-fē] Suture of the tongue.

glottis [GLŎT-ĭs] {glotis} Part of the larynx consisting of the vocal folds of mucous membrane and muscle.

glucagon [GLŪ-kō-gŏn] {glucagon} Hormone released by the pancreas to increase blood sugar.

glucocorticoids [glū-kō-KŌR-tĭ-kŏydz] Hormones released by the adrenal cortex.

glucose [GLŪ-kōs] {glucosa} Form of sugar found in the blood; may indicate diabetes when found in the urine; sugar found in fruits and plants and in various parts of the body.

glucose tolerance test (GTT) Blood test for body's ability to metabolize carbohydrates; taken after a 12-hour fast, then repeated every hour for 4 to 6 hours after ingestion of a sugar solution.

glucosuria [glū-kō-SŪ-rē-ă] Glucose in the urine.

glycated hemoglobin Blood test for an average of glucose levels over the previous 2-3 months.

glycogen [GLĪ-kō-jĕn] {glucógeno} Converted glucose stored in the liver for future use; starch that can be converted into glucose.

glycosuria [glī-kō-SŪ-rē-ă] Glucose in the urine.

goiter [GŎY-tĕr] {bocio} Abnormal enlargement of the thyroid gland as a result of its overactivity or lack of iodine in the diet.

gonad [GŌ-năd] {gónada} Male or female sex organ; *see* ovary.

goniometer [gŏ-nē-ŎM-ĕ-tĕr] {goniómetro} Instrument that measures angles or range of motion in a joint.

gonorrhea [gŏn-ō-RĒ-ă] {gonorrea} Sexually transmitted inflammation of the genital membranes.

gouty arthritis, gout [GŎWT-ē, gŏwt] Inflammation of the joints, present in gout; usually caused by uric acid crystals.

graafian follicle [gră-FĒ-ăn FŎL-ĭ-kl] Follicle in the ovary that holds an oocyte during development and then releases it.

grade Maturity of a tumor.

graft Any tissue or organ implanted to replace or mend damaged areas.

grand mal [măhl] **seizure** *See* tonic-clonic seizure.

granulocyte [GRĂN-yū-lō-sīt] Leukocyte with granular cytoplasm.

granulocytosis [GRĂN-yū-lō-sī-TŌ-sĭs] {granulocitosis} Condition with an abnormal number of granulocytes in the bloodstream.

Graves' [grāvz] **disease** Overactivity of the thyroid gland.

gravida [GRĂV-ĭ-dă] {grávida} Pregnant woman.

gray (gy) Unit of measure equal to 100 rads.

greenstick fracture Fracture with twisting or bending of the bone but no breaking; usually occurs in children.

group therapy Talk therapy under the leadership of a psychotherapist in which the members of the group discuss their feelings and try to help each other improve.

growth hormone (GH) Hormone released by the anterior pituitary.

gums [gŭmz] {encía} Dense fibrous tissue that forms a protective covering around the sockets and the part of the jawline inside the oral cavity; fleshy sockets that hold the teeth.

gynecologist [gī-nĕ-KŎL-ō-jĭst] {ginecólogo} Specialist who diagnoses and treats the processes and disorders of the female reproductive system.

gyrus (*pl.*, **gyri**) [JĪ-rŭs (JĪ-rĭ)] {circunvolución} *See* convolution.

H

hair follicle [FŎL-ĭ-kl] Tubelike sac in the dermis out of which the hair shaft develops.

hair root {raiz de pelo} Portion of the hair beneath the skin surface.

hair shaft Portion of the hair visible above the skin surface.

hairline fracture Fracture with no bone separation or fragmentation.

halitosis [hăl-ĭ-TŌ-sĭs] {halitosis} Foul mouth odor.

hard palate [PĂL-ăt] Hard anterior portion of the palate at the roof of the mouth; hardening of the arteries.

hearing {audición} Ability to perceive sound.

heart [hărt] {corazón} Muscular organ that receives blood from the veins and sends it into the arteries.

heart block *See* atrioventricular block.

heart transplant Implantation of the heart of a person who has just died into a person whose diseased heart cannot sustain life.

heel [hēl] {talon} Back, rounded portion of the foot.

helper cell T cell that stimulates the immune response.

hematemesis [hē-mă-TĔM-ē-sĭs] {hematemesis} Blood in vomit.

hematochezia [HĒ-mă-tō-KĒ-zē-ă] Red blood in stool.

hematocrit [HĒ-mă-tō-krĭt, HĔM-ă-tō-krĭt] {hematócrito} Measure of the percentage of red blood cells in a blood sample.

hematocytoblast [HĒ-mă-tō-SĪ-tō-blăst] {hematocitoblasto} Most immature blood cell.

hematuria [hē-mă-TŪ-rē-ă] {hematuria} Blood in the urine.

heme [hēm] Pigment containing iron in hemoglobin.

hemochromatosis [HĒ-mō-krō-mă-TŌ-sĭs] Hereditary condition with excessive iron buildup in the blood.

hemodialysis [HĒ-mō-dī-ĂL-ĭ-sĭs] {hemodiálisis} Dialysis performed by passing blood through a filter outside the body and returning filtered blood to the body.

hemoglobin [hē-mō-GLŌ-bĭn] {hemoglobina} Protein in red blood cells essential to the transport of oxygen.

hemolysis [hē-MŎL-ĭ-sĭs] {hemolisis} Disorder with breakdown of red blood cell membranes.

hemophilia [hē-mō-FĬL-ē-ă] {hemofilia} Hereditary disorder with lack of clotting factor in the blood.

hemoptysis [hē-MŎP-tĭ-sĭs] Lung or bronchial hemorrhage resulting in the spitting of blood.

hemorrhagic [hĕm-ō-RĂJ-ĭk] **stroke** Stroke caused by blood escaping from a damaged cerebral artery.

hemorrhoidectomy [HĔM-ō-rŏy-DĔK-tō-mē] {hemorroidectomía} Surgical removal of hemorrhoids.

hemorrhoids [HĔM-ō-rŏydz] {hemorroides} Varicose condition of veins in the anal region; swollen, twisted veins in the anus.

hemostatic [hē-mō-STĂT-ĭk] Agent that stops bleeding.

hemothorax [hē-mō-THŌ-răks] {hemotórax} Blood in the pleural cavity.

heparin [HĔP-ă-rĭn] {heparina} Anticoagulant present in the body; also, synthetic version administered to prevent clotting; substance in blood that prevents clotting.

hepatic lobectomy [hĕ-PĂT-ĭk lō-BĔK-tō-mē] Removal of one or more lobes of the liver.

hepatitis [hĕp-ă-TĪ-tĭs] {hepatitis} Inflammation or disease of the liver.

hepatomegaly [HĔP-ă-tō-MĔG-ă-lē] {hepatomegalia} Enlarged liver.

hepatopathy [hĕp-ă-TŎP-ă-thē] {hepatopatía} Liver disease.

hernia [HĔR-nē-ă] {hernia} Abnormal protrusion of tissue through muscle that contains it.

herniated [HĔR-nē-ā-tĕd] **disk** Protrusion of an intervertebral disk into the neural canal.

herpes [HĔR-pēz] {herpes} An inflammatory skin disease caused by viruses of the family Herpesviridae.

herpes simplex virus Type 1 Herpes that recurs on the lips and around the area of the mouth, usually during viral illnesses or states of stress.

herpes simplex virus Type 2 Herpes that recurs on the genitalia; can be easily transmitted from one person to another through sexual contact.

herpes zoster [ZŎS-tĕr] Painful herpes that affects nerve roots; shingles.

heterograft [HĔT-ĕr-ō-grăft] {heterinjerto} Skin graft using donor skin from one species to another; xenograft.

heteroplasia [HĔT-ĕr-ō-PLĀ-zē-ă] Dysplasia.

hiatal hernia [hī-Ā-tăl HĔR-nē-ă] Protrusion of the stomach through an opening in the diaphragm.

high blood pressure {presión arterial alta} *See* hypertension.

hilum (*also* hilus) [HĪ-lŭm (HĪ-lŭs)] {hilio} 1. Portion of the kidney where blood vessels and nerves enter and exit. 2. Midsection of the lung where the nerves and vessels enter and exit.

hirsutism [HĔR-sū-tĭzm] {hirsutismo} Abnormal hair growth due to an excess of androgens.

histamine [HĬS-tă-mēn] {histamine} Substance released by basophils and eosinophils; involved in allergic reactions.

histiocytic [HĬS-tē-ō-SĬT-ĭk] **lymphoma** Lymphoma with malignant cells that resemble histiocytes.

hives {urticaria} *See* urticaria.

Hodgkin's lymphoma, Hodgkin's disease Type of lymph cancer of uncertain origin that generally appears in early adulthood.

Holter [HŌL-tĕr] **monitor** Portable device that provides a 24-hour electrocardiogram.

homeopathic [hō-mē-ō-PĂTH-ĭk] **medicine** Medical system that uses diluted doses of substances to stimulate immunity.

homograft [HŌ-mō-grăft] {homoinjerto} Skin graft using donor skin from one person to another; allograft.

hordeolum [hōr-DĒ-ō-lŭm] {orzuelo} Infection of a sebaceous gland of the eyelid; sty.

hormone [HŌR-mōn] {hormona} Chemical secretion from glands such as the ovaries; substance secreted by glands and carried in the bloodstream to various parts of the body; chemical substance in the body that forms in one organ and moves to another organ or part on which the substance has an effect; manufactured version of that chemical substance.

hormone replacement therapy (HRT) Treatment with hormones when the body stops or decreases the production of hormones by itself; ingestion of hormones to replace missing (or increase low levels of needed) hormones.

human growth hormone (HCG) Naturally occurring substance in the body that promotes growth; synthesized substance that serves the same function.

human immunodeficiency [ĬM-yū-nō-dē-FĬSH-ĕn-sē] **virus (HIV)** Virus that causes AIDS; spread by sexual contact and exchange of body fluids, and shared use of needles.

humerus [HYŪ-mĕr-ŭs] {húmero} Long bone of the arm connecting to the scapula on top and the radius and ulna at the bottom.

humoral [HYŪ-mōr-ăl] **immunity** Resistance to disease provided by plasma cells and antibody production.

Huntington's chorea [kōr-Ē-ă] Hereditary disorder with uncontrollable, jerking movements.

hydrocele [HĪ-drō-sēl] {hidrocele} Fluid-containing hernia of the testis.

hydrocephalus [hī-drō-SĔF-ă-lŭs] {hidrocefalia} Overproduction of fluid in the brain.

hydronephrosis [HĪ-drō-nĕ-FRŌ-sĭs] Abnormal collection of urine in the kidneys due to a blockage.

hymen [HĪ-mĕn] {himen} Fold of mucous membranes covering the vagina of a young female; usually ruptures during first intercourse.

hyperadrenalism [HĪ-pĕr-ă-DRĔN-ă-lĭzm] Overactivity of the adrenal glands.

hyperbilirubinemia [HĪ-pĕr-BĬL-i-rū-bĭ-NĒ-mē-ă] Excessive bilirubin in the blood.

hypercapnia [hī-pĕr-KĂP-nē-ă] Excessive buildup of carbon dioxide in lungs, usually associated with hypoventilation.

hyperchromatic [HĪ-pĕr-krō-MĂT-ĭk] Intensely colored.

hyperopia [hī-pĕr-Ō-pē-ă] Focusing behind the retina causing vision distortion; farsightedness.

hyperparathyroidism [HĪ-pĕr-pă-ră-THĪ-rŏyd-izm] {hiperparatiroidismo} Overactivity of the parathyroid glands.

hyperplastic [hī-pĕr-PLĂS-tĭk] Excessive in development (of cells).

hyperpnea [hī-pĕrp-NĒ-ă] Abnormally deep breathing.

hypersecretion [HĪ-pĕr-sē-KRĒ-shŭn] Abnormally high secretion, as from a gland.

hypersensitivity [HĪ-pĕr-sĕn-sĭ-TĬV-ĭ-tē] {hipersensibilidad} Abnormal reaction to an allergen.

hypersplenism [hī-pĕr-SPLĔN-ĭzm] Overactive spleen.

hypertension [HĪ-pĕr-TĔN-shŭn] Chronic condition with blood pressure greater than 140/90.

hypertensive heart disease Heart disease caused, or worsened, by high blood pressure.

hyperthyroidism [HĪ-pĕr-THĪ-rŏyd-ĭzm] {hipertiroidismo} Overactivity of the thyroid gland.

hypertrophy [hī-PĔR-trō-fē] Abnormal increase as in muscle size.

hyperventilation [HĪ-pĕr-vĕn-tĭ-LĀ-shŭn] {hiperventilación} Abnormally fast breathing in and out, often associated with anxiety.

hypnosis [hĭp-NŌ-sĭs] State of semiconsciousness.

hypnotic [hĭp-NŎT-ĭk] Agent that induces sleep.

hypoadrenalism [HĪ-pō-ă-DRĔN-ă-lĭzm] {hipoadrenalismo} Underactivity of the adrenal glands.

hypochondria [hī-pō-KŎN-drē-ă] Condition of preoccupation with imagined illnesses in the patient's body.

hypochondriac [hī-pō-KŎN-drē-ăk] **regions** Left and right regions of the body just below the cartilage of the ribs and immediately above the abdomen.

hypodermis [hī-pō-DĔR-mĭs] {hipodermis} Subcutaneous skin layer; layer below the dermis.

hypogastric [hī-pō-GĂS-trĭk] **region** Area of the body just below the umbilical region.

hypoglycemia [HĪ-pō-glī-SĒ-mē-ă] {hypoglucemia} Abnormally low level of glucose in the blood.

hypoglycemic [HĪ-pō-glī-SĒ-mĭk] {hipoglucémico} Agent that lowers blood glucose.

hypoparathyroidism [HĪ-pō-pă-ră-THĪ-rŏyd-ĭzm] {hipoparatiroidismo} Underactivity of the parathyroid glands.

hypopharynx [HĪ-pō-FĂR-ĭnks] {hipofaringe} Laryngopharynx.

hypophysectomy [hī-pŏf-ĭ-SĒK-tō-mē] Removal of the pituitary gland.

hypophysis [hī-PŎF-ĭ-sĭs] {hipófisis} Pituitary gland.

hypoplastic [HĪ-pŏ-PLĂS-tĭk] Underdeveloped, as tissue.

hypopnea [hī-PŎP-nē-ă] Shallow breathing.

hyposecretion [HĪ-pō-sē-KRĒ-shŭn] Abnormally low secretion, as from a gland.

hypospadias [HĪ-pō-SPĀ-dē-ǎs] {hipospadias} Birth defect with abnormal opening of the urethra on the bottom side of the penis.

hypotension [HĪ-pō-TĚN-shǔn] {hipotensión} Chronic condition with blood pressure below normal.

hypothalamus [HĪ-pō-THĂL-ǎ-mǔs] {hipotálamo} One of the parts of the diencephalon; serves as a sensory relay station; gland in the nervous system that releases hormones to aid in regulating pituitary hormones.

hypothyroidism [HĪ-pō-THĪ-rǒyd-izm] {hipotiroidismo} Underactivity of the thyroid gland.

hypotonia [HĪ-pō-TŌ-nē-ǎ] Abnormally reduced muscle tension.

hypoventilation [HĪ-pō-věn-tǐ-LĀ-shǔn] {hipoventilación} Abnormally low movement of air in and out of the lungs.

hypoxemia [hī-pǒk-SĒ-mē-ǎ] {hipoxemia} Deficient amount of oxygen in the blood.

hypoxia [hī-PŎK-sē-ǎ] {hipoxia} Deficient amount of oxygen in tissue.

hysterectomy [hǐs-těr-ĚK-tō-mē] {histerectomía} Removal of the uterus.

hysterosalpingography [HĬS-těr-ō-sǎl-pǐng-GŎG-rǎ-fē] {histerosalpingografía} X-ray of the uterus and uterine tubes after a contrast medium has been injected.

hysteroscopy [hǐs-těr-ŎS-kō-pē] {histeroscopia} Examination of the uterus using a hysteroscope.

I

icterus [ĬK-těr-ǔs] {icterus} Jaundice.

ileitis [ĬL-ē-Ī-tǐs] {ileitis} Inflammation of the ileum.

ileostomy [ĬL-ē-ŎS-tō-mē] {ileostomía} Creation of an opening into the ileum.

ileum [ĬL-ē-ǔm] {íleon} Bottom part of the small intestine that connects to the large intestine.

ileus [ĬL-ē-ǔs] {íleo} Intestinal blockage.

iliac [ĬL-ē-ǎk] **regions** Left and right regions of the body near the upper portion of the hip bone.

ilium [ĬL-ē-ǔm] {ileum} Wide portion of the hip bone.

imaging [ĬM-ǎ-jǐng] Production of a visual output using x-rays, sound waves, or magnetic fields.

immunity [ǐ-MYŪ-nǐ-tē] {inmunidad} Resistance to particular pathogens.

immunization [ĬM-yū-nǐ-ZĀ-shǔn] Vaccination.

immunoglobulin [ĬM-yū-nō-GLŎB-yū-lǐn] {inmunoglobina} Antibody.

immunosuppressive [ĬM-yū-nō-sǔ-PRĚS-ǐv] **disease** Disease that flourishes because of lowered immune response.

impacted fracture Fracture in which a fragment from one part of the fracture is driven into the tissue of another part.

impetigo [ǐm-pě-TĪ-gō] {impétigo} A type of pyoderma.

implant 1. To attach to the lining of the uterus in the first stage of pregnancy. 2. Artificial replacement tooth that has an extension set into bone.

impotence [ĬM-pō-těns] {impotencia} Inability to maintain an erection for ejaculation.

in utero [ǐn YŪ-těr-ō] Within the uterus; unborn.

incisional [ǐn-SĬZH-shǔn-l] **biopsy** Removal of a part of a tumor for examination.

incisor [ǐn-SĪ-zhūr] First and second tooth next to the median of the jawline.

incomplete fracture Fracture that does not go entirely through a bone.

incontinence [ǐn-KŎN-tǐ-něns] {incontinencia} Inability to prevent excretion of urine or feces.

incus [ĬN-kǔs] {incus} One of the three auditory ossicles; the anvil.

indwelling [ĬN-dwě-lǐng] Of a type of catheter inserted into the body.

infarct [ĬN-fǎrkt] {infarto} Area of necrosis caused by a sudden drop in the supply of arterial or venous blood.

infarction [ǐn-FĂRK-shǔn] {infarto} Sudden drop in the supply of arterial or venous blood, often due to an embolus or thrombus.

infectious mononucleosis [MŎN-ō-nū-klē-Ō-sǐs] Acute infectious disease caused by the Epstein-Barr virus.

inferior [ǐn-FĒR-ē-ōr] Below another body structure.

inferior lobe [ǐn-FĒ-rē-ōr lōb] Bottom lobe of the lung.

inferior vena cava [VĒ-nǎ KĂ-vǎ, KĀ-vǎ] Large vein that draws blood from the lower part of the body to the right atrium.

infertility [ǐn-fěr-TĬL-ǐ-tē] {infertilidad} Inability to fertilize ova.

inflammatory [ǐn-FLĂM-ǎ-tōr-ē] Having an inflamed appearance (red and swollen).

infusion [ǐn-FYŪ-zhǔn] Administration of a fluid through an intravenous tube at a slow and steady rate.

inguinal [ĬN-gwǐ-nǎl] **regions** Left and right regions of the body near the upper portion of the hip bone.

inhalation [ǐn-hǎ-LĀ-shǔn] {inhalación} 1. Breathing in. 2. Taking in of drugs in a fine spray of droplets.

inhibiting factor Substance in a hormone that prevents the secretion of other hormones.

insertion {inserción} Point at which a muscle attaches to a movable bone.

inspiration [ǐn-spǐ-RĀ-shǔn] {inspiración} Inhalation.

insulin [ĬN-sū-lǐn] {insulina} Substance released by the pancreas to lower blood sugar.

insulin-dependent diabetes mellitus (IDDM) See Type I diabetes.

integument [ǐn-TĚG-yū-měnt] {integumento} Skin and all the elements that are contained within and arise from it.

integumentary [ǐn-těg-yū-MĚN-tǎ-rē] **system** Body system that includes skin, hair, and nails.

intercostal muscles [ǐn-těr-KŎS-tǎl MŬS-ělz] Muscles between the ribs.

interferon [ǐn-těr-FĒR-ǒn] Protein produced by T cells and other cells; destroys disease-causing cells with its antiviral properties.

interleukin [ǐn-těr-LŪ-kǐn] {interleucina} Protein produced by T cells; helps regulate immune system.

intermittent claudication Attacks of limping, particularly in the legs, due to ischemia of the muscles.

internal fixation device Device, such as a pin, inserted in bone to hold it in place.

internal respiration Exchange of oxygen and carbon dioxide between the cells.

interneuron [ĬN-těr-NŪ-rǒn] {interneurona} Neuron that carries and processes sensory information.

interstitial [ĭn-tĕr-STĬSH-ăl] **therapy** Brachytherapy in which the radioactive substance is placed within the tissue or tumor.

intervertebral [ĭn-tĕr-VĔR-tĕ-brăl] **disk** *See* cartilaginous disk.

intra-arterial [ĬN-tră-ăr-TĒ-rē-ăl] Injected directly into an artery.

intracardiac [ĬN-tră-KĂR-dē-ăk] Injected directly into heart muscle.

intracardiac [ĭn-tră-KĂR-dē-ăk] **tumor** A tumor within one of the heart chambers.

intracavitary [ĬN-tră-CĂV-ĭ-tăr-ē] **therapy** Brachytherapy in which the radioactive substance is placed in a cavity near a cancerous lesion.

intracorporeal electrohydraulic lithotripsy [ĬN-tră-kŏr-PŌ-rē-ăl ē-LĔK-trō-hī-DRŎ-lĭk LĬTH-ō-trĭp-sē] Use of an endoscope to break up stones.

intracutaneous [ĬN-tră-kyū-TĀ-nē-ŭs] Injected just beneath the outer layer of skin.

intradermal [ĬN-tră-DĔR-măl] {intradérmico} From within the skin, particularly from the dermis; *See* intracutaneous.

intradermal [ĬN-tră-DĔR-măl] **test** Test that injects antigen or protein between layers of skin.

intramuscular [ĬN-tră-MŬS-kyū-lăr] Injected deep into muscle tissue.

intraosseus [ĬN-tră-ŎS-ē-ŭs] Injected directly into bone.

intraspinal [ĬN-tră-SPĪ-năl] Injected directly into spinal spaces.

intrathecal [ĬN-tră-THĒ-kăl] *See* intraspinal.

intrauterine [ĬN-tră-YŪ-tĕr-ĭn] **device (IUD)** Contraceptive device consisting of a coil placed in the uterus to block implantation of a fertilized ovum.

intravascular stent Stent placed within a blood vessel to allow blood to flow freely.

intravenous (IV) [ĬN-tră-VĒ-nŭs] {intravenoso (IV)} Administered through a tube into a vein.

introitus [ĭn-TRŌ-ĭ-tŭs] {introito} External opening or entrance to a hollow organ, such as a vagina.

intussusception [ĬN-tŭs-sŭ-SĔP-shŭn] Prolapse or collapse of an intestinal part into a neighboring part. One section collapses into another like a telescope.

invasive [ĭn-VĀ-sĭv] Infiltrating other organs; spreading.

involuntary muscle Muscle not movable at will.

iodine [Ī-ō-dīn] Substance used in radiopharmaceuticals for contrast medium and radiation therapy.

ion [Ī-ŏn] Positively charged particle used to ionize tissue.

ionize [Ī-ŏn-īz] To destroy cells by changing neutral particles to ions using x-rays.

iridectomy [ĭr-ĭ-DĔK-tō-mē] {iridectomía} Removal of part of the iris.

iridotomy [ĭr-ĭ-DŎT-ō-mē] Incision into the iris to relieve pressure.

iris [Ī-rĭs] {iris} Colored part of the eye; contains muscles that expand and contract in response to light.

iritis [ī-RĪ-tĭs] {iritis} Inflammation of the iris.

irradiated [ĭ-RĀ-dē-āt-ĕd] Treated with radiation.

irregular bones Any of a group of bones with a special shape to fit into certain areas of the skeleton, such as the skull.

ischemia [ĭs-KĒ-mē-ă] {isquemia} Localized blood insufficiency caused by an obstruction.

ischium [ĬS-kē-ŭm] {isquión} One of three fused bones that form the pelvic girdle.

islets of Langerhans [LĂN-gĕr-hănz] Specialized cells in the pancreas that release insulin and glucagon.

isthmus [ĬS-mŭs] {istmo} Narrow region at the bottom of the uterus opening into the cervix; narrow band of tissue connecting the two lobes of the thyroid gland.

J

jaundice [JĂWN-dĭs] {ictericia} Excessive bilirubin in the blood causing yellowing of the skin.

jejunum [jĕ-JŪ-nŭm] {yeyuno} Middle section of the small intestine.

joint [jŏynt] {empalme} Place of joining between two or more bones.

K

Kaposi's sarcoma [KĂ-pō-sēz săr-KŌ-mă] Skin cancer associated with AIDS.

Kegel [KĒ-gĕl] **exercises** Exercises to strengthen pubic muscles.

keloid [KĒ-lŏyd] {queloide} Thick scarring of the skin that forms after an injury or surgery.

keratin [KĔR-ă-tĭn] {queratina} Hard, horny protein that forms nails and hair.

keratitis [kĕr-ă-TĪ-tĭs] {queratitis} Inflammation of the cornea.

keratolytic [KĔR-ă-tō-LĬT-ĭk] Agent that aids in the removal of warts and corns.

keratoplasty [KĔR-ă-tō-plăs-tē] {queratoplastia} Corneal transplant.

keratosis [kĕr-ă-TŌ-sĭs] {queratosis} Lesion on the epidermis containing keratin.

ketoacidosis [KĒ-tō-ă-sĭ-DŌ-sĭs] {cetoacidosis} Condition of high acid levels caused by the abnormal release of ketones in the body.

ketone [KĒ-tōn] {cetona} Substance that results from the breakdown of fat; indicates diabetes or starvation when present in the urine.

ketonuria [kē-tō-NŪ-rē-ă] {cetonuria} Increased urinary excretion of ketones, usually indicative of diabetes or starvation.

ketosis [kē-TŌ-sĭs] {cetosis} Condition caused by the abnormal release of ketones in the body.

kidney [KĬD-nē] {riñón} Organ that forms urine and reabsorbs essential substances back into the bloodstream.

kidney failure Loss of kidney function.

kidney, ureter, bladder (KUB) X-ray of three parts of the urinary system.

kyphosis [kī-FŌ-sĭs] {cifosis} Abnormal posterior spine curvature.

L

labia majora [LĀ-bē-ă mă-JOR-ă] Two folds of skin that form the borders of the vulva.

labia minora [mī-NOR-ă] Two folds of skin between the labia majora.

labor [LĀ-bŏr] Process of expelling the fetus and placenta from the uterus.

labyrinthitis [LĂB-ĭ-rĭn-THĪ-tĭs] {laberintitis} Inflammation of the labyrinth.

lacrimal [LĂK-rĭ-măl] **bone** Thin, flat bone of the face.

lacrimal [LĂK-rĭ-măl] **glands** Glands that secrete liquid to moisten the eyes and produce tears.

lacrimation [lăk-rĭ-MĀ-shŭn] {lagrimeo} Secretion of tears, usually excessively.

lactation [lăk-TĀ-shŭn] {lactación} Production of milk from the breasts following delivery.

lactiferous [lăk-TĬF-ĕr-ŭs] {lactifero} Producing milk.

lamina (*pl.*, **laminae**) [LĂM-ĭ-nă (LĂM-ĭ-nē)] {lámina} Thin, flat part of either side of the arch of a vertebra.

laminectomy [LĂM-ĭ-NĔK-tō-mē] Removal of part of an intervertebral disk.

laparoscopy [lăp-ă-RŎS-kō-pē] {laparoscopia} Use of a lighted tubular instrument inserted through a woman's navel to perform a tubal ligation or to examine the fallopian tubes.

large intestine Passageway in the intestinal tract for waste received from the small intestine to be excreted through the anus; also, the place where water reabsorption takes place.

laryngectomy [LĂR-ĭn-JĔK-tō-mē] Removal of the larynx.

laryngitis [lăr-ĭn-JĪ-tĭs] {laringitis} Inflammation of the larynx.

laryngocentesis [lă-rĭng-gō-sĕn-TĒ-sĭs] Surgical puncture of the larynx.

laryngopharynx [lă-RĬNG-gō-făr-ĭnks] Part of the pharynx below and behind the larynx.

laryngoplasty [lă-RĬNG-gō-plăs-tē] {laringoplastia} Repair of the larynx.

laryngoscopy [LĂR-ĭng-GŎS-kō-pē] {laringoscopia} Visual examination of the mouth and larynx using an endoscope.

laryngospasm [lă-RĬNG-gō-spăsm] Sudden contraction of the larynx, which may cause coughing and may restrict breathing.

laryngostomy [LĂR-ĭng-GŎS-tō-mē] {laringostomía} Creation of an artificial opening in the larynx.

laryngotracheobronchitis [lă-RĬNG-gō-TRĀ-kē-ō-brŏng-KĪ-tĭs] Inflammation of the larynx, trachea, and bronchi.

laryngotracheotomy [lă-RĬNG-gō-trā-kē-ŎT-ō-mē] Incision into the larynx and trachea.

larynx [LĂR-ĭngks] {laringe} Organ of voice production in the respiratory tract, between the pharynx and the trachea; voice box.

lateral [LĂT-ĕr-ăl] To the side.

lateral incisor Second tooth from the median of the jawline.

lateral plane Imaginary line that divides the body perpendicularly to the medial plane.

laxative [LĂX-ă-tĭv] Agent that induces bowels to move in order to relieve constipation.

left atrium Upper left heart chamber.

left lower quadrant Quadrant on the lower left anterior side of the patient's body.

left upper quadrant Quadrant on the upper left anterior side of the patient's body.

left ventricle Lower left heart chamber.

leiomyoma [LĪ-ō-mĭ-Ō-mă] Benign tumor of smooth muscle.

leiomyosarcoma [LĪ-ō-MĪ-ō-săr-KŌ-mă] Malignant tumor of smooth muscle.

lens [lĕnz] {lens, lente} Colorless, flexible transparent body behind the iris.

lesion [LĒ-zhŭn] {lesión} Wound, damage, or injury to the skin.

leukemia [lū-KĒ-mē-ă] General term for a number of disorders with excessive white blood cells in the bloodstream and bone marrow.

leukocyte [LŪ-kō-sīt] Mature white blood cell.

leukoderma [lū-kō-DĔR-mă] {leucoderma} Absence of pigment in the skin or in an area of the skin.

leukoplakia [lū-kō-PLĀ-kē-ă] {leucoplaquia} White patch of mucous membrane on the tongue or cheek.

leukorrhea [lū-kō-RĒ-ă] {leucorrea} Abnormal vaginal discharge; usually whitish.

ligament [LĬG-ă-mĕnt] {ligamento} Sheet of fibrous tissue connecting and supporting bones; attaches bone to bone.

lingual tonsils [LĬNG-gwăl TŎN-sĭls] Two mounds of lymph tissue at the back of the tongue.

lipase [LĬP-ās] {lipasa} Enzyme contained in pancreatic juice.

lipid [LĬP-ĭd] **profile** Laboratory test that provides the levels of lipids, triglycerides, and other substances in the blood.

lipid-lowering Helpful in lowering cholesterol levels.

lips {labio} Two muscular folds formed around the outside boundary of the mouth.

lithotomy [lĭ-THŎT-ō-mē] Surgical removal of bladder stones.

liver [LĬV-ĕr] {hígado} Organ important in digestive and metabolic functions; secretes bile.

liver biopsy Removal of a small amount of liver tissue to examine for disease.

lobectomy [lō-BĔK-tō-mē] {lobectomía} 1. Removal of one of the lobes of a lung. 2. Removal of a portion of the brain to treat certain disorders.

lobotomy [lō-BŎT-ō-mē] {lobotomía} Incision into the frontal lobe of the brain.

long bone Any bone of the extremities with a shaft.

lordosis [lōr-DŌ-sĭs] {lordosis} Abnormal anterior spine curvature resulting in a sway back.

Lou Gehrig's disease *See* amyotrophic lateral sclerosis.

low blood pressure {presión arterial baja} *See* hypotension.

lumbar [LŬM-băr] **(spinal) puncture** Withdrawal of cerebrospinal fluid from between two lumbar vertebrae.

lumbar [LŬM-băr] **regions** Left and right regions of the body near the abdomen.

lumbar [LŬM-băr] **vertebrae** Five vertebrae of the lower back.

lumen [LŪ-mĕn] {lumen} Channel inside an artery through which blood flows.

lumpectomy [lŭm-PĔK-tō-mē] {nodulectomía} Surgical removal of a localized breast tumor.

lung [lŭng] {pulmón} One of two organs of respiration (left lung and right lung) in the thoracic cavity where oxygenation of blood takes place.

lunula (*pl.*, **lunulae**) [LŪ-nū-lă (LŪ-nū-lē)] {lúnula} Half-moon shaped area at the base of the nail plate.

luteinizing [LŪ-tē-ĭn-ĪZ-ĭng] **hormone (LH)** Hormone essential to ovulation; hormone released to aid in maturation of ova and ovulation.

lymph [lĭmf] {linfa} Fluid that contains white blood cells and other substances and flows in the lymphatic vessels.

percutaneous transluminal [pĕr-kyū-TĂ-nē-ŭs trăns-LŪ-mĭn-ăl] **coronary angioplasty** See balloon catheter dilation.

perfusion deficit Lack of flow through a blood vessel, usually caused by an occlusion.

pericarditis [PĔR-ĭ-kăr-DĪ-tĭs] {pericarditis} Inflammation of the pericardium.

pericardium [pĕr-ĭ-KĂR-dē-ŭm] {pericardio} Protective covering of the heart.

perilymph [PĔR-ĭ-lĭmf] Liquid secreted by the walls of the osseus labyrinth.

perimenopause [pĕr-ĭ-MĔN-ō-păws] Three- to five-year period of decreasing estrogen levels prior to menopause.

perimetrium [pĕr-ĭ-MĒ-trē-ŭm] {perimetrio} Outer layer of the uterus.

perineum [PĔR-ĭ-NĒ-ŭm] {perineo} Space between the labia majora and the anus; area between the penis and the anus.

periodontist [PĔR-ē-ō-DŎN-tĭst] Dentist who specializes in the treatment of gum disease.

periosteum [pĕr-ē-ŎS-tē-ŭm] {periostio} Fibrous membrane covering the surface of bone.

peripheral vascular disease Vascular disease in the lower extremities, usually due to blockages in the arteries of the groin or legs.

peristalsis [pĕr-ĭ-STĂL-sĭs] {peristaltismo} Coordinated, rhythmic contractions of smooth muscle that force food through the digestive tract.

peritoneal [PĔR-ĭ-tō-NĒ-ăl] **dialysis** Type of dialysis in which liquid that extracts substances from blood is inserted into the peritoneal cavity and emptied outside the body.

peritoneoscopy [PĔR-ĭ-tō-nē-ŏS-kō-pē] {peritoneoscopia} Examination of the abdominal cavity using a peritoneoscope.

peritonitis [PĔR-ĭ-tō-NĪ-tĭs] {peritonitis} Inflammation of the peritoneum.

permanent teeth Second set of teeth that erupt at regular intervals starting at around age six.

pertussis [pĕr-TŬS-ĭs] {pertussis} Severe infection of the pharynx, larynx, and trachea caused by bacteria; whooping cough.

PET (positron emission tomography) scan [PŎZ-ĭ-trŏn ē-MĬ-shŭn tō-MŎG-ră-fē] {TEP} Imaging of the brain using radioactive isotopes and tomography; a series of images that shows the distribution of substances through tissue.

petechia (*pl.*, **petechiae**) [pĕ-TĒ-kē-ă, pĕ-TĔK-ē-ă (pĕ-TĒ-kē-ē, pĕ-TĔK-ē-ē)] {petequia} A tiny hemorrhage beneath the surface of the skin; minute hemorrhages in the skin.

petit mal [PĔ-tē măhl] **seizure** See absence seizure.

Peyronie's [pă-RŌN-ēz] **disease** Abnormal curvature of the penis caused by hardening in the interior of the penis.

pH Measurement of the acidity or alkalinity of a solution such as urine.

phacoemulsification [FĀ-kō-ē-mŭls-ĭ-fĭ-KĀ-shŭn] Use of ultrasound to break up and remove cataracts.

phagocytosis [FĂG-ō-sī-TŌ-sĭs] {fagocitosis} Ingestion of foreign substances by specialized cells.

phalanges (*sing.*, **phalanx**) [fă-LĂN-jēz (FĂ-lăngks)] {falange} Long bones of the fingers and toes.

phantom limb, phantom pain Pain felt in a paralyzed or amputated limb.

pharmacist [FĂR-mă-sĭst] Person licensed to dispense medications.

pharmacodynamics [FĂR-mă-kō-dī-NĂM-ĭks] Study of how drugs affect the body.

pharmacokinetics [FĂR-mă-kō-kĭ-NĔT-ĭks] Study of how the body absorbs, metabolizes, and excretes drugs.

pharmacology [făr-mă-KŎL-ō-jē] {farmacología} Science that studies, develops, and tests new drugs.

pharyngeal tonsils [fă-RĬN-jē-ăl TŎN-sĭlz] Adenoids.

pharyngitis [făr-ĭn-JĪ-tĭs] {faringitis} Inflammation of the pharynx.

pharynx [FĂR-ĭngks] {faringe} Passageway at back of mouth for air and food; throat; tube through which food passes to the esophagus.

phenylketones [FĔN-ĭl-KĒ-tōns] Substances that, if accumulated in the urine of infants, indicate phenylketonuria (PKU), a disease treated by diet.

phimosis [fĭ-MŌ-sĭs] {fimosis} Abnormal narrowing of the opening of the foreskin.

phlebitis [flĕ-BĪ-tĭs] {flebitis} Inflammation of a vein.

phlebography [flĕ-BŎG-ră-fē] {flebografía} Viewing of a vein by x-ray after injection of a contrast medium.

phlebotomy [flĕ-BŎT-ō-mē] {flebotomía} Drawing blood from a vein via a small incision; See venipuncture.

phobia [FŌ-bē-ă] Irrational or obsessive fear of something.

phosphorus [FŎS-fōr-ŭs] {fósforo} Mineral important to the formation of bone.

photophobia [fō-tō-FŌ-bē-ă] {fotofobia} Extreme sensitivity to light.

physical therapy Movement therapy to restore use of damaged areas of the body.

pia mater [PĪ-ă, PĒ-ă MĀ-tĕr, MĂH-tĕr)] {piamadre} Innermost layer of meninges.

pica [PĪ-kă] Eating disorder in which the patient compulsively eats nonnutritive substances, such as clay and paint.

pilonidal [pī-lō-NĪ-dăl] **cyst** Cyst containing hair, usually found at the lower end of the spinal column.

pineal [PĬN-ē-ăl] **gland** Gland located above pituitary gland; secretes melatonin.

pinkeye Conjunctivitis.

pinna [PĬN-ă] Auricle.

pituitary [pĭ-TŪ-ĭ-tăr-ē] **gland** Major endocrine gland; secretes hormones essential to metabolic functions.

placenta [plă-SĔN-tă] {placenta} Nutrient-rich organ that develops in the uterus during pregnancy; supplies nutrients to the fetus.

placenta previa [plă-SĔN-tă PRĒ-vē-ă] Placement of the placenta so it blocks the birth canal.

plantar [PLĂN-tăr] **wart** Wart on the sole of the foot.

plaque [plăk] {placa} Microorganisms that grow on the crowns along the roots of teeth causing decay of teeth and breakdown of gums; see patch; buildup of solid material, such as a fatty deposit, on the lining of an artery.

plasma [PLĂZ-mă] Liquid portion of unclotted blood.

plasma [PLĂZ-mă] {plasma} **cell** Specialized lymphocyte that produces immunoglobulins.

plasmapheresis [PLĂZ-mă-fō-RĒ-sĭs] {plasmaféresis} Process of removing blood from a person, centrifuging it, and returning only red blood cells to that person.

plastic surgery Repair or reconstruction (as of the skin) by means of surgery.

platelet [PLĀT-lĕt] {plaqueta} Thrombocyte; part of a megakaryocyte that initiates clotting.

platelet count (PLT) Measurement of number of platelets in a blood sample.

play therapy Revealing of feelings through play with a trained therapist.

pleomorphic [plē-ō-MŌR-fĭk] Having many types of cells.

pleura (*pl.*, **pleurae**) [PLŪR-ă (PLŪR-ē)] {pleura} Double layer of membrane making up the outside of the lungs.

pleural cavity [PLŪR-ăl KĂV-ĭ-tē] Space between the two pleura.

pleural effusion [PLŪR-ăl ĕ-FYŪ-zhŭn] Escape of fluid into the pleural cavity.

pleuritis, pleurisy [plū-RĪ-tĭs, PLŪR-ĭ-sē] {pleuritis} Inflammation of the pleura.

pleurocentesis [PLŪR-ō-sĕn-TĒ-sĭs] Surgical puncture of pleural space.

pleuropexy [PLŪR-ō-PĔK-sē] Fixing in place of the pleura surgically, usually in case of injury or deterioration.

pneumobronchotomy [NŪ-mō-brŏng-KŎT-ō-mē] Incision of the lung and bronchus.

pneumoconiosis [NŪ-mō-kō-nē-Ō-sĭs] {neumoconiosis} Lung condition caused by inhaling dust.

pneumonectomy [NŪ-mō-NĔK-tō-mē] {neumonectomía} Removal of a lung.

pneumonia [nū-MŌ-nē-ă] {neumonía} Acute infection of the alveoli.

pneumonitis [nū-mō-NĪ-tĭs] {neumonitis} Inflammation of the lung.

pneumothorax [nū-mō-THŌR-ăks] {neumotórax} Accumulation of air or gas in the pleural cavity.

podagra [pō-DĂG-ră] {podagra} Pain in the big toe, often associated with gout.

podiatrist [pō-DĪ-ă-trĭst] {podiatra} Medical specialist who examines, diagnoses, and treats disorders of the foot.

poikilocytosis [PŎY-kĭ-lō-sī-TŌ-sĭs] {poiquilocitosis} Disorder with irregularly shaped red blood cells.

polarization [pō-lăr-ĭ-ZĀ-shŭn] {polarización} Resting state of the myocardial tissue in the conduction system of the heart.

polycystic [pŏl-ē-SĬS-tĭk] **kidney disease** Condition with many cysts on and within the kidneys.

polycythemia [PŎL-ē-sī-THĒ-mē-ă] {policetemia} Disorder with an abnormal increase in red blood cells and hemoglobin.

polydipsia [pŏl-ē-DĬP-sē-ă] {polydipsa} Excessive thirst.

polyp [PŎL-ĭp] {pólipo} Bulging mass of tissue that projects outward from the skin surface.

polypectomy [pŏl-ĭ-PĔK-tō-mē] {polipectomía} Removal of polyps.

polypoid [PŎL-ĭ-pŏyd] Containing polyps.

polyposis [PŎL-ĭ-PŌ-sĭs] {poliposis} Condition with polyps, as in the intestines.

polysomnography (PSG) [PŎL-ē-sŏm-NŎG-ră-fē] Recording of electrical and movement patterns during sleep.

polyuria [pŏl-ē-YŪ-rē-ă] {poliuria} Excessive urination; excessive amount of water in the urine.

pons [pŏnz] {pons} Part of the brainstem that controls certain respiratory functions.

popliteal [pŏp-LĬT-ē-ăl] **artery** An artery that supplies blood to the cells of the area behind the knee.

pore {poro} Opening or hole, particularly in the skin.

positron emission tomography [tō-MŎG-ră-fē] **(PET) scan** Type of nuclear image that measures movement of areas of the heart.

posterior At or toward the back side (of the body).

postprandial [pōst-PRĂN-dē-ăl] **blood sugar** Test for glucose in blood, usually about two hours after a meal.

post-traumatic stress disorder (PTSD) Condition of extreme traumatic stress that may occur and last for years after a traumatic time or incident.

PPD Purified protein derivative of tuberculin.

preeclampsia [prē-ĕ-KLĂMP-sē-ă] Toxic infection during pregnancy.

premature [PRĒ-mă-chūr] Born before 37 weeks gestation.

premature atrial contractions (PACs) Atrial contractions that occur before the normal impulse; can be the cause of palpitations.

premature ventricular contractions (PVCs) Ventricular contractions that occur before the normal impulse; can be the cause of palpitations.

premolar [prē-MŌ-lăr] Molar in primary teeth.

presbyacusis [prĕz-bē-ă-KŪ-sĭs] {presbiacusia} Age-related hearing loss.

presbyopia [prĕz-bē-Ō-pē-ă] {presbiopía} Age-related diminished ability to focus or accommodate.

prescription [prē-SKRĬP-shŭn] {prescripción} Order given by a doctor for medication dosage, route, and timing of administration.

pressure sore *See* decubitus ulcer.

preventative [prē-VĔN-tă-tĭve] Designed to stop or prevent disease.

preventive medicine Medical specialty concerned with preventing disease.

priapism [PRĪ-ă-pĭzm] {priapismo} Persistent, painful erection of the penis.

primary teeth First set of teeth that erupt at regular intervals between six months and age four.

probe Sharp device for exploring body cavities or clearing blockages.

process [PRŎ-sĕs, PRŎS-ĕs] Bony outgrowth or projection.

proctitis [prŏk-TĪ-tĭs] {proctitis} Inflammation of the rectum and anus.

proctoplasty [PRŎK-tō-plăs-tē] Repair of the rectum and anus.

proctoscopy [prŏk-TŎS-kō-pē] {proctoscopia} Examination of the rectum and anus using a proctoscope.

progesterone [prō-JĔS-tĕr-ŏn] {progesterona} One of the primary female hormones.

prone Lying on the stomach with the face down.

proprietary [prŏ-PRĪ-ĕ-tăr-ē] **name** *See* trade name.

prostate [PRŎS-tāt] {próstata} **gland** Gland surrounding the urethra that emits a fluid to help the sperm move and contracts its muscular tissue during ejaculation to help the sperm exit the body.

prostatectomy [prŏs-tă-TĔK-tō-mē] {prostatectomía} Removal of the prostate.

prostate-specific antigen [ĂN-tĭ-jĕn] **(PSA) test** Blood test for prostate cancer.

prostatitis [prŏs-tă-TĪ-tĭs] {prostatitis} Inflammation of the prostate.

prosthetic [prŏs-THĔT-ĭk] **device** Artificial device used as a substitute for a missing or diseased body part.

proteinuria [prō-tē-NŪ-rē-ă] Abnormal presence of protein in the urine.

prothrombin [prō-THRŎM-bĭn] {protrombina} Type of plasma protein that aids in clotting.

prothrombin time (PT) Test for ability of blood to coagulate.

protocol [PRŌ-tō-kōl] Course of treatment.

proximal [PRŎK-sĭ-măl] At or near the point of attachment to the trunk.

pruritus [prū-RĪ-tĭs] {prurito} Itching.

pseudophakia [sū-dō-FĀ-kē-ă] {seudofaquia} Eye with an implanted lens after cataract surgery.

psoriasis [sō-RĪ-ă-sĭs] {psoriasis} Chronic skin condition accompanied by scaly lesions with extreme pruritus.

psychiatry [sĭ-KĪ-ă-trē] Medical specialty concerned with the diagnosis and treatment of mental disorders.

psychoanalysis [sī-kō-ă-NĂL-ĭ-sĭs] Therapy that attempts to have patients bring unconscious emotions to the surface to deal with them.

psychology [sī-KŎL-ō-jē] Profession that studies human behavior and treats mental disorders.

psychopharmacology [sī-kō-FĂR-mă-KŎL-ō-jĕ] Science that deals with medications that affect the emotions.

psychosis [sī-KŌ-sĭs] Extreme disordered thinking.

psychotherapy [sī-kō-THĂR-ă-pē] Treatment of mental disorders with verbal and nonverbal communication.

puberty [PYŪ-bĕr-tē] {pubertad} Pre-teen or early teen period when secondary sex characteristics develop and menstruation begins.

pubes [PYŪ-bĭs] {pubis} Anteroinferior portion of the hip bone.

pubic symphysis [PYŪ-bĭk SĬM-fă-sĭs] Joint between the two pubic bones.

pulmonary abscess [PŬL-mō-năr-ē ĂB-sĭs] Large collection of pus in the lungs.

pulmonary [PŬL-mō-năr-ē] **artery** {arteria pulmunar} One of two arteries that carry blood that is low in oxygen from the heart to the lungs.

pulmonary artery stenosis Narrowing of the pulmonary artery, preventing the lungs from receiving enough blood from the heart to oxygenate.

pulmonary edema Abnormal accumulation of fluid in the lungs.

pulmonary edema [PŬL-mō-năr-ē ĕ-DĒ-mă] Fluid in the air sacs and bronchioles usually caused by failure of the heart to pump enough blood to and from lungs.

pulmonary function tests Tests that measure the mechanics of breathing.

pulmonary valve Valve that controls the blood flow between the right ventricle and the pulmonary arteries.

pulmonary vein One of four veins that bring oxygenated blood from the lungs to the left atrium.

pulp [pŭlp] Connective tissue, blood vessels, and nerves that fill the pulp cavity.

pulp cavity Center portion of a tooth.

pulse [pŭls] {pulso} Rhythmic expansion and contraction of a blood vessel, usually an artery.

pupil [PYŪ-pĭl] {pupila} Black circular center of the eye; opens and closes when muscles in the iris expand and contract in response to light.

purpura [PŬR-pū-ră] {púrpura} Skin condition with extensive hemorrhages underneath the skin covering a wide area.

pustule [PŬS-tūl] {pústula} Small elevation on the skin containing pus.

pyelitis [pī-ĕ-LĪ-tĭs] {pielitis} Inflammation of the renal pelvis.

pyeloplasty [PĪ-ĕ-lō-PLĂS-tē] Surgical repair of the renal pelvis.

pyelotomy [pī-ĕ-LŎT-ō-mē] Incision into the renal pelvis.

pylorus [pī-LŌR-ŭs] {píloro} Narrowed bottom part of the stomach.

pyoderma [pī-ō-DĔR-mă] {pioderma} Any inflammation of the skin that produces pus.

pyrogenic [pī-rō-JĔN-ĭk] **meningitis** Meningitis caused by bacteria; can be fatal; bacterial meningitis.

pyuria [pī-YŪ-rē-ă] {piuria} Pus in the urine.

R

rad [răd] **(radiation absorbed dose)** Unit of radioactive substance that can be absorbed in a particular period of time.

radiation [RĀ-dē-Ā-shŭn] Bombarding of tumors with rays that damage the DNA of cells.

radiation [RĀ-dē-Ā-shŭn] Energy carried by a stream of particles from a substance.

radiation therapy Treatment of cancer that uses ionizing radiation to destroy malignant cells.

radiculitis [ră-dĭk-yū-LĪ-tĭs] {radiculitis} Inflammation of the spinal nerve roots.

radioactive immunoassay (RIA) Test for measuring hormone levels in plasma; taken after radioactive solution is ingested.

radioactive iodine therapy Use of radioactive iodine to eliminate thyroid tumors.

radioactive iodine uptake Test for how quickly the thyroid gland pulls in ingested iodine.

radiography [RĂ-dē-ŎG-ră-fē] Production of diagnostic images.

radioimmunoassay (RIA) [RĂ-dē-ō-ĬM-ū-nō-ĂS-sā] In vitro test to determine the amount of drugs or medication left in the body.

radiology [RĀ-dē-ŎL-ō-jē] Medical specialty in diagnostic imaging and radiation treatment.

radiolucent [RĀ-dē-ō-LŪ-sĕnt] Able to be easily penetrated by x-rays.

radionuclide [RĀ-dē-ō-NŪ-klīd] Radioactive substance.

radiopaque [RĀ-dē-ō-PĀK] Not able to be easily penetrated by x-rays.

radiopharmaceutical [RĀ-dē-ō-făr-mă-SŪ-tǐ-kăl] Chemical substance containing radioactive material.

radioresistant [RĀ-dē-ō-rē-ZĬS-tănt] Not greatly affected by radiation.

radiosensitive [RĀ-dē-ō-SĔN-sǐ-tǐv] Easily affected by radiation.

radius [RĀ-dē-ŭs] Shorter bone of the forearm.

rales [rāhlz] {rales} *See* crackles.

Raynaud's phenomenon [rā-NŌZ] Spasm in the arteries of the fingers causing numbness or pain.

reabsorption [rē-ăb-SŎRB-shun] Process of returning essential elements to the bloodstream after filtration.

receptor [rē-SĔP-tōr] {receptor} Tissue or organ that receives nerve impulses; part of a target cell with properties compatible with a particular substance (hormone).

reconstructive [rĕ-cŏn-STRŬC-tǐv] Designed to restore a body part to its original state or appearance.

rectum [RĔK-tŭm] {recto} Bottom portion of large intestine; connected to anal canal.

red blood cell One of the solid parts of blood formed from stem cells and having hemoglobin within; erythrocyte.

red blood cell count Measurement of red blood cells in a cubic millimeter of blood.

red blood cell morphology Observation of shape of red blood cells.

reduction {reducción} Return of a part to its normal position.

reflex [RĒ-flĕks] {reflejo} Involuntary muscular contraction in response to a stimulus.

reflux [RĒ-flŭks] {reflujo} *See* regurgitation.

refraction [rē-FRĂK-shŭn] {refracción} Process of bending light rays.

regurgitation [rē-GŬR-jǐ-TĀ-shŭn] {regurgitación} Backward flow from the normal direction.

reiki [RĒ-kī] Therapy that uses touch from a healer.

relapse [RĒ-lăps] Recurrence of a disease.

releasing factor Substance in a hormone that allows secretion of other hormones.

remission [rĕ-MĬSH-ŭn] Disappearance of a disease for a time.

renal pelvis Collecting area for urine in the center of the kidney.

renin [RĒ-nǐn] {renina} Enzyme produced in the kidneys to regulate the filtration rate of blood by increasing blood pressure as necessary.

renogram [RĒ-nō-grăm] {renograma} Radioactive imaging of kidney function after introduction of a substance that is filtered through the kidney while it is observed.

repolarization [rē-pō-lăr-ĭ-ZĀ-shŭn] {repolarización} Recharging state; transition from contraction to resting that occurs in the conduction system of the heart.

reproductive [RĒ-prō-DŬK-tǐv] **system** Either the male or female body system that controls reproduction.

resectioning [rē-SĔK-shŭn-ĭng] Removal of a tumor and a large amount of surrounding tissue.

resectoscope [rē-SĔK-tō-skōp] {resectoscopio} Type of endoscope for removal of lesions.

respiratory [RĔS-pǐ-rā-tōr-ē, rĕ-SPĪR-ă-tōr-ē] **system** Body system that includes the lungs and airways and performs breathing; body's system for breathing.

respiratory [RĔS-pǐ-ră-tōr-ē, rĕ-SPĪR-ă-tōr-ē] **tract** Passageways through which air moves into and out of the lungs.

reticular [rĕ-TĬK-ū-lăr] **layer** Bottom sublayer of the dermis containing reticula (network of structures with connective tissue between).

reticulocytosis [rĕ-TĬK-yū-lō-sǐ-TŌ-sǐs] {reticulocitosis} Disorder with an abnormal number of immature erythrocytes.

retina [RĔT-ǐ-nă] {retina} Oval, light-sensitive membrane in the interior layer of the eye; decodes light waves and transmits information to the brain.

retinitis [rĕt-ǐ-NĪ-tǐs] {retinitis} Inflammation of the retina.

retinitis pigmentosa [pǐg-mĕn-TŌ-să] Progressive, inherited disease with a pigmented spot on the retina and poor night vision.

retractor [rē-TRĂK-tōr] An instrument used to hold back edges of tissue and organs to expose other tissues or body parts; especially used in surgery.

retroflexion [rĕ-trō-FLĔK-shŭn] {retroflexión} Bending backward of the uterus.

retrograde pyelogram [RĔT-rō-grād PĪ-ĕl-ō-grăm] **(RP)** X-ray of the bladder and ureters after a contrast medium is injected into the bladder.

retroperitoneal [RĔ-trō-PĔR-ǐ-tō-nē-ăl] {retroperitoneal} Posterior to the peritoneum.

retroversion [rē-trō-VĔR-shŭn] {retroversión} Backward turn of the uterus.

retrovirus [rē-trō-VĪ-rŭs] {retrovirus} Type of virus that spreads by using DNA in the body to help it replicate its RNA.

Rh factor Type of antigen in blood that can cause a transfusion reaction.

rhabdomyoma [RĂB-dō-mī-Ō-mă] {rabdomioma} Benign tumor in striated muscle.

rhabdomyosarcoma [RĂB-dō-mī-ō-săr-KŌ-mă] {rabdomiosarcoma} Malignant tumor in striated muscle.

rheumatic heart disease Heart valve and/or muscle damage caused by an untreated streptococcal infection.

rheumatoid [RŪ-mă-tŏyd] **arthritis** Autoimmune disorder affecting connective tissue.

rheumatoid factor test Test used to detect rheumatoid arthritis.

rheumatologist [rū-mă-TŎL-ō-jǐst] {reumatólogo} Physician who examines, diagnoses, and treats disorders of the joints and musculoskeletal system.

rhinitis [rī-NĪ-tǐs] {rinitis} Nasal inflammation.

rhinoplasty [RĪ-nō-plăs-tē] {rinoplastia} Surgical repair of the nose.

rhinorrhea [rī-nō-RĒ-ă] {rinorrea} Nasal discharge.

Rh-negative Lacking Rh factor on surface of blood cells.

rhonchi [RŎNG-kī] {ronquidos} *See* wheezes.

Rh-positive Having Rh factor on surface of blood cells.

rib {costilla} One of twenty-four bones that form the chest wall.

rickets [RĬK-ĕts] {raquitismo} Disease of the skeletal system, usually caused by vitamin D deficiency.

right atrium Upper right chamber of the heart.

right lower quadrant Quadrant on the lower right anterior side of the patient's body.

right upper quadrant Quadrant on the upper right anterior side of the patient's body.

right ventricle Lower right chamber of the heart.

rigidity {rigidez} Stiffness.

rigor [RĬG-ōr] {rigor} Stiffening.

ringworm {tiña} Fungal infection; tinea.

risk factor Any of various factors considered to increase the probability that a disease will occur; for example, high blood pressure and smoking are considered risk factors for heart disease.

rods [rŏdz] {bastoncillos} Specialized receptor cells in the retina that perceive black to white shades.

roentgenology [RĔNT-gĕn-ŎL-ō-jē] Radiology.

root [rūt] Portion of the tooth that lies below the jawline.

root canal Tubular structure holding blood vessels and nerves between the pulp cavity and the jawline.

rosacea [rō-ZĀ-shē-ă] {rosácea} Vascular disease that causes blotchy, red patches on the skin, particularly on the nose and cheeks.

roseola [rō-ZĒ-ō-lă] Skin eruption of small, rosy patches, usually caused by a virus.

rub {roce} Frictional sound heard between heartbeats, usually indicating a pericardial murmur.

rubella [rū-BĔL-ă] {rubéola} Disease that causes a viral skin rash; German measles.

rubeola [rū-BĒ-ō-lă] {rubéola} Disease that causes a viral skin rash; measles.

rugae [RŪ-gē] {rugae} Folds in stomach lining.

S

sacrum [SĀ-krŭm] {sacro} Next-to-last spinal vertebra made up of five fused bones; vertebra that forms part of the pelvis.

sagittal [SĂJ-ĭ-tăl] **plane** Imaginary line that divides the body into right and left portions.

saliva [să-LĪ-vă] {saliva} Fluid secreted by salivary glands; contains amylase.

salivary [SĂL-ĭ-văr-ē] **glands** Glands in the mouth that secrete fluids that aid in breaking down food.

salpingectomy [săl-pĭn-JĔK-tō-mē] {salpingectomía} Removal of a fallopian tube.

salpingitis [săl-pĭn-JĪ-tĭs] {salpingitis} Inflammation of the fallopian tubes.

salpingotomy [săl-pĭng-GŎT-ō-mē] Incision into the fallopian tubes.

saphenous [să-FĒ-nŭs] **vein** Any of a group of veins that transport deoxygenated blood from the legs.

sarcoidosis [săr-kŏy-DŌ-sĭs] {sarcoidosis} Inflammatory condition with lesions on the lymph nodes and other organs.

sarcoma [săr-KŌ-mă] Relatively rare tumor that originates in muscle, connective tissue, and lymph.

scabies [SKĀ-bēz] {sarna} Skin eruption caused by a mite burrowing into the skin.

scale {escala, costra} Small plate of hard skin that falls off.

scalpel [SKĂL-pl] Knife used in surgery or dissection.

scan Image obtained from the interior of the body.

scapula [SKĂP-yū-lă] {escápula} Large flat bone that forms the shoulder blade.

Schick [shĭk] **test** Test for diphtheria.

schizophrenia [skĭz-ō-FRĒ-nē-ă] Condition with recurring psychosis, often with hallucinations.

sciatica [sī-ĂT-ĭ-kă] {ciática} 1. Pain in the lower back, usually radiating down the leg, from a herniated disk or other injury or condition. 2. Inflammation of the sciatic nerve.

scirrhous [SKĬR-ŭs] Hard, densely packed.

sclera (*pl.*, **sclerae**) [SKLĒR-ă (SKLĒR-ē)] {esclerótica} Thick, tough membrane in the outer eye layer; supports eyeball structure.

scleritis [sklĕ-RĪ-tĭs] {escleritis} Inflammation of the sclera.

scleroderma [sklĕr-ō-DĔR-mă] {esclerodermia} Thickening of the skin caused by an increase in collagen formation.

scoliosis [skō-lē-Ō-sĭs] {escolisis} Abnormal lateral curvature of the spinal column.

scotoma [skō-TŌ-mă] {escotoma} Blind spot in vision.

scratch test Test for allergic sensitivity in which a small amount of antigen is scratched onto the surface of the skin.

scrotum [SKRŌ-tŭm] {escroto} Sac outside the body containing the testicles.

sebaceous [sĕ-BĀ-shŭs] **cyst** Cyst containing yellow sebum.

sebaceous [sĕ-BĀ-shŭs] **glands** Glands in the dermis that open to hair follicles and secrete sebum.

seborrhea [sĕb-ō-RĒ-ă] {seborrea} Overproduction of sebum by the sebaceous glands.

sebum [SĒ-bŭm] {sebo} Oily substance, usually secreted into the hair follicle.

second bicuspid Fifth tooth from the median of the jawline.

second molar Second to last tooth at the back of the mouth.

secondary hypertension Hypertension having a known cause, such as kidney disease.

secondary teeth Permanent teeth.

second-degree burn Moderately severe burn that affects the epidermis and dermis; usually involves blistering.

sedative [SĔD-ă-tĭv] Agent that relieves feelings of agitation.

sedimentation rate (SR) *See* erythrocyte sedimentation rate.

sella turcica [SĔL-ă TŬR-sĭ-kă] {silla turcica} Bony depression in the sphenoid bone where the pituitary gland is located.

semen [SĒ-mĕn] {semen} Thick, whitish fluid containing spermatozoa and secretions from the seminal vesicles, Cowper's glands, and prostate; ejaculated from the penis.

semen analysis Observation of semen for viability of sperm.

semicircular canals Structures in the inner ear important to equilibrium.

semilunar [sĕm-ē-LŪ-năr] **valve** One of the two valves that prevent the backflow of blood flowing out of the heart into the aorta and the pulmonary artery.

seminoma [sĕm-ĭ-NŌ-mă] Malignant tumor of the testicle.

sensory receptors Specialized tissue containing cells that can receive stimuli.

sensory [SĔN-sō-rē] **system** Body system that includes the eyes and ears and those parts of other systems involved in the reactions of the five senses; organs or tissue that perceive and receive stimuli from outside or within the body.

septal defect Congenital abnormality consisting of an opening in the septum between the atria or ventricles.

septoplasty [SĔP-tō-plăs-tē] {septoplastia} Surgical repair of the nasal septum.

septostomy [sĕp-TŎS-tō-mē] {septostomía} Creation of an opening in the nasal septum.

septum (*pl.*, **septa**) [SĔP-tŭm (SĔP-tă)] {tabique} 1. Partition between the left and right chambers of the heart. 2. Cartilaginous division, as in the nose or mediastinum.

sequestrum [sĕ-KWĔS-trŭm] {secuestro} Piece of dead tissue or bone separated from the surrounding area.

serum [SĒR-ŭm] {suero} The liquid left after blood has clotted.

serum calcium Test for calcium in the blood.

serum creatine phosphokinase [KRĒ-ă-tēn fŏs-fō-KĪ-năs] Enzyme active in muscle contraction; usually phosphokinase is elevated after a myocardial infarction and in the presence of other degenerative muscle diseases.

serum enzyme tests Laboratory tests performed to detect enzymes present during or after a myocardial infarction; cardiac enzyme studies.

serum phosphorus [FŎS-fōr-ŭs] Test for phosphorus in the blood.

sesamoid [SĔS-ă-mŏyd] **bone** Bone formed in a tendon over a joint.

sessile [SĔS-īl] **polyp** Polyp that projects upward from a broad base.

shin [shĭn] {espinilla} Anterior ridge of the tibia.

shingles [SHĬN-glz] {culebrilla} Viral disease affecting the peripheral nerves and caused by herpes zoster.

short bones Square-shaped bones with approximately equal dimensions on all sides.

sialoadenitis [SĪ-ă-lō-ăd-ĕ-NĪ-tĭs] Inflammation of the salivary glands.

sight {vista} Ability to see.

sigmoid [SĬG-mŏyd] **colon** S-shaped part of large intestine connecting at the bottom to the rectum.

sigmoidoscopy [SĬG-mŏy-DŎS-kō-pē] {sigmoidoscopia} Examination of the sigmoid colon using a sigmoidoscope.

silicosis [sĭl-ĭ-KŌ-sĭs] Lung condition caused by silica dust from grinding rocks or glass or other materials used in manufacturing.

simple fracture Fracture with no open skin wound.

singultus [sĭng-GŬL-tŭs] {singulto} Hiccuping.

sinoatrial [sī-nō-Ā-trē-ăl] **(SA) node** Region of the right atrium containing specialized tissue that sends electrical impulses to the heart muscle, causing it to contract.

sinus [SĪ-nŭs] {seno} 1. Hollow cavity, especially either of two cavities on the sides of the nose. 2. Space between the lactiferous ducts and the nipple.

sinusitis [sī-nū-SĪ-tĭs] {sinusitis} Inflammation of the sinuses.

sinusotomy [sĭn-ū-SŎT-ō-mē] {sinusotomía} Incision of a sinus.

sinus rhythm Normal heart rhythm.

skeleton [SKĔL-ĕ-tŏn] {esqueleto} Bony framework of the body.

skin graft Placement of fresh skin over a damaged area.

SMA (sequential multiple analyzer) Original blood chemistry machine; now a synonym for blood chemistry.

small intestine Twenty-foot long tube that continues the process of digestion started in the stomach; place where most absorption takes place.

smell {olfacción, oler} Ability to perceive odors.

smooth muscle Fibrous muscle of internal organs that acts involuntarily.

social worker Nonmedical professional who is trained as an advocate for people (such as the elderly or children) and may also be trained in the treatment of mental disorders.

sociopathy [SŌ-sē-ŏ-păth-ē] Extreme callous disregard for others.

socket Space in the jawline out of which teeth erupt above the jawline.

soft palate [PĂL-ăt] Soft posterior part of the palate in the mouth; flexible muscular sheet that separates the nasopharynx from the rest of the pharynx.

solid tumor Carcinoma; most common type of tumor.

somatic [sō-MĂT-ĭk] **nervous system** Part of the peripheral nervous system that receives and processes sensory input from various parts of the body.

somatoform [SŌ-mă-tō-fŏrm] **disorders** Mental disorders including physical symptoms that have a psychological base.

somatotrophic [SŌ-mă-tō-TRŌF-ĭk] **hormone (STH)** Hormone secreted by anterior pituitary gland; important in growth and development.

somnambulism [sŏm-NĂM-byū-lĭzm] {sonambulismo} Sleepwalking.

somnolence [SŎM-nō-lĕns] {somnolencia} Extreme sleepiness caused by a neurological disorder.

sonogram [SŎN-ō-grăm] Ultrasound image.

sonography [sŏ-NŎG-ră-fē] {sonografía} Production of images based on the echoes of sound waves against structures.

spasm [spăzm] {espasmo} Sudden, involuntary muscle contraction.

spastic [SPĂS-tĭk] Tending to have spasms.

specific gravity Measurement of the concentration of wastes, minerals, and solids in urine.

SPECT (single photon emission computed tomography) brain scan Brain image produced by the use of radioactive isotopes.

sperm [spĕrm] {esperma} Male sex cell that contains chromosomes.

spermatogenesis [SPĔR-mă-tō-JĔN-ĕ-sĭs] Production of sperm.

spermatozoon(*pl.*, **spermatozoa**) [SPĔR-mă-tō-ZŌ-ŏn (SPĔR-mă-tō-ZŌ-ă)] {espermatozoo} *See* sperm.

spermicide [SPĔR-mĭ-sīd] {espermicida} Contraceptive chemical that destroys sperm; usually in cream or jelly form.

sphenoid [SFĔ-nŏyd] **bone** Bone that forms the base of the skull.

sphenoid sinus Sinus above and behind the nose.

sphygmomanometer [SFĬG-mō-mă-NŎM-ĕ-tĕr] {esfigmomanómetro} Device for measuring blood pressure.

spina bifida [SPĪ-nă BĬF-ĭ-dă] {espina bífida} Congenital defect with deformity of the spinal column.

spinal [SPĪ-năl] **cavity** Body space that contains the spinal cord.

spinal column Column of vertebrae at the posterior of the body, from the neck to the coccyx.

spinal cord Ropelike tissue that sits inside the vertebral column and from which spinal nerves extend.

spinal curvature Abnormal curvature of the spine.

spinal nerves Any of 31 pairs of nerves that carry messages to and from the spinal cord and the torso and extremities.

spinous [SPĪ-nŭs] **process** Protrusion from the center of the vertebral arch.

spirometer [spī-RŎM-ĕ-tĕr] {espirómetro} Testing machine that measures the lungs' volume and capacity.

spleen [splēn] {bazo} Organ of lymph system that filters, stores, and removes blood, and activates lymphocytes.

splenectomy [splĕ-NĔK-tō-mē] {esplenectomía} Removal of the spleen.

splenomegaly [splĕn-ō-MĔG-ă-lē] Enlarged spleen.

splinting {ferulización} Applying a splint to immobilize a body part.

spondylolisthesis [SPŎN-dĭ-lō-lĭs-THĒ-sĭs] {espondilolistesis} Degenerative condition in which one vertebra misaligns with the one below it; slipped disk.

spondylolysis [spŏn-dĭ-LŎL-ĭ-sĭs] {espodilolisis} Degenerative condition of the moving part of a vertebra.

spondylosyndesis [SPŎN-dĭ-lō-sĭn-DĒ-sĭs] {espondilosindesis} Fusion of two or more spinal vertebrae.

sponge {esponja} Polyurethane contraceptive device filled with spermicide and placed in vagina near cervix.

spongy bone Bone with an open latticework filled with connective tissue or marrow.

sprain [sprān] Injury to a joint without dislocation or fracture.

spur [spŭr] Bony projection growing out of a bone; calcar.

sputum [SPŪ-tŭm] **sample or culture** Culture of material that is expectorated (or brought back up as mucus).

squamous cell carcinoma [SKWĂ-mŭs sĕl kăr-sĭn-NŌ-mă] Cancer of the squamous epithelium.

squamous epithelium [SKWĂ-mŭs ĕp-ĭ-THĒ-lē-ŭm] Flat, scaly layer of cells that makes up the epidermis.

stage Degree of tumor spread.

standard precautions Guidelines issued by the Centers for Disease Control for preventing the spread of disease.

stapedectomy [stā-pĕ-DĔK-tō-mĕ] Removal of the stapes to cure otosclerosis.

stapes (*pl.,*** stapes, stapedes)** [STĀ-pēz (STĀ-pĕ-dēz)] {estribo} One of the three auditory ossicles; the stirrup.

staples Metal devices used to suture surgical incisions.

statins [STĂ-tĭnz] A class of lipid-lowering agents that are the most frequently used today.

steatorrhea [STĒ-ă-tō-RĒ-ă] {esteatorrea} Fat in the blood.

stem cell Immature cell formed in bone marrow that becomes differentiated into either a red or a white blood cell.

stenosis [stĕ-NŌ-sĭs] {estenosis} Narrowing, particularly of blood vessels or of the cardiac valves.

stent [stĕnt] Surgically implanted device used to hold something (as a blood vessel) open.

stereotactic [STĔR-ē-ō-TĂK-tĭk] **frame** Headgear worn by patients needing pinpoint accuracy in the treatment of brain anomalies.

stereotaxy [STĔR-ē-ō-TĂK-sē], **stereotactic** [STĔR-ē-ō-TĂK-tĭk] **surgery** Destruction of deep-seated brain structures using three-dimensional coordinates to locate the structures.

sternum [STĔR-nŭm] {esternón} Long, flat bone that forms the midline of the anterior of the thorax.

steroid [STĔR-ŏyd, STĒR-ŏyd] A hormone or chemical substance released by several endocrine glands or manufactured in various medications.

stimulus (*pl.,*** stimuli)** [STĬM-yū-lŭs (STĬM-yū-lī)] {estimulo} Anything that arouses a response.

stomach [STŎM-ăk] {estómago} Large sac between the esophagus and small intestine; place where food is broken down.

stool [stūl] {heces} Feces.

strabismus [stră-BĬZ-mŭs] {estrabismo} Eye misalignment.

strain [strān] {distender} Injury to a muscle as a result of improper use or overuse.

stratified squamous epithelium Layers of epithelial cells that make up the strata of epithelium of the epidermis.

stratum (*pl.,*** strata)** [STRĂT-ŭm (STRĂ-tă)] {estrato} Layer of tissue, especially a layer of the skin.

stratum corneum [KŌR-nē-ŭm] Top sublayer of the epidermis.

stratum germinativum [jĕr-mĭ-NĂT-ĭ-vŭm] Bottom sublayer of the epidermis.

stress test Test that measures heart rate, blood pressure, and other body functions while the patient is exercising on a treadmill.

striae [STRĪ-ē] {estrías} Stretch marks made in the collagen fibers of the dermis layer.

striated [strī-ĀT-ĕd] **muscle** Muscle with a ribbed appearance that is controlled at will.

stridor [STRĪ-dŏr] {estridor} High-pitched crowing sound heard in certain respiratory conditions.

stroke [strōk] {accidente cerebrovascular} *See* cerebrovascular accident (CVA).

sty, stye [stī] {orzuelo} Hordeolum.

styloid [STĬ-lŏyd] **process** Peg-shaped protrusion from a bone.

subcutaneous [sŭb-kyū-TĀ-nē-ŭs] Injected into the fatty layer of tissue beneath the outer layer of skin.

subcutaneous [sŭb-kyū-TĀ-nē-ŭs] **layer** Bottom layer of the skin containing fatty tissue.

subdural [sŭb-DŪR-ăl] **space** Area between the dura mater and the pia mater across which the arachnoid runs.

sublingually [sŭb-LĬNG-gwă-lē] Under the tongue.

subluxation [sŭb-lŭk-SĀ-shŭn] {subluxación} Partial dislocation, as between joint surfaces.

sudden infant death syndrome (SIDS) Death of an infant, usually while sleeping, of unknown cause.

sulcus (*pl.*, **sulci**) [SŬL-kŭs (SŬL-sī)] {surco} Groove or furrow in the surface of bone; *see* fissure.

superficial [sū-pĕr-FĬSH-ăl] At or near the surface (of the body).

superior [sū-PĒR-ē-ōr] Above another body structure.

superior lobe Topmost lobe of each lung.

superior vena cava Large vein that transports blood collected from the upper part of the body to the heart.

supine [sū-PĪN] Lying on the spine facing upward.

suppository [sū-PŎZ-ĭ-tōr-ē] {supositorio} Drug mixed with a semi-solid melting substance meant for administration by insertion into the vagina, rectum, or urethra.

suppressor [sū-PRĔS-ōr] **cell** T cell that suppresses B cells and other immune cells.

suprarenal [SŪ-pră-RĒ-năl] **gland** Adrenal gland.

surgery [SĔR-jer-ē] Removal, transplant, or manipulation of tissue.

surgical scissors Scissors used for cutting and dissecting tissue during surgery.

suture [SŪ-chūr] {sutura} Joining of two bone parts with a fibrous membrane.

suture [SŪ-chūr] **needles** Needles used in closing surgical wounds by sewing.

sweat glands Coiled glands of the skin that secrete perspiration to regulate body temperature and excrete waste products.

sweat test Test for cystic fibrosis that measures the amount of salt in sweat.

sympathetic [sĭm-pă-THĔT-ĭk] **nervous system** Part of the autonomic nervous system that operates when the body is under stress.

sympathomimetic [SĬM-pă-thō-mĭ-MĔT-ĭk] {simpatomimético} Mimicking functions of the sympathetic nervous system.

symphysis [SĬM-fĭ-sĭs] {sinfisis} Type of cartilaginous joint uniting two bones.

synapse [SĬN-ăps] {sinapsis} Space over which nerve impulses jump from one neuron to another.

synarthrosis [SĬN-ăr-THRŌ-sĭs] {sinartrosis} Fibrous joint with no movement.

syncope [SĬN-kō-pē] {síncope} Loss of consciousness due to a sudden lack of oxygen in the brain.

syndrome of inappropriate ADH (SIADH) Excessive secretion of antidiuretic hormone.

synovectomy [sĭn-ō-VĔK-tō-mē] {sinovectomía} Removal of part or all of a joint's synovial membrane.

synovial [sĭ-NŌ-vē-ăl] **fluid** Fluid that serves to lubricate joints.

synovial joint A joint that moves.

synovial membrane Connective tissue lining the cavity of joints and producing the synovial fluid.

syphilis [SĬF-ĭ-lĭs] {sífilis} Sexually transmitted infection.

syringe [sĭ-RĬNJ] {jeringa} Instrument used for injection or withdrawal of fluids.

system [SĬS-tĕm] Any group of organs and ancillary parts that work together to perform a major body function.

systemic lupus erythematosus (SLE) Most severe form of lupus, involving internal organs.

systole [SĬS-tō-lē] {systole} Contraction phase of the heartbeat.

T

tachycardia [TĂK-ĭ-KĂR-dē-ă] {taquicardia} Heart rate greater than 100 beats per minute.

tachypnea [tăk-ĭp-NĒ-ă] {taquipnea} Abnormally fast breathing.

talipes calcaneus [TĂL-ĭ-pēz kăl-KĀ-nē-ŭs] Deformity of the heel resulting from weakened calf muscles.

talipes valgus [VĂL-gŭs] Foot deformity characterized by eversion of the foot.

talipes varus [VĂ-rŭs] Foot deformity characterized by inversion of the foot.

target cell Cell with receptors that are compatible with specific hormones.

tarsus, tarsal [TĂR-sŭs, TĂR-săl] **bones** Seven bones of the instep (arch of the foot).

taste Ability to perceive the qualities of ingested matter.

taste buds Organs that sense the taste of food.

taste cells Specialized receptor cells within the taste buds.

Tay-Sachs [TĀ-săks] **disease** Hereditary disease that causes deterioration in the central nervous system and, eventually, death.

T cells Specialized cells that develop in the thymus and are responsible for cellular immunity, and assist with humoral immunity.

tears [tĕrz] {lágrimas} Moisture secreted from the lacrimal glands.

telangiectasia [tĕl-ĂN-jē-ĕk-TĀ-zhē-ă] A permanent dilation of the small blood vessels.

temporal [TĔM-pō-răl] **bone** Large bone forming the base and sides of the skull.

temporal lobe [TĔM-pō-ral lōb] One of the four parts of each hemisphere of the cerebrum.

temporomandibular [TĔM-pō-rō-măn-DĬB-yū-lăr] **joint (TMJ)** Joint of the lower jaw between the temporal bone and the mandible.

temporomandibular [TĔM-pō-rō-măn-DĬB-yū-lăr] **joint (TMJ) dysfunction** Pain in the jawline due to dislocation of the joint.

tendinitis, tendonitis [tĕn-dĭn-ĪT-ĭs] {tendonitis} Inflammation of a tendon.

tendon [TĔN-dŏn] {tendon} Fibrous band that connects muscle to bone or other structures.

tenotomy [tĕ-NŎT-ō-mē] {tenotomía} Surgical cutting of a tendon.

teratoma [tĕr-ă-TŌ-mă] Growth containing several types of tissue and various types of cells.

terminal end fibers Group of fibers at the end of an axon that passes the impulses leaving the neuron to the next neuron.

testicle [TĔS-tĭ-kl] {testículo} See testis.

testis (*pl.*, **testes**) [TĔS-tĭs (TĔS-tēz)], **testicle** [TES-ti-kl] {testículo} Male organ that produces sperm and is contained in the scrotum; one of two male organs that secrete hormones in the endocrine system.

testosterone [tĕs-TŎS-tĕ-rōn] {testosterona} Primary male hormone.

tetany [TĔT-ă-nē] {tetania} Painfully long muscle contraction. Muscle paralysis, usually due to decreased levels of ionized calcium in the blood.

tetralogy of Fallot [fă-LŌ] Set of four congenital heart abnormalities appearing together that cause deoxygenated blood to enter the systemic circulation: ventricular septal-defect, pulmonary stenosis, incorrect position of the aorta, and right ventricular hypertrophy.

thalamus [THĂL-ă-mŭs] {tálamo} One of the four parts of the diencephalon; serves as a sensory relay station.

thalassemia [thăl-ă-SĒ-mē-ă] {talasemia} Hereditary disorder characterized by inability to produce sufficient hemoglobin.

therapeutic drug monitoring (TDM) Taking of regular blood or urine tests to track drug use and effectiveness of medication.

therapeutic massage Stimulates the skin, muscles, and tissue to promote healing.

therapeutic touch The laying on of hands to promote healing.

therapist [THĂR-ă-pĭst] Nonmedical professional trained in the treatment of mental disorders through talk therapy.

third molar Molar furthest from the median of the jawline.

third-degree burn Most severe type of burn; involves complete destruction of an area of skin.

thoracic [thō-RĂS-ĭk] **cavity** Body space above the abdominal cavity that contains the heart, lungs, and major blood vessels.

thoracic [thō-RĂS-ĭk] **surgeon** Surgeon who specializes in surgery of the thorax.

thoracic [thō-RĂS-ĭk] **vertebrae** Twelve vertebrae of the chest area.

thoracocentesis [THŌR-ă-kō-sĕn-TĒ-sĭs] {toracocentesis} Surgical puncture of the chest cavity.

thoracostomy [thŏr-ă-KŎS-tō-mē] {toracostomía} Establishment of an opening in the chest cavity.

thoracotomy [thŏr-ă-KŎT-ō-mē] {toracotomía} Incision into the chest cavity.

thorax [THŌ-răks] {tórax} Part of the trunk between the neck and the abdomen; chest; chest cavity.

throat [thrōwt] {garganta} *See* pharynx.

throat culture Test for streptococcal or other infections in which a swab taken on the surface of the throat is placed in a culture to see if certain bacteria grow.

thrombectomy [thrŏm-BĔK-tō-mē] {trombectomia} Surgical removal of a thrombus.

thrombin [THRŎMB-ĭn] {trombina} Enzyme that helps in clot formation.

thrombocyte [THRŎM-bō-sĭt] {trombocito} Platelet; cell fragment that produces thrombin.

thrombocytopenia [THRŎM-bō-sĭ-tō-PĒ-nē-ă] Bleeding condition with insufficient production of platelets.

thrombolytic [thrŏm-bō-LĬT-ĭk] Agent that dissolves a thrombus; agent that dissolves blood clots.

thrombophlebitis [THRŎM-bō-flĕ-BĪ-tĭs] {tromboflebitis} Inflammation of a vein with a thrombus.

thromboplastin [thrŏm-bō-PLĂS-tĭn] Protein that aids in forming a fibrin clot.

thrombosis [thrŏm-BŌ-sĭs] {trombosis} Presence of a thrombus in a blood vessel.

thrombotic [thrŏm-BŎT-ĭk] **stroke** Stroke caused by a thrombus.

thrombotic [thrŏm-BŎT-ĭk] **occlusion** Narrowing caused by a thrombus.

thrombus [THRŎM-bŭs] {trombo} Blood clot; stationary blood clot in the cardiovascular system, usually formed from matter found in the blood.

thymectomy [thī-MĔK-tō-mē] {timectomía} Removal of the thymus gland.

thymoma [thī-MŌ-mă] {timoma} Tumor of the thymus gland.

thymosin [THĪ-mō-sĭn] {timosina} Hormone secreted by the thymus gland that aids in distribution of thymocytes and lymphoctyes.

thymus [THĪ-mŭs] **gland** Soft gland with two lobes that is involved in immune responses; located in mediastinum; gland that is part of the immune system as well as part of the endocrine system; aids in the maturation of T and B cells.

thyroid [THĪ-rŏyd] **gland** Gland with two lobes located on either side of the trachea; helps control blood calcium levels and metabolic functions.

thyroid cartilage *See* Adam's apple.

thyroid function test or study Test for levels of TSH, T_3, and T_4 in blood plasma to determine thyroid function.

thyroid scan Imaging test for thyroid abnormalities.

thyroidectomy [thī-rŏy-DĔK-tō-mē] {tiroidectomía} Removal of the thyroid.

thyroid-stimulating hormone (TSH) Hormone secreted by anterior pituitary gland; stimulates release of thyroid hormones.

thyrotoxicosis [THĪ-rō-tŏk-sĭ-KŌ-sĭs] Overactivity of the thyroid gland.

thyroxine [thī-RŎK-sĕn, -sĭn] **(T_4)** Compound found in or manufactured for thyroid gland; helps regulate metabolism.

tibia [TĬB-ē-ă] {tibia} Larger of the two lower leg bones.

tic {tic} Twitching movement that accompanies some neurological disorders.

tine [tīn] **test, TB tine** Screening test for tuberculosis in which a small dose of tuberculin is injected into a series of sites within a small space with a tine (instrument that punctures the surface of the skin).

tinea [TĬN-ē-ă] {tiña} Fungal infection; ringworm.

Tinel's [tĭ-NĔLZ] **sign** "Pins and needles" sensation felt when an injured nerve site is tapped.

tinnitus [tĭ-NI-tŭs, TĬ-nĭ-tŭs] {tinnitus} Constant ringing or buzzing in the ear.

tissue [TĬSH-ū] Any group of cells that work together to perform a single function.

tissue-type plasminogen [plăz-MĬN-ō-jĕn] **activator (tPA, TPA)** Agent that prevents a thrombus from forming.

T lymphocytes *See* T cells.

TNM system Tumor, node, metastasis system of categorizing tumors.

tocolytic [tŏ-kō-LĬT-ĭk] **agent** Hormone given to stop labor.

tomography [tō-MŎG-ră-fē] Type of imaging that produces three-dimensional images.

tongue [tŭng] {lengua} Fleshy part of the mouth that moves food during mastication.

tonic-clonic seizure Severe epileptic seizure accompanied by convulsions, twitching, and loss of consciousness.

tonometry [tō-NŎM-ĕ-trē] {tonometría} Measurement of tension or pressure within the eye.

tonsillectomy [TŎN-sĭ-LĔK-tō-mē] {tonsilectomía} Removal of the tonsils.

tonsillitis [TŎN-sĭ-LĪ-tĭs] {tonsillitis} Inflammation of the tonsils.

topical anesthetic Anesthetic applied to the surface of the skin.

topically [TŎP-ĭ-căl-lē] On the surface of the skin.

touch {tacto} Ability to perceive sensation on the skin.

Tourette [tū-RĔT] **syndrome** Neurological disorder that causes uncontrollable speech sounds and tics.

toxicology [tŏk-sĭ-KŎL-ō-jē] {toxicología} Study of harmful effects of drugs.

trabeculectomy [tră-BĔK-yū-LĔK-tō-mē] Removal of part of the trabeculum to allow aqueous humor to flow freely around the eye.

tracer study Image that traces the passage of a radiopharmaceutical through an organ or tissue.

trachea [TRĀ-kē-ă] {tráquea} Airway from the larynx into the bronchi; windpipe.

tracheitis [trā-kē-Ī-tĭs] Inflammation of the trachea.

tracheoplasty [TRĀ-kē-ō-PLĂS-tē] {traqueoplastia} Repair of the trachea.

tracheostomy [TRĀ-kē-ŎS-tō-mē] {traqueostomía} Creation of an artificial opening in the trachea.

tracheotomy [trā-kē-ŎT-ō-mē] {traqueotomia} Incision into the trachea.

traction [TRĂK-shŭn] {tracción} Dragging or pulling or straightening of something, as a limb, by attachment of elastic or other devices.

trade name Name copyrighted by the manufacturer for a particular version of a drug.

traditional Chinese medicine Various practices that promote balance between yin and yang to promote and maintain health.

tranquilizer [TRĂNG-kwĭ-lĭ-zĕr] Medication used to relieve anxiety.

transcranial sonogram [trăns-KRĀ-nē-ăl SŎN-ō-grăm] Brain images produced by the use of sound waves.

transfusion [trăns-FYŪ-zhŭn] {transfusión} Injection of donor blood into a person needing blood.

transient ischemic [ĭs-KĒ-mĭk] **attack** Short neurological incident usually not resulting in permanent injury, but usually signaling that a larger stroke may occur.

transverse plane Imaginary line that intersects the body horizontally.

transverse process Protrusion on either side of the vertebral arch.

tremor [TRĔM-ōr] {tremblor} Abnormal, repetitive muscle contractions.

trephination, trepanation [trĕf-ĭ-NĀ-shŭn, trĕp-ă-NĀ-shŭn] Circular incision into the skull.

trichiasis [trĭ-KĪ-ă-sĭs] Abnormal growth of eyelashes in a direction that causes them to rub on the eye.

tricuspid [trĭ-KŬS-pĭd] **valve** Atrioventricular valve on the right side of the heart.

tricuspid stenosis Abnormal narrowing of the opening of the tricuspid valve.

triglyceride [trĭ-GLĬS-ĕr-ĭd] {triglicérido} Fatty substance; lipid.

trigone [TRĪ-gōn] {trígono} Triangular area at the base of the bladder through which the ureters enter and the urethra exits the bladder.

triiodothyronine [trĭ-Ī-ō-dō-THĪ-rō-nēn] **(T₃)** Thyroid hormone that stimulates growth.

trochanter [trō-KĂN-tĕr] {trocánter} Bony protrusion at the upper end of the femur.

true ribs Seven upper ribs of the chest that attach to the sternum.

tubercle [TŪ-bĕr-kl] {tubérculo} Slight bony elevation to which a ligament or muscle may be attached.

tuberculosis [tū-bĕr-kyū-LŌ-sĭs] {tuberculosis} Acute infectious disease caused by bacteria called bacilli.

tuberosity [TŪ-bĕr-ŎS-ĭ-tē] {tuberosidad} Large elevation in the surface of a bone.

tumor [TŪ-mōr] {tumor} Any mass of tissue; swelling; growth made up of cells that reproduce abnormally.

tylectomy Surgical removal of a localized tumor.

tympanic [tĭm-PĂN-ĭk] **membrane** Eardrum.

tympanitis [tĭm-pă-NĪ-tĭs] Inflammation of the eardrum.

tympanoplasty [TĬM-pă-nō-plăs-tē] Repair of an eardrum.

Type I diabetes Endocrine disorder with abnormally low levels of insulin; also known as insulin-dependent diabetes mellitus (IDDM).

Type II diabetes Disease caused by failure of the body to recognize insulin that is present or by an abnormally low level of insulin; also known as noninsulin-dependent diabetes mellitus (NIDDM); usually adult onset.

U

ulcer [ŬL-sĕr] {úlcera} Open lesion, usually with superficial loss of tissue.

ulcerating [ŬL-sĕr-ā-tĭng] Having open wounds.

ulcerative colitis [kō-LĪ-tĭs] Inflammation of the colon with ulcers.

ulna [ŬL-nă] {ulna} Larger bone of the forearm.

ultrasonography [ŬL-tră-să-sō-NŎG-ră-fē] Use of sound waves to produce images of the interior of a body.

ultrasound [ŬL-tră-sŏwnd] Image resulting from ultrasonography; produced by sound waves.

ultraviolet [ŭl-tră-VĪ-ō-lĕt] **light** Artificial sunlight used to treat some skin lesions.

umbilical [ŭm-BĬL-ĭ-kăl] **cord** Cord that connects the placenta in the mother's uterus to the navel of the fetus during gestation for nourishment of the fetus.

umbilical [ŭm-BĬL-ĭ-kăl] **region** Area of the body surrounding the umbilicus.

undiffferentiated [ŬN-dĭf-ĕr-ĔN-she-ā-tĕd] Lacking a defined cell structure.

upper respiratory infection Infection of all or part of upper portion of respiratory tract.

uptake [ŭp-TĀK] Speed of absorption of a radio-pharmaceutical by a particular organ or body part.

urea [yū-RĒ-ă] {urea} Waste product of nitrogen metabolism excreted in normal adult urine.

uremia [yū-RĒ-mē-ă] {uremia} Excess of urea and other wastes in the blood.

ureter [yū-RĒ-tĕr] {uréter} One of two tubes that conducts urine from the kidney to the bladder.

ureterectomy [yū-rē-tĕr-ĔK-tō-mē] Surgical removal of all or some of a ureter.

ureteroplasty [yū-RĒ-tĕr-ō-plăs-tē] Surgical repair of a ureter.

ureterorrhaphy [yū-rē-tĕr-ŌR-ă-fē] Suturing of a ureter.

urethra [yū-RĒ-thră] {uretra} Tube through which urine is transported from the bladder to the exterior of the body.

urethrogram [yū-RĒ-thrō-grăm] X-ray of the urethra and prostate.

urethropexy [yū-RĒ-thrō-pĕx-ē] Surgical fixing of the urethra.

urethroplasty [yū-RĒ-thrō-plăs-tē] Surgical repair of the urethra.

urethrorrhaphy [yū-rē-THRŌR-ă-fē] Suturing of the urethra.

urethrostomy [yū-rē-THRŌS-tō-mē] Establishment of an opening between the urethra and the exterior of the body.

urethrotomy [yū-rē-THRŎT-ō-mē] Surgical incision of a narrowing in the urethra.

uric [YŪR-ĭk] **acid** Nitrogenous waste excreted in the urine.

uric [YŪR-ĭk] **acid test** Test for acid content in urine; elevated levels may indicate gout.

urinalysis [yū-rĭ-NĂL-ĭ-sĭs] {análisis de orina} Examination of the properties of urine.

urinary [YŪR-ĭ-nār-ē] **bladder** *See* bladder.

urinary [YŪR-ĭ-nār-ē] **system** Body system that includes the kidneys, ureters, bladder, and urethra and helps maintain homeostasis by removing fluid and dissolved waste; body system that forms and excretes urine and helps in the reabsorption of essential substances.

urinary tract infection (UTI) Infection of the urinary tract.

urine [YŪR-ĭn] {orina} Fluid excreted by the urinary system.

urine sugar Test for diabetes; determined by presence of ketones or sugar in urine.

urology [yū-RŎL-ō-jē] {urología} Medical specialty that diagnoses and treats the urinary system and the male reproductive system.

urostomy [yū-RŎS-tō-mē] Establishment of an opening in the abdomen to the exterior of the body for the release of urine.

urticaria [ŬR-tĭ-KĂR-ē-ă] {urticaria} Group of reddish wheals, usually accompanied by pruritus and often caused by an allergy.

uterine [YŪ-tĕr-ĭn] **tube** One of two tubes through which ova travel from an ovary to the uterus.

uterus [YŪ-tĕr-ŭs] {útero} Female reproductive organ; site of implantation after fertilization or release of the lining during menstruation.

uvea [YŪ-vē-ă] {úvea} Region of the eye containing the iris, choroid membrane, and ciliary bodies.

uvula [YŪ-vyū-lă] {uvula} Cone-shaped projection hanging down from soft palate.

V

vaccination [VĂK-sĭ-NĀ-shŭn] {vacunación} Injection of an antigen from a different organism to cause active immunity.

vaccine [VĂK-sēn] {vacuna} Antigen developed from a different organism that causes active immunity in the recipient.

vagina [vă-JĪ-nă] {vagina} Genital canal leading from the uterus to the vulva.

vaginitis [văj-ĭ-NĪ-tĭs] {vaginitis} Inflammation of the vagina.

vagotomy [vă-GŎT-ō-mē] Surgical cutting off of the vagus nerve.

valve [vălv] {válvula} Any of various structures that slow or prevent fluid from flowing backward or forward.

valve replacement Surgical replacement of a coronary valve.

valvotomy [văl-VŎT-ō-mē] Incision into a cardiac valve to remove an obstruction.

valvulitis [văl-vyū-LĪ-tĭs] {valvulitis} Inflammation of a heart valve.

valvuloplasty [VĂL-vyū-lō-PLĂS-tē] {valvuloplastia} Surgical reconstruction of a cardiac valve.

varicella [văr-ĭ-SĔL-ă] {varicela} Contagious skin disease, usually occurring during childhood, and often accompanied by the formation of pustules; chicken pox.

varicocele [VĂR-ĭ-kō-sēl] {varicocele} Enlargement of veins of the spermatic cord.

varicose [VĂR-ĭ-kōs] **vein** Dilated, enlarged, or twisted vein, usually on the leg.

vas deferens [văs DĔF-ĕr-ĕns] Narrow tube through which sperm leave the epididymis and travel to the seminal vesicles and into the urethra.

vascular [VĂS-kyū-lăr] **lesion** Lesion in a blood vessel that shows through the skin.

vasectomy [vă-SĔK-tō-mē] {vasectomía} Removal of part of the vas deferens to prevent conception.

vasoconstrictor [VĀ-sō-kŏn-STRĬK-tōr] Agent that narrows the blood vessels.

vasodilator [VĀ-sō-dĭ-LĀ-tōr] Agent that dilates or widens the blood vessels.

vasopressin [vā-sō-PRĔS-ĭn] Hormone secreted by pituitary gland; raises blood pressure.

vasovasostomy [VĀ-sō-vă-SŎS-tō-mē] {vasovasostomía} Reversal of a vasectomy.

vegetation [vĕj-ĕ-TĀ-shŭn] {vegetación} Clot on a heart valve or opening, usually caused by infection.

vein [vān] {vena} Any of various blood vessels carrying deoxygenated blood toward the heart, except the pulmonary vein.

vena cava (*pl.*, **venae cavae**) [VĒ-nă KĂ-vă (VĒ-nă KĂ-vē)] *See* superior vena cava and inferior vena cava.

venipuncture [VĔN-ĭ-pŭnk-chŭr, VĒ-nĭ-pŭnk-chŭr] {venipuntura} Small puncture into a vein, usually to draw blood or inject a solution; insertion of a needle into a vein, usually for the purpose of extracting a blood sample.

venography [vē-NŎG-ră-fē] {venografía} Viewing of a vein by x-ray after injection of a contrast medium.

ventilators [VĔN-tĭ-lā-tōrz] Mechanical breathing devices.

ventral [VĔN-trăl] At or toward the front (of the body).

ventral [VĔN-trăl] **cavity** Major cavity in the front of the body containing the thoracic, abdominal, and pelvic cavities.

ventral thalamus One of the four parts of the diencephalon; serves as a sensory relay station.

ventricle [VĔN-trĭ-kl] {ventrículo} 1. Either of the two lower chambers of the heart. 2. Cavity in the brain for cerebrospinal fluid.

ventriculogram [věn-TRĬK-yū-lō-grăm] X-ray of a ventricle taken after injection of a contrast medium.

venule [VĔN-yūl, VĒ-nūl] {vénula} A tiny vein connecting to a capillary.

verruca (*pl.*, **verrucae**) [vě-RŪ-kă (vě-RŪ-kē)] Flesh-colored growth, sometimes caused by a virus; wart.

verrucous [vě-RŪ-kōs] {verruga} Wartlike in appearance.

vertebra (*pl.*, **vertebrae**) [VĔR-tě-bră (VĔR-tě-brē)] {vertebra, *pl.*, vertebras} One of the bony segments of the spinal column.

vertebral body Main portion of the vertebra, separate from the arches of the vertebra.

vertebral column Spinal column.

vertigo [VĔR-tĭ-gō, věr-TĬ-gō] {vértigo} Dizziness.

vesicle [VĔS-ĭ-kl] {vesicular} Small, raised sac on the skin containing fluid.

vestibule [VĔS-tĭ-būl] {vestíbulo} Bony chamber between the semicircular canal and the cochlea.

vial [VĪ-ăl] {vial} A small receptacle for holding liquid or pill medications.

villus (*pl.*, **villi**) [VĬL-ŭs (VĬL-ī)] {vellosidad} Tiny, fingerlike projection on the lining of the small intestine with capillaries through which digested nutrients are absorbed into the bloodstream and lymphatic system.

viral meningitis Meningitis caused by a virus and not as severe as pyrogenic meningitis.

virilism [VĬR-ĭ-lĭzm] {virilismo} Condition with excessive androgen production, often resulting in the appearance of mature male characteristics in young.

visceral [VĬS-ěr-ăl] **muscle** Smooth muscle.

visceral pleura [VĬS-ěr-ăl PLŪR-ă] Inner layer of the pleura.

vitamin [VĪT-ă-mĭn] {vitamina} Organic substance found in food.

vitamin D Vitamin important to the formation of bone.

vitiligo [vĭt-ĭ-LĬ-gō] {vitiligo} Condition in which white patches appear on otherwise normally pigmented skin.

vocal cords Strips of epithelial tissue that vibrate and play a major role in the production of sound.

voice box *See* larynx.

voiding (urinating) cystourethrogram [sĭs-tō-yū-RĒ-thrō-grăm] **(VCU, VCUG)** X-ray image made after introduction of a contrast medium and while urination is taking place.

voluntary muscle Striated muscle.

volvulus [VŎL-vyū-lūs] {vólvulo} Intestinal blockage caused by the intestine twisting on itself.

vomer [VŌ-měr] {vómer} Flat bone forming the nasal septum.

von Willebrand's [vŏn WĬL-lě-brăndz] **disease** Hemorrhagic disorder with tendency to bleed from mucous membranes.

vulva [VŬL-vă] {vulva} External female genitalia.

W

wart [wōrt] {varruga} *See* verruca.

Western blot Test primarily used to check for antibodies to HIV in serum.

wheal [hwēl] {roncha} Itchy patch of raised skin.

wheezes [HWĒZ-ěz] {sibilancias} Whistling sounds heard on inspiration in certain breathing disorders, especially asthma.

white blood cell One of the solid parts of blood from stem cells that plays a role in defense against disease; leukocyte.

whitehead [WHĬT-hěd] {punto blanco} Closed comedo that does not contain the dark bacteria present in blackheads.

whooping cough [HOŌP-ĭng kăwf] *See* pertussis.

Wilms' tumor Malignant kidney tumor found primarily in young children; nephroblastoma.

windpipe *See* trachea.

X

xenograft [ZĚN-ō-grăft] {xenoinjerto} *See* heterograft.

x-ray [ěks-rā] High-energy particles of radiation from the interior of a substance.

Z

zygomatic [ZĪ-gō-MĂT-ĭk] **bone** Bone that forms the cheek.

APPENDIX D

Normal Laboratory Values

The table below lists a number of common laboratory tests taken either in normal CBCs (complete blood counts) or a urinalysis or as separate diagnostic tools. Page number references to the text are given so that you may look up the discussion of a particular test in the text.

Abbreviations used in table:

W	women	mol	mole
M	men	l	liter
d	deci	m	milli
g	gram	μ	micro
k	kilo	n	nano
kat	katal (unit of catalytic activity)	p	pico

Note that "normal" values can vary depending on a variety of factors, including the patient's age or gender, time of day test was taken, and so on. In addition, as new medical advances are made, the understanding of what is the best range for some readings has changed. For example, optimal blood pressure readings are now lower than they were ten years ago.

Laboratory Test (page number in text)	Normal Range in US Units	Normal Range in SI Units	To Convert US to SI Units
ALT (Alanine aminotransferase) (475)	W 7-30 units/liter M 10-55 units/liter	W 0.12-0.50 μkat/liter M 0.17-0.92 μkat/liter	x 0.01667
Albumin (314)	3.1–4.3 g/dl	31–43 g/liter	x 10
Alkaline Phosphatase (475)	W 30-100 units/liter M 45-115 units/liter	W 0.5-1.67 μkat/liter M 0.75-1.92 μkat/liter	x 0.01667
Aspartate aminotransferase (475)	W 9-25 units/liter M 10-40 units/liter	W 0.15-0.42 μkat/liter M 0.17-0.67 μkat/liter	x 0.01667
Basophils (400)	0-3% of lymphocytes	0.0-0.3 fraction of white blood cells	x 0.01
Bilirubin – Direct (314)	0.0-0.4 mg/dl	0-7 μmol/liter	x 17.1
Bilirubin – Total (314)	0.0-1.0 mg/dl	0-17 μmol/liter	x 17.1

Laboratory Test (page number in text)	Normal Range in US Units	Normal Range in SI Units	To Convert US to SI Units
Blood pressure (170)	120/80 millimeters of mercury (mmHg). Top number is systolic pressure, when heart is pumping. Bottom number is diastolic pressure when heart is at rest. Blood pressure can be too low (hypotension) or too high (hypertension).		No conversion
Cholesterol, total Desirable Marginal High (182)	<200 mg/dL 200–239 mg/dL >239 mg/dL	<5.17 mmol/liter 5.17–6.18 mmol/liter >6.18 mmol/liter	x 0.02586
Cholesterol, LDL Desirable Marginal High Very high (182)	<100 mg/dL 100–159 mg/dL 160–189 mg/dL >190 mg/dL	<2.59 mmol/liter 2.59–4.14 mmol/liter 4.14–4.89 mmol/liter >4.91 mmol/liter	x 0.02586
Cholesterol, HDL Desirable Moderate Low (heart risk) (182)	>60 mg/dL 40-60 mg/dL <40 mg/dL	>1.55 mmol/liter 1.03–1.55 mmol/liter <1.03 mmol/liter	x 0.02586
Eosinophils (400)	0-8% of white blood cells	0.0–0.8 fraction of white blood cells	x 0.01
Erythrocytes RBC (412)	4.0–6.0 ml (females slightly lower than males)	4.0–6.0 10^{12} /liter	
Glucose, urine (314)	<0.05 g/dl	<0.003 mmol/liter	x 0.05551
Glucose, plasma fasting reading—often in self-test (512)	70–110 mg/dl (nonfasting not to exceed 140 mg/dl)	3.9–6.1 mmol/liter	x 0.05551
Hematocrit (412)	W 36.0%–46.0% of red blood cells M 37.0%–49.0% of red blood cells	W 0.36–0.46 fraction of red blood cells M 0.37–0.49 fraction of red blood cells	x 0.01
Hemoglobin (412)	W 12.0–16.0 g/dl M 13.0–18.0 g/dl	W 7.4–9.9 mmol/liter M 8.1–11.2 mmol/liter	x 0.6206
Leukocytes (WBC) (412)	4.5–11.0x10^3/mm^3	4.5–11.0x10^9/liter	x 10^6
Lymphocytes (401)	16%–46% of white blood cells	0.16–0.46 fraction of white blood cells	x 0.01
Mean corpuscular hemoglobin (MCH) (412)	25.0–35.0 pg/cell	25.0–35.0 pg/cell	No conversion
Mean corpuscular hemoglobin concentration (MCHC) (412)	31.0–37.0 g/dl	310–370 g/liter	x 10

Laboratory Test (page number in text)	Normal Range in US Units	Normal Range in SI Units	To Convert US to SI Units
Mean corpuscular volume (MCV) (412)	W 78–102 μm^3 M 78–100 μm^3 M 78–100 fl	W 78–102 fl	No conversion
Monocytes (401)	4–11% of white blood cells	0.04–0.11 fraction of white blood cells	x 0.01
Neutrophils (400)	45%–75% of white blood cells	0.45–0.75 fraction of white blood cells	x 0.01
Potassium	3.4–5.0 mmol/liter	3.4–5.0 mmol/liter	No conversion
Prostate specific antigen (PSA) (381)	0–2.5 ng/ml		
Serum calcium (131)	8.5–10.5 mg/dl	2.1–2.6 mmol/liter	x 0.25
Sodium	135–145 mmol/liter	135–145 mmol/liter	No conversion
Testosterone, total (morning sample)	W 6–86 ng/dl M 270-1070 ng/dl	W 0.21–2.98 nmol/liter M 9.36-37.10 nmol/liter	x 0.03467
Testosterone, unbound Age 20–40 Age 41–60 Age 61–80	W 0.6–3.1, M 15.0–40.0 pg/ml W 0.4–2.5, M 13.0–35.0 pg/ml W 0.2–2.0, M 12.0–28.0 pg/ml	W 20.8–107.5, M 520–1387 pmol/liter W 13.9–86.7, M 451–1213 pmol/liter W 6.9–69.3, M 416–971 pmol/liter	x 34.67
Triglycerides, fasting Normal Borderline High Very high (182)	40–150 mg/dl 150–200 mg/dl 200–500 mg/dl >500 mg/dl	0.45–1.69 mmol/liter 1.69–2.26 mmol/liter 2.26-–5.65 mmol/liter >5.65 mmol/liter	x 0.01129
Urea, plasma (BUN) (314)	8–25 mg/dl	2.9–8.9 mmol/liter	x 0.357
Urinalysis: pH Specific gravity (312)	5.0–9.0 1.001–1.035	5.0–9.0 1.001–1.035	No conversion
WBC (White blood cells, leukocytes) (412)	4.5–11.0x10^3/mm^3	4.5–11.0x10^9 liter	x 10^6

Table adapted from www.aidsinfonet.org

APPENDIX

E

Medical Terminology Style

Government agencies, national organizations, and educational institutions vary the rules set up for style of medical terminology. One area with great variation is the spelling of *eponyms*, terms derived from proper names. For example, Alzheimer's disease was named after Alois Alzheimer, a German neurologist. Several major organizations (especially the AMA—American Medical Association and AHDI—American Association for Healthcare Documentation Integrity) have decided to simplify eponyms by dropping the apostrophe S, so that Alzheimer's disease is known by some as Alzheimer disease. The national charitable organizations and the governmental health organizations currently retain the use of the possessive.

The list below shows examples of medical eponyms in the two different styles.

U. S. Government	AMA and AHDI
Alzheimer's disease	Alzheimer disease
Babinski's reflex	Babinski reflex
Bartholin's glands	Bartholin glands
Bell's palsy	Bell palsy
Cooley's anemia	Cooley anemia
Cushing's syndrome	Cushing syndrome
Fontan's operation	Fontan operation
Meniere's disease	Meniere disease
non-Hodgkin's lymphoma	non-Hodgkin lymphoma
Parkinson's disease	Parkinson disease
Raynaud's phenomemon	Raynaud phenomenon
Tinel's sign	Tinel sign
Wilm's tumor	Wilm tumor

For the name of the disease, structure, condition, and so on, the initial capital remains style. However, for words derived from eponyms, some organizations recommend the use of lowercase; for example, *parkinsonian symptom*.

Photo Credits

Index

A

a-, 24
aa, 657
AA, 622
AAMR, 622
AAMT, 5
A/G, 297
AB, 338
ab-, abs-, 24
abbreviations, 21, 74, 126, 169, 219–220,
    262, 297, 338, 363, 391, 423, 454,
    495, 534–535, 575, 607–608, 622,
    636, 657–658
abdomin(o), 51
abdominal cavity, 41
abdominal hysterectomy, 348
abdominal sonogram, 304
abdominal ultrasonography, 456
abdominocentesis, 466, 468
abducens, 255
abduction, 113
ABG, 219
abnormal growths in the nervous
    system, 270
abnormalities in the female cycle, 343
abortifacient, 350, 351
abortion, 342, 345, 347
abruptio placentae, 342, 345
abscess, 81, 84, 640
absence seizure, 270, 272
absorb, 653
absorption, 439, 447
a.c., 657
acanth(o), 7
acanthoid, 7
acc., 534
accessory organ, 325
accessory, 255
accommodation, 525
ACE inhibitors, 194, 196
acetabul(o), 51, 123
acetabulectomy, 51, 123
acetabulum, 111, 115
acetone, 306
acetylcholine, 251, 256
AcG, 169
Ach, 251, 262
achalasia, 459, 462
acidosis, 504, 506
acne, 81, 84
    treatment of, 89
acne vulgaris, 81, 84

acquired active immunity, 418, 420
acquired immunodeficiency
    syndrome, 426, 429
acquired passive immunity, 419, 420
acromi(o), 123
acromion, 110, 115
acromioscapular, 123
ACTH, 486, 490, 495
actin(o), 7
actinic keratosis, 83, 84
actinotherapy, 7
acoustic neuroma, 541
acromegaly, 500, 506
acupuncture, 666, 670
acute lymphocytic leukemia, 399
acute myelogenous leukemia, 398
ad, 657
a.d., 657
ad-, 24
-ad, 27
AD, 534, 657
Adam's apple, 211, 213, 485, 489
ADD, 618, 622
addict, 617, 619
addictive, 646
Addison's disease, 504, 506
adduction, 113
aden(o), 51, 422, 495
adenectomy, 509, 510
adenocarcinoma, 422, 581
adenohypophysis, 485, 486, 489
adenoid(o), 218
adenoidectomy, 218, 234, 235
adenoiditis, 227, 229
adenoma, 503, 581
adenopathy, 495
ADH, 297, 486, 490, 495
adip(o), 51, 73
adipose, 67, 69
adipose tissue, 326
ad lib, 657
adolescence, 557, 559, 562
adren(o), adrenal(o), 51, 495
adrenal cortex, 486, 487, 489
adrenal disorders, 503–504
adrenalectomy, 509, 510
adrenal gland, 483, 487–488, 489
adrenaline, 490
adrenal medulla, 486, 488, 490
adrenocorticotropic hormone,
    486, 490
adrenogenital syndrome, 504

adrenomegaly, 495
adult ADD, 618
adulthood, 559
    diseases of, 563
adult respiratory distress syndrome, 228
advanced directive, 560
aer(o), 7
aerogen, 7
aerotitis media, 541
AF, 169
AFB, 219
afferent neuron, 251, 256
AFP, 338, 577
afterbirth, 331, 332
agglutin(o), 390
agglutination, 386, 387
agglutinogen, 386, 387
agglutinogenic, 390
aggressiveness, 616, 619
agitation, 616, 619
AGN, 297
agnosia, 269, 272
agranulocyte, 384, 387
AH, 338
AIDS, 344, 423, 426–427, 429
AIH, 363
airway, 209
alanine transaminase, 456
albinism, 81, 84
albumin, 303, 306, 379, 387
albuminuria, 309, 310
alcohol/substance abuse, 617
aldosterone, 487, 490
alge, algesi, algio, algo, 7
-algia, 27
algospasm, 7
alimentary canal, 439, 447
A-K, 126
alkaline phosphatase, 457
ALL, 399, 423, 575
allergen, 76, 428, 429
allergy, 428, 429
allograft, 91, 92
alopecia, 68, 69, 598
alopecia areata, 83, 84
alpha cell, 488
alphafetoprotein test, 577
alpha-hydroxy acid, 95
alpha ray, 594
ALS, 262, 269, 272
ALT, 454, 456
alternative medical system, 666–667, 670

alternative medicine, 665-666, 670
  coding in, 669
  manipulation and body-based
      methods of, 668–669
  terms in, 665–670
alveol(o), 51, 218
alveolar, 578, 579
alveolitis, 51, 218
alveolus (*pl.*, alveoli), 212, 213
Alzheimer's disease, 269, 272
AM, 656
AMA, 5, 665
amalgam, 637, 640
ambi-, 24
ambivalence, 616, 619
ambulatory, 603
amenorrhea, 343, 345
American Psychiatric Association, 616
amino acid, 251, 441, 448
AML, 398, 423, 575
amnesia, 270, 272
amni(o), 336
amniocentesis, 336, 347, 349, 606
amnion, 331, 332
amniotic fluid, 332
amphiarthrosis (*pl.*, amphiarthroses), 111, 115
amputation, 142, 143
amyl(o), 7
amylase, 441, 447, 448
amylophagia, 7
amyotrophic lateral sclerosis, 269, 272
an(o), 452
an-, 24
ana-, 24
anabolic steroid, 114, 371
anacusis, 541
anal canal, 440, 446, 448
anal fistula, 461, 462
anal fistulectomy, 467, 468
analgesic, 145, 146, 278, 279, 316, 649, 653
anaphylaxis, 429
anaplasia, 570, 572
anaplastic, 578, 579
anastomosis, 190, 191, 467, 468
andr(o), 362
andro, 7
androblastoma, 7
androgen, 487, 490
andropathy, 362
anemia, 28, 397, 399
anesthetic, 94, 95, 278, 279, 649, 653
  given generally, 278, 279
  given locally, 278, 279
aneurysm, 181, 183, 272
angi(o), 51, 168
angina, 181, 183
angina pectoris, 181, 183
angiocardiogram, 173
angiocardiography, 173, 176
angiogram, 168, 173
angiography, 173, 176, 595
angioplasty, 190, 191
angioscopy, 190, 191
angiotensin converting enzyme inhibitor, 195, 196
anisocytosis, 398, 399
ankle, 111, 115

ankyl(o), 123
ankyloglossia, 459, 462
ankylosis, 123, 134, 136
anoplasty, 452
anorchia, 365, 367
anorchism, 365, 367
anorexia, 459
anorexia nervosa, 459, 462, 617, 619
anovulation, 343, 345
antacid, 470, 471, 649, 653
ante-, 24
anteflexion, 343, 345
anterior, 44, 48
anterior chamber, 525
anthracosis, 229
anti-, 24
antianemic, 649
antianginal, 195, 196, 649
antianxiety agent, 625, 626, 649
antiarrhythmic, 194, 196, 649
antibacterial, 24, 93, 94, 95, 649, 653
antibiotic, 93, 95, 315, 316, 649, 653
antibiotic ophthalmic solution, 547
antibody, 386, 420
anticholinergic, 649
anticlotting, 195, 196
anticoagulant, 195, 196, 403, 404, 649
anticonvulsant, 278, 279, 649
antidepressant, 625, 626, 649
antidiabetic, 649, 653
antidiarrheal, 470, 471, 649
antidiuretic, 315, 316
antidiuretic hormone, 484, 486, 490
antidote, 647, 653
antiemetic, 470, 471, 649
antifungal, 93, 94, 95, 650, 653
antigen, 76, 386, 420
antiglobulin test, 395
antihistamine, 93, 94, 95, 650, 653
antihyperglycemic, 511, 512
antihypertensive, 194, 195, 196, 650
antihypoglycemic, 511, 512, 513
anti-infective, 648, 649, 653
anti-inflammatory, 93, 94, 95, 145, 146, 650
antineoplastic, 650
antiparkinson, 650
antiplatelet, 195
antipruritic, 94, 95
antipsychotic, 625, 626, 650
antipyretic, 650
antiseptic, 93, 95
antisocial, 618
antispasmodic, 316, 470, 471
antitoxin, 419, 420
antitubercular, 650, 653
antitussive, 237, 238, 650
antiulcer, 650
antiviral, 650, 653
anuria, 297, 309, 310
anus, 325, 328, 446, 448, 461
anxiety, 616, 619
anxiety disorder, 616
aort(o), 51, 168
aorta, 157, 158, 160, 163
aortic regurgitation, 182, 183
aortic stenosis, 181, 183
aortic valve, 156, 157, 158, 160

aortitis, 51, 168
aortogram, 173
aortography, 173, 176
A&P, 219
AP, 219
APA, 622
apex, 212, 214
Apgar score, 558, 560
aphagia, 459, 462
aphakia, 540, 541
aphasia, 30, 271, 272
aplastic anemia, 397
apnea, 226, 229
apo-, 24
apocrine gland, 69
apoptosis, 569, 572
append(o), appendic(o), 51, 452
appendage, 445, 448
appendectomy, 28, 466–467, 468, 606
appendicitis, 51, 452, 460, 462
appendicular, 105
appendix, 444, 445, 448
apraxia, 269, 272
APTT, 391
aqueous humor, 525, 526
arachnoid, 254, 256
ARD, 219
ARDS, 219, 228
areola, 327, 332
ARF, 219, 297
ARMID, 545
arrhythmias, 179, 183
ARRT, 593
arteri(o), arter(o), 51, 168
arterial blood gases, 223, 224
arteriogram, 173
arteriography, 173, 176, 595
arteriol(o), 51
arteriole, 159, 163, 291
arteriosclerosis, 51, 168, 183, 271
arteriotomy, 190, 191
arteritis, 181, 183
artery, 156–159, 161, 163, 379
arthr(o), 51, 123
arthralgia, 51, 134, 136
arthritis, 135, 136
arthrocentesis, 142, 143
arthrodesis, 28, 143, 143
arthrogram, 123
arthrography, 129, 130, 595
arthroplasty, 142, 143
arthroscopy, 129, 130
articular cartilage, 106, 115
articulation, 111, 115
artificial insemination, 331
AS, 169, 534, 657
asbestosis, 229, 230
ascending colon, 446
ascites, 461, 462
ASCVD, 169
ASD, 169
ASHD, 169
aseptic, 603, 604
aspartate transaminase, 456
aspartic acid, 251
aspermia, 366, 367
aspirate, 210

cerebrum, 252–253, 257
cerumen, 69, 526
cerumen impacion, 541
ceruminous gland, 69
cerumin(o), 533
ceruminolytic, 533
cervic(o), 52, 123, 336
cervical, 255
cervical os, 326
cervical polyps, 343
cervical vertebrae, 110, 115
cervicitis, 336, 343, 345
cervicodynia, 52, 123
cervix, 325, 326, 328, 332
cesarean section, 556, 560
chalazion, 540, 542
chambers, 525
chancroid, 366, 367
CHD, 169
cheek, 441, 448
cheil(o), chil(o), 52
cheilitis, 459, 462
cheiloplasty, 466, 468
chem(o), 7, 656
chemical digestion, 439
chemical phase, 302
chemical test of a stool specimen, 456
chemistry profile, 393, 396
chemolysis, 7
chemotherapy, 93, 95, 586, 656
cherry angioma, 79, 80, 85
Cheyne-Stokes respiration, 226, 230
CHF, 169
chicken pox, 80
childhood, 562
chir(o), 52
chiropractic, 668, 670
chiropractor, 129, 130
chlamydia, 344, 345
chloasma, 81, 85
chlor(o), 7
chloruresis, 7
choking, 442
chol(e), cholo, 52, 452
cholangi(o), 452
cholangiogram, 452, 456
cholangiography, 456, 457, 595
cholangitis, 460, 462
choleic, 452
cholecyst(o), 452
cholecystectomy, 452, 467, 468
cholecystitis, 460, 462
cholecystogram, 456
cholecystography, 456, 457, 595
choledoch(o), 452
choledocholithiasis, 460
choledocholithotomy, 466, 468
choledochotomy, 452
cholesteatoma, 541, 542
cholesterol, 175, 177
cholelithiasis, 460, 462
cholelithotomy, 466, 468
cholelithotripsy, 466, 468
chondrio, chondr(o), 7, 52, 123
chondrocyte, 7
chondromalacia, 135, 136
chondroplasty, 123

chondrosarcoma, 581
chore(o), 7
choreoathetosis, 7
chorion, 331, 332
choroid, 524, 526, 529
chrom, chromat, chromo, 7
chromatogenous, 7
chromosomes, 38, 360
chronic bronchitis, 227, 228, 230
chronic lymphocytic leukemia, 399
chronic myelogenous leukemia, 399
chronic obstructive pulmonary
       disease, 228, 230
chronic pneumonia, 229
chrono, 7
chronometry, 7
chyl(o), 8
chylopoiesis, 8
chym(o), 8
chyme, 444, 448
chymopoiesis, 8
cicatrix, 80, 85
-cidal, 27
-cide, 27
cilia, 210, 214
ciliary body, 524, 526, 529
cine(o), 8, 606
cineradiography, 8, 593, 599, 606
circum-, 24
circumcision, 368, 370
cirrhosis, 460, 462
CIS, 338
clamp, 603, 604
-clasis, 28, 606
-clast, 28, 606
claudication, 180, 184
claustrophobia, 27, 622
claustrophobic, 27
clavicle, 110, 115
climacteric, 331, 332
clitoris, 325, 327, 328, 332
CLL, 399, 423, 575
closed, 602, 604
closed fracture, 133, 136
closed head trauma, 268
closed reduction, 142
clotting, 378, 380, 385, 403
CML, 399, 423, 575
CMV, 423
CNS, 252, 262
CO, 169, 174
CO(2), 159, 163
co-, col-, com-, con-, cor-, 24
coagulant, 403, 404
coagulation, 378, 380, 387
coarctation of the aorta, 181, 184
coccygeal, 255
coccyx, 110, 116, 255
cochle(o), 533
cochlea, 527, 528, 529
cochleovestibular, 533
coitus, 331, 332
coitus interruptus, 370
col(o), colon(o), 52, 452
cold sore, 81, 85
COLD, 219
colectomy, 467, 468

collagen, 67, 70
Colles' fracture, 133, 136
colectomy, 452, 467, 468
colic, 461, 462
colitis, 460, 463
colon, 446, 448, 467
colonic polyposis, 461
colonoscopy, 456, 457, 458
colorectal cancer, 461
colostomy, 468, 469, 607
colp(o), 52, 337
colporrhagia, 337
colposcope, 340
colposcopy, 340, 341
coma, 268, 273
combining forms, 6–13
comedo (pl., comedos, comedones), 82, 85
comminuted fracture, 133, 136
common bile duct, 447
comp., 657
compact bone, 106, 116
complementary medicine, 665, 670
     coding in, 669
     manipulation and body-based
          methods of, 668–669
     terms in, 665–670
complete blood count, 394, 396
complex fracture, 133, 137
complicated fracture, 133, 137
compound fracture, 133, 137
compression fracture, 133, 137
computed tomography, 129, 595, 599
computerized (axial)
          tomography, 265, 595, 599
concussion, 268, 273
condom catheter, 301, 306
condom, 330, 332, 370
conduction system, 160–161, 164
conductive hearing loss, 541
conductive tissue, 160
conductivity, 250, 257
condyl(o), 123
condyle, 107, 116
condylectomy, 123
condyloma, 343, 345
cone, 525, 529
connective tissue, 39, 42
congenital disorders, 268
congenital heart condition, 183
congenital heart disease, 183, 184
congenital hypothyroidism, 502
congestive heart failure, 182, 184
coni(o), 8
coniometer, 8
conization, 347, 349
conjunctiv(o), 533
conjunctiva, 524, 529, 540
conjunctivitis, 540, 542
conjunctivoplasty, 533
constipation, 461, 463, 470
constriction, 180, 184
contact lens, 539, 542
contra-, 24
contraception, 330, 332
contracture, 134, 137
contraindicated, 647, 653
contrast medium, 595

conventional medicine, 665
convolution, 252, 253, 257
Cooley's anemia, 398
Coombs' test, 395
COPD, 219, 228
copulation, 331, 332
cor(o), core(o), 52, 533
cordotomy, 277
coreoplasty, 533
corium, 66–67, 70
corn, 83, 85
corne(o), 533
cornea, 524, 526, 529
corneal transplant, 545
corneoscleral, 533
coronal plane, 45, 48
coronary, 182
coronary angioplasty, 190, 191
coronary artery, 157
coronary artery disease, 181, 184, 195
coronary bypass surgery, 190, 191
coronary circulation, 157–158
corpus callosum, 253, 257
corpus luteum, 329, 332
cortex, 291, 292, 294
cortic(o), 52
corticosteroid, 94, 95, 145, 146, 490
corticosterone, 486
cortisol, 487, 490
cosmesis, 91
cosmetic, 602, 604
cost(o), costi, 52, 123
costiform, 123
Cowper's glands, 359, 360
CP, 262
CPK, 169, 176
CPR, 169, 219
crackles, 226, 230
crani(o), 53, 123, 261
cranial cavity, 40, 42
cranial nerve, 255, 257
craniectomy, 277
craniofacial, 261
craniotomy, 123, 277
cranium, 253, 257
creatine phosphokinase, 176
creatine, 291, 294
creatinine clearance test, 303
creatinine, 291, 294
crepitation, 135, 137
crepitus, 135, 137
crest, 107, 116
cretinism, 502
CRF, 297
CRH, 495
crin(o), 8
-crine, 28
crinogenic, 8
-crit, 28
Crohn's disease, 460, 463
cross-sectional plane, 45, 48
crown, 633, 634
croup, 226, 230
crust, 79, 80, 85
cry(o), 8
cryocautery, 8
cryogenic, 603, 604

cryopexy, 546
cryoretinopexy, 546
cryosurgery, 91, 92, 347, 349, 584
crypt(o), 8
cryptogenic, 8
cryptorchism, 365, 367
CS, 338
C-section, 338
CSF, 253, 257, 262
C-spine, 607
CT, 129, 607
CT scan, 262, 265, 595, 599
CTA, 220
CTS, 126
culdocentesis, 347, 349
culdoscopy, 340, 341
Cushing's syndrome, 503, 506
curet, 603
curettage, 91, 92
curette, 603, 604
cusp, 633, 634
cuspid, 633, 634
cuticle, 68, 70
CVA, 169, 262, 271, 273
CVD, 169, 179, 262
Cx, 338, 657
CXR, 220, 607
cyan(o), 8
cyanopsia, 8
cyanosis, 180, 184
cycl(o), 8, 533
cyclectomy, 8
cyclodialysis, 533
cyst(o), cysti, 8, 53, 296
cyst, 79, 85
cystectomy, 313
cystic, 578, 579
cystic fibrosis, 228, 230
cystic duct, 447
cystitis, 296, 309, 310
cystocele, 309, 310
cystoid, 8
cystolith, 309, 310
cystopexy, 313
cystoplasty, 313
cystorrhaphy, 313
cystoscope, 304, 306
cystoscopy, 304, 306
cyt(o), 8, 53
-cyte, 28
cytoarchitecture, 8
cytomegalovirus, 427
cytoplasm, 38, 572
-cytosis, 28
cytotoxic cell, 419, 420

D

D, 534
D1, 126
dacry(o), 533
D & C, 338, 347
dacryoadenitis, 540, 542
dacryocystectomy, 545, 546
dacryocystitis, 542, 540
dacryolith, 533
dactyl(o), 53, 123

dactylitis, 123
dandruff, 82
DAW, 657
dB, 534
DDS, 636
de-, 24
deafness, 541, 542
death, 557
debridement, 91, 92
decibel, 527, 529
deciduous teeth, 631, 634
decongestant, 237, 238, 650
decubitus ulcers, 80, 85
dedifferentiated, 570, 572
deep, 45, 48
deep vein thrombosis, 180, 184
def, 636
DEF, 636
defecation, 439, 446, 448
defensiveness, 616
degenerative arthritis, 135, 137
degenerative diseases, 269
deglutition, 441, 448
deliriousness, 616, 619
delusional, 616, 619
dementia, 269, 273, 616, 619
dementia symptoms, 616
demyelination, 269, 273
dendrite, 249, 257
densitometer, 129, 130
dent(o), denti, 53, 636
dental assistant, 631
dental care
    terms in, 631–635
dental hygienist, 631
dental practice,
    abbreviations in, 636
    combining forms relating to, 636
    diagnostic pathological, and treatment
        terms relating to, 637–640
    pharmacological terms
        relating to, 641–642
    terms in, 631–645
dental technician, 631
dentilabial, 636
dentin, 633, 634
dentist, 631, 634
dentistry, 631
denture, 638, 640
deoxyribonucleic acid, 571
dependency, 618
depigmentation, 81, 85
depilation, 68
depolarization, 160, 164
depression, 616, 619
derm(o), derma, 53, 74
-derma, 28
dermabrasion, 91, 92
dermat(o), 53, 73
dermatitis, 81, 85
dermatochalasis, 540, 542
dermatology, 76, 77
dermatome, 91
dermis, 66, 67, 70
    inflammation of, 81
dermoid cyst, 343
DES, 338, 575

descending colon, 446
-desis, 28
dextr(o), 8
dextrocardia, 8
di-, dif-, dir-, dis-, 24
dia-, 24
diabetes, 498, 504–505, 506
diabetes insipidus, 501, 506
diabetes mellitus, 501, 507
diabetic nephropathy, 505, 507
diabetic neuropathy, 505, 507
diabetic retinopathy, 505, 507, 540
diacritical marks, 5
diagnostic, 602, 604
*Diagnostic and Statistical Manual of
    Mental Disorders*, 616
diagnostic imaging, 593–598, 599
    abbreviations relating to, 607–608
    combining forms relating to, 606
    suffixes relating to, 606–607
dialysis, 304, 306
diaphoresis, 68, 70
diaphragm, 41, 42, 212, 214, 330, 332
diaphysis, 106, 116
diarrhea, 461, 463, 598
diarthrosis, (*pl.*, diarhtroses), 111, 116
diastole, 160, 164
diencephalon, 253, 257
diff, 391
differential, 382
differentiated, 381, 570, 572
diffuse, 578, 579
digestion, 439, 440, 448
digestive system, 40, 42, 439–481
    abbreviations relating to, 454
    combining forms relating to, 452–454
    diagnostic, procedural, and laboratory
        terms relating to, 455–458
    pathological terms relating to, 458–465
    pharmacological terms
        relating to, 470–471
    structure and function of, 439–451
    surgical terms relating to, 466–469
digital rectal exam, 364, 577
digital subtraction angiography, 174, 177, 595
dil., 657
dilation & curettage, 347
dilator, 603, 604
diopter, 536, 538
diphtheria, 226, 230
diplopia, 540, 542
dips(o), 8
dipsomania, 8
directional terms, 44–45
disc, 657
discoid lupus erythematosus, 81, 85
disk, 109, 116
diskography, 129, 130
dislocation, 134, 137
disp., 657
dissociative disorder, 617, 619
distal, 45, 48
distal epiphysis, 106
distal surface, 633
diuretic, 194, 196, 316, 650
div., 657
diverticula, 461, 463

diverticulitis, 461, 463
diverticulectomy, 467, 469
diverticulosis, 461, 463
DJD, 126
DLE, 74, 81, 85
DM, 495
DNA, 571, 575
DNR, 560
documentation, 18
    chronological method of, 19
    SOAP method of, 18
DOE, 220
dopamine, 251, 269, 273
Doppler ultrasound, 174, 177
dors(o), dorsi, 8
dorsal, 44, 48
dorsal cavity, 40, 42
dorsal vertebrae, 110, 116
dorsalgia, 8
dorsiflexion, 113
double pneumonia, 229
DPT, 219, 227
DRE, 364, 575, 577
drilling, 637, 640
drug, 646–655
drug-eluting stent, 190
druggist, 647, 654
DSA, 169, 174, 595, 607
DSM, 622
DT, 622
DTC, 620
DTR, 126
DUB, 338
ductless gland, 482, 490
ductus arteriosus, 161, 162, 164
ductus venosus, 161, 162, 164
duoden(o), 53, 452
duodenal ulcer, 460, 463
duodenitis, 452
duodenum, 440, 443, 444, 448
dura mater, 254, 257
durable power of attorney, 560
duritis, 270, 273
DVA, 534
DVT, 169
DW, 657
D₅W, 657
dwarfism, 483, 500, 507
dx, 657
dynamo, 8
dynamometer, 8
-dynia, 28
dys-, 25
dyscrasia, 397, 399
dysentery, 461, 463
dysmenorrhea, 343, 345
dyspareunia, 343, 345
dyspepsia, 460, 463
dysphagia, 271, 459, 463
dysphasia, 271, 273
dysphonia, 226, 230
dysplasia, 570, 572, 575, 577
dysplastic, 578, 579
dyspnea, 226, 230
dysrhythmia, 179, 184
dystonia, 135, 137
dysuria, 309, 310

E

ear, 526–528, 529
    diagnosing, 537
    disorders of, 541
eating disorder, 459, 617
EBV, 423
ECC, 338
ECCE, 534
ecchymosis (*pl.*, ecchymoses),
        79, 81, 85
eccrine gland, 69, 70
ECG, EKG, 169, 173
ECHO, 169
echo, 8
echocardiogram, 8, 174
echocardiography, 174, 177, 596
echoencephalography, 265
eclampsia, 342
ECT, 622, 623, 624
ect(o)-, 25
-ectasia, 28
-ectasis, 28
-ectomy, 28, 606
ectopic pregnancy, 342
eczema, 81, 85
EDC, 338
-edema, 28
edema, 309, 310, 540
EEG, 264, 266
EENT, 534
efferent neuron, 251, 257
egg cell, 324, 327
egg nucleus, 327
EGD, 454
EIA, 423, 424, 425
ejaculation, 360
ejaculatory duct, 358, 359
ejection fraction, 174, 177
elbow, 111, 116
electr(o), 8, 606
electrocauterization, 584
electrocardiogram, 8, 173, 174, 606
electrocardiography, 173, 177
electroconvulsive therapy, 623, 624
electrodesiccation, 92
electroencephalogram, 264, 266
electrolyte, 490
electromyogram, 129, 130
electrophoresis, 379, 387
electroshock therapy, 623, 624
elimination, 439, 448
ELISA, 423, 424, 425
elix., 657
elixir, 651
-ema, 28
EMB, 338
embolectomy, 190, 191
embolic stroke, 271, 273
embolus, 180, 184, 271, 273
embryo, 556, 560
emesis, 443, 448
-emesis, 28
EMG, 126
-emia, 28
-emic, 28
emollient, 94, 95

e.m.p., 657
emphysema, 228, 230
empyema, 229, 230
emulsification, 447, 448
enamel, 633, 634
encapsulated, 569, 572
encephal(o), 53, 261
encephalitis, 261, 270, 273
encephalogram, 265, 266
encephalography, 265
end(o)-, 25
endarterectomy, 190, 191
endocarditis, 182, 185
endocardium, 155, 164
endocrine gland, 482, 486, 490
endocrine system, 40, 42, 482–522
    abbreviations relating to, 495
    combining forms relating to, 495
    diagnostic and procedural terms
        relating to, 496–498
    pathological terms relating to, 499–508
    pharmacological terms
        relating to, 511–513
    structure and function of, 482–492
    surgical terms relating to, 509–510
endodontist, 638, 640
endolymph, 527, 529
endometrial cancer, 344
endometriosis, 344, 345
endometrium, 326, 327, 328, 332
endorphin, 251
endoscope, 223, 224
endoscopic, 603
endoscopic retrograde
    cholangiopancreatography, 456
endoscopy, 223
endosteum, 106, 116
endothelium, 156, 164
endotracheal intubation, 235
endovascular surgery, 190, 191
end-stage renal disease, 309, 310
end-to-side anastomosis, 467
energy therapy, 669, 670
ENT, 219, 234, 534
enter(o), 53, 453
enteric-coated, 648, 654
enteritis, 460, 463
enteropathy, 453
enucleation, 545, 546
enuresis, 309, 310
enzyme, 441, 448
enzyme-linked immunosorbent
    assay, 424, 425
eos, 391
eosin(o), 8, 390
eosinopenia, 390
eosinophil, 384, 387
eosinophilia, 399
eosinophilic, 8
epi-, 25
epicardium, 155, 164
epidermis, 66–67, 70
epidermoid, 578, 579
epididym(o), 362
epididymectomy, 368, 370
epididymis, 358, 359, 360
epididymitis, 366, 367

epididymoplasty, 362
epidural hematomas, 268
epidural space, 254, 257
epigastric region, 47, 48
epiglott(o), 218
epiglottis, 210, 214, 442, 449
epiglottitis, 218, 227, 230
epilation, 68
epilepsy, 270, 273
epinephrine, 486, 488, 490
epiphora, 540, 542
epiphyseal plate, 106, 116
epiphysitis, 135, 137
episi(o), 53, 337
episiotomy, 327
epispadias, 365, 366, 367
epistaxis, 227, 231
epithalamus, 253, 257
epithelial tissue, 39, 42
EQ, 622, 624
equilibrium, 526–527, 530
ER, 575
ERCP, 454, 456, 607
ergo, 8
ergograph, 8
erosion, 79, 80, 85
ERT, 338
eructation, 460, 463
erythr(o), 8, 391
erythroblastosis fetalis, 342, 399
erythroclasis, 8
erythrocyte sedimentation rate, 394, 396
erythrocyte, 380, 382, 383, 387, 391
erythrocytopenia, 398
erythropenia, 398, 400
erythropoietin, 383, 387
esophag(o), 453
esophageal reflux, 459
esophageal varices, 459
esophagitis, 459, 463
esophagoplasty, 466, 469
esophagoscope, 456
esophagoscopy, 453, 456, 457
esophagus, 210, 440, 442–443, 449
    disorders of, 459
esotropia, 539, 542
ESR, 391, 394, 396
ESRD, 297, 309, 310
essential hypertension, 180, 185
EST, 615, 622, 623, 624
-esthesia, 28
esthesio, 9
esthesiometry, 9
estrogen, 328, 329, 332
ESWL, 297, 305, 306
ET, 235
ET tube, 219
ethmo, 9
ethmoid bone, 108, 109, 116
ethmoid sinus, 108, 116
ethmonasal, 9
etio, 9
etiopathology, 9
ETT, 169, 173
etymology, 2
eu-, 25
EUD, 301

euphoria, 31, 622
eupnea, 226, 231
eustachian tube, 526, 530
euthanasia, 559, 560
eversion, 132
evoked potential, 264, 266
Ewing's sarcoma, 581
ex-, 25
exanthematous viral diseases, 80, 85
ex aq., 657
excisional biopsy, 583, 584
excitability, 250, 257
excoriation, 79, 80, 85
excrete, 654
excretory system, 290
exenteration, 584
exercise tolerance test, 173
exfoliative biopsy, 584
exhalation, 210, 212, 213, 214
exo-, 25
exocrine gland, 68, 70, 428, 490
exophthalmos, 502, 507, 540, 542
exophthalmus, 540, 542
exostosis, 135, 137
exotropia, 539, 542
expectorant, 237, 238, 650
expiration, 212, 214
ext., 657
extension, 113
external beam machine, 598
external fixation device, 142, 143
external nares, 210, 214
external respiration, 209, 214
external urinary drainage catheter, 301
extra-, 25
extracorporeal circulation, 190
extracorporeal shock wave
    lithotripsy, 305, 306
extracranial MRA, 265
exudate, 76, 77
eye, 524–526, 530
    diagnosing, 535–536
    disorders of, 539–541
eye color, 525
eyebrow, 526, 530
eyelash, 526, 530
eyelid, 526, 530
    conditions of, 540
eyestrain, 539, 542
eyeteeth, 633

F

facial cranial nerve, 255
Factor VIII, 398
failure of the beta cells, 504
fainting, 271, 273
fallopian tubes, 325, 333
false ribs, 110
farsightedness, 539, 542
fasci(o), 123
fascia (pl., fasciae), 114, 116
fasciotomy, 123
fasting blood sugar, 496, 497
fatty acid, 441, 449
FDA, 646, 657
feces, 445, 449

gonadotropin, 495
gonio, 9
goniometer, 9, 129, 130
gonorrhea, 344, 345
GOT, 169, 176
gout, 135, 137
gouty arthritis, 135, 137
gr, 657
graafian follicle, 324, 333
grade, 577, 579
graft, 190, 191
-gram, 29, 606
grand mal seizure, 270, 273
granulo, 9
granulocyte, 384, 388
granulocytosis, 399, 400
granuloma, 9
-graph, 29, 607
-graphy, 29, 607
Graves' disease, 502, 507
gravida, 331, 333, 352
gray, 598, 599
great toe, 142
greenstick fracture, 133, 137
growth hormone, 486, 491
group therapy, 623, 624
gtt, 657
GTT, 342, 495, 497
gums, 441, 449, 631, 634, 635
gy, 598, 599, 607
gyn(o), gyne, gynec(o), 9, 337
gynecologist, 340, 341
gynecology, 337
gynopathy, 9
gyrus (pl., gyri), 252, 253, 257

H

H, 657
h., 657
habitual abortion, 342
hair, 65, 67–68
hair follicle, 66, 67, 70
hair root, 67, 70
hair shaft, 67, 70
hairline fracture, 133, 137
halitosis, 459, 464
hallucinogen, 625
hammer toe, 142
hard palate, 441, 449
hardening of the arteries, 182
HBOT, 219
HCG, 329, 338, 340, 495, 577
HCT, Hct, 391, 395
HD, 297
HDL, 169, 175
healing touch, 669
health care proxy, 560
hearing, 523, 526–527, 530
heart, 155–199
    general diseases of, 181–182
heart attack, 181, 182
heart block, 180, 185
heartburn, 444
heart failure, 182
heart rhythm, 179–180
heart transplant, 190, 191

heel, 111, 117
Heimlich maneuver, 211
helper cell, 419, 420
hem(a), 53
hemangi(o), 168
hemangioma, 168
hematochezia, 461, 464
hematocrit, 380, 388, 395
hematocytoblast, 381, 388
hematemesis, 460, 464
hematopoietic system, 417
hematuria, 310, 311
heme, 383, 388
hemi-, 23, 25
hemiplegia, 23
hemo, hemat(o), 53, 391
hemoccult, 456
hemochromatosis, 398, 400
hemodialysis, 304, 306, 391
hemoglobin, 383, 388, 395, 405
hemolysis, 398, 400
hemolytic anemia, 398
hemophilia, 398, 400
hemoptysis, 228, 231
hemorrhage, 27
hemorrhagic stroke, 271, 273
hemorrhoid, 181, 185, 461, 464
hemorrhoidectomy, 190, 191, 467, 469
hemostatic, 403, 404, 650
hemothorax, 229, 231
heparin, 195, 196, 380, 388
hepat(o), hepatic(o), 53, 453
hepatic duct, 447
hepatic flexure, 446
hepatic lobectomy, 467, 469
hepatic portal system, 447
hepatitis, 453, 460, 464
hepatomegaly, 460, 464
hepatopathy, 460, 464
hernia, 366, 367, 373, 461
herniated disk, 132, 137
herniorrhaphy, 607
herpes simplex virus Type 1, 81, 86
herpes simplex virus Type 2, 81, 86
herpes zoster, 81, 86
herpes, 81, 86
heterograft, 91, 92
heteroplasia, 570, 572
HGB, Hgb, HB, 391, 395
hiatal hernia, 460, 461, 464
hidr(o), 53, 74
high blood pressure, 162, 180, 185, 195
high-density lipoprotein, 175
hilum, 212, 214, 291, 294
hilus, 212, 214
HIPAA (Health Insurance Portability and
    Accountability Act of 1996), 16–17
Hippocrates, 1
Hippocratic oath, 1–2
hirsutism, 504, 507
histamine, 93, 251, 384, 388
histi(o), histo, 53
histiocyte, 428
histiocytic lymphoma, 428, 429
histrionic, 618
HIV, 344, 423, 424, 426, 427
hives, 81, 86

Hodgkin's disease, 428, 429, 582
Hodgkin's lymphoma, 428, 429
Holter monitor, 173, 177
home(o), homo, 9
homeopathic medicine, 666
homeoplasia, 9
homeostasis, 292, 378, 571
homograft, 91, 92
hordeolum, 540, 543
hormone, 324, 328–329, 333, 482,
    486, 491, 648, 654
hormone replacement therapy, 350, 351,
    511, 513, 514–515
hospice, 560
Hospital Formulary, 646
HPV, 343, 344
HRT, 338, 350, 511, 513
h.s., 657
HSG, 338
HSO, 338
HSV, 423
human chorionic gonadotropin, 340, 577
human development, 556–565
    stages of, 556–561
human growth hormone, 512, 513
human immunodeficiency virus, 426, 430
human papilloma virus, 344
humer(o), 124
humeroscapular, 124
humerus, 111, 112, 117
humoral immunity, 418, 420
humoral response, 417
Huntington's chorea, 269, 274
hyaline membrane disease, 228
hydr(o), 9
hydrocele, 366, 367
hydrocephalus, 268, 274
hydrocephaly, 9
hydrochloric acid, 443
hydronephrosis, 309, 311
hymen, 326, 328, 333
hyper-, 25
hyperadrenalism, 503, 507
hyperbilirubinemia, 460, 464
hypercapnia, 226, 231
hyperchromatic, 578, 579
hyperinsulinism, 504
hypermania, 621
hypernephroma, 582
hyperopia, 539, 540, 543
hyperparathyroidism, 503, 507
hyperplasia, 114
hyperplastic, 578, 579
hyperpnea, 226, 231
hypersecretion, 484, 499, 507
hypersensitivity, 429, 430
hypersplenism, 428, 430
hypertension, 180, 185
hypertensive heart disease, 180, 185
hyperthyroidism, 502, 507
hypertrophy, 137
hyperventilation, 226, 231
hypn(o), 9, 621
hypnogenesis, 9
hypnosis, 623, 624
hypnotic, 278, 279, 651
hypo-, 25

microcytosis, 398, 400
microorganism, 10
microphage, 417, 421
microscope, 607
microscopic capillaries, 414
microscopic laser surgery, 545
microscopic phase, 303
microscopy, 607
microsurgery, 545, 606
micturition, 293
midbrain, 252, 258
middle age, 559
middle lobe, 212
midsagittal plane, 45, 252
mind-altering substance, 627
mind-body intervention, 666, 667
mineralocorticoid, 486, 491
minimally invasive, 189, 602, 604
mio, 11
miopragia, 11
miotic, 547, 548
miscarriage, 342, 346
missed abortion, 342
mitochondria, 38
mitosis, 571, 573
mitral insufficiency, 182, 185
mitral reflux, 182, 185
mitral stenosis, 182
mitral valve, 156-157, 164
mitral valve prolapse, 182, 185
mixed-episode disorder, 617, 619
ml, 657
modality, 587
modified radical mastectomy, 348
Mohs' surgery, 603
molar, 634
mon(o)-, 26
mono, 391
monoamine, 251
monocyte, 384
mons pubis, 327, 334
mood disorder, 617
morning-after pill, 351
morph(o), 11
morphology, 11
motile, 358
motor neuron, 250, 251, 257
mouth, 441, 450, 453
  disorders of, 459
MR, 169
MRA, 265, 607
MRI, 129, 174, 265, 596-597, 600, 607
MS, 169, 269, 274
MSH, 486, 491, 495
MUGA, 169, 174, 177, 608
multi-, 26
multip, 338
multiple myeloma, 399, 400
multiple sclerosis, 269, 274
multiple-gated acquisition
    angiography, 174, 177
murmur, 173, 185
muscle, 105, 113–114, 118
muscle relaxant, 145, 146
muscles for breathing, 213
muscle tissue, 39
muscular dystrophy, 135, 138

musculoskeletal system, 40, 105–147
muta, 574
mutagen(o), 574
mutagenic, 574
mutation, 571, 574
mydriatic, 547, 548
MVP, 169
my(o), 55, 124
myalgia, 134, 138
myasthenia gravis, 269, 274
myc(o), 74
mycobacterium avium-intracellulare, 427
myel(o), 55, 124
myelin sheath, 258
myelitis, 274
myeloblast, 398, 400
myelocyst, 124
myelogram, 265, 266
myelography, 129, 130, 596
myeloma, 135, 138
myelomalacia, 261
myocardial infarction, 181, 186
myocarditis, 182, 186
myocardium, 124, 155, 164
myodynia, 134, 138
myoma, 30, 135, 138
myomectomy, 348, 349
myometrium, 327, 334
myopia, 539, 543
myoplasty, 142, 143
myositis, 135, 138
myring(o), 534
myringitis, 534, 541, 543
myringotomy, 546
myxedema, 502, 508

N

n, noct., 657
nail, 55, 68, 70
  health conditions of, 69
NAMH, 622
NARC, 622
narcissism, 618
narco, 11
narcolepsy, 11, 271, 274
narcotic, 145, 146, 274, 279
nas(o), 218, 534
nasal bone, 108, 118
nasal cavity, 118, 215
nasal septum, 210, 215
nasogastric, 218
nasogastric intubation, 457
nasopharyngitis, 227, 231
nasopharyngoscopy, 223, 224
nasopharynx, 210, 215
nasosinusitis, 534
nausea, 460, 464, 598
natural immunity, 418, 421
naturopathic medicine, 667
nearsightedness, 539, 543
nebulizer, 237, 239
necr(o), 11
necrology, 11
necrophilia, 621
necrosis, 180, 186
necrotic, 578, 579

needle biopsy, 584
needle holder, 603, 604
neonate, 557, 558
neonatologists, 558
neonatology, 558, 561
neoplasm, 83, 86, 573, 575
neoplastic, 575
nephr(o), 55, 297
nephrectomy, 314
nephritis, 29, 308, 311
nephroblastoma, 309, 311
nephrolithiasis, 308
nephrolithotomy, 313, 314
nephrologist, 301
nephrolysis, 313, 314
nephroma, 309, 311
nephron, 291, 294
nephron disease, 303
nephropexy, 30, 314, 607
nephrorrhaphy, 313, 314
nephrosarcoma, 582
nephrosis, 309, 311
nephrostomy, 313, 314
nerve, 258
nerve cell, 249, 258
nerve conduction velocity, 264, 266
nerve impulse, 258
nervous system, 40, 42, 249–281
  diagnostic, procedural, and laboratory
      terms for, 264-265
  infectious diseases of, 270
nervous tissue, 39, 42
neur(o), neuri, 261, 621
neural canal, 110, 118
neural transmitter, 258
neurectomy, 277
neurilemma, 258
neuritis, 261, 270, 274
neuroblastoma, 582
neuroglia, 251, 261, 273
neuroglial cells, 258
neurohypophysis, 485, 491
neuron, 249, 258
neuropeptide, 251
neuroplasty, 277
neuroretina, 530
neurosis, 619, 621
neurosurgeon, 276
neurotomy, 277
neurotransmitter, 250, 258, 274
neutropenia, 399
neutrophil, 384
nevus (pl., nevi), 81, 86
NHL, 575
NIDDM, 495, 508
NIMH, 622
nipple, 334
nitrate, 196
nitrous oxide, 641
NMR, 608
noct(i), 11
nocturia, 11, 311
nocturnal enuresis, 311
nodular, 578, 579
nodule, 79, 86
nondegenerative disorders, 269

pachyonychia, 11
pain, 527-529
palatine bone, 109
palatine tonsils, 210, 215
palliation, 560
palliative care, 560
palpitation, 180, 186
palsy, 274
pan, pant(o)-, 26
pancreas, 449, 453, 464, 469, 486,
      488-489, 491, 495
  disorders of, 460, 504-505
pancreatectomy, 467, 469, 510
pancreatic juice, 447
pancreat(o), 453, 495
pancreatitis, 464
pancytopenia, 400
panic attack, 617
panic disorder, 616
pansinusitis, 227, 232
PAP smear, 340-341
Papanicolaou smear, 340-341
papilledema, 540
papilla (*pl.*, papillae), 327, 449, 531
papillary, 578-579
papillary layer, 67, 70
papule, 79, 87
par(a)-, 26
-para, 30
para, 331, 334
paracentesis, 466, 469
paracusis, 543
paralysis, 254
paranasal sinus, 210, 215
paranoia, 616, 620
paraplegia, 23
parasiticide, 95
parasympathetic nervous system, 256, 258
parathormone, 492
parathyroid, 492
  disorders of, 503
parathyroid(o), 495
parathyroidectomy, 509-510
parathyroid gland, 487, 492, 503
parathyroid hormone, 487, 492, 503
parenteral administration, 652
-paresis, 30
paresthesia, 269, 274
parietal bone, 108, 118
parietal lobe, 253, 258
parietal pericardium, 155
parietal pleura, 212, 215
Parkinson's disease, 269, 274
paronychia, 87
parotid gland, 441
parotiditis, 459, 464
parotitis, 459, 464
-parous, 30
paroxysmal, 232
partial, 640
partial thromboplastin time, 394, 396
parturition, 334
patch, 78-79
patch test, 77
patell(o), 124
patella, 111, 118
patellectomy, 124

patent ductus arteriosus, 183, 186
path(o), 11
pathogen, 11, 421
pathological fracture, 133, 138
-pathy, 30
Patient's Bill of Rights (American Hospital
      Association), 16
pattern baldness, 68
p.c., 657
PCP, 220, 423, 427
PCV, 391
PDR, 646, 657
PE tube, 534
peak flow meter, 223-224
peau d'orange, 97
ped(i), pedo-, 124
PED, 363
pediatrician, 558
pediatrics, 558, 561
pediculated polyp, 79, 87
pediculosis capitis, 83
pediculosis pubis, 83
pediculosis, 83, 87
pedodontist, 631, 634
pedometer, 124
PEEP, 220
pelv(i), pelvo, 55, 124
pelvic cavity, 41, 42, 111
pelvic girdle, 110-111, 118
pelvic inflammatory disease, 338
pelvic ultrasonography, 340
pelvimetry, 340-341
pelvis, 111, 118
pelviscope, 124
pemphigus, 81, 87
-penia, 30
penile erectile dysfunction, 363, 366
penile prosthesis, 364
penis, 361, 365, 366
-pepsia, 30
pepsin, 443, 450
peptic ulcer, 460, 464
per-, 26
percussion, 223-224
percutaneous transluminal coronary
      angioplasty, 169, 189, 192
perfusion deficit, 180, 186
perfusion study, 598
peri-, 26
pericardi(o), 168
pericardial cavity, 155
pericardial fluid, 155
pericarditis, 33, 168, 182, 186
pericardium, 6, 155, 165
perilymph, 527, 531
perimenopause, 331, 334
perimetrium, 327, 334
perine(o), 337
perineocele, 337
perineum, 327, 334, 359, 361
periodontal ligament, 633
periodontist, 638, 640
periosteum, 106, 118
peripheral nervous system, , 249,
      254-255, 259, 262
peripheral vascular disease, 180, 186
peristalsis, 293, 441-442, 450

peritoneal dialysis, 297, 304-305
periton(eo), 453
peritoneoscope, 456
peritoneoscopy, 456, 458
peritonitis, 461, 465
permanent teeth, 632-635
pernicious anemia, 397
PERRL, PERRLA, 534
personality disorder, 616, 618
perspiration, 68
pertussis, 227, 232
PET, 174, , 177, 265-266, 595-596, 600, 608
petechia (*pl.*, petechiae), 87, 181, 186, 398
petit mal seizure, 270, 274
-pexy, 30, 607
Peyronie's disease, 366, 367
PFT, 220
pH, 297, 302, 306
phacoemulsification, 545, 546
phac(o), phak(o), 534
phacoma, 534
phag(o), 391
-phage, -phagia, -phagy, 30
phago, 11
phagocyte, 11, 251, 391, 417
phagocytic system, 417
phagocytosis, 417-418, 421
phalang(o), 124
phalangectomy, 124
phalanx (*pl.*, phalanges), 111, 118
  distal segment of, 111
  middle segment of, 111
  proximal segment of, 111
phantom limb, 135, 138
phantom pain, 135, 138
pharmacist, 647, 654
pharmaco, 11
pharmacodynamics, 647, 655
pharmacokinetics, 625, 647, 655
pharmacology, 11, 647, 655
  abbreviations relating to, 656-658
  combining terms relating to, 656-658
  terms in, 646-659
pharyng(o), 55, 218, 453
pharyngeal tonsils, 210, 215
pharyngitis, 55, 218, 227, 232
pharyngotonsillitis, 453
pharynx, 210, 215, 441, 450
  disorders of, 459
-phasia, 30
phenylketones, 303, 306
-pheresis, 30
-phil, 30
-philia, 30, 621
phimosis, 365, 367
phleb(o), 56, 168
phlebitis, 56, 168, 181, 186
phlebogram, 173
phlebography, 173, 177
phlebotomy, 2, 190, 192, 392, 396
phobia, 616, 620
-phobia, 30, 616, 622
phon(o), 11, 219
-phonia, 30
phonometer, 11, 219
-phoresis, 30
-phoria, 31, 622

phosphorus, 105, 118
phot(o), 11
photometer, 11
photophobia, 268, 540, 544
phren(o), 56, 219
-phrenia, 31
phrenitis, 219
-phthisis, 31
-phylaxis, 31
physi, physio, 11
physical phase, 302
physical therapy, 135, 138
Physician's Desk Reference, 646, 657
physiotherapy, 11
-physis, 31
physo, 11
physocele, 11
phyt(o), 11
phytoxin, 11
pia mater, 254, 258
pica, 617, 620
PID, 338, 343
pigment, 525
pil(o), 56, 74
pilonidal cyst, 79, 87
pimple, 79
pineal gland, 484, 486, 491
pinkeye, 540, 544
pinna, 526, 529, 531
pituitary, 485, 486, 489-492
    disorders of, 500-501
PKU, 297, 306
placenta previa, 346
placenta, 326, 331, 334, 345
-plakia, 31
planes of the body, 45–46
plantar flexion, 113
plantar wart, 81, 87
plaque, 79, 86-87, 175, 180, 183, 186, 640
-plasia, 31, 575
-plasm, 31, 575
plasma, 388
plasma, plasmat(o), plasmo, 11, 56
plasma cell, 418, 419
plasmapheresis, 11, 379, 388
plastic surgery, 91, 92, 545
-plastic, 31, 575
-plasty, 31, 607
platelet count, 394, 396
platelet, , 378, 384-385, 388
play therapy, 623, 624
-plegia, 27, 31
-plegic, 31
pleomorphic, 578, 579
pleur(o), 56, 219
pleura (*pl.*, pleurae), 212, 215
pleural cavity, 212, 215
pleural effusion, 229, 232
pleurisy, 227, 232
pleuritis, 219, 227, 232
pleurocentesis, 235, 236
pleurography, 56
pleuropexy, 235, 236
PLT, 391, 394, 396
pluralizing of terms, 3
pluri-, 26
pluriglandular, 26

p.m., 657
PMN, 391
PMP, 338
PMS, 329, 338
PND, 220
-pnea, 31
pneum(o), pneuma, pneumat(o),
    pneumon(o), 56, 219
pneumobronchotomy, 234, 236
pneumoconiosis, 229, 232
pneumocystis carinii pneumonia, 427
pneumolith, 219
pneumoncystis carinii pneumonia, 229
pneumonectomy, 234, 236
pneumonia, 228, 229, 232
pneumonitis, 56, 219, 227, 232
pneumothorax, 229, 232
PNS, 262
p.o., 657
pod(o), 56, 124
podagra, 135, 138
podalgia, 124
podiatrist, 56, 129, 130
-poiesis, 31
-poietic, 31
-poietin, 31
poikilo, 12
poikilocyte, 12
poikilocytosis, 398, 400
polarization, 160, 165
poly-, 26
poly, 391
polyarteritis, 26
polycystic kidney disease, 311, 309
polycystic ovaries, 343
polycythemia, 398, 400
polydipsia, 501, 508
polymorphonucleated cell, 417
polyp, 79, 87
polypectomy, 466, 469
polypoid, 578, 579
polyposis, 461, 465
polysomnography, 264, 266
polyunsaturated fat, 175
polyuria, 309, 311, 501, 508
pons, 252, 258
popliteal artery, 159, 165
pore, 68, 70
-porosis, 31
positron emission tomography, 265, 266
positron emission tomography scan, 174,
    177, 595, 600
post-, 26
posterior, 44, 49
posterior chamber, 525
posterior pituitary gland, 485
posthemorrhagic anemia, 398
postmortem, 26
postprandial blood sugar, 497
post-traumatic stress disorder, 617, 620
PPD, 74, 77
pre-, 26
preeclampsia, 342, 346
prefix, 6
    in medical terms 23–27
pregnancy, 331, 556-558
    complications during, 342, 343

premature, 342, 563, 564
premature atrial contraction, 180, 186
premature ventricular contraction, 180, 186
premenstrual syndrome, 329
prenatal, 26
prepuce, 359
premature, 563, 564
premolar, 633, 635
presbyacusis, 541, 544
presbycusis, 541
presbyopia, 539, 544
prescription, 647, 655
pressure sore, 80, 87
preventative, 602, 604
preventive medicine, 563, 564
priapism, 366, 367
primary teeth, 631, 635
primip, 338
privacy, 16-17
    rights, 16-17
    violations of, 17
PRL, 495
PRN, 657
pro-, 26
probe, 603, 604
process, 107, 119
proct(o), 56, 453
proctitis, 461, 465
proctologist, 453
proctoplasty, 466, 469
proctoscope, 456
proctoscopy, 456, 458
prodrome, 26
progesterone, 328, 329, 334, 486
prolactin, 329
prolapsed uterus, 343
pronation, 113
prone, 45, 49
proprietary name, 647, 655
prostat(o), 363
prostate, 293, 294, 358, 359, 361, 364
prostate cancer, 364, 366
prostatectomy, 368, 370
prostate-specific antigen test, 364, 577
prostatic fluid, 359
prostatitis, 363, 366, 367
prosthetic devices, 142, 143
protein, 379
proteinuria, 309, 311
prothrombin, 380, 388
prothrombin time, 394, 396
protocol, 578, 579
proximal, 45, 46, 49
proximal epiphysis, 106
pruritus, 80, 87
PSA, 363, 365, 575, 577
pseud(o), 12
pseudodiabetes, 12
pseudophakia, 540, 544
PSG, 264, 266
psoriasis, 82, 87
psych(o), psyche, 56, 621
psychedelic, 625
psychiatric treatment,
    terms in, 623
psychiatrist, 615
psychiatry, 615, 620

rhabdomyolysis, 125
rhabdomyoma, 135, 138
rhabdomyosarcoma, 135, 139, 582
rhabdosphincter, 125
rheumatic heart disease, 183, 187
rheumatoid arthritis, 129, 135
rheumatoid factor test, 129, 130
rheumatologist, 129, 130
rhin(o), 56, 219
rhinitis, 219, 227, 232
rhinoplasty, 234, 236, 607
rhinorrhea, 227, 232
Rh-negative, 386, 388
rhonchi, 226. 232
Rh-positive, 386, 388
rhythm method, 330
RIA, 498, 597, 600, 607
rib, 110, 119, 326
ribonucleic acid, 572
ribosome, 38, 39
rickets, 132, 139
right atrium, 156, 157, 158,
        160, 161, 162, 165
right lower quadrant, 44, 47, 49
right upper quadrant, 46, 47, 49
right ventricle, 156, 157, 158,
        160, 161, 162, 165
rigidity, 135, 139
rigor, 135, 139
ringworm, 80, 87
risk factor, 179, 187
RLL, 220
RLQ, 44, 47, 49
RNA, 426, 572, 575
rod, 525, 531
roentgenology, 593, 600
ROM, 126, 129
root, 633, 635
root canal, 633, 635
root canal work, 638
rosacea, 81, 87
roseola, 81, 87
rotation, 113
RP, 297, 304
-rrhage, 31
-rrhagia, 31
-rrhaphy, 31, 607
-rrhea, 31
-rrhexis, 32
RT, 575
rub, 180, 187
rubella, 80, 87
rubeola, 80, 87
rugae, 326, 441, 443, 444, 450
RUL, 220
RUQ, 46, 49
Rx, 658

S

s, 658
SA, 169
sacr(o), 56
sacral, 255
sacrum, 110, 119
sagittal plane, 45, 49
saliva, 439, 441, 450

salivary gland, 441, 450
salping(o), 12, 337
salpingectomy, 12, 348, 349
salpingitis, 343, 346
salpingo-oophorectomy, 348
salpingoplasty, 337
salpingotomy, 347, 348, 349
saphenous vein, 159, 165
sarco, 56
sarcoidosis, 428, 430
sarcoma, 569, 573, 582
SARS, 220, 227, 228
saturated fat, 175
scabies, 83, 88
scale, 79, 80, 88
scalpel, 603, 605
scan, 597, 600
scanner, 597
scapula, 110, 119
scapul(o), 125
scapulodynia, 125
Schick test, 77
-schisis, 32
schisto, 12
schistocytosis, 12
schiz(o), 13, 621
schizophasia, 621
schizophrenia, 12, 618, 620
sciatica, 132, 139, 270, 275
scirrhous, 578, 580
scler(o), 12, 56, 534
sclera, 524, 531
sclerectasia, 534
scleritis, 541, 544
scleroderma, 12, 82, 88
scoli(o), 12, 125
scoliokyphosis, 125
scoliometer, 12
scoliosis, 135, 139
-scope, 32, 607
-scopy, 32, 607
scot(o), 12, 534
scotograph, 12
scotoma, 540, 544
scotometer, 534
scratch test, 76, 77
scrotum, 358, 359, 361
seb(o), 74
sebaceous cyst, 79, 88
sebaceous gland, 65, 66, 69, 71
seborrhea, 82, 88
seborrheic dermatitis, 82
sebum, 69, 71
secondary hypertension, 180, 187
secondary oocyte, 327
secondary teeth, 632, 633, 635
second bicuspid, 633, 635
second-degree burn, 82, 88
second molar, 633, 635
sedative, 278, 279, 626
sedimentation rate, 394, 396
seg, 391
sella turcica, 108, 119, 485
semen analysis, 364, 365
semen, 359, 361
semi-, 26
semicircular canal, 527, 531

semilunar valve, 157, 165
seminal vesicle, 358, 359
seminiferous tubules, 358
seminoma, 366, 367
sensorineural, 541
sensory neuron, 250, 251, 256
sensory receptors, 524, 531
sensory system, 40, 42, 523–550
    abbreviations relating to, 534–535
    combining forms relating to, 533–534
    diagnostic, procedural, and laboratory
        terms relating to, 536–538
    pathological terms relating to, 539–544
    pharmacological terms relating to, 547–548
    structure and function of, 523–532
    surgical terms relating to, 545–546
septal defect, 183, 187
septoplasty, 234, 236
septostomy, 234, 236
septum (pl., septa), 156, 165, 211, 215
sequential multiple analyzer, 395, 396
sequestrum, 135, 139
serology, 378
serotonin, 251
serous otitis media, 541
serum, 378, 380, 389, 497
serum bilirubin, 456
serum calcium, 129, 130
serum creatine phosphokinase
        (CPK), 129, 131
serum enzyme test, 176, 177
serum glutamic oxaloacetic transaminase, 456
serum glutamic pyruvic transaminase, 456
serum phosphorus, 129, 131
sesamoid bone, 107, 119
sessile polyp, 79, 88
sexually transmitted disease, 344, 366
SG, 297
SGOT, 454, 456
SGPT, 454, 456
shave biopsy, 92
shin, 111, 119
shingles, 81, 88, 270, 275
short bone, 107, 119
SIADH, 501, 508
sial(o), 56, 453
sialaden(o), 453
sialism, 453
sialoadenitis, 453, 459, 465
sickle cell anemia, 398
sidero, 12
sideropenia, 12
SIDS, 220, 563, 564
Sig., 658
sight, 524–526, 531
sigmoid(o), 56, 453
sigmoid colon, 446, 450, 456
sigmoidoscopy, 453, 456, 458
silicosis, 229, 232
simple fracture, 133, 139
single photon emission computed
        tomography brain scan, 265, 266
singultus, 226, 232
sinoatrial (SA) node, 160, 165
sinus, 107, 119, 327, 334
sinusitis, 227, 232
sinusotomy, 234, 236

sinus rhythm, 161, 165
sito, 12
sitotoxin, 12
skeletal muscle, 113
skeleton, 105, 119
skin, 527–528
skin grafts, 91, 92
skull, 107–108, 254
SL, 658
SLE, 74, 81, 88, 423
sleep apnea, 264
SMA, 395, 396
small intestine, 439, 440, 444–445, 450
smell, 523, 528, 531
smooth muscle, 119
SNOMED CT® (Systematized Nomenclature
    of Medicine Clinical Terms), 20
SOAP method, 18–19
SOB, 220
socket, 631, 635
social worker, 615, 620
sociopathy, 618, 620
soft palate, 210, 215, 441, 450
solid tumor, 569, 573
sol., 658
solution, 651
SOM, 534
somat(o), 12, 56
somatic nervous system, 255, 259
somatoform disorder, 618, 620
somatogenic, 12
somatostatin, 251
somatotrophic hormone, 492
somn(o), somni, 12
somnambulism, 12, 271, 275
-somnia, 32
somnolence, 271, 275
son(o), 12, 606
sonogram, 596, 601, 606
sonography, 181, 184, 606
sonomotor, 14
s.o.s., 658
sp., 658
spasm, 139
-spasm, 32
spasmo, 12
spasmolytic, 12
spastic, 134, 139
specific gravity, 302, 307
SPECT, 265, 266, 608
speculum, 340
sperm nucleus, 327
sperm(o), sperma, spermat(o), 57, 363
sperm, 358, 361
spermatogenesis, 358, 361
spermatozoon (pl., spermatozoa), 358, 361
spermicide, 330, 334
sphenoid bone, 108, 119
sphenoid sinus, 108, 119
spher(o), 12
spherocyte, 12
sphygm(o), 168
sphygmomanometer, 173, 177
spin(o), 261
spina bifida cystica, 268, 274
spina bifida occulta, 268
spina bifida, 132, 139, 268

spinal cavity, 41
spinal column, 109-110, 119
spinal cord, 254, 259
    diseases of, 268–271
spinal curvature, 135, 139
spinal nerve, 254, 259
spinoneural, 261
spinous process, 110
spir(o), 12, 219
spirometer, 219, 223, 225
spirometry, 223
spiroscope, 12
splanchn(o), splanchni, 57
splanchnolith, 57
spleen, 415, 421
splen(o), 57, 423
splenectomy, 431, 432
splenomegaly, 430
splenic flexure, 446
splinting, 142, 143
spondyl(o), 57, 125
spondylitis, 57, 125
spondylolisthesis, 135, 139
spondylolysis, 139
spondylosyndesis, 142, 143
sponge, 330, 335
spongy bone, 106, 119
spontaneous abortion, 342
SPP, 363
sprain, 134, 139
spur, 132, 136
sputum culture, 223, 225
sputum sample, 223
squamo, 12
squamofrontal, 12
squamous cell carcinoma, 83, 88
squamous epithelium, 66, 71
SR, 391, 394
ss, 658
stage, 580
standard precaution, 603
-stalsis, 32
stapes, 526, 531
staple, 603
staphyl(o), 13
staphylococcus (pl., staphylococci), 13, 74
stapedectomy, 564
-stasis, 32
stat, 658
-stat, 32
-static, 32
statins, 195, 196
STD, 344
steat(o), 74, 454
steatorrhea, 454, 461
stem cell, 381, 389
steno, 13
stenocephaly, 13
stenosis, 183, 187
-stenosis, 32
stent, 190, 192
stere(o), 13
stereology, 13
stereotactic frame, 598
stereotactic surgery, 277
stereotaxy, 277
stern(o), 57, 125

sternodynia, 125
sternum, 110, 119
steroid, 513
steth(o), 57, 219
stethoscope, 219
STH, 492, 495
stillbirth, 342
stimulus (pl., stimuli), 259
St John's Wort, 648
stomach, , 439, 443-444, 450
    disorders of, 459-460
stomach ulcer, 464
stomat(o), stom(a), 57, 454
stomatitis, 454
-stomy, 32, 607
stone basket, 313
stool, 450
stool culture, 456
stool guaiac, 456
strabismus, 539, 544
strain, 134, 139
strangulated hernia, 461
stratified squamous epithelium, 71
stratum corneum, 66, 71
stratum germinativum, 71
stratum, 71
strepto, 13
streptococcus, 13
stress test, 173, 177
striae, 67
striated muscle, 120, 125
stridor, 226, 232
stroke volume, 169
stroke, 275
sty, stye, 540, 544
styl(o), 13
styloid process, 108
styloid, 13
sub-, 26
subc, 658
subcutaneous, 655
subdural space, 254
sublingual gland, 441
sublingually, 648, 655
subluxation, 134, 139
submandibular gland, 442
sudden infant death syndrome, 220, 564
suffixes, 6
    in medical terms 23–33
sugar, 449
sulcus (pl., sulci), 119, 259
super-, 26
superficial, 45, 49
superior, 45, 49
superior lobe, 212, 215
superior vena cava, 159, 165
supination, 113
supine, 45, 49
supp., 658
supperative otitis media, 541
suppository, 655, 658
supra-, 26
supraglottis, 235
suprarenal gland, 487, 492
surgery, 602–605
    abbreviations relating to, 607-608
    combining forms relating to, 606

toxicology, 647, 655
toxicogenic, 656
toxicosis, 423
toxic shock syndrome, 343
toxipathy, 13
tPA, TPA, 169, 195, 196
TPN, 454, 658
TPR, 220, 658
trabeculae, 525
trabeculectomy, 545, 546
tracer study, 597, 601
trache(o), 57, 219
trachea, 210, 211, 216
tracheitis, 227, 233
trachel(o), 57
trachelophyma, 57
tracheoplasty, 234, 236
tracheoscopy, 219
tracheostomy, 235, 236
tracheotomy, 57, 235, 236
traction, 142, 143
trade name, 647-648, 655
traditional Chinese medicine, 667, 670
tranquilizer, 625, 626
trans-, 27
transcranial sonogram, 265, 266
trans-fats, 175
transfusion, 385-386, 389
transient ischemic attack, 271, 275
transient vasoconstrictors, 371
transocular, 27
transurethral resection of the prostate, 368
transvaginal ultrasound, 340
transverse, 557
transverse colon, 446
transverse plane, 45, 49
transverse process, 110, 120
trauma disorders, 268
tremor, 135, 139
trepanation, 277, 278
trephination, 277, 278
trich(o), trichi, 57, 74
trichiasis, 540, 544
trichoid, 57
trichomoniasis, 344
trichopathy, 74
tricuspid stenosis, 182, 187
tricuspid valve, 156, 165
trigeminal, 255
triglyceride, 175, 177
trigon(o), 297
trigone, 293, 294
trigonitis, 297
triiodothyronine, 485, 492
trochanter, 107, 120
trochlear, 255
-trophic, 32
tropho, 13
trophocyte, 13
-trophy, 32
-tropia, 32
-tropic, 32
troponin I, 175
troponin T, 175
-tropy, 32
true ribs, 110, 120
TSH, 486, 495

tsp., 658
TSS, 338
tubal ligation, 347
tubal pregnancy, 342
tubercle, 107, 120
tuberculosis, 228, 233
tuberosity, 107, 120
tumor, 79, 88, 569, 573
    types and causes of, 569-571
TURP, 363, 368
Tx, 575
tylectomy, 584
tympan(o), 534
tympanic membrane, 526, 532
tympanitis, 541, 544
tympanoplasty, 534, 545, 546
Type I diabetes, 504, 508
Type II diabetes, 504, 508

U

U, 658
UA, 297
UC, 338
u.d., 658
UGI(S), 454
ulcer, 80, 81, 90
ulcerating, 578, 580
ulcerative colitis, 460, 465
uln(o), 125
ulna, 111, 120
ulnocarpal, 125
ultra-, 27606
ultrasonic, 27
ultrasonography, 174, 596, 601, 607
ultrasound, 596, 601, 606
ultraviolet light, 93, 95
umbilical cord, 331, 335
umbilical hernia, 462
umbilical region, 48, 49
un-, 27
undifferentiated, 570, 578, 580
ung., 657, 658
uni-, 27
unconscious, 27
United States Pharmacopeia, 646
uniglandular, 27
universal donor, 386
universal recipient, 386
upper GI series, 456
upper respiratory infection, 226, 233
uptake, 598, 601
ur(o), urin(o), 297
urea, 302, 306
uremia, 297, 309, 311
ureter(o), 297
ureter, 290, 293, 295, 376
ureterectomy, 313, 314
ureteritis, 309
ureteroplasty, 313, 314
ureterorrhaphy, 313, 314
ureterostenosis, 297
urethr(o), 297
urethra, 290, 293, 295, 339, 376, 386
urethral stenosis, 309
urethritis, 309
urethrocystitis, 309

urethrogram, 364, 365
urethropexy, 313, 314
urethroplasty, 313, 314
urethrorrhaphy, 313, 314
urethrorrhea, 297
urethrostomy, 313, 314
urethrotomy, 313, 314
URI, 220
-uria, 32, 297
uric acid, 291, 295
uric acid test, 129, 131
urinalysis, 301–303, 307
urinary bladder, 293, 295
urinary catheterization, 301
urinary system, 40, 43, 290, 295
urinary tract infection, 308, 311
urinary tract procedure, 304-305
urine, 291, 295
urine sugar, 497, 498
urologist, 301
urology, 312, 314
urostomy, 313, 314
urticaria, 81, 88
U/S, 608
U.S.P., 646, 658
uter(o), 337
uterine tube, 325, 335
uterine wall, 342
uteroplasty, 337
uterus, 325, 335
UTI, 297, 308, 311
uve(o), 534
uvea, 525, 532
uveitis, 534
uvula, 441, 450

V

VA, 534
vaccination, 418, 421
vaccine, 418, 421
vag(o), 261
vagectomy, 261
vagin(o), 337
vagina, 325, 335
vaginal hysterectomy, 348
vaginitis, 337, 343, 346
vagotomy, 261, 277, 278
vagus, 255
valve, 156, 165
valve replacement, 190, 192
valvotomy, 190, 192
valvulitis, 183, 187
valvuloplasty, 190, 192
varicella, 80, 88
varico, 57
varicocele, 366, 367
varicophlebitis, 57
varicose vein, 181, 187
vas deferens, 358, 361
vas(o), 57, 169
vascular disorder, 271
vascular lesion , 78, 88
vasculo, 57
vasculopathy, 57
vasectomy, 369, 370
vasoconstrictor, 195, 196

vasodepressor, 169
vasodilator, 195, 196, 651
vasopressin, 486, 492
vasovasostomy, 369, 370
VC, 220
VCU, VCUG, 297, 304, 307
vegetation, 183, 187
vein stripping, 182
vein, 156, 166
ven(o), veni, 57, 169
vena cava, 159, 166
venipuncture, 190, 192, 392, 396
venogram, 173
venography, 169, 173, 177, 596
ventilator, 237, 239
ventral, 44, 49
ventral cavity, 41, 43
ventral thalamus, 253, 259
ventricle, 156, 166, 253, 259
ventricul(o), 57, 261
ventriculitis, 261
ventriculogram, 173, 177
venule, 159, 166
vermiform appendix, 445, 446
verrucous, 578, 580
-version, 32
vertebr(o), 58, 125
vertebra (pl., vertebrae), 109 , 120, 266
vertebral body, 110, 120
vertebral column, 109, 120
vertebroarterial, 125
vertigo, 541, 544
very low-density lipoprotein, 175
vesic(o), 58, 297
vesicle, 79, 88
vesicoabdominal, 297
vesicoprostatic, 58
vestibule, 527, 532
vestibulocochlear, 255
VF, 546
   violations of, 16
vial, 662, 666

villus (pl., villi), 463, 469
viral meningitis, 280, 285
viral pneumonia, 237
virilism, 516, 519
visceral muscle, 113, 120
visceral pericardium, 163, 165
visceral pleura, 221, 224
vision correction, 557
visual field examination, 547
vitamin, 658, 666
vitamin D, 105, 120
vitligo, 82, 90
vitreous, 536, 537
vitreous chamber, 536
vitreous humor, 536
vivi, 15
viviparous, 15
VLDL, 177, 182
vocal cord, 219, 224
voice box, 219, 224
voiding, 304
voiding (urinating)
         cystourethrogram, 304, 307
voluntary muscle, 113, 120
volvulus, 479, 483
vomer, 108, 120
vomiting, 610
Von Willebrand's disease, 415, 417
V/Q, 229, 619
V/Q perfusion scan, 231
VSD, 177
VT, 177
vulv(o), 351
vulva, 339, 341, 349
vulvitis, 351

W

Wart, 81, 88
WBC, 391, 395
western blot, 424
wheal, 79, 88

wheezes, 226, 233
white blood cell, 378, 384, 389
white blood cell differential and red blood
         cell morphology, 394
white blood count, 395
whitehead, 82, 88
whooping cough, 227, 233
Wilms"s tumor, 309, 311
windpipe, 210, 216
wisdom tooth, 633
word root, 6

X

xanth(o), 134, 74
xanthoderma, 134
xanthoma, 74
xeno, 13
xenophobia, 13
xer(o), 13, 74
xerasia, 13
xeroderma, 74
xiph(o), 13
xiphocostal, 13
x-ray, 456, 594-595, 601
x-ray technology, 594
XRT, 575, 608

Y

yellow bone marrow, 107

Z

ZDV, 423
zo(o), 13
zooblast, 13
zygomatic bone, 10, 120
zygote, 556
zym(o), 13
zymogram, 13